FISH DISEASE
Diagnosis and Treatment

FISH DISEASE

Diagnosis and Treatment

EDWARD J. NOGA, M.S., D.V.M.

Professor of Aquatic Medicine,
Department of Companion Animal and Special Species Medicine,
North Carolina State University,
College of Veterinary Medicine,
Raleigh, North Carolina

with 316 *illustrations, including* 176 *in color*

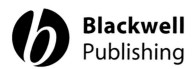

© 2000 Iowa State University Press

Blackwell Publishing Professional
2121 State Avenue, Ames, Iowa 50014

Orders: 1-800-862-6657
Office: 1-515-292-0140
Fax: 1-515-292-3348
Web site: www.blackwellprofessional.com

First edition, 1996 (© Mosby–Year Book, Inc.)
First Iowa State University Press edition, 2000

Library of Congress Cataloging-in-Publication Data
Noga, Edward J.
    Fish disease: diagnosis and treatment / Edward J. Noga.
        p. cm.
    Includes bibliographical references (p.).
    ISBN-13: 978-0-8138-2558-8
    ISBN-10: 0-8138-2558-X
        1. Fishes—Diseases. I. Title.

SH171 .N64 1999
639.3—dc21   99-058466

The last digit is the print number: 9 8 7 6 5

Preface

Over 70 percent of the earth's surface is covered with water. Fish are ubiquitous inhabitants of this ecosystem. With over 30,000 named species and many more that may yet be discovered, fish are the most successful vertebrate group and play an extremely important ecological role. In both natural environments and culture, disease has a serious impact on fish. There is an acute awareness of and concern for the diseases affecting our fishery stocks (Noga, 1988). Fish health experts are increasingly called on to provide answers about disease outbreaks in fishery populations. Largely because of the decline in fishery stocks and the increase in consumer demand, fish culture, both for food and as pets, has been the fastest growing segment of animal agriculture in the United States and worldwide. Disease is universally recognized as one of the most serious threats to the commercial success of aquaculture (U.S.D.A., 1991).

This book is intended to guide you, the reader, through the most commonly encountered fish diseases and to provide you with the knowledge to manage these problems effectively. While the focus of this work is on cultured fish, most of the information also applies to wild populations.

Many readers will immediately notice that this book is not designed like traditional textbooks that cover fish disease. I have used a systems-based approach to describe fish diseases rather than the taxonomic approach, where all virus diseases are covered as a group, then all bacterial diseases, then all fungal diseases, then all parasitic diseases. In my experience, diagnosticians mainly identify problems by systems rather than by taxonomic groups. For example, water quality is examined (environmental system), then the skin (dermal system), then the gills, then the internal organs. I believe that design of a diagnostic guide along these lines makes for a much more understandable and user-friendly method for diagnoses because you, the reader, can literally *follow along* with the flow of the book and identify problems as they are encountered during the clinical work-up.

Another feature that I believe is important is detailed descriptions of pathogens. Diagnosis of most of the common fish disease problems involves fairly simple techniques; this is in part due to our relatively unsophisticated methods used to identify problems, which are heavily based on the morphologic recognition of a pathogen. For example, diagnosis of parasites, a common problem, is made by identifying the parasite in a tissue sample; this necessitates that high-quality, representative examples be provided as illustrative material. I have tried to do this.

Finally, to identify and manage the problems, the clinician needs an adequate understanding of the methods used for disease diagnosis and treatment. Thus, I have included detailed explanations and illustrations of common procedures.

The end result is what I hope will be for you a useful, practical, and valuable guide for everyday problems that you might encounter in working with this fascinating group of animals.

Edward J. Noga, M.S., D.V.M.

Acknowledgments

This work would not have been possible without the invaluable assistance of many people. Notable among these are the medical illustrators. I would especially like to thank Anne Runyon, who did a marvelous job in creating almost all of the line drawings in the text. Brenda Bunch also contributed significantly to the illustrations by producing the computer-generated composite photographs. Bruce Kendall, Susan Rosenvinge, Melinda Fine, and Helen Bolen also helped in this effort. I would also like to thank the entire photography staff of the N.C.S.U. Biomedical Communications Center, especially Wendy Savage, for assistance with production of most of the photographs that I have accumulated over the years. Douglas Wagner and Bruce Kendall created the cover design.

Many persons and organizations generously provided photographs, including Andrew Mitchell, Glenn Hoffman, Heino Moller, Angelo Colorni, Charlie Smith, Todd Wenzel, Jiri Lom, George Blasiola, Michael Kent, Doug Mitchum, Stephen Spotte, Ronald Roberts, David Demont, Carl Sindermann, Richard Callinan, Marshall Beleau, Richard Wolke, Hsu-Tien Huang, Fred Meyer, Ronald Hedrick, Chien Tu, Ruth Floyd, Sherwood Johnson, Arik Diamant, Lester Khoo, the CL Davis Foundation for Veterinary Pathology, the Armed Forces Institute of Pathology, the American Fisheries Society, and the U.S. National Fish Health Research Laboratory. Lester Khoo also took many of the photomicrographs.

Several reviewers provided useful comments that significantly improved early drafts of the manuscript, including Angelo Colorni, Jiri Lom, George Blasiola, Gigi Davidson, Ruth Floyd, Ron Hedrick, Gregory Lewbart, Christine Moffitt, Karen Steidinger, Darryl Baker, Susan Homire and two anonymous reviewers. Ethylyn Spencer, Margaret Hemingway, and Deborah Collins greatly assisted in production of the tables used in the text.

I also wish to thank Ms. Linda Duncan and her staff at Mosby-Year Book, especially Ms. Melba Steube, for their patience and perseverance. Ms. Duncan's predecessors in this endeavor, Robert Reinhardt and William Lamsback, got this project started and fought for my concept. Gail Morey Hudson created a superb book design.

While many people made important contributions to this book, any errors of omission or commission remain entirely my responsibility.

Edward J. Noga, M.S., D.V.M.

Anne Runyon drew Figures II-13A, II-13B, II-14D, II-15C,D, II-16A,B, II-17A, II-20C, II-21A, II-22A, II-24A, II-25A, II-28A, II-29A, II-30A, II-31A, II-32A, II-43A, II-55A, II-55I, II-56A, II-57E,F, II-58A, II-59A,B, II-66I, II-69B, II-70AB, III-2C. Brenda Bunch produced the computerized composite photographs (Figures II-13C-J, II-16C-I, II-19A-F, II-33B-F, II-55B-H, II-56B-G, II-57A-D, II-59C-J, II-66A-H, II-70C-H, II-72A-H). The cover is a computer-generated composite photograph of a striped bass with skin ulcers. The original subject was laser-scanned, using a flatbed scanner, and modified, using a Macintosh computer and then with Adobe Photoshop. Computer-generated montages were created by Douglas Wagner and the cover design was created by Bruce Kendall, both of Bio-Medical Communications, North Carolina State University College of Veterinary Medicine.

Contents

Before reading the text, familiarize yourself with the flow diagram of a clinical case work-up (Fig. I-I). The book is organized exactly as shown in the flow diagram.

The book is divided into three major parts: (Part I) *METHODS FOR DIAGNOSING FISH DISEASES,* (Part II) *PROBLEM LIST,* and (Part III) *METHODS FOR TREATING FISH DISEASES.* Part I provides a detailed guide to the methods used to diagnose fish diseases. The methods are covered in the order in which they would be performed during a case work-up (see Fig. I-I, STEPS IN WORKING UP A FISH DISEASE CASE).

Part II (*PROBLEM LIST*) is a comprehensive coverage of fish diseases. Note that the problems are listed in the order in which they are encountered in the clinical work-up, as described in Part I. For example, water quality problems that are routinely identified in the clinical work-up are listed first, followed by problems that are identified from examining the skin and gills, followed by internal and systemic diseases, and then, problems that cannot be definitively diagnosed in a routine clinical work-up but are suspected to be the cause based on the clinical work-up and rule-out of other problems (Fig. I-I, RULE-OUT DIAGNOSES). Confirmation of a rule-out diagnosis usually requires submission of samples to a specialized reference laboratory to obtain a definitive diagnosis. The last group of rule-out diagnoses are of unknown cause (*idiopathic*) and are also diagnosed by ruling out all other possible causes. This sequential arrangement of problems allows you to *follow along* through the problem list as you do the clinical work-up, facilitating diagnosis.

Part III (*METHODS FOR TREATING FISH DISEASES*) provides a detailed description of how hish are treated and the drugs that are effective for various problems.

FISH DISEASE
Diagnosis and Treatment

PART I

METHODS FOR DIAGNOSING FISH DISEASES

CHAPTER 1

Major Cultured Species

Before discussing methods used for diagnosing fish diseases, it is important to have an understanding of the numerous types of fish species that are cultured, as well as the diversity of culture systems. Understanding the different requirements for maintaining these different groups is essential to both short- and long-term health management.

AQUARIUM FISH

Aquarium (*pet*) fish constitute an extremely large segment of the pet animal industry (Winfree, 1989). An estimated $350 million is spent annually on fish in the United States in stores that sell aquariums and/or pet fish; even more is spent on supplies. Recent statistics indicate that annual sales of fish in pet stores constitute over 65% of the revenue generated by pet animal sales. While some fish, such as the common goldfish, cost less than a dollar, many fish command high prices—some cost as much as several hundred dollars. The average freshwater aquarium fish probably costs somewhere between $2 and $10; marine fish are usually considerably more expensive, averaging $15 to $20. Expensive and highly sophisticated marine aquaria are becoming increasingly more common, and it is not unusual for an owner to have several hundred dollars invested in fish alone. Some pet fish owners, like owners of other animals, also become emotionally attached to their pets and are willing to spend considerable sums for proper medical care. It is also interesting to note that over 80% of pet fish owners also own other pets.

Thousands of types of pet fish (from the commonplace guppy to the more exotic and the often more expensive species) are kept by hobbyists. The reader should refer to Axelrod et al. (1980); Bower (1983); Moe (1992a, 1992b); and other reference texts for specific details on taxonomy, biology, and husbandry. Many hobbyists specialize in a single group of fish (e.g., African cichlids), and there are a number of local, national, and international breed associations for these various groups.

Freshwater Aquarium Fish

The largest segment of the aquarium fish industry is the freshwater aquarium fish. Major groups include the poeciliids and the egg-layers.

Poeciliids (guppies, mollies, swordtails, platies) — These are also known as livebearers because they are viviparous. (A few other nonpoeciliid fish are also viviparous.) They are prolific, with many inbred strains. These fish are often relatively inexpensive, although certain strains may be expensive.

The so-called egg-layers encompass all other freshwater aquarium fish. Major groups include the following:

Characins (tetras) — These are active, schooling fish that usually stay in the upper water column. Some species may be a bit aggressive and nip fins or chase tankmates. Most make good members of a *community tank*. This group also includes the piranhas, but the latter are not good for the community tank (see *oddball fish*).

Tropical Cyprinids (barbs, danios) — These are active, schooling fish that usually stay in the upper water column. Like the characins, they may be a bit aggressive and nip fins or chase tankmates. Most make good members of a community tank.

Cool Water Cyprinids (goldfish, koi, carp, etc.) — These are hardy fish that are popular for both aquarium and pond culture. They are not truly tropical fish but can thrive in a wide range of temperatures. They do best in slightly cooler water.

Anabantids (Siamese fighting fish, gouramies, paradise fish, etc.) — These are generally peaceful fish that are good candidates for a community tank, except for the popular Siamese fighting fish, which, although aggressive toward conspecifics, are shy toward unrelated species. Anabantids breathe air by using an accessory organ modified from gill tissue (labyrinth).

Cyprinodonts (killifishes, topminnows) — These are generally small, often brilliantly colored fish, many of which have short natural life spans (e.g., annual fish). They are often shy among other types of fish and do best in a separate aquarium. There is usually marked sexual dimorphism.

Catfish (*Corydoras, Pimelodella, Plecostomus*, etc.) **and Loaches** (clown loach, kuhli loach, etc.) — These are generally peaceful, bottom-feeding fishes that are usful as *scavengers* to keep the gravel clean. Most make good members of a community tank.

Cichlids (freshwater angelfish, discus, oscar, African rift lake cichlids, etc.) — These are a popular group of fish that include a wide range of species having diverse behaviors. Some make excellent members for a community tank (e.g., angelfish), while others are extremely territorial and can only be kept with equally aggressive species (e.g., oscar). Some species have marked sexual dimorphism.

Oddball Fish (archerfish, piranha, freshwater butterfly fish, etc.) — These are species that are occasionally kept by aquarists as novelties. They include a diverse array of species.

Marine Aquarium Fish

Marine fish are becoming an increasingly larger component of the pet fish industry. At least part of this growth is because of the recent strides that have been made in successfully keeping these fish in captivity. Better tank design, such as the introduction of all-glass aquaria, and more reliable and efficient pumps, filters, and other apparatus have helped to greatly improve water quality, which is essential for marine fish health. Another factor that may contribute to the surge in marine aquarium keeping relates to the greater amount of disposable income in many households, which has allowed more people to afford these beautiful but expensive creatures. Many marine hobbyists have *reef* tanks, which are elaborate and usually expensive setups, that are used for the display of live invertebrates (corals, anemones, etc.) as well as fish. When a dozen or more such animals are kept in a single tank, this can become a sizable economic investment.

Important ecological differences between the marine and the freshwater fish have a direct bearing on their health in captivity (Table I-1). Compared with freshwater ecosystems, the tropical marine environment has little natural fluctuation in temperature, oxygen, or other water quality conditions. Thus, marine reef fish are not adapted to withstand the poor water conditions to which they are often exposed in captivity; this is exacerbated by the fact that almost all marine aquarium fish are wild-caught and must also acclimate to the confines of culture. Reef fish are highly territorial, adding to the stress of capture. They can carry latent infections, which recrudesce under captive conditions. Many reef fish have specialized diets, such as feeding on sponges or corals. Many cannot adapt to standard aquarium food and starve to death in captivity. Unfortunately, certain reef fish are imported and sold in stores with little regard for

Table I-1 Differences between tropical marine and freshwater aquarium fish.

	Freshwater	Marine
Many inbred strains	Yes	No
Many bred in captivity	Yes	No
Specialized feeding habits or nutritional requirements	Relatively few	Relatively many
Sensitivity to environmental changes	Relatively small	Relatively great
Territorial	Many	Almost all

From Noga, 1992.

whether they will ever accept food. All of these factors add up to an increased susceptibility to disease and the marine fishes' deserved reputation for being more difficult to keep than their freshwater counterparts. This emphasizes the need for competent health care.

Fish chosen for a marine aquarium should be species with histories of successful maintenance in captivity, and the fish should be eating well. To avoid aggression problems, a good rule of thumb is to have only one fish of any color, color pattern, or shape. Bower (1983) and Moe (1992a, 1992b) provide an excellent discussion on choosing fish and proper management of the marine aquarium. In general the best families for the home aquarium are, in descending order, the following: anemonefish, damselfish, angelfish, gobies, wrasses, parrotfish, and butterflyfish. Note that there are *many* exceptions to this rule of thumb.

It is becoming extremely popular for invertebrates to be kept with marine fish in reef tanks or other less elaborate setups. Anemones, sea urchins, starfish, shrimps, crabs, and even corals are commonly sold in aquarium stores.

Aquarium fish include a diverse array of species from many different habitats, and while they can often withstand a wide range of environments, they do best under more defined conditions (see *PROBLEMS 6* through *9*).

BAIT FISH

Several species comprise an important industry that produces bait fish for sport fishermen. Included in this group are various minnow species (Cyprinidae, Cyprinodontidae), such as the fathead minnow and golden shiner. Farms are concentrated in the southeast United States, especially Arkansas. Fish are typically raised in small ponds.

FOOD FISH

Aquaculture is the fastest growing segment of American agriculture (Lovell, 1979; U.S.D.A., 1991). Similar rapid growth is occurring worldwide (Pillay, 1993). This is not just one industry but actually an amalgamation of many different industries that culture many different species of aquatic animals (Brown, 1983; Pillay, 1993). The most commonly cultured fish include carp (family Cyprinidae), trout and salmon (Salmonidae), catfish (Ictaluridae, Clariidae, Pangasidae, Siluridae), eel (Anguillidae), tilapia (Cichlidae), mullet (Mugiludae), milkfish (Chanidae), yellowtail (Carangidae), sea bass (Serranidae, Centropomidae), and sea bream (Sparidae). Pillay (1993) provides a good introduction to culture of various groups. With such a diverse enterprise, only generalizations can be made about the types of fish and culture systems. Only representative species cultured in the United States are covered below.

Warm Water Food Fish

This category includes fish that thrive at high temperatures, generally greater than about 15° C (about 60° F). In the United States the most important member of the warm water food fish is the channel catfish (Ictaluridae). Annual U.S. production is over 136 million kg (300 million lb), having a farm value of nearly 250 million dollars. This translates into over half of all aquaculture production in the United States. Major producing states are concentrated in the Southeast, especially in the southern Mississippi River floodplain, because of an ample clean water supply and a long growing season. However, significant catfish production also exists in other areas, ranging from California to North Carolina and Missouri to Florida.

Most catfish are less demanding of water quality conditions than cold water species and are usually raised in earthen ponds. Catfish are typically spawned in late spring or summer, with the young fish being kept in small ponds or other small facilities until they reach an adequate size (usually 13 to 20 cm or 5 to 8 inches) to fend for themselves in larger ponds, where they remain until they are harvested.

Many catfish farms are vertically integrated, with broodstock for spawning, hatchery and nursery facilities, and grow-out operations on the same farm. Some farms specialize in supplying fingerlings to other producers. Commercial catfish farms typically raise fish in 2 to 8 ha (5 to 20 ac) ponds. Annual yields average 6500 kg/ha (5800 lb/acre). This represents an annual harvest income of $9750 to $11,375/ha ($4060 to $4640/ac) at the current farm price of catfish ($1.50 to 1.75/kg = $0.70 to $0.80/lb). With such a substantial investment at stake, proper medical care is a worthwhile expenditure.

Tilapias are also raised on a limited basis where high tropical temperatures can be maintained (far southern states or areas having geothermal well water) or in intensive, closed culture systems. Redfish (Sciaenidae) is a marine species that is cultured extensively in states that border the Gulf of Mexico.

Cold Water Food Fish

This category includes fish that thrive at low temperatures, generally less than about 15° C (about 60° F). The principal members of this group in the United States and worldwide are the salmon and trout. Rainbow trout is the most important cultured species in the United States, but many others (Atlantic salmon, brown trout, various Pacific salmon) are also valuable. Annual farm value of U.S.-produced trout and salmon is over $70 million.

Salmonids are anadromous (spawn in freshwater and then migrate to the sea to mature) and can be grown in both freshwater and seawater. Because they are demanding in their water quality requirements, most salmonids are raised in open or semiopen systems. Most commercial salmonid production in the United States is in freshwater raceways, but increasing numbers of salmon are being raised in marine net-pens.

Other species of growing importance in the United States include sturgeon (Acipenseridae) and hybrid striped bass, especially striped bass × white bass hybrids (Percichthyidae). Hybrid striped bass are more appropriately considered a cool water group, since they can tolerate much higher temperatures than salmonids.

CHAPTER 2

Types of Culture Systems

Environment has a major influence on virtually every important disease affecting cultured fish (Snieszko, 1974; Smart, 1981), and thus it is only appropriate that a treatise on fish diseases include a discussion of culture systems. The following four major types of systems are used to culture fish: aquaria, ponds, cages, and raceways. The major difference among these types of systems is simply how quickly water *turns over* (i.e., how quickly it is exchanged with new water). This ranges from aquaria and ponds, where no water is exchanged, to flow-through systems, where new water is being added continuously. This dictates the fish density that can be kept in each system, unless the culturist provides additional life-support systems.

All basic life-support processes, including providing oxygen and removing toxins, are performed by properly designed culture systems. In flow-through systems, such as raceways, these processes are accomplished by the constant addition of new, well-oxygenated water, which dilutes out toxins. Constant addition of new water allows for high fish densities. Ponds have virtually no regular water exchange, and aside from rainfall, no new water is added naturally. Thus, ponds must rely on resident biological processes to provide oxygen and remove toxins (see *CLOSED CULTURE SYSTEMS: PONDS*). These biological processes occur in all bodies of water but have a certain finite capacity to support a fish population. This *carrying capacity* dictates the number of fish that a pond can sustain. Aquaria can typically hold higher fish densities than ponds because supplemental life-support systems, including air pumps for oxygen and filters for toxin removal, are normally used in aquaria.

The amount of water turnover also tremendously influences the available therapeutic options. Systems with high water turnover are difficult to manipulate environmentally (e.g., to change temperature, salinity, etc.), mainly because of economic costs and environmental concerns. Also, water-borne medication, which is the most common method of treating fish disease, is more difficult in flow-through systems for the same reasons.

CLOSED CULTURE SYSTEMS: AQUARIA

Aquaria are mainly used for maintaining pet fish, although some food fish are also cultured in these *intensive* systems. Space does not permit a detailed discussion of the types of aquarium culture systems used for maintaining fish. The reader is referred to standard texts (Axelrod et al., 1980; Spotte, 1979a, 1979b, 1992; Moe, 1992a, 1992b) for details. The purpose of this discussion is to describe the basic components that are needed for aquarium culture, with emphasis on pet fish.

An aquarium is analogous to a spaceship in that all essential life-support systems must be provided; this includes removing toxins and supplying oxygen, proper temperature, and food. The basic components include the following:

1. Aquarium (*tank*) — It is usually made entirely of glass (*all-glass aquarium*). Tanks are less frequently made of plastic or fiberglass. Sizes typically range from 1 gallon to over 50,000 (4 to 200,000 liters) gallons in large public aquaria. Most hobbyists have aquaria ranging from 5 to 125 gallons (20 to 500 liters).

2. Substrate — This consists of various types of gravel, sand, or limestone. Some substrates are inert, while others may leach minerals (e.g., crushed coral reacts with acids in the tank to release calcium and magnesium, increasing the hardness) or other substances. Some types of gravels may also leach toxins, such as heavy metals; these should not be used in aquaria. The most inert types of minerals are quartz, granite, and mica.

3. Filters — The major types of filters are corner, undergravel, and outside types. Some have a water pump for increased circulation (*power filter*). Some may be elaborate (*wet-dry filter* for marine reef tanks). Filters usually perform multiple functions; the two most important functions are to circulate the water for oxygenation and to remove nitrogenous waste products via the bacteria that colonize the filter bed. Filters also remove particulate and/or colored materials, which reduce the aesthetics of the tank and may also be harmful to fish. Along with the tank size, the size and type of filters are primary factors that dictate the

amount of fish biomass that can be held in any given aquarium.

4. Aerators — These include airstones and other devices driven by pneumatic pumps that increase circulation and thus oxygen levels.

5. Live plants — Many different types of plants are maintained in aquaria, including mainly vascular plants (i.e., higher plants) in freshwater tanks and macroalgae in marine aquaria. Plants provide oxygen, remove nutrients, and act as refuges for shy fish.

6. Decorations — These include coral, ornaments, and various types of artificial plants. All items should have been tested safe for use in aquaria.

7. Heater — This is a thermostatically controlled electrical unit that maintains a constant temperature. Some are only partly submerged, while others are completely submersible.

8. Disinfection units — These are used to remove pathogens from the water. Most popular are units that produce ozone or ultraviolet light to kill microorganisms. While they are useful when water is being recirculated among multiple aquaria, their utility, when used for only one aquarium, is questionable.

CLOSED CULTURE SYSTEMS: PONDS
The Pond as an Ecosystem

Many of the principles that apply to aquarium ecology also apply to pond ecology. It is useful to consider the pond itself as a single, functioning entity, since the pond's health is vital to the fish's health. In many ways the pond's vital functions are similar to that of a single organism (Noga & Francis-Floyd, 1991). Respiration, acid-base balance, elimination of nitrogenous wastes, and other biological functions must be maintained. Some factors, such as temperature, are beyond control; however, others can be modified considerably through active intervention of the farmer and as an indirect consequence of management practices. It is also important to realize that changing a single parameter, such as increasing pH, can have a profound effect on many other variables (Table I-2).

Thus, it is not possible to treat the pond without affecting the fish, and conversely, it is not possible to treat the fish without affecting the pond ecosystem (Tucker, 1985; Tucker et al., 1979). This makes water quality analysis as important to assessing a fish disease problem as the physical examination is to routine clinical assessment of land animals. Adjacent ponds may be identical in size, soil substrate, source of water, and number of fish stocked, but each will develop as a unique ecosystem and must be treated as such.

Several routine management practices are performed to maintain proper pond health, including the following:

1. Fertilization — May be used to stimulate growth of algae, which is the major producer of oxygen in the pond and which removes much of the ammonia.

2. Aerators — Supplemental aeration is used when oxygen is low. Paddlewheels, diffusers, and other devices may be used.

3. Liming — Is used to neutralize acids and to maintain a proper pH. It also provides carbonate ion needed for algal growth and calcium and magnesium needed by fish. Liming is often done after draining a pond at the end of a production cycle (see *PROBLEM 6*).

In addition, algicide treatment has been used to control excessive algal growth but is usually not recommended (see PROBLEM 1).

Commercial Ponds

Commercial fish ponds are typically earthen, rectangular, 0.9 to 1.2 m (3 to 4 feet) deep, and 0.4 to 8 hectares (1 to 20 acres) in size. Commercial pond fish production faces problems that are similar to those in other forms of intensive animal agriculture. High stocking densities mandate high nutrient input from feed, which in turn causes the buildup of toxic wastes. High nutrient levels also stimulate algae growth, causing large fluctuations in dissolved oxygen. These suboptimal conditions place considerable stress on the fish; water is an excellent medium for the transmission of infectious agents, and diseases can spread rapidly through susceptible populations. Diseases must be

Table I-2 Interrelationships between some important water quality factors in a fish pond.

Factor	Effect* of increase in factor on:			
	Dissolved oxygen	Dissolved CO_2	Ammonia toxicity	Copper toxicity
Temperature	Decrease	Decrease	Increase	Increase[†]
pH	No direct effect	Decrease	Increase	Decrease
Alkalinity	No direct effect	Decrease	No direct effect	Decrease
Phytoplankton[‡]	Increased fluctuation	Increased fluctuation	Complicated effect	Complicated effect
Hardness[§]	No direct effect	No direct effect	No direct effect	No direct effect

From Noga & Floyd, 1991
*Only direct causal relationships are presented. These relationships hold if all other factors remain constant. For example, only the direct effect of alkalinity is considered, although methods used to increase alkalinity (buffering capacity) may also increase pH.
[†]Fish become ill or succumb more quickly when the temperature is higher.
[‡]Increases in the duration or intensity of light may have similar effects because of increased photosynthesis.
[§]if attributable mainly to calcium carbonate.

diagnosed rapidly and accurately; even a matter of several hours can be crucial to the outcome of an epidemic. Thus, herd health management with proper intervention to prevent problems is the best approach.

Some ponds are also stocked with fish that the owners then charge customers to fish (*fee-fishing ponds*). These ponds are frequently restocked with large fish. Owners must keep fish actively feeding to provide a quality experience for customers.

Farm Ponds

Many landowners raise fish in *farm ponds* that are stocked with channel catfish, as well as game fish (e.g. bass, bluegill). In the state of North Carolina alone, it is estimated that over 100,000 farm ponds exist. While such ponds usually do not constitute a primary source of income for the owner, they often represent a significant investment in time and/or money, and provide a considerable amount of enjoyment, as well as a source of food. Some individuals start out with such small production units, hoping to expand later if the business is profitable. While these systems are usually not as intensively managed as the larger commercial operations, the concepts regarding proper management are the same. Medical advice for these fish could be incorporated into routine calls that are made to care for other farm animals.

Farm ponds vary greatly in size and depth but are usually relatively small; they may be deep, leading to stratification problems (see *PROBLEM 3*).

Pet Fish Ponds

Ponds are also popular for keeping some pet fishes (e.g., goldfish and koi). These ponds may have no filtration or aeration (Andrews et al., 1988). Filtration or aeration is not needed if the fish are in a low enough density, but the owners must be aware that fish may quickly outgrow a small pond.

FLOW-THROUGH CULTURE SYSTEMS

In the United States, flow-through (also known as *open* culture) systems are primarily used to raise salmonids. General characteristics include a high water turnover rate and the dependence on a flushing effect to maintain water quality. A flow-through system is any system that uses continuously flowing water, which enters at one point in the system and exits at another point. The major

limitation to flow-though culture is the amount of water available for use. While small systems can rely on dechlorinated tap water or low-capacity wells, larger systems usually need a source of surface water (e.g., stream, impounded lake).

The most common type of flow-through system is the raceway, a long, narrow *ditch* made of concrete, earth (e.g., *Danish pond*), or fiberglass (Stevenson, 1987). Raceways are often longitudinally divided into compartments, with a 0.3 m (1 foot) deep *waterfall* between each compartment. This waterfall adds more oxygen to the water; oxygen is the major limiting factor to the number of fish (and thus number of compartments) possible. Some farms have begun to use liquid oxygen to increase stocking densities; in such cases, ammonia toxicity and low pH become the major concerns (see *PROBLEMS 4* through *6*). It is usually not feasible to control other water quality variables, such as temperature, pH, or hardness, in flow-through systems.

The major advantage to a flow-through system is the ability to have a high stocking density and still have high-quality water (see Table III-1). However, disadvantages include the need for a large amount of high-quality water, which severely restricts the sites suitable for this type of culture. Increasingly stringent local and national regulations restrict the type and amount of effluents that can be released by such farms.

Many flow-through systems must use surface (e.g., stream) water, whose quality and quantity are highly dependent on rainfall (runoff). This can cause overcrowding and stressfully high temperatures in summer or during droughts.

Many diseases are transmitted via water, and important pathogens are often endemic in feral fish populations that inhabit the water source. This also makes the system susceptible to pathogens or toxins that may originate upstream of the system. An exception to this environmental variability is flow-through systems that use a ground water (i.e., well or spring) source. Ground water is usually free of pathogens and not chemically influenced by rainfall. Ground water sources are chemically stable and vary little over time.

SEMIOPEN CULTURE SYSTEMS

Cages and net-pens are intermediate in water exchange between open and closed systems. In the United States, cages and net-pens primarily are used to raise salmonids in seawater.

CHAPTER 3

Equipping a Fish Disease Diagnostic Facility

BASIC DIAGNOSTIC TOOLS

Most of the equipment required for fish disease diagnosis is inexpensively available. The only major piece of equipment that is absolutely needed is a high-quality microscope having 10X, 40X, and 100X (oil immersion) objectives (giving final magnifications of 100X, 400X, and 1000X with a 10X ocular). Other basic, required equipment includes disposable latex gloves, simple surgical instruments (scalpel, fine and coarse forceps, and fine and coarse scissors); 10% neutral, buffered formalin; microscope slides; and coverslips (all available from companies such as Baxter Diagnostics, Inc., Carolina Biological Supply Company, or Fisher Scientific).

In addition, water testing kits (available from companies such as Chemetrics, Inc., Hach Company, LaMotte Company, Marine Enterprises International, Ltd., or Tetra

Sales, USA), disinfectant/antiseptic (see *PHARMA-COPOEIA*), anesthetic (see *PHARMACOPOEIA*), several clean 20 and 40 liter (5 and 10 gallon) plastic buckets, a supply of various-sized aquarium bags, various-sized nets, and several airstones connected to a small air pump (available from companies such as Aquatic Ecosystems, Inc., Argent Chemical Laboratories, or Aquacenter or from a local pet shop) are all that are usually needed.

It is also helpful to have media available for bacterial culture (sold by companies such as Baxter Diagnostics, Inc. or Fisher Scientific), depending on the number and types of cases seen. Addresses for suppliers are listed in *APPENDIX II*. Details about choosing specific items for the clinic are described in *THE CLINICAL WORK-UP*. See the *PHARMACOPOEIA* for items needed for treating diseases.

CHAPTER 4

The Clinical Work-Up

CASE SUBMISSIONS
Submissions to the Clinic

The basic steps that should be followed in the clinical work-up of a fish disease case are illustrated in Fig. I-1. If fish are submitted to the clinic, virtually all procedures can be handled on an outpatient basis, eliminating the need to keep fish overnight. Most cases will be initiated by a telephone call from an owner who is having a problem. The owner should be asked to bring in one to several representative fish for examination. It is important to determine whether the owner is amenable to the euthanization of any fish for the determination of a diagnosis. Hobbyists who are breeders are usually willing to sacrifice some fish, unless the fish are rare or expensive brood stock. While a complete postmortem examination is superior to performing only biopsies, this will not be possible in many pet fish cases; this can usually be discerned during the conversation with the owner.

If the client is submitting the fish to the clinic, the owner should be advised to bring both the fish and a water sample in *separate* clean containers. The best containers are a clean plastic bucket (never exposed to soap or other toxic chemical), plastic-lined cooler, styrofoam cooler, or a plastic aquarium bag. However, a *well-washed and rinsed* glass food container is also acceptable. Half a liter (one pint) of water is adequate for core water quality analysis.

To transport the fish (assuming the trip to the clinic will be less than 30 minutes), a good rule of thumb is to have about one liter of water for every one centimeter of fish (or one-half gallon of water for every 1 inch of fish) to be transported. Much higher densities can be used if supplemental oxygenation is provided. It is best to place the container of fish in a cooler to prevent temperature shock. Fish may also be transported directly in the cooler. For longer journeys, it is best to provide supplemental oxygen during transport. Oxygen cylinders or portable aerators (Baitsaver or equivalent) can be used to provide oxygenation. Alternatively, small fish can be shipped in a sealed plastic aquarium bag that has an oxygen-enriched atmosphere. The *Fish Disease Diagnosis Form (APPENDIX I)* provides details on various methods of shipment.

The ability to diagnose a problem is directly related to the quality of the samples submitted. Live fish that show typical clinical signs of the problem provide the best samples. Preserved material is least useful for most, but not all, diagnoses. Different methods of tissue storage are more useful for certain problems. Water samples also have a finite storage time (Table I-3).

Commercial Producers

While most individual pet fish cases are best submitted directly to the clinic, it is often important to visit the facilities of commercial growers, such as pet fish breeders, retailers, wholesalers, or commercial food fish producers. A visit allows a more thorough evaluation of the facilities and management, which are often the root cause of a disease complaint. The procedures used for diagnostic work-up are the same as for individual aquarium fish (see Fig. I-1).

Since more fish are usually involved in commercial producers' cases, more fish can be examined, which strengthens the diagnosis. Generally, four to six fish should be examined during epidemics. Live fish should be used whenever possible. The only exception is when all of the live fish appear healthy; in this case, the freshest dead fish should also be examined.

If fish are being certified for presence or absence of certain diseases, the number examined depends on the total population size, the prevalence of the disease to be surveyed, and the level of confidence desired (Sims & Schill, 1984). Amos (1985) and Thoesen (1994) provide detailed methods for certifying fish to be free of specific diseases.

WATER QUALITY ANALYSIS
Core Water Quality Parameters

Core water quality parameters are tests that should be run when **any** fish disease case is submitted. They include ammonia, nitrite, and pH (and salinity in a marine or brackish water system). Oxygen and temperature are also part of this core list but should be measured on site (i.e.,

Steps in working up a fish disease case

Client submits fish and water sample

Client

Take case history
Oxygen
Temperature
Additional information

Water sample

Measure
Oxygen (only on site)
Temperature (only on site)
Ammonia
Nitrite
pH
Hardness
Salinity

1-9*

Fish
Place in aerated container

Examine for
Behavioral abnormalities
Physical abnormalities
Sedate fish
Make blood smear
  (only if grossly anemic)
Biopsy skin, gills
Fecal smear
Identify
Metazoan ectoparasites
Protozoan ectoparasites
Skin/gill bacteria
Skin/gill fungi
Lymphocystis
Epitheliocystis
Hemopathies

10-43

Euthanize fish

Culture
Kidney, other organs for systemic bacterial infections

44-54

Necropsy fish

Identify
Metazoan endoparasites
Protozoan endoparasites
Systemic fungal infections
Idiopathic epidermal proliferation
Neoplasia

55-72

Do identified problems sufficiently explain morbidity and mortality?

Yes

No

Rule-out diagnoses
All presumptive diagnoses
Definitive diagnosis via specialized tests+
Identify
Systemic viral infections   Generic anomalies
Nutritional deficiency   Noxious algae
Miscellaneous poisoning   Idiopathic diseases
Traumatic lesions

73-92

Prioritize problems

Threat to life
Primary cause
Treatment priority

Treatment / follow-up

Short-term therapy — medication
Long-term therapy — management

*Refer to work problems

+Not all rule-out problems can be definitively diagnosed

Fig. 1-1   Steps in working up a fish disease case.

Table I-3   Recommended sampling containers and storage procedures for water samples.

Variable	Container	Volume (ml)	Handling procedure	Analyze within
All	Clean or new			ASAP
Oxygen	Glass stoppered glass	300	Fill totally, 4° in dark	6 hours
Temperature	N/A	N/A	N/A	None; must do on site
pH	Polyethylene	100	4° C in dark	6 hours
Ammonia; nitrate; nitrite	Polyethylene or glass (**NOT** HNO_3-washed)	500	Acidify with 1 ml concentrated H_2SO_4/L (to pH <2.0); store on ice or freeze 4° C	24 hours 24 hours
Metals	Polyethylene, HNO_3-washed	500	Acidify with analytical HNO_3 to pH <2.0; freeze if analysis delayed	24 hours
Pesticides, other organochemicals	Glass- or Teflon-stoppered glass, hexane-washed (**no** plastics)	500	Fill totally	24 hours
Solids (dissolved; suspended; settleable)	Glass or plastic	500	4° C	
Cyanides	Glass or plastic	100	Add 0.2 ml of 10 M NaOH, to pH 12	24 hours
Algae	Glass or plastic	100	Fresh chilled, or add Lugol's iodine to color of weak tea or add 10% formalin 1 : 1	24 hours
Summary (agents unknown)	Polyethylene; HNO_3-washed	500	Add HNO_3 to pH <2.0	24 hours
	Glass or plastic; (2 samples)	500	Freeze one	24 hours
	Glass; hexane-washed	500	Fill totally	24 hours
	Glass; hexane-washed	500	Fill totally, 4° C in dark	6 hours

From Langdon, 1988; Hill, 1983; Boyd, 1979. Suggested time intervals should be considered liberal estimates. Samples may be less stable under some conditions. HNO_3 = nitric acid; H_2SO_4 = sulfuric acid; NaOH = sodium hydroxide.

at the pond, aquarium) to be accurate; this can be done only if the clinician visits the site. Otherwise, oxygen and temperature must be assessed from the history (i.e., the client has measured the oxygen or temperature; or, a problem with oxygen or temperature is discerned from the client interview).

While it is not part of the core list, it is often advisable to measure alkalinity and hardness in commercial ponds and nitrate in aquaria (especially marine aquaria). Chloride should also be measured in commercial ponds when nitrite levels are high (see *PROBLEM 5*).

Special (Noncore) Water Quality Sampling

Many other water quality changes besides the core list can affect fish health (see *PROBLEMS 80* through *86*). While not routinely measured, some cases may warrant examining these other factors (see *RULE-OUT DIAGNOSES* and Fig. I-1). Specific recommendations for sample collection vary with the type of substance being measured and with how quickly the sample can be submitted (i.e., will preservative be added?). Also, different types of samples need to be collected in different types of sample containers (plastic, glass). After determining that certain measurements should be taken, the clinician should contact the laboratory where the samples are to be submitted to obtain specific information on methods of collec-

tion. The American Public Health Association (A.P.H.A., 1992) also provides extensive details on water sampling.

Water Quality Testing

Many manufacturers produce simple test kits for measuring core water quality parameters and other water quality variables. Most tests are based on adding a known amount of the water sample to a vial and then adding chemicals, which react with the substance to be measured, producing a colored reaction. The amount of substance present is proportional to the intensity of the color change. Most tests take less than 5 minutes to run. It is important to realize that special procedures are sometimes required to test substances in seawater; thus, while most kits for measurements in seawater are also usable for freshwater samples, the converse is not always true.

The accuracy of commercial water test kits is related to the cost of the kit. Inexpensive kits that use a color chart for measurement are available from aquarium wholesalers or retailers (e.g., Marine Enterprises). These water test kits are only semiquantitative but give a general indication of water quality and are often sensitive enough to diagnose most water quality problems encountered in routine clinical cases. More expensive kits designed specifically for water quality testing on commercial farms (e.g., FF-1A Kit [approximately $90]; FF-2 Kit [approximately $350];

Hach Company) are more accurate and acceptable for all routine diagnostic procedures; these also have the advantage of combining most routine tests into one kit. Even more sophisticated colorimetric kits use a spectrophotometer for measurements (e.g., Hach DREL 2000, approximately $3000) and are usually accurate to within 20% of the so-called *standard methods* (Boyd, 1979).

The most accurate methods for water quality analyses are the standard methods. In the United States, most standard methods are developed and sanctioned under the auspices of either the American Public Health Association (A.P.H.A., 1992) or the United States Environmental Protection Agency (U.S.E.P.A., 1979). Standard methods of analytical accuracy are not needed for clinical diagnoses, unless a particular case may eventually involve litigation or is involved in certain research protocols. Samples taken for regulatory compliance monitoring or collected as evidence during enforcement investigations must also conform to well-defined procedures regarding sample handling, shipment, and chain-of-custody documentation. The clinician should refer to EPA guidelines or contact the appropriate environmental agency (e.g., U.S.E.P.A or regional or state environmental agency) for assistance in collecting such samples.

If frequent visits to culture facilities are anticipated, it is also advisable to purchase a dissolved oxygen meter (e.g., YSI about $600). Electronic probes are also available for measuring temperature, pH, nitrite, chloride, and conductivity (salinity). The major advantage of electronic probes is that measurements can be taken quickly and accurately. However, probes are expensive, must be calibrated regularly, and are subject to failure if they are not maintained properly. It is also desirable that probes withstand disinfection, reducing the potential transmission of disease. For example, YSI dissolved oxygen probes can be left in disinfectant indefinitely, including 70% ethanol, povidone-iodine, quaternary ammonium, or just about any chemical that does not damage the housing (e.g., does not chemically react with the plastic housing; the probe itself is inert, being Teflon). Details of various water sampling devices are described with specific water quality problems.

Water Samples Submitted to the Clinic

The water sample should be immediately examined for core water quality parameters because changes can occur within a short time after collection (see Table I-3). If it cannot be examined immediately but will be examined within 1 hour, it should be left at room temperature. If it will not be examined for over an hour, it should be refrigerated but should be tested for ammonia, nitrite, and pH within 24 hours. The water should be allowed to come back to room temperature before doing any measurements.

Water Sampling on Site

Water samples may vary tremendously from one part of a culture system to the other. For example, oxygen and pH are highest, while carbon dioxide and ammonia are lowest, at the inflow of a flow-through system. The opposite is true at the outflow. Thus, flow-through systems should be sampled for oxygen, pH, and ammonia at both the inflow and the effluent.

Ponds should be sampled for dissolved oxygen and temperature at both the windward and leeward sides to account for wind-induced mixing (Boyd, 1990). Samples should be taken at 0.5 to 1.0 m (1.5 to 3 feet) in waters less than 2.0 m (6 feet) deep. Both surface and water samples should be taken to assess variability. Different bodies of water can have markedly different water quality characteristics, even with identical stocking densities, feeding rates, etc. (Noga & Francis-Floyd, 1991). Thus, each system should be treated as an individual unit in terms of water quality sampling.

TAKING THE HISTORY

When ready to see the client, a thorough history should be taken (see *Fish Disease Diagnosis Form, APPENDIX I*) (Stoskopf, 1988). It can be useful to try to determine whether the problem is acute or chronic, since this can help to eliminate some differentials (Fig. I-2). Acute problems are typically those that have developed within a matter of only a few days and have resulted in considerable morbidity and/or mortality within that time. Conversely, chronic problems typically develop over several weeks or more and may only result in an occasional mortality. Also, such fish are often in poor condition and may be anorexic.

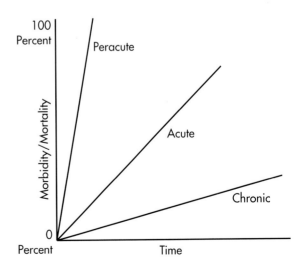

Fig. I-2 Typical morbidity and/or mortality rates with peracute, acute, or chronic disease.

Important questions to ask include the following:
- How long has the culture system (aquarium, pond, etc.) held fish?
- Are all fish affected?
- If not, which are not?
- Do the fish display any behavioral signs, such as *flashing* (rubbing against objects suggesting skin problems) or *piping* (staying near the air-water interface to obtain more oxygen, suggesting gill problems)? Low oxygen is common; unfortunately, oxygen can only be accurately measured on site (i.e., at the pond), so the history may be crucial to assessment.

It is often best to ask the client to describe the usual routine for feeding, water changes, and other management procedures to discern an accurate history. It is also important to determine what prior treatments, including medications, have been given.

THE PHYSICAL EXAM

When a client submits live fish to the clinic, aeration should be immediately placed into the container that holds the fish. Once a thorough history has been taken, the fish should be closely examined for behavioral abnormalities (e.g., increased respiration, suggesting possible gill problems or nitrite toxicity) (Francis-Floyd, 1988) and external lesions (e.g., ulcers, masses, *cloudiness* of the skin caused by increased mucus production, erosion or irregularities of the fins, etc.). Examining gills is most easily done when taking biopsies (see *GILL BIOPSIES*).

Color Change as an Indicator of Fish Health

The melanin pigmentation in fish's skin is under neuroendocrine control and is thus affected by hormones, such as epinephrine. When fish are sick, maintenance of a normal pigmentation pattern presumably takes less precedence than homeostasis of more vital body functions. Thus, sick fish are often abnormally colored, compared with the healthier tankmates. This is a common response of salmonids to disease, with sick fish being typically darker than normal. A color change can also be caused by blindness, which eliminates the normal visual cues that are needed to maintain a normal color pattern in daylight (Fig. I-3, *A*). Fish in breeding condition often have more brilliant colors than nonbreeding fish (Axelrod et al., 1980). Since the chemical signals that control pigmentation are transmitted via the nerves, peripheral nerve damage, such as from vertebral instability, can cause a focal change in pigmentation pattern (see *PROBLEM 64*). Focal color change can also be caused by local tissue irritation/damage, such as parasite feeding, chronic wounds, or healing wounds, which cause a change in the pigment cell distribution at that site (see *PROBLEMS 53* and *55*).

Reddening of the body is usually caused by hemorrhage, which can result from systemic bacterial or viral infections (see *PROBLEMS 44* and *73*), or skin wounds. Loss of fin tissue most often results from poor water quality (see *PROBLEM 36*). Parasites may also incite a thickening of the skin, which leads to a whitish cast or white foci (see *PROBLEM 19*). See *EVALUATION OF SKIN BIOPSIES*, p. 21, for a further discussion of gross lesions affecting the skin. Observations of color pattern are best made while the fish is in its culture system, since the pattern can also be affected by acute stress (e.g., confinement).

Other Common Gross Signs of Disease

Sick fish often congregate together, separating themselves from their healthier cohorts (Fig. I-3, *A*). Weak fish in raceways or other systems with flowing water will often be found near the water outlet. Sick fish may also exhibit other behavioral signs, including staying near the surface of the water because of hypoxia (see *PROBLEM 1*), scraping the body because of parasite irritation, or showing various behavioral abnormalities because of nervous system involvement (see *PROBLEM 74*).

Another common clinical sign is abdominal swelling (Fig. I-3, *B*), which is most commonly caused by an infectious peritonitis (viral, bacterial, or parasitic) but can also be caused by a metabolic disturbance (e.g., renal failure), neoplasia, or obesity. This clinical sign is often referred to as *dropsy* in the aquarium literature. Abdominal swelling may also be a normal sign of sexual maturity in female fish that are ready to spawn.

Eye lesions, such as exophthalmos (Fig. I-3, *C*) are common in several infectious diseases, including several viral and bacterial infections. Unilateral lesions often indicate a possible traumatic cause, especially in large fish. Many nutritional deficiencies are also associated with ocular pathology.

Skeletal deformities (Fig. I-3, *D*), especially of the vertebral column, are also seen in several types of diseases, ranging from certain parasitic infections to nutritional deficiencies to toxicoses.

See *GILL BIOPSY PROCEDURE*, p. 23, and *COMMON LESIONS FOUND IN THE VISCERA*, p. 41, for other gross signs of disease.

PREPARING FISH FOR BIOPSY

Latex gloves should be worn when handling fish for disease diagnosis. Fish skin is not keratinized and thus is susceptible to iatrogenic damage. (**A dry paper towel should never be used to grab a fish for biopsy!**) Latex gloves are soft and slippery when wet, reducing possible skin damage and preventing the loss of surface-dwelling

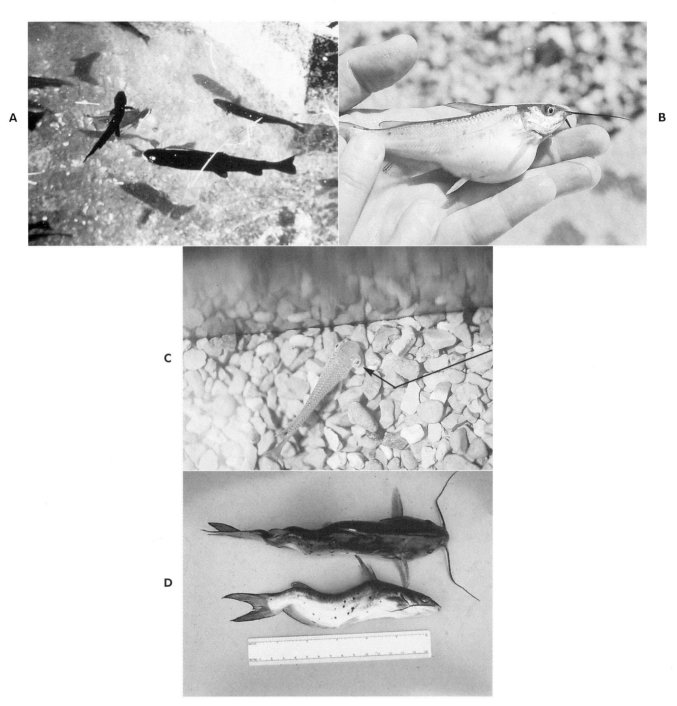

Fig. I-3   Common gross signs of disease in fish. **A,** Salmonids congregating near the outlet screen of a raceway. In this case the dark color is caused by blindness. But, color change is a general indicator of ill health. The segregation of these fish away from the rest of the fish population is also characteristic of sick fish. **B,** Massive swelling in a channel catfish caused by fluid accumulation in the peritoneal cavity. **C,** Exophthalmos (*arrow*) in a killifish. **D,** Spinal curvature, including scoliosis (*lateral curvature*) and lordosis (*forward curvature*).

(*A* photograph courtesy of C.L. Davis, Foundation for Veterinary Pathology; *B* and *C* photographs courtesy of T. Wenzel; *D* photograph courtesy of A. Mitchell.)

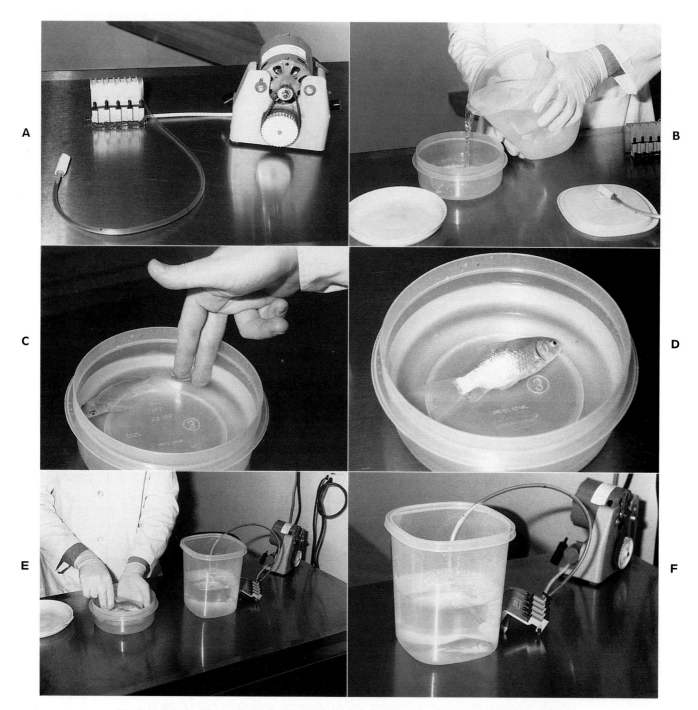

Fig. 1-4 Method for sedating fish before a clinical procedure. **A,** A simple device for providing aeration during a clinical visit. An electrical air pump is attached to a gang valve having five outlets, so that up to five containers can be aerated at once. **B,** Adding some water from the container in which the fish was submitted to another container to be used for sedation. **C,** Mixing the tranquilizer/anesthetic before adding the fish. **D,** Fish is responding to sedation (losing balance). **E,** Fish is being removed for a clinical procedure. **F,** Fish placed in aerated water after completion of the clinical procedure.

parasites when handling the fish. Also, some zoonotic pathogens can be contracted by handling infected fish (see *PROBLEMS 45, 48, 49,* and *53*). Many disposable gloves are coated with talc, so gloved hands should be rinsed in water before handling the fish to prevent talc crystals from contaminating biopsies (see Fig. II-42, *C*).

After the visual examination, the skin and gills should be biopsied to look for pathogens. Skin biopsies usually can be taken from any fish larger than 25 mm (1 inch), and a gill biopsy can usually be taken from any fish larger than 50 mm (2 inches). These techniques are valuable because many of the diseases that affect fish are confined to the skin or gills.

Sedation / Anesthesia

The same drugs are used for both sedation and anesthesia in fish. The only difference between sedation and anesthesia is the dosage of drug and/or the length of time that the fish is exposed. Since these drugs are all administered through the water, the dosage is directly proportional to both the amount of drug in the water and how long the fish has been left in the solution.

For biopsy, a portion of the water used to transport the fish is placed into an aquarium bag or other suitable container and a small amount of anesthetic (and buffer, if necessary) is added (see the *PHARMACOPOEIA* for types of anesthetics available) (Fig. I-4, *A* through *F*). The fish is then placed in the anesthetic bath and watched carefully. The *PHARMACOPOEIA* provides a range of doses that have been used for various fish species. Response to a given dosage varies considerably, depending on fish species and environmental conditions. When these drugs are used on a fish species with unknown susceptibility, start with the lower recommended dose and gradually add more if needed, until the desired effect is reached.

Fish exhibit planes of anesthesia that are similar to mammals. The first stage is excitation; some fish, such as eels, struggle violently during this stage and may attempt to escape. The container that holds such fish should be well covered. After excitation the fish becomes depressed (less response to touch), loses equilibrium (lies increasingly on its side), and respiration slows (gilling, the opening and closing of the gill covers, becomes slower and weaker). If the fish is left in the anesthetic bath long enough, breathing will stop. Fish should not be left in anesthetic long enough to stop breathing; however, many fish will recover even after breathing has stopped for several minutes.

If the proper amount of anesthetic is added, the fish should be immobilized in less than 5 minutes. If the fish remains alert after this time, a bit more anesthetic should be added. Once the fish has ceased to struggle and can be handled, a fin clip should be taken with fine forceps and a skin scrape should be taken with a scalpel. These

biopsies should be placed immediately on a slide with a drop of aquarium water, a coverslip should be added, and then the specimen can be examined. A gill biopsy should then be taken, using fine scissors.

Anesthesia often causes involuntary defecation, allowing the collection of a fecal sample (see *FECAL EXAM*). Sedation or anesthesia may also cause some loosely attached ectoparasites, such as monogeneans or leeches, to detach from the fish (Noga et al., 1990; Svendsen & Haug, 1991). It could interfere with diagnosis of these problems by biasing the number of organisms observed on wet mounts. However, the importance of parasite narcotization on making a clinical diagnosis has not been studied. With practice, many fish can be biopsied without sedation. If the fish can be euthanized, pithing or cervical severance can be used for immobilization rather than chemical overdose (see *PHARMACOPOEIA*).

USING THE MICROSCOPE

Next to water testing, examining tissues by wet mount is the most informative technique in fish disease diagnosis. In fact, the majority of fish disease cases can be diagnosed by using just the water quality tests outlined and by an examination of skin and gill wet mounts.

The microscope used for diagnosis should have a range of objectives, including at least 10X, 40X (low and high dry) and 100X (oil immersion, high power). A low-power (4X) objective is also useful for rapidly scanning a sample. Close down the iris diaphragm to exclude much of the light and increase contrast. When wet mounts are examined, it is important to determine the size of various objects in the microscope's field because the proper identification of a parasite or other organism is much easier when its size is known.

The most accurate way to measure an object's size is to use an ocular micrometer. This micrometer is placed into the eyepiece of the microscope and can then be superimposed over the organism in question to measure its size. Another way to measure the size of an object is to compare it to the size of a red blood cell (RBC) in the same field. Fish RBCs usually range from about 6 to 9 μm on the long axis. They can be identified on a wet mount by their platter-shaped or fried-egg appearance (see Fig. I-11). Because the RBCs are fairly consistent in size, they can be used to estimate the dimensions of an object. Latex beads can also be used for size estimation.

BIOPSY PROCEDURES: PREPARING SLIDES

Immediately before performing any biopsies, a drop of water (seawater, if it is a marine fish) is added to a slide for every biopsy that is to be performed on the fish. Water from the container that holds the fish can be used (Fig. I-

5, *A*). One of the quickest ways to transfer the water is to dip the tip of your finger into it and then touch your finger to the slide. This will leave a small drop of water on the slide. A pipet can also be used. The biopsy should be placed immediately in the water drop to prevent any organisms in the sample from drying out and thus dying.

SKIN BIOPSY

Skin biopsy is the single most useful tool available for diagnosing diseases in fish because the skin is a primary target organ for a number of common infectious agents. The skin of fish has layers analogous to those present in mammals, including the hypodermis, dermis, basement membrane, epidermis, and cuticle (Fig. I-6, *B*). The dermis contains pigment cells and the scales, which are embedded in connective tissue and overlap one another like shingles on a roof. Some species, such as catfish, lack scales, while others, such as eels, have small scales.

Covering the scales is the epidermis, a stratified squamous epithelium with goblet (mucus-producing) cells. The epidermis is covered by the cuticle, a thin layer of mucus that contains sloughed epithelial cells and many protective substances, such as antibody, lysozyme, and C-reactive protein (Alexander & Ingram, 1992). In almost all fish, the epithelium is not keratinized, and living cells are present in all layers. This makes fish skin susceptible to both acute and chronic injury.

The skin performs the following three functions in all fish: (1) it reduces drag by providing a smooth friction-free surface for locomotion; (2) it acts as a first line of defense against the invasion of infectious agents; and (3) it makes an impermeable barrier to the movement of fluids and salts. In some species (e.g., eels, catfish), it also acts as an accessory site for respiration. Its critical importance in maintaining internal homeostasis is a major reason why skin damage, exclusive of other organ involvement, can kill fish.

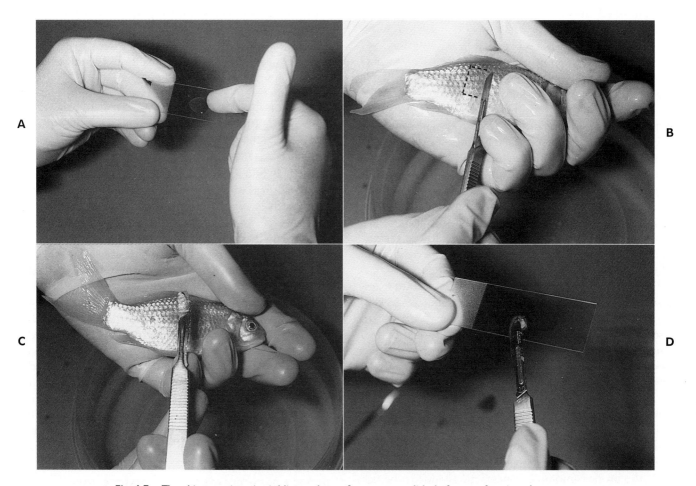

Fig. I-5   The skin scraping. **A,** Adding a drop of water to a slide before performing the biopsy. Dip a finger in water, and then touch the finger to the slide. **B,** Scraping the skin with a scalpel to obtain a biopsy sample. Note that the back side of the blade is used for scraping. Only a relatively small area (*dotted line*) should be scraped. **C,** Biopsy material on the scalpel blade. Note that scales (flat, refractile) have been included in the biopsy, indicating that the entire epithelial layer has been removed. **D,** Scraping the biopsy material onto the slide.

Continued.

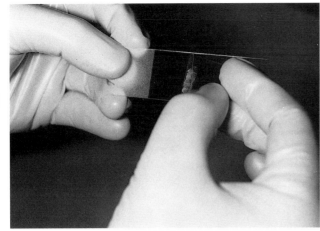
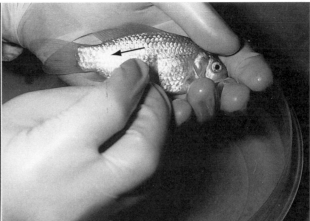
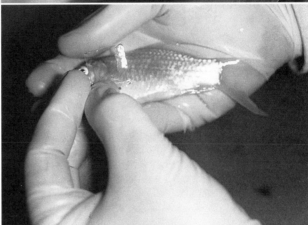

Fig. I-5—cont'd. E, Covering the sample with a coverslip. F, Using a coverslip to make a skin scraping (glass is best). Arrow points in direction of the scraping. G, Biopsy material, including scales, on the coverslip.

SKIN BIOPSY PROCEDURES: SCRAPING

Two major methods are used to obtain skin biopsies: skin scraping and fin clipping. Skin scraping is performed by taking a spatula or a scalpel and gently scraping along the side of the body or fins while the fish is adequately restrained (Fig. I-5, B through G). Lightly sedated fish can usually be prevented from struggling by enclosing the body with a loosely clasped hand. Avoid damaging the skin when performing any procedures by not exposing the fish to dry or rough surfaces. For example, fish should not be held with paper towels, even if the towels are moistened. This rough surface can easily remove the cuticle. Latex rubber gloves moistened with water are especially good for handling fish.

Only gentle pressure is necessary when taking a scraping because most pathogens are found near the surface. Much less pressure is required than that used in performing skin scrapings of mammals. Overzealous sampling does more harm than good. Even light scrapings usually remove the epidermis and dermis from small fish (see Figs. I-5, C, and I-6, A). Large areas of skin should not be scraped because the resulting open wound may become secondarily infected or cause serious fluid imbalance.

Scrapings should be taken where obvious lesions are present. The smaller wounds should be examined carefully since older lesions are often overgrown by oppor-

tunistic bacteria (e.g., *Aeromonas hydrophila*, see *PROBLEM 45*) or water molds (see *PROBLEM 33*). The leading edge of a lesion should always be examined because this area is most likely to harbor the inciting pathogen(s). To determine the initiating etiological agent may require sampling sites other than obvious lesions to discover which pathogens are present and also examining other fish in the same group. When pathogens are not detected by wet mount, bacterial culture of lesions is warranted.

The scraping should be immediately transferred to a glass slide, applying a drop of water (seawater, if a marine fish) and a plastic coverslip. Plastic coverslips are preferred to glass, since they are inexpensive and are less easily broken when crushing wet mounts from viscera. The wet mount should be examined immediately, since many parasites, especially the protozoa, will die soon after being removed from their hosts. Most parasites are difficult to identify when dead. It can be helpful to apply a drop of methylcellulose solution (Carolina Biological Supply Company) to slow the movement of protozoa, but this is almost never needed for identification of parasites.

Fungal hyphae, granulomas, and most protozoa are visible at low (40X to 100X) magnification under the microscope. The definitive identification of protozoa and bacteria usually requires high dry magnification (400X) and sometimes oil immersion (1000X).

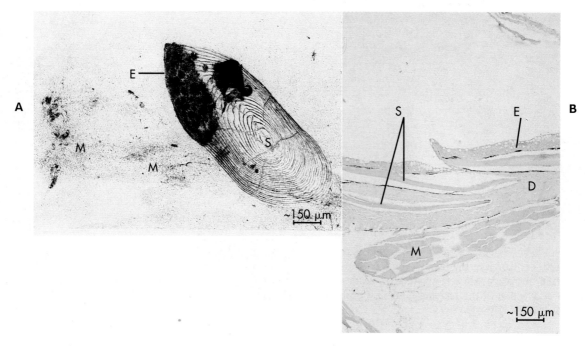

Fig. I-6   A, Low-power photomicrograph of a scraping from normal skin of a black-pigmented fish showing a scale (*S*), dark epithelium (*E*) covering the posterior part of the scale and mucus, and epithelium (*M*) scraped from the skin. **B,** Histological section of normal skin. The space between the scale and dermis is an artifact caused by shrinkage during histological preparation. *S* = scale; *E* = epithelium; *D* = dermis; *M* = muscle; hematoxylin and eosin.

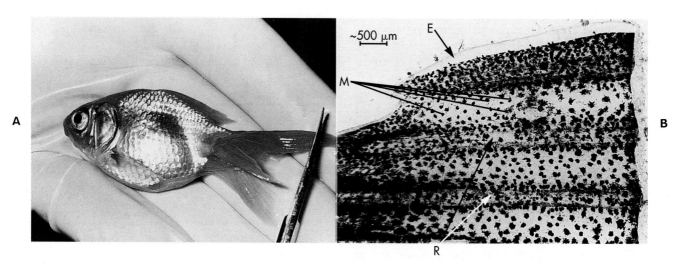

Fig. I-7   The fin clip. A, Clipping the fin. **B,** Microscopic features in normal, black-pigmented fin, including fin rays (*R*) and epithelium (*E*), which covers the entire fin but is most easily seen on the edge of the fin. Numerous melanocytes (*M*) are also present. The cut edge of the fin is on the right in the *original* photo.

SKIN BIOPSY PROCEDURES: FIN CLIP

To fin clip (Fig. I-7, *A* and *B*), simply snip a small piece of one of the fins (the tail fin is usually the easiest) and prepare it as described for the skin scraping. This procedure is less traumatic than skin scraping because a cleaner and much smaller wound is produced; however, it is usually not as useful as a skin scrape. It may be difficult to see small pathogens such as *Ichthyobodo*, since the thick, hard fin rays prevent the preparation of a thin smear. The thinner parts of the smear should be searched.

EVALUATION OF SKIN BIOPSIES

Like all organ systems, the skin has a characteristic repertoire of reactions to injury. These can include hemorrhage, erosion, and ulceration (Fig. I-8, *A* and *B*). Fin ulceration (often termed *fin erosion* or *fin rot*) is actually a gangrenous loss of tissue. It usually presents as a progressive necrosis starting at the tip of the fin. The leading edge of the lesion is often hyperemic or hemorrhagic. The necrotic tissue loses its normal color and often becomes white. Fragments of the fin rays may remain after the epithelium has sloughed, leaving a ragged appearance to the fin. Proliferation of epithelium may also occur concurrently with the progressive necrosis.

Another common response of the skin is hyperactivity of epithelium and goblet cells, which results in a thickening of the epithelium or increased mucus production that can give a cloudy appearance to the skin (Fig. I-8, *C*). Also, because the epidermis is not vascularized in small fish, there can be extensive epidermal damage without any bleeding. This may appear as depigmentation (Fig. I-8, *D*).

Numerous ectoparasites, bacteria, and other agents can incite these responses and often act together to produce lesions. Thus, the diagnosis of skin lesions can be complicated by the presence of several agents. Most ectoparasites can be present in low numbers on fish without causing

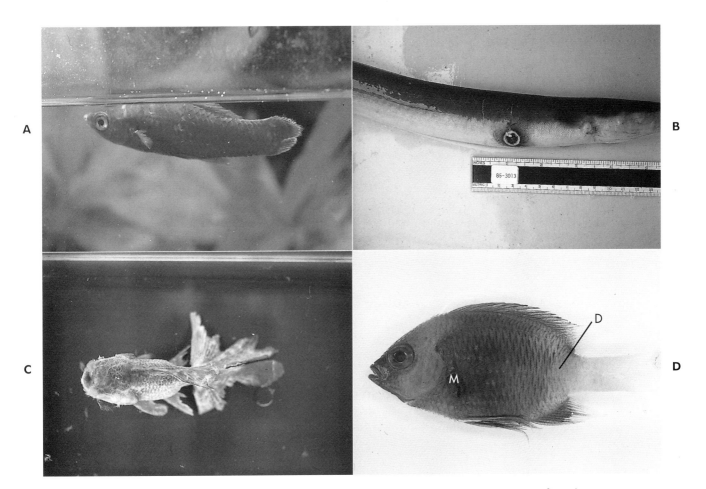

Fig. I-8 Common responses of the skin to damage. All of these responses are nonspecific and are thus only suggestive of certain problems. **A,** Caudal fin erosion and ulceration (*fin rot*). **B,** Skin ulcer. Note the hemorrhage around the ulcer. **C,** Cloudy appearance of the skin, with white flecks of detaching tissue; this may be due to epithelial hyperplasia and/or increased mucus production. **D,** Depigmentation (*D*) and melanization (*M*).

disease. For example, normal and apparently healthy channel catfish frequently have one or two trichodinids per low power field (MacMillan, 1985). Even such virulent pathogens as *Ichthyophthirius* (see *PROBLEM 19*) and *Amyloodinium* (see *PROBLEM 26*) can be carried asymptomatically. Conversely, heavy ectoparasitemia may be associated with systemic bacterial infections or other debilitating conditions. Thus, their significance depends on their concentration relative to other clinical findings.

It is important to determine the agent responsible for *initiating* a skin lesion to provide proper treatment. For example, water molds can colonize open skin wounds, and chronic ulcers often have many bacteria, especially motile rods, regardless of their primary etiology. However, even opportunists can kill fish, so treatment of secondary infections also is often advisable.

Many systemic diseases can have dermatological manifestations, although the etiological agents will often not be detectable in these dermatological lesions. Reddening of the fins and body (caused by congestion or hemorrhage) can be caused by gram negative bacteremias/septicemias, virus infections, or stressful environmental conditions (Smith & Ramos, 1976). Fish with mycobacteriosis (see *PROBLEM 53*) often have fin ulceration and faded coloration (Fig. I-8, *D*) (Reichenbache-Klinke, 1973).

Traumatic damage, such as that caused by aggressive tankmates (see *PROBLEM 87*), may mimic an infectious fin ulceration. Trauma is more likely to affect the more submissive members of a tank. Infectious agents are not present in purely traumatic lesions, although these may become secondarily infected.

Abnormal pigmentation may arise because of metacercarial infections (see *PROBLEM 55*) or other inflammatory lesions (e.g., *Ichthyophonus* (see *PROBLEM 67*) or *Mycobacterium* (see *PROBLEM 53*), or it may be a healing response to injury (Fig. I-8, *D*). Chronic inflammatory lesions often have large numbers of melanin-containing cells, including normal pigment cells (melanocytes) and inflammatory cells (melanomacrophages). These lesions should not be mistaken for melanotic cancers, which are much less common in fish.

GILL BIOPSY

Gill biopsy is a useful diagnostic tool in fish medicine. Many infectious agents that affect the skin can also infect the gills. Like the skin, the gill is a multifunctional organ; it is the major respiratory organ, is the primary site of nitrogenous waste excretion, and plays an important role in ionic balance. The complexity of the gill is reflected in its anatomical structure. Each gill arch has rows of macroscopically visible finger-like processes—the primary lamellae (Fig. I-9, *A* through *D*). Each primary lamella has rows of microscopic secondary lamellae. A capillary-like network of vessels in the secondary lamellae moves blood countercurrent to the water flow, facilitating gas exchange.

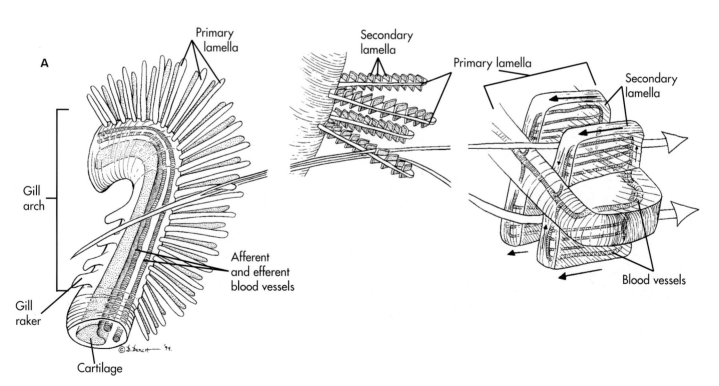

Fig. I-9   A, Diagram of normal gill. *Light arrows* indicate direction of water flow; *dark arrows* indicate blood flow.

Continued.

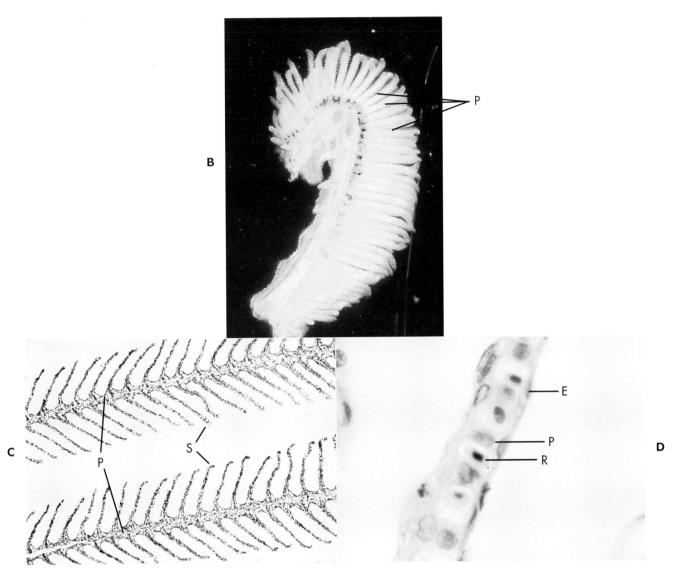

Fig. I-9—cont'd.   B, Low-power microscopic view of a formalin-fixed gill arch, showing primary lamellae (*P*), each having rows of secondary lamellae. (Compare with Fig. I-10, *C.*) C, Low-power histological section of normal gill. *P* = primary lamella; *S* = secondary lamella; hematoxylin and eosin. D, High-power histological section of normal gill secondary lamella. *R* = red blood cell; *P* = pillar cell; *E* = epithelial cell; hematoxylin and eosin.

GILL BIOPSY PROCEDURE

Immediately before biopsy the gills should be examined grossly. Healthy gills are bright red. Pale pink gills suggest anemia, while pale tan gills suggest methemoglobin formation (see *PROBLEM 5*). Do not confuse anemia with postmortem change (gills quickly become pale pink after death because of passive drainage of blood from the gills). Because the thymus is grossly visible in the gill chamber, it can also be evaluated at the same time. It should be glistening white (see Fig. I-32). Thymic hemorrhage has been associated with stress in salmonids (Goede & Barton, 1990).

Gill biopsy (Fig. I-10, *A* through *H*; Fig. I-11, *A* and *B)* is performed by inserting the tip of a pair of fine (e.g.,

iridectomy) scissors into the gill chamber. The scissors are then gently opened, lifting the operculum until the gill arches can be seen. The tips of several primary lamellae are then cut and transferred to a slide; a coverslip is then applied. Only the tips of the lamellae should be cut; bleeding should be minimal.

EVALUATION OF GILL BIOPSIES

The most common response of the gill to damage is hyperplasia and hypertrophy of epithelial cells, which can eventually lead to fusion of adjacent secondary or even primary lamellae. This severely reduces gas exchange at the wound site and can lead to respiratory distress. This can occur because of injury from bacteria or parasites or

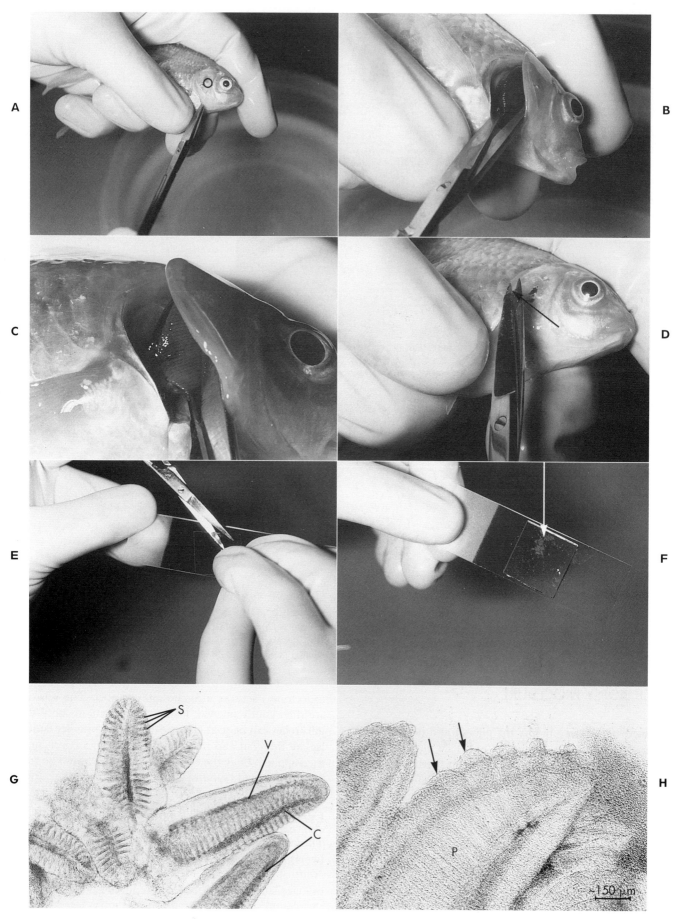

Fig. I-IO   *For legend see opposite page.*

Fig. I-10   The gill biopsy. **A,** Using a fine pair of scissors to pry open the gill cover, or operculum (*O*). **B,** Inserting the scissors under the tips of the gills just before cutting the tips. **C,** Close-up of Fig. I-10, *B.* Each horizontal, finger-like strip of tissue is a primary lamella. Only the distal tips of the primary lamella should be cut. **D,** Gill tissue on the scissor (*arrow*) after being excised from the gill. **E,** Scraping the biopsy material onto the slide with a coverslip. **F,** Gill tissue (light material at the *arrow*) covered with the coverslip. **G,** Low-power photomicrograph of biopsy of a normal gill. The large finger-like structures are primary lamellae. *S* = secondary lamellae; *C* = cartilage support of primary lamella; *V* = blood vessels. **H,** High-power view of normal gill, showing secondary lamellae (*arrows*). Individual secondary lamellae may not be visible in some squashes of normal gill, depending on how the tissue lies. *P* = primary lamella.

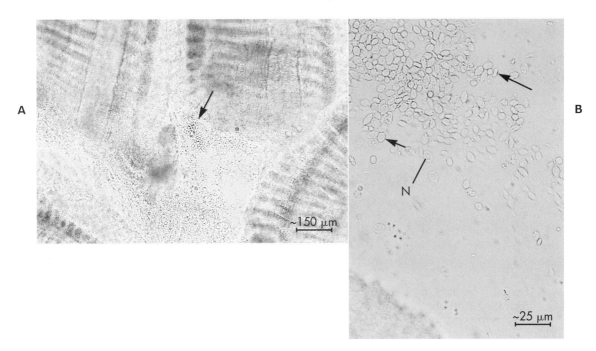

Fig. I-11   Blood cells in a wet mount of gill. **A,** The cells (*arrow*) are streaming from the cut surface of the gill. **B,** High-power view showing individual red blood cells. Key characteristics include oval shape in top view (*small arrow*) and laterally compressed in side view (*large arrow*). Nucleus (*N*) gives cells a fried-egg appearance.

(*A* and *B* photographs by L. Khoo and E. Noga.)

from poor water quality. Hyperplasia and hypertrophy can result from the feeding activity of protozoa such as *Trichodina* (see *PROBLEM 21*), *Chilodonella* (see *PROBLEM 22*), or *Ichthyobodo* (see *PROBLEM 28*) (Wooten, 1989). Some parasites, such as *Ichthyophthirius* (see *PROBLEM 19*) and *Amyloodinium* (see *PROBLEM 26*), induce focal hyperplasia at their attachment sites (see Fig. II-19, *D*). Some bacterial pathogens produce substances that stimulate epithelial proliferation. Epithelial hyperplasia and lamellar fusion have also been documented in vitamin deficiencies (see *PROBLEM 79*). Changes in gill structure are most easily recognized in histological sections, but if gill hyperplasia is detected on a wet mount it indicates that serious damage is present (Fig. I-12, *A* and *B*).

As on the skin, many pathogens may be present in low numbers on the gill without causing clinical disease;

thus, interpretation of their significance depends upon other clinical findings.

A common sequela of gill infections is telangiectasis, or the dilatation of groups of small blood vessels on the secondary lamellae (Fig. I-12, *C*). This condition can also result from a number of environmental toxins. Telangiectasis can also be iatrogenically induced in some fish by cranial concussion (Herman & Meade, 1985). Frank necrosis of gill tissue (*gill rot*) is characterized by the destruction of secondary lamellae and, in severe cases, the stripping of gill tissue down to the cartilaginous skeleton of the primary lamellae. It can be caused by pigmented bacteria and various toxins.

Because the gill is highly vascularized, lamellar biopsy can also be used to examine the blood in fish that are too small to be bled by conventional means (Fig. I-11), allowing the detection of hemoparasites or other pathogens.

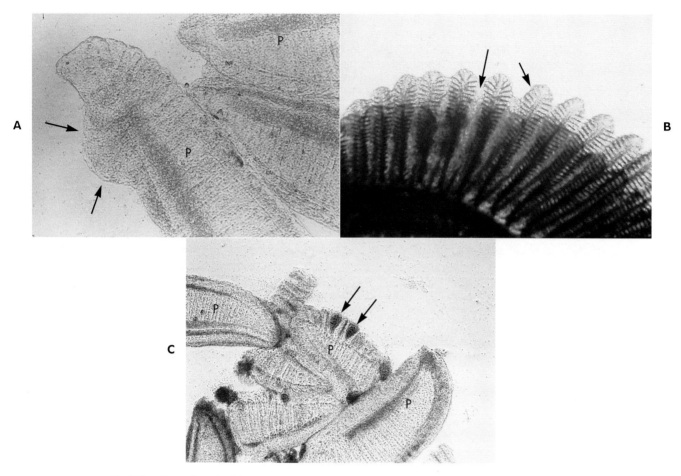

Fig. 1-12 Examples of gill lesions visible in wet mounts. **A,** Focal epithelial hyperplasia (*arrows*), protruding above the surface of the primary lamella (*P*). **B,** Severe epithelial hyperplasia, with resultant fusion of lamellae to one another. There is both fusion of adjacent secondary lamellae (*small arrow*) and fusion of adjacent primary lamellae (*large arrow*). **C,** Telangiectases (*arrows*) or weakening of blood vessel wall of a secondary lamella, causing vessel dilation. *P* = primary lamella. (*B* photograph courtesy of A. Mitchell.)

FECAL EXAM

A fecal exam may identify helminth ova (especially nematodes and also digeneans) and some protozoans (e.g., *Hexamita*). Fecal material can be obtained by siphoning debris from the bottom of the tank. This is not stressful to the fish; however, it is least sensitive for diagnosis. Samples are also contaminated with many nonpathogenic organisms. A fecal sample can often be obtained by anesthetizing a fish. Standard sodium nitrate flotation can be used for concentrating samples from fecal matter or aquarium debris (Langdon, 1992a).

BLEEDING FISH

Hematology and clinical chemistry are not routinely used for fish disease diagnosis, although they can be useful in some circumstances. Anemia in fish is often easily detected by examining the gills, which are a pale pink color (rather than a normally bright red color) if anemia is present. Blood samples should always be taken if fish are anemic.

Fish that are less than 8 cm (3 inches) usually cannot be bled without risk of killing them, so this technique is not feasible for small fish that cannot be sacrificed.

Anticoagulants

If blood is to be obtained for simply determining hematocrit or for making routine blood smears to look for hemoparasites or bacteremia, standard mammalian blood collection procedures are satisfactory. Heparin is usually an effective anticoagulant when used at ~50 to 100 USP Units/mL. However, heparin, which inhibits thrombin, will not prevent coagulation if clotting has begun (i.e., if a small clot is present in the sample because of blood vessel damage during sampling), because coagulation can proceed via an alternate pathway; this is a common problem in fish because of their small vessels. Ethylenediamine tetraacetic acid (EDTA) at 4 to 5 mg/ml final concentration will totally prevent clotting by chelating required divalent cations. However, using EDTA in combination with tricaine sedation is not recommended because it inexplicably causes hemolysis in many cases. This hemolysis problem can be reduced by cooling the blood to 4° C and/or rapidly preparing smears and removing plasma from the cells.

Blood Separation and Analysis

If detailed cellular or chemical analyses are to be performed (e.g., differential counts, enzyme measurements, etc.), the clinician should optimize the conditions for the fish species that are being examined because various researchers have noted problems under a wide range of conditions that are routinely used in mammalian hematology. The most important variables are type and concentration of anticoagulant and type of anesthetic. It is best to avoid using chemical anesthesia. Stun fish if possible. Samples should be analyzed as quickly as possible. Significant changes often occur in whole blood after 1-hour storage at room temperature and can occur 1 to 3 hours after refrigeration (Houston, 1990).

Plasma and/or serum should be rapidly separated from cells and frozen at the lowest possible temperature. For serum, it is usually best to allow the sample to clot at room temperature for 5 minutes, refrigerate it for 1 to 2 hours, rim the clot, and then centrifuge to separate the serum from cells. Pediatric serum separator tubes

(Becton-Dickinson) are useful because they handle small volumes.

All fish blood cells, including erythrocytes and thrombocytes (platelet analogue) are nucleated, which prevents the use of automated white cell counting or differentiation. Total white cell counts must be done by staining the white cells and then counting them with a hemacytometer (see Box I-1). Differential counts are obtained from blood smears.

Preparing Blood Smears

Blood smears are prepared as are routinely done for mammals. Smears should be made quickly; drying smears with a hair dryer is desirable. Commercial differential stains (e.g., Diff-Quik, Baxter Diagnostics, Inc.) are suitable for most diagnostic purposes (Fig. I-13). White blood cell morphology varies greatly between different fish species.

Bleeding with Needle and Syringe

For larger fish, a needle and syringe with anticoagulant can be used to bleed the fish from one of several sites. One of the least traumatic sites for collecting blood is the caudal vessels. This site can be approached laterally or ventrally. After the fish is sedated, the needle is gently pushed through the skin near the base of the caudal peduncle. After contact is made with the vertebral column, which is felt as firm resistance, the needle is directed slightly ventrally and lateral to the vertebral

---

❧ BOX I-1 ❧

METHOD FOR STAINING BLOOD
FOR WHITE BLOOD CELL COUNTING*

Step 1. Prepare Natt-Herrick's stain as follows:
Sodium chloride (NaCl) . . . . 3.88 g
Sodium sulfate (NaSO$_4$) . . . . 2.50 g
Sodium phosphate (Na$_2$HPO$_4$) . . . . 1.74 g
Potassium phosphate (KH$_2$PO$_4$) . . . . 0.25 g
Formalin (37 percent) . . . . 7.50 ml
Methyl violet . . . . 0.10 g
Bring to 1000 ml with distilled water and filter through Whatman #10 medium filter paper.
Step 2. Prepare a 1:200 dilution of blood with Natt-Herrick's stain (add 20 μl blood to 4 ml of Natt-Herrick's stain).
Step 3. Mix well, and leave at room temperature for 5 minutes; then fill both sides of a hemocytometer with the stained blood.

Step 4. After 5 more minutes, perform a white blood cell count, using the 10X objective. That is, count all white blood cells in the 4 large corner squares on both sides of the hemocytometer chamber (the counts within each square should be within 10 percent of each other). Add all 8 counts together and use this total count to calculate:

$$\frac{\text{Total \# WBCs counted}}{8} \times 2000 = \text{\#WBCs/μl of blood.}$$

All white blood cells (leucocytes + thrombocytes) will stain dark violet, distinguishing them from red blood cells. It is usually not possible to easily distinguish thrombocytes from leucocytes.

*Modified from procedure of T. Laws. Personal Communication.

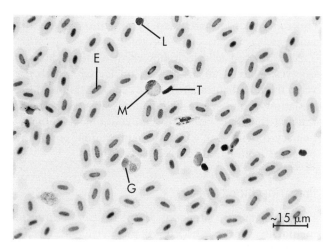

Fig. I-13   Blood smear from a normal goldfish. Blood cell morphology varies greatly among different species. If used, smears must be compared with those from known, healthy individuals. Erythrocyte (*E*); thrombocyte (*T*); lymphocyte (*L*); monocyte (*M*); granulocyte (*G*). Modified Wright's stain.

[Photograph by L. Khoo and E. Noga.]

column, while the syringe gently aspirates (Fig. I-14, *A* and *B*). It may be necessary to slowly rotate the needle before blood can be withdrawn. When one of the caudal vessels is entered (either artery or vein; they run closely together), blood is aspirated. Filling the hub of the needle is a sufficient amount for making a blood smear.

Larger fish may also be bled from the heart. The heart is usually located near the posterior edge of the gill chambers (Fig. I-15). The heart may also be approached dorsally by directing the needle into the posterior portion of the gill chamber. Bleeding the heart is probably more traumatic and potentially more dangerous than bleeding the caudal vessels. Less commonly used anatomical approaches are discussed by Houston (1990).

Bleeding by Capillary Tube

This method is used to bleed small fish (less than 8 cm or 3 inches). The fish is anesthetized and then placed on a smooth, flat surface. The base of the tail is then severed with a scalpel blade (Fig. I-16). A heparinized capillary tube is quickly applied to the caudal vessels, and the blood is collected in the tube by capillary action. A blood smear is then made immediately and is stained, using standard methods. This method probably results in significant tissue fluid contamination, which should be considered if samples are used for clinical chemistry. The fish should be euthanized immediately.

BIOPSY OF INTERNAL ORGANS

The kidney is the preferred site for isolation of many viral and bacterial diseases in fish (Amos, 1985;

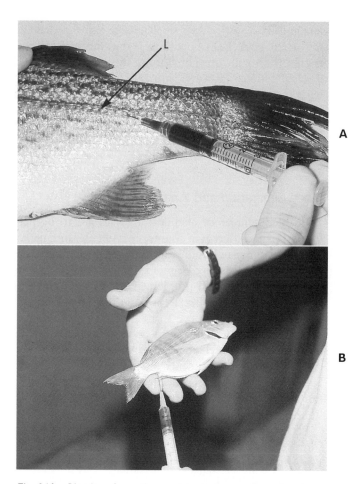

Fig. I-14   Bleeding from the caudal vein by needle and syringe. **A,** Location for inserting the needle, using the lateral approach. *L* = lateral line. **B,** Location for inserting the needle, using the ventral approach.

Thoesen, 1994). However, if valuable fish are involved (e.g., broodstock), it may not be desirable to sacrifice such fish to determine their health status. An alternative, nonlethal method involves biopsy (Noga et al., 1988, *B*). In teleost fish, the kidney is a long, ribbon-shaped organ that runs retroperitoneally along the length of the peritoneal cavity. Because it is composed of hematopoietic, as well as excretory tissues, the kidney does not have the solid structure of normal mammalian renal parenchyma; instead it has the consistency of bone marrow. At its cranial limit, the kidney curves ventrally and lies just beneath the medial surface of the branchial chamber. This makes it accessible to needle aspiration.

The fish to be biopsied either is anesthetized or is restrained by another person. The gill operculum is lifted, and a 3 cc syringe with a 22 gauge, 1.5 inch needle is directed dorsally and then dorsocaudally into the kidney, just caudal to the last branchial arch (Fig. I-17, *A*). The syringe is then aspirated until 0.10 ml of kidney tissue is collected, filling the hub of the syringe. In

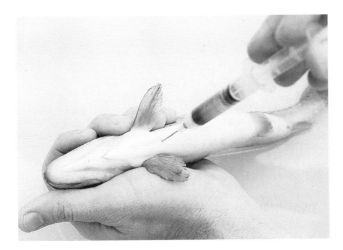

Fig. I-15 Bleeding a rainbow trout from the heart.

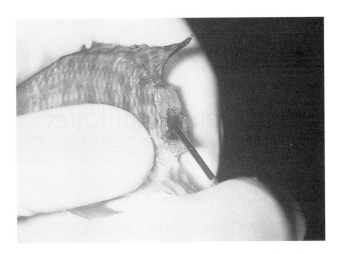

Fig. I-16 Bleeding from the caudal vein by severing the tail. After anesthetization, a sharp scalpel is used to cut off the base of the tail. A heparinized capillary tube is immediately applied to the vessel until sufficient blood is obtained.

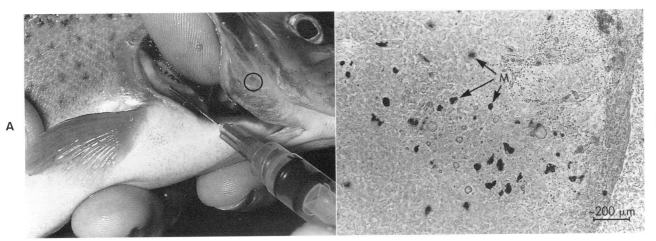

Fig. I-17 Anterior kidney biopsy technique. **A,** Inserting a needle through the medial membrane of the gill chamber and into the kidney. O = operculum. **B,** Confirmation that kidney material has been obtained as indicated by the presence of melanocytes (M) in a wet mount of biopsy material.

(From Noga et al., 1988.)

salmonids, the presence of kidney tissue can be rapidly confirmed by examining a small portion of the aspirate microscopically and confirming that tissue fragments and melanocytes are present (Fig. I-17, *B*).

This technique is as effective as standard necropsy culture in diagnosing enteric redmouth disease in rainbow trout (Noga et al., 1988b) and would probably be useful for diagnosing other infectious diseases in salmonids.

Its usefulness in other fish species remains to be determined and is probably limited to fairly large fish (probably those that are at least 15 cm or 6 inches long). Note that not all fish have melanocytes in the anterior kidney, and thus only tissue fragments may be seen. Other techniques that involve minor surgical procedures to nonlethally sample posterior kidney and liver have also been developed. See Wooster et al. (1993) for details.

CHAPTER 5

Postmortem Techniques

EUTHANASIA

Proper methods for euthanasia are given in the *PHAR-MACOPOEIA*.

PRESERVING PARASITES

Live specimens are always preferable for diagnosis, but if assistance is needed for identification and live material cannot be sent to a reference laboratory, samples need to be properly preserved. Table I-4 describes procedures for properly preparing specimens.

Many protozoa can be identified in histological sections, but many can detach from skin or gills with fixation and processing. It is best to fix the gills together, rather than cutting them into individual filaments, especially when loosely attached parasites (e.g., *Chilodonella*, *Trichodina*) may be present. Protozoa can be smeared on a slide, air dried, and stained—the same as for blood smears (see Fig. II-20, *E*), but this technique is rarely used for identifying protozoa in clinical material. Techniques for preserving metazoan parasites are more commonly used.

CULTURING FOR BACTERIA

It is often desirable to refer fish to a regional reference laboratory if bacterial disease is suspected because the techniques required to properly identify bacterial pathogens of fish are somewhat specialized. Samples should be submitted to a laboratory that is familiar with culturing bacteria from aquatic species because many aquatic pathogens have special requirements. For example, it is best to culture fish isolates at room temperature (22° to 25° C), not 37° C, as is routinely done in commercial microbiology labs, since some fish pathogens grow poorly or not at all at 37° C. For *Vibrio salmonicida*, samples should be incubated at 17° C. Samples from marine fish should be cultured on a medium that has a high salt content (e.g., trypticase soy agar with 2% NaCl) or on a nutrient-rich blood agar, such as Columbia agar with 5% defibrinated sheep blood (CBA). CBA is a good general-purpose medium for both freshwater and marine bacterial pathogens.

Some bacteria require other, specialized media, but these media are not routinely used in the clinical work-up. Selective media can also be used to enhance the isolation of certain pathogens but would not be routinely used in a clinical work-up unless prior knowledge of pathogens likely to be encountered warranted it. Not all differential media used for freshwater organisms may be reliable in estuarine environments. For example, Rimmler-Shotts (Shotts & Rimmler, 1973), a useful, selective medium for identifying *Aeromonas hydrophila* in freshwater, cannot differentiate between *A. hydrophila* and non-01 vibrios in estuarine waters (Kaper et al., 1981). See Shotts and Teska (1989) for various selective media used for bacterial isolation.

Samples may be submitted to a laboratory in one of several ways (Table I-5). Live specimens should be used for culture whenever possible. The only exception is when the only fish displaying clinical signs are dead (i.e., all of the live fish appear healthy). Identification of an obligate pathogen (e.g., *Aeromonas salmonicida*) in a dead fish is a stronger diagnosis than the isolation of an opportunist (e.g., *Aeromonas hydrophila*), especially if large numbers are present.

Whole fish may be frozen and shipped to the laboratory on dry ice. The recoverability of many common bacterial fish pathogens ranges from 20 to 60 days when samples are frozen at −20° C, which is the temperature of a home freezer (Brady & Vinitnantharat, 1990). Immunodiagnosis is increasingly being used for rapid, presumptive identification of pathogens (e.g., bacterial kidney disease [BKD]; see *PROBLEM 52*). While spleen, liver, and peritoneal fluids are common culture sites, the organ of choice for isolating systemic bacterial pathogens in fish is the kidney, which can be approached dorsally or ventrally (Figs. I-18, *A* through *H*, and I-19, *A* through *D*).

Dorsal Approach to Kidney

The fish is euthanized and the dorsal fin is clipped off. The surface of the back is decontaminated either by swabbing the area with antiseptic (e.g., quaternary ammonium or 70% alcohol) or by searing the skin with a

Table I-4 Recommended methods of preserving parasites for future identification.

Parasite group	Relaxation procedure	"Relaxed" parasite	Fixation	Storage	Final preparation for identification
Monogeneans/ digeneans*	None usually needed for small worms; gently flatten under a coverslip, and flood slide with fixative for 5 minutes	Not contracted; allows some expulsion of eggs from uterus	Hot (55° to 65° C) AFA or hot NBF	AFA or ETOH	Stained and permanently mounted in mounting medium
Cestodes*	Cold (4° to 8° C) water or saline for 1 to 12 hours; gently flatten under a coverslip, and flood slide with fixative for 5 minutes	Not contracted; allows some expulsion of eggs from uterus	Hot AFA or hot NBF or hot ETOH	AFA or ETOH	Stained and permanently mounted in mounting medium
Nematodes*	None usually needed for small worms; stretch large worms by holding each end of the worm with forceps, and add fixative for 5 minutes	Completely uncoiled	Hot AFA or hot ETOH	AFA or ETOH or glycerol: ETOH	Small nematodes can be cleared in glycerol: ETOH and mounted permanently in glycerol jelly; large nematodes are cleared and temporarily mounted in glycerol: ETOH
Acanthocephalans	Cold (4° to 8° C) water or saline for 1 to 12 hours	Proboscis fully extruded	Hot AFA or hot HBF or hot ETOH (puncture cuticle)	AFA or ETOH	Small: stained and mounted; large: unstained and mounted in glycerol: ETOH
Hirudineans	Tricaine; sodium pentobarbitol	Not contracted	Hot ETOH	ETOH	Small: stained and mounted; large: glycerol: ETOH
Arthropods	Not required	Not required	Cold (4° to 8°C) ETOH	ETOH	Unstained and cleared in 10% KOH or Hoyer mounting medium
Ciliates†	N/A	N/A	Air-dry smear‡	Stain immediately	Stained with Wright's or Klein's silver stain (Lom and Dykova, 1993) and permanently coverslipped with mounting medium (Permount or equivalent)
Flagellates†	N/A	N/A	Air-dry smear‡	Stain immediately	Stained with Wright's, and permanently coverslipped with mounting medium (Permount or equivalent)
Amoebae†	N/A	N/A	Air-dry smear‡	Stain immediately	Stained with Wright's, and permanently coverslipped with mounting medium (Permount or equivalent)
Myxozoa†	N/A	N/A	Air-dry smear‡	Stain immediately	Stained with Wright's, and permanently coverslipped with mounting medium (Permount or equivalent)
Microsporidians†	N/A	N/A	Air-dry smear‡	Stain immediately	Stained with Wright's, or Gram's, and permanently coverslipped with mounting medium (Permount or equivalent)

Modified from Smith & Noga, 1993.
AFA=alcohol-formalin-acetic acid; NBF=10% neutral buffered formalin; ETOH=70% ethanol; glycerol: ETOH=100% glycerol: 70% ethanol.
*Before beginning preservation procedures, encapsulated larvae should be manually dissected out of the capsule or the capsule should be digested with 0.2% pepsin in 0.1 M HCl.
†See problem list for other techniques used in diagnosis.
‡Note that this procedure is less reliable for protozoan identifcation than routine histopathology but can be useful when submitting specimens to reference laboratories for identification.

Table 1-5 Diagnostic usefulness of different tissue preservation techniques for identifying fish pathogens.*

Specimen	Protozoan ectoparasites[†]	Monogenean ectoparasites[+]	Metazoan parasites (except Monogenea)[†]	Myxozoa and Microspore[†]	Viral isolation	Bacterial isolation	Histologic value
Live fish	+++	+++	+++	+++	+++	+++	+++
Dead fish[‡]	−	−	++	++	+	−	−
Iced fish[§]	+	++	+++	+++	++	+	+
Frozen fish[‖]	+	+	++	++	++	++	+
Fixed fish[¶]	++	+	+	++	−	−	+++

*The ability to recover various pathogens varies greatly; these comparisons are only intended as general guidelines. +++ = best; − = virtually useless.
[†]Comparisons between live, dead, iced, and frozen fish are based upon the ability to identify parasites in wet mounts; diagnostic usefulness of fixed fish is based upon the ability to identify pathogens in histological sections.
[‡]Dead fish left in water at room temperature for 6 to 12 hours.
[§]Live fish placed in a plastic bag on wet ice for 6 to 12 hours.
[‖]Live fish placed in a plastic bag frozen at −20° C.
[¶]Tissues from live fish immediately placed in 10% neutral buffered formalin.

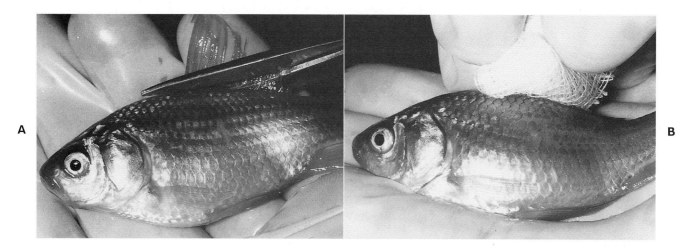

A

B

Fig. 1-18 Culturing for bacteria, using the dorsal approach. **A,** After anesthetization the dorsal fin is clipped to reduce possible contamination. **B,** The surface of the back is decontaminated with antiseptic and then dried with a dry, sterile gauze pad.

Continued.

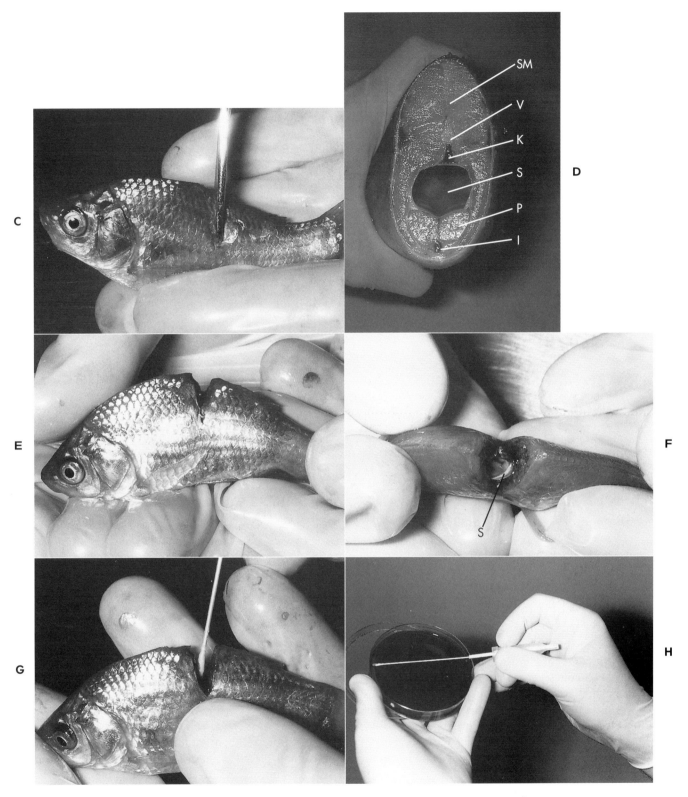

Fig. 1-18—cont'd.   C, The back is cut with sterile scissors. Care is taken not to cut so far as to enter the peritoneal cavity. This step is the most likely time for contamination to occur. D, Whole-body cross-section through a fish. Note that the kidney (*K*) is ventral to the vertebral column (*V*), which must be severed before reaching the kidney. The swim bladder (*S*) is ventral to the kidney. *P* = viscera in the peritoneal cavity, including intestine (*I*). *SM* = skeletal muscle. E, Reflecting the body ventrally (fish in Fig. 1-18, *C*) to expose the kidney for culture. F, Entrance into the kidney is indicated by the appearance of a large amount of hemorrhage because of the highly vascular nature of the kidney. The collapsed, white swim bladder (*S*) lies ventral to the kidney; it is not clearly visible on all fish. G, Touching a sterile Culturette to the kidney and being careful not to touch other areas, which would cause sample contamination. H, Inoculating a Columbia blood agar plate with the sample, using a Mini-tip Culturette (Becton-Dickinson) and spreading the inoculum.

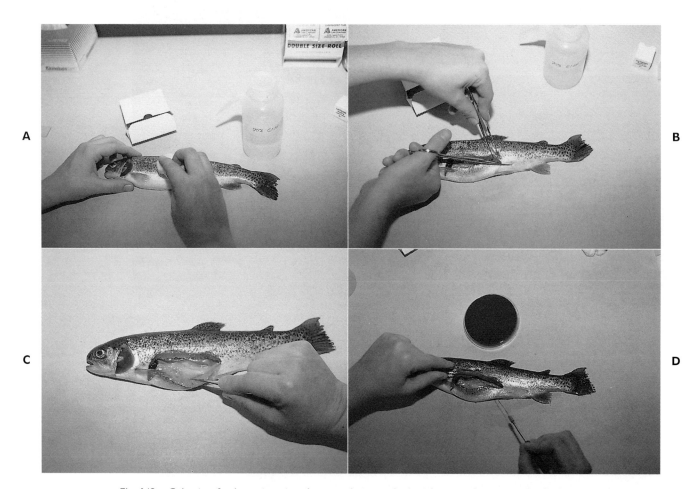

Fig. I-I9 Culturing for bacteria, using the ventral approach. **A,** After anesthetization the flank is swabbed with antiseptic, avoiding the anus and any skin lesions. The area is then dried with a dry sterile gauze pad. **B,** The body wall is cut with sterile scissors. Care is taken to avoid the anus and to cut close to the body wall to prevent severing the intestine. **C,** Viscera are aseptically reflected, exposing the swim bladder (also see Fig. I-18, *E*). The swim bladder must be cut or reflected to reach the kidney. **D,** The kidney is often covered by a tough fibrous capsule, which must be severed to enter the parenchyma.

flat, metal object (e.g., knife or spatula) heated in a flame. If an antiseptic is used, the skin should be wiped dry with sterile gauze. Sterile scissors are then used to cut into the decontaminated area. The incision should be made just deep enough to cut through the vertebral column. Cutting deeper may enter the peritoneal cavity, possibly rupturing the intestines and contaminating the sample.

The exact incision site varies slightly, depending on the species, but generally, an incision is made just posterior to the dorsal fin. Another useful landmark is to cut at one quarter of the distance from the anus to the posterior edge of the operculum. Once the incision has been made, the head and tail of the fish should be bent downward (ventrally) to expose the kidney (see Fig. I-18, *E*). The kidney lies immediately beneath the vertebral column and appears as a dark red, bloody area (see Fig. I-18, *F*). If the incision is not deep enough, that is, if the incision is only into the epaxial (upper body) muscles, almost no blood will be present, since muscle has much less blood

supply than the kidney. Once the kidney is exposed, a sample then can be taken with a sterile loop or a Culturette (Becton-Dickinson Microbiological Systems).

Ventral Approach to Kidney

The fish is swabbed with antiseptic, avoiding the anal area, and placed in lateral recumbency. The peritoneal cavity is opened, using aseptic technique, and the body wall is cut away (see Fig. I-19, *B*). The kidney is reached by **gently** pushing the viscera in the peritoneal cavity to one side and deflecting the swim bladder away from the vertebral column. This part of the procedure is best done with a sterile, blunt probe. The kidney runs the entire length of the peritoneal cavity, just ventral to the vertebral column. Note that on large fish, you may need to use a scalpel to cut the membrane that separates the kidney from the swim bladder. A loop or swab may be used for culture. This material can then be immediately streaked onto a culture plate or shipped on ice to a diagnostic laboratory if it is placed in a transport medium. Alternatively, a piece of kidney may be removed and placed in a sterile syringe barrel or red-top Vacutainer (Becton-Dickinson) tube; unless it is plated immediately, the specimen should be frozen for shipment to the laboratory.

Culturing Other Viscera

The ventral approach can also be used for sampling other organs, such as spleen and liver. If the peritoneal cavity has not been entered aseptically, the surface of the organ to be sampled can be seared with a hot scalpel blade and then a loop can be inserted through the seared tissue until unheated tissue is reached; this is only possible with large fish. For smaller fish, whole organs are removed aseptically, and a loop is used to streak the tissue across a plate.

Culturing Skin Lesions

Skin lesions are common in many bacterial diseases, and some bacterial diseases begin as primary skin infections. It can be difficult to determine the initiating agent because lesions are often overgrown by secondary invaders. It is important to sample early lesions whenever possible to determine the predominant organism, since the latter is often the initiating agent.

To avoid contamination of the sample, it is best to culture skin lesions on fish that have not yet had any other clinical procedures performed. Skin lesions can be cultured with a loop, but it is easier to isolate single colonies when the following procedure is used:

1. Place a sterile, 1 µl volume loop into the leading edge of the skin lesion. It can be useful to aseptically remove some scales from the edge of the lesion to be

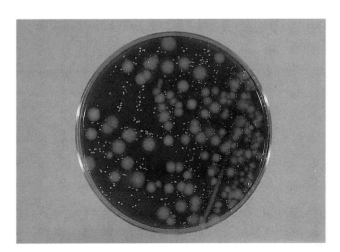

Fig. I-20 A blood agar plate from a skin lesion of a fish having well-isolated bacterial colonies.

sure that the leading edge is sampled; however, this is usually not needed.

2. Immediately inoculate the material on the loop into a small, 4 mm² area on the periphery of a culture plate.
3. Using a sterile Mini-Tip Culturette (Becton-Dickinson), immediately swab the inoculated area onto half of the plate; then pull the streak across one quarter of the plate and then across the final quarter of the plate. This procedure almost always results in the isolation of single colonies and also allows you to estimate the number of bacteria present in the lesion (Fig. I-20).

Rapid Screening for Antibiotic Susceptibility

Bacterial infections can spread rapidly through a population, and it is important to treat fish with an appropriate antibiotic as soon as possible, since a matter of a day or two can be crucial. It can thus be useful to rapidly screen for antibiotic susceptibility. This is only a *qualitative* test at best and does *not* substitute for a properly performed sensitivity assay. However, it can provide some indication of the best antibiotic to use while the proper test is being performed. A simplified test for determining bacterial susceptibility follows (adapted from Collins, 1993):

1. Dampen the tip of a sterile swab with sterile saline. (The condensation water on the lid of a sterile bacterial culture plate can be used if it is not contaminated.)
2. Pick a single bacterial colony with the tip of the swab, and spread it as evenly as possible across the whole surface of the test medium.
3. Use a sterile forceps, and evenly distribute antibiotic sensitivity discs on the surface of the agar. Be sure the discs are firmly placed on the agar.
4. Replace the lid on the agar plate, and let it stand for a few minutes to ensure that the discs adhere. Then carefully invert the plate and incubate.
5. An inhibition zone of ≤ 15 to 16 mm suggests resistance; sensitive fish pathogens typically have clearing zones of at least 20 mm. These results may vary with the type of disc and/or antibiotic used. Testing three to four isolates is advisable.

SAMPLING FOR FUNGI

Fungal culture is rarely needed in routine fish disease diagnoses because the most common fungal pathogens, the Oomycetes (see *PROBLEM 33*), can be diagnosed without culture. However, some rarer fungal diseases (see *PROBLEM 68*) require culture for definitive diagnosis. Culture for non-Oomycetes is not usually done unless typical fungal organisms are seen either in wet mounts or via histopathology (see *PROBLEM 68*).

For fungal culture, plates should be inoculated with a small (approximately 12 mm³) mass of fungus-infected tissue and incubated at room temperature. Once growth of the fungus is noticeable (usually within several days), it is advisable to transfer the growing edge of the mycelium to a fresh culture plate by aseptically excising a small portion of the agar containing the leading edge of growth. This procedure will help to eliminate any bacterial contaminants that were introduced with the tissue sample.

For non-Oomycetes, Sabouraud dextrose agar (SDA) is a good, commercially available, general-purpose medium for isolating almost all of these pathogens. If a non-Oomycete fungal pathogen is suspected, tissue samples should be inoculated onto SDA slants and incubated at room temperature. Be aware that airborne fungal spores can often contaminate cultures; thus, be certain that the type of fungus isolated in culture is morphologically similar to the type of fungus present in the lesions. If the fungus will not grow on SDA, other, more specialized media can be tried (see Hatai, 1989), or samples can be referred to a specialized laboratory.

Oomycetes are best isolated by using cornmeal agar, YpSs, or another nutrient-poor medium to inhibit growth of contaminating bacteria (Seymour & Fuller, 1987). While Oomycetes are usually easily isolated, culturing Oomycetes from bacteria-infected lesions may be difficult because bacteria inhibit Oomycetes, especially slow-growing forms, such as *Aphanomyces* (see *PROBLEM 34*). In heavily contaminated lesions, adding penicillin (approximately 500 U/ml) and/or streptomycin (approximately 0.2 µg/ml) may improve yields; however, some Oomycetes (especially *Aphanomyces*) are significantly inhibited by antibiotics. *Saprolegnia* and *Achlya*, the two genera most commonly isolated from fish, are usually not significantly inhibited.

SAMPLING FOR VIRUSES

Definitive identification of viral infection relies on cell culture and immunological identification of the pathogen. Such procedures are best left to competent laboratory personnel who specialize in such techniques. However, reliable use of those techniques depends upon the submission of high-quality samples. Different viruses vary in their abilities to survive preservation procedures; specific recommendations are given for specific viral diseases in the problem list. However, in general, live fish are best submitted when a virus is suspected and the specific agent is uncertain. Otherwise, fish on wet ice or dry ice should be sent immediately by overnight mail. Fish that cannot be sent immediately should usually be frozen at the lowest temperature possible, although it is best for some viruses to store samples at 4° C if processing will occur in a few days.

EXAMINING TISSUES POSTMORTEM

Circumstances permitting, it is always desirable to do a complete necropsy on selected individuals. Four to six fish showing clinical signs that are typical of the outbreak should be necropsied, if possible. While necropsy may not be possible with highly valuable fish, it is mandatory when a clinician performs an examination of a large fish population that includes expendable fish.

Condition of Tissue

The diagnostic usefulness of the postmortem examination is highly dependent upon the quality of specimens presented (see Table I-3). Whenever possible, live fish should be examined. Owners may present fish for diagnosis that have recently died; however, such fish are often of no diagnostic value. Fish decompose much more rapidly than mammals under similar conditions; this is especially true for small fish. Most ectoparasitic protozoa and Monogenea (see *PROBLEMS 16, 18*) die within minutes to hours of host death, depending on temperature and parasite species. Larger parasites, such as copepods (see *PROBLEM 13*) or branchiurans (see *PROBLEM 14*), may be detectable for longer periods.

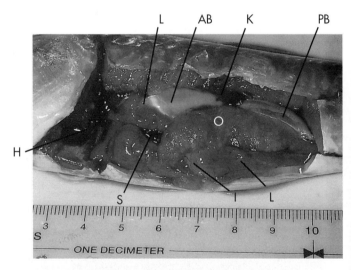

Fig. I-21 Gross anatomy of the viscera of a fish (koi). *H* = heart; *L* = liver, which has several lobes covering the intestine (*I*); *O* = ovary, which is large because this fish was almost ready to spawn; *K* = kidney; *S* = spleen. Note that the swim bladder has an anterior (*AB*) and posterior (*PB*) chamber. This is characteristic of cyprinid fish, but other fish have a single chamber.

Bacterial invasion of both skin and internal organs occurs rapidly after death, making interpretation of culture results difficult. Finally, because fish tissues autolyze rapidly, histological evaluations are compromised.

If submitting live fish is not an option, animals can be put in a plastic bag and placed on wet ice. Again, the diagnostic value of the tissues will deteriorate with time; fish should be examined within several hours of death.

If fish cannot be submitted within several hours, euthanized fish should be frozen immediately ($-20°$ C). Most ectoparasitic protozoa and Monogenea will usually not be recognizable after freezing, but the macroscopic host response to some protozoa may be visible (e.g., white cysts of *Ichthyophthirius*).

Protozoan ectoparasites and Monogenea usually cannot be identified from wet mounts of chemically preserved (fixed) tissue. Most parasites are recognizable in histological sections, but many ectoparasites detach from the skin and gills during processing, so they may be difficult to find in sections. Granulomas (see Fig. I-33) are easily seen in wet mounts of fixed tissues. Affected tissues can then be histologically processed for a diagnosis. Histology is useful for differentiating many of the diseases affecting internal organs.

Necropsy Procedures

Skin and gill examinations should be done as described for biopsy procedures. It is often advisable not to euthanize fish until the skin and gill examinations have been completed because of the aforementioned problems with decomposition. If bacterial cultures are to be taken, these should be done next, as described previously.

After euthanization, place the fish in lateral recumbency, and make a longitudinal incision along the ventral midline from the anal opening to just ventral to the gill chamber. This incision will exend from the posterior peritoneal cavity into the pericardial sac. Make latitudinal incisions at both ends of this previous incision that extend to the dorsal aspect of the body cavity. Reflect the body wall dorsally, exposing the viscera (Fig. I-21).

If fluid is present, make smears as described for blood sampling. Identify and examine the intestines, liver, spleen, gonads, and heart. Reflect the swim bladder ventrally and examine the anterior kidney and posterior kidney (Fig. I-22). The braincase is entered by using a pair of sharp scissors to reflect the dorsal cranium anteriorly (Fig. I-23, *A* and *B*). After visual inspection, fine scissors and forceps are used to remove the brain in toto (Fig. I-23, *C*). Direct smears of various tissues can be stained for bacteria, although it is best to stain histological sections appropriately (e.g., Brown and Brenn's Gram stain) so that host response and tissue damage can also be evaluated.

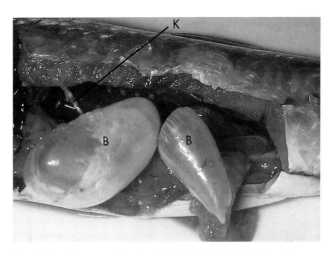

Fig. I-22 Viscera and swim bladder (*B*) in Fig. I-21 have been reflected, revealing the kidney (*K*).

Fixation Procedures

A 1 cm^2 portion of each lesion and of each organ should be placed in fixative. Even small fish should be dissected to expose internal organs to fixative, although very small fish (<5 mm or 0.2 inch) can be usually be fixed in toto without autolysis artifacts. The fixative of choice for routine diagnosis is 10% neutral buffered formalin. Bouin's fluid is considered by some to provide better fixation, but it has several disadvantages (potentially explosive when dry, difficult to remove totally from fixed tissues, and damages fixed tissues if not completely removed) that reduce its attractiveness.

Tissues can be processed routinely using standard histological techniques and embedded in paraffin (Bucke, 1989). Note that gills and scaled skin must be decalcified before sectioning. Hematoxylin and eosin and other standard stains can be used on fish tissues. Thus, samples can be submitted to mammalian histopathology laboratories.

Wet Mount Procedures

It is often useful to also make tissue squashes, especially of kidney, spleen, liver, or any lesions. Small fish can be squashed whole or the entire viscera can be removed and squashed. To make a tissue squash, excise a small (approximately 8 mm^3) piece of tissue and place it on a slide with a drop of water or normal saline. Place the edge of a plastic coverslip near the tissue, and then gently squash it (Fig. I-24). Examine the tissue architecture under low (100X) magnification and look for parasites and granulomas; then crush the tissue into a thin smear, and examine it at 100X and high dry (400X) power to identify protozoa and bacteria.

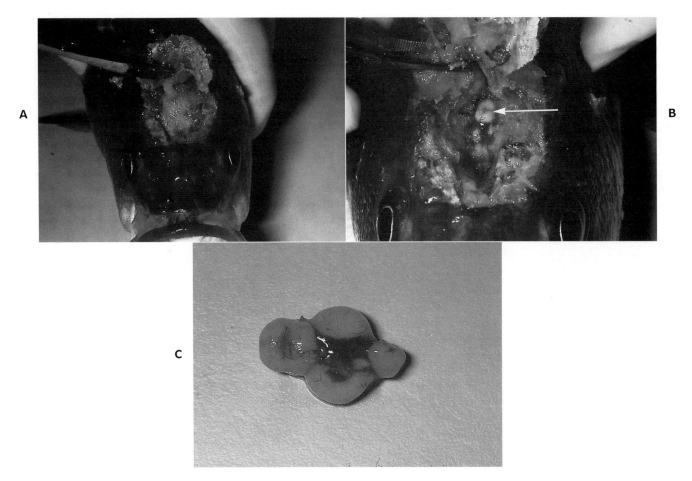

Fig. I-23   Brain necropsy. **A,** Exposing the brain by using rongeurs to reflect the dorsal portion of the skull posteriorly. **B,** The brain in situ (*arrow*). **C,** Intact brain removed.

(*A, B,* and *C* photographs by L. Khoo and E. Noga.)

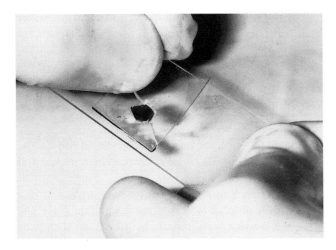

Fig. I-24   Squashing tissue for a wet mount.

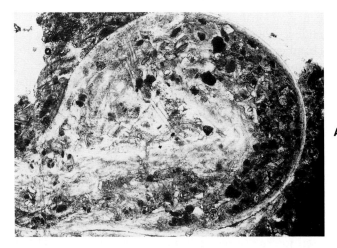

Fig. I-25   A, Wet mount of normal intestine of a small (~2.5 cm) fish. The intestine is thin-walled, and the luminal contents are easily seen.

Continued.

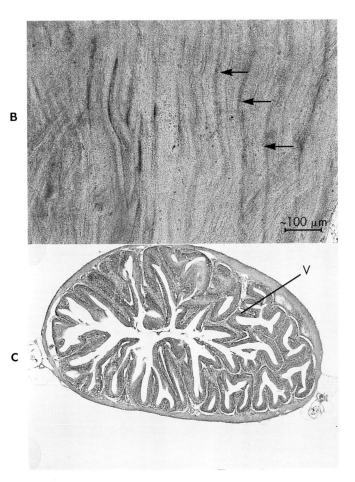

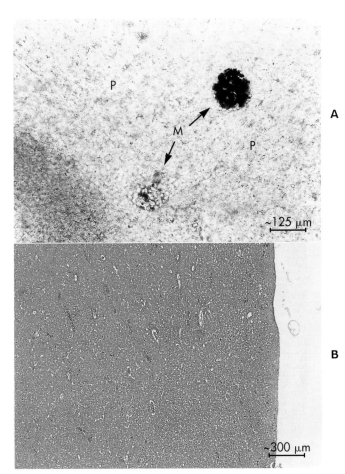

Fig. I-25—cont'd.   B, Wet mount of intestine showing rugae, or folds (*arrows*), which are composed of villi. C, Histological cross-section of normal intestine. *V* = villi. Hematoxylin and eosin.

(*B* photograph by L. Khoo and E. Noga.)

Fig. I-26   A, Wet mount of normal liver. Note homogeneous parenchyma (*P*) and aggregates of pigmented macrophages, the melanomacrophage centers (*M*). B, Histological section of normal liver. Hematoxylin and eosin.

(*B* photograph by L. Khoo and E. Noga.)

Structure of Normal Tissues

The viscera of fish are generally similar to those of mammals, but certain peculiarities should be recognized. Small fish, such as most aquarium fish, have little connective tissue stroma, making the viscera flaccid and coincidentally facilitating the preparation of wet mounts. Note that squashes are most easily made from (and thus most useful in) organs of small fish. Organs of large fish ($\geq$ 20 to 25 cm or 8 to 10 inches) have more connective tissue and are harder to squash. Pigmented cells are a normal finding in virtually all organs and are especially common in hematopoietic tissues. The peritoneum of many fish is lined with melanocytes. Aggregates of pigmented cells, the melanomacrophage centers, are also common (see Fig. I-27).

Key Features of Internal Organs

Intestine — The intestinal tract is usually the first organ seen when the peritoneal cavity is opened. However, body fat is most commonly deposited in the peritoneal cavity and may obscure the viscera. The intestinal tract is a straight, thin-walled tube. In many aquarium fish the lumen is too small to be easily cut open, but in such fish the intestinal contents can often be seen through the wall (Fig. I-25, *A* through *C*). The intestine should be opened *after* the other viscera have been examined to reduce contamination by bacteria and other organisms. The stomach is larger than the intestines. The presence or absence of food in the intestinal tract is easily assessed.

Liver — The liver is a brown to red-brown to tan organ in the anterior portion of the peritoneal cavity. Microscopically, normal liver has a homogeneous appearance; an occasional melanomacrophage center may be seen (Fig. I-26, *A* and *B*).

Gall Bladder — The gall bladder is a large, translucent sac with green or yellowish fluid. It lies close to the liver and is often large (i.e., it is often larger than the spleen).

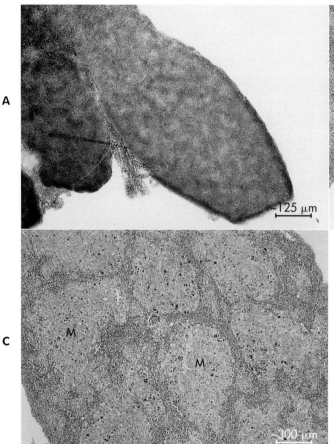

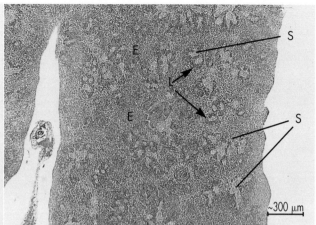

Fig. I-27   **A,** Wet mount of normal spleen. Note the lighter areas of *white pulp*, which give the tissue a reticulated appearance. **B,** Histological section of normal spleen, having concentrations of leucocytes (*L,* white pulp) surrounding splenic ellipsoids (*S*), having phagocytic cells. *E* = erythrocytes (red pulp). Hematoxylin and eosin. **C,** Histological section of abnormal spleen, having abnormally large melanomacrophage centers (*M*), with golden brown-to-black pigment, consisting of ceroid, lipofuscin, and melanin. Hematoxylin and eosin.

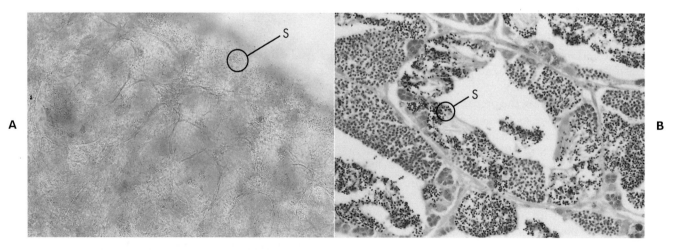

Fig. I-28   **A,** Wet mount of normal testis. Note individual spermatozoa (*S*) visible on the edge of the cut tissue. **B,** Histological section of normal testis filled with spermatozoa. *S* = spermatozoa. Hematoxylin and eosin.

(*A* and *B* photographs by L. Khoo and E. Noga.)

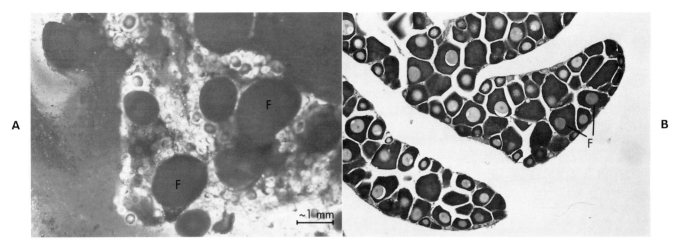

Fig. I-29   A, Wet mount of normal ovary. Compare with testes (Fig. I-28, A and B). Do not confuse follicles (F) with granulomas (see Fig. I-33). B, Histological section of normal ovary. F = follicles. Hematoxylin and eosin.

(*A* photograph by L. Khoo and E. Noga.)

It may be accidentally ruptured when the peritoneal cavity is opened, tainting the viscera yellow-green.

Spleen — The spleen is a bright red to black organ located in the mesentery. Microscopically, normal spleen has a reticulated appearance because of the network of ellipsoids that are the sites of blood filtration (Fig. I-27, *A* through *C*).

Gonad — The reproductive organs may be difficult to see in fish that are not sexually mature. In immature fish, the reproductive organs are ribbon-like, grey-white or yellow strips that usually lie just ventral to the swim bladder. In some fish that are ready to spawn, the ovaries may occupy most of the peritoneal cavity and cause gross abdominal distension. Even in immature fish, sex can often be determined by examining a wet mount, which may reveal the presence of sperm (Fig. I-28, *A* and *B*) in a male or follicles (Fig. I-29, *A* and *B*) in a female.

Swim Bladder — The swim bladder is a white, shiny organ that lies near the back (dorsum), just ventral to the kidney. Filled with gas, its primary function is to maintain buoyancy.

Kidney — The kidney is a retroperitoneal organ that is functionally (and often morphologically) divided into two segments. The anterior kidney is the primary site of hematopoiesis; it is a dark red to black, soft amorphous tissue that has the consistency of bone marrow (Fig. I-30, *A* and *D*). The posterior kidney has a similar gross appearance but has renal excretory tissue as well (Fig. I-30, *B*, *C*, and *E*).

Heart/Skeletal Muscle — The heart lies in the pericardial cavity, which is just anterior to the peritoneal cavity in the *throat* region of the fish. It is a red, highly muscular, two-chambered organ. It empties into the ventral aorta via the white, elastic, bulbus arteriosus. Wet mounts of normal skeletal or cardiac muscle will reveal individual muscle fibers with striations (Fig. I-31).

Brain — The brain is superficially similar to those of mammals, with morphological differentiation of various neural centers. Microscopically, it appears as a grey-white organ that has an amorphous appearance on wet mount.

Glands — Most of the major glandular tissues found in mammals occur in fish; they are only detectable histologically, except for thymus (Fig. I-32). Analogues of the adrenal cortex (interrenal cells) and adrenal medulla (chromaffin cells) are found in the anterior kidney. Pancreatic exocrine and endocrine tissues are usually dispersed throughout the mesentery or may be associated with the liver or spleen. Thyroid tissue is usually dispersed around the ventral aorta but may also be found in the kidney, spleen, or mesentery.

Common Lesions Found in the Viscera

Necropsy can provide information on nutritional status. Aquarium fish are often overfed, resulting in excessive accumulation of fat in the peritoneal cavity. In fish that are fed unbalanced diets, the liver may be pale yellow because of lipidosis. The significance of obesity in pet fish is uncertain, but excessive lipid deposition is commonly associated with clinical disorders in food fish, such as trout (see *PROBLEM 79*). However, note that normal liver color varies considerably among species; it also varies seasonally, so it is necessary to be aware of the normal physiological color variation for a particular species.

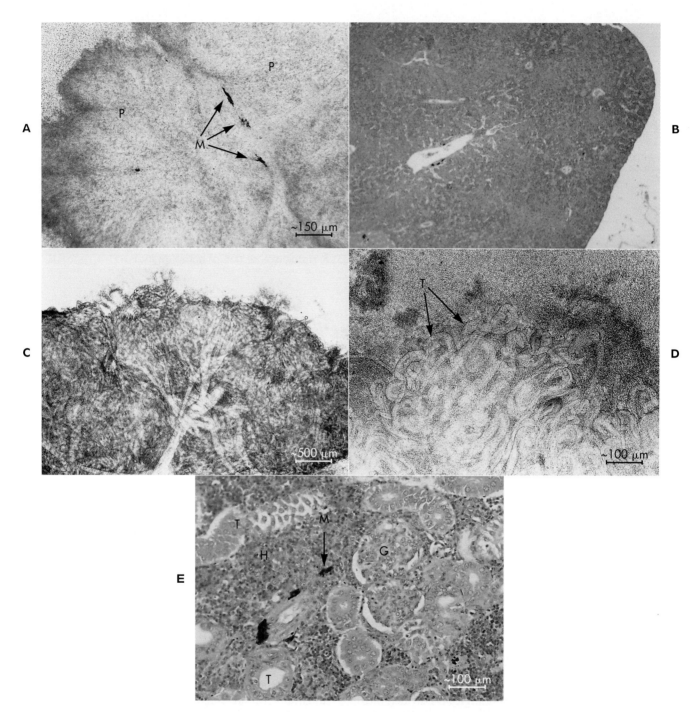

Fig. I-30   **A,** Wet mount of normal anterior kidney. Note the homogeneous parenchyma (*P*). Most of the cells are hematopoietic elements. The absence of renal excretory tissue is a normal finding. *M* = melanocytes. **B,** Histological section of normal anterior kidney. Hematoxylin and eosin. **C,** Wet mount of normal posterior kidney. Low-power view showing dendritic collecting duct. **D,** Wet mount of normal posterior kidney. Higher-power view, showing renal tubules (*T*). Most of the interstitial tissue surrounding the tubules is hematopoietic. **E,** Histological section of normal posterior kidney. *G* = glomeruli; *T* = renal tubules; *H* = hematopoietic tissue; *M* = melanocyte. Hematoxylin and eosin.

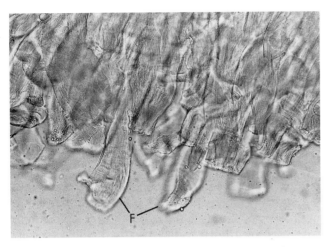

Fig. I-31 Wet mount of normal skeletal (striated) muscle. Note the individual fibers (*F*) with striations.

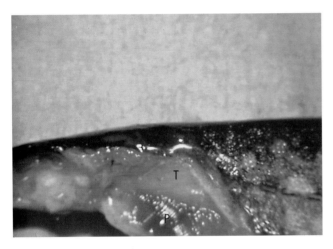

Fig. I-32 Thymus (*T*), located at the dorsomedial aspect of the gill chamber. Head is to the left. *P*=pseudobranch.

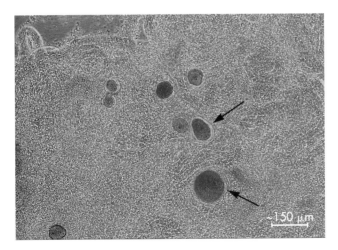

Fig. I-33 Granulomas in a wet mount. Note the dark, necrotic center (*C*) surrounded by lighter, viable, inflammatory cells (*arrows*).

Fluid accumulation in the abdomen (*dropsy*) (see Fig. I-3, *B*) is a common clinical presentation. It can result from infection by viruses, bacteria, or parasites. Examination of abdominal fluid may reveal bacteria or parasites (e.g., *Hexamita*). Ascitic fluid may also form from osmoregulatory dysfunction. Hemorrhages in the viscera can be caused by systemic viral or bacterial infections.

Several chronic inflammatory diseases can affect internal organs. Among the most important is mycobacteriosis, which can affect virtually any internal organ. Granulomas produced by this pathogen must be differentiated from neoplasia (see *PROBLEM 72*) (foreign-body reactions produced against protozoan or metazoan parasites) and from melanomacrophage centers.

Melanomacrophage centers (MMC) are usually solid foci of cells that have varying amounts of pigment (see Fig. I-27). While these are common in healthy fish, they increase in number with chronic stress (Wolke, 1992). Thus, MMC are an indicator of chronic stress; however, it is necessary to know the normal prevalence in a particular fish species to make an accurate diagnosis of chronic stress.

In contrast to melanomacrophages, granulomas are usually multilayered structures having a central zone of necrotic debris (Fig. I-33). This necrotic center is the most useful feature for identifying granulomas. It is important to recognize that granulomas may contain pigment and melanomacrophage centers accumulate in many disease states. Thus, in some cases, histology may be needed for differentiation, especially if other tests are negative.

Trematodes, nematodes, and cestodes, especially larvae, occur in the mesentery or viscera. Compared with mammals, internal helminths are much less serious problems in fish. However, some internal helminths can cause serious disease.

ZOONOTIC DISEASES

Several zoonotic helminths can infect humans but can only be contracted after ingestion of infected fish. A few fish pathogens can infect the clinician during a clinical work-up. Aeromonads, vibrios, and *Edwardsiella tarda* (see *PROBLEMS 45, 48,* and *49*) can infect the skin or cause gastroenteritis or systemic infections. However, the agent of most concern is *Mycobacterium* (see *PROBLEM 53*). Only atypical mycobacteria infect fish; these are the least pathogenic mycobacteria for humans, but they can cause *fish tank granuloma*, a chronic infection that is usually limited to the extremities (i.e., fingers and hands). Fortunately, incidences of zoonotic infections with these pathogens appear to be uncommon events when compared with the relative risk of exposure to these agents. However, appropriate caution is warranted, especially in immunosuppressed individuals (Angulo et al., 1994).

CHAPTER 6

Guidelines for Interpreting Clinical Findings

STRESS AND FISH DISEASE

The metabolic, biochemical, and physiological processes of fish are basically similar to those of mammals. Fish are susceptible to the same types of agents that affect warm-blooded animals, including viruses, bacteria, fungi, parasites, as well as various noninfectious problems. However, stress appears to play a considerably larger role in causing disease in fish (Walters & Plumb, 1980; Collins et al., 1976). Stress can be considered as a continuum of insults, varying from mild to severe (Fig. I-34). How much of an impact stress has on a fish depends on the severity of the stress, its duration, and the physiological state of the fish, among other considerations. Thus, many disease problems in fish stem from poor management; this important principle should always be kept in mind when trying to identify the true cause of a fish disease.

ENVIRONMENT AND FISH HEALTH

Good water quality is the key to successful fish production. Water quality includes all physical, chemical, and biological factors that influence the use of water for fish culture. Any characteristic of water that affects the survival, reproduction, growth, or management of fish is a water-quality variable. An abundant water supply solves many problems associated with intensive fish culture by diluting out accumulated wastes and toxic

products, as well as by maintaining optimal water conditions. However, water is a precious and often limiting resource in aquaculture, and thus many methods have been developed to increase the holding capacity of culture systems.

ACCLIMATION: ITS RELATIONSHIP TO INTERPRETING WATER QUALITY AND OTHER ENVIRONMENTAL INFLUENCES

Acclimation is the physiological adaptation of an animal to a new environment. Acclimation is an important concept to understand in fish health because it helps explain why fish may get sick under one set of circumstances but may be perfectly healthy under exactly the same conditions at some other time.

A tank of fish in which the pH has slowly dropped from 7.0 to 5.5 over several months may appear normal; however, if the water is rapidly adjusted back to 7.0, many of the fish may die. Even though pH 5.5 is stressful and not healthy, many fish can tolerate such conditions if they are introduced to the environment slowly. Whereas, even though a pH of 7.0 is within the normal range for most freshwater fish, too rapid a return to normal will be dangerous.

With the chronic low pH stress described above, where environmental conditions gradually deteriorate, indirect effects of the stress are often seen; these may include failure to reproduce, poor growth, developmental anomalies,

Relationship between environmental stress
and the health status of fish

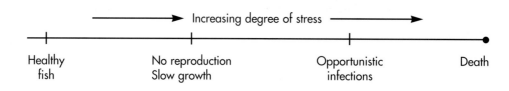

Fig. I-34   Relationship between environmental stress and fish health.

or, commonly, the presence of what are referred to as opportunistic infections; that is, diseases that develop when the fish's defenses are not up to par. As you review the problems in the diagnostic guide, you will notice that most of the environmental (water quality) problems often occur concurrently with opportunistic infections. Most infectious diseases of fish probably take advantage, in one way or another, of compromised defenses; however, some pathogens readily do this. These particular agents are generally considered to have a relatively low pathogenicity for fish and thus can only flourish under immunocompromising conditions. Classical examples of such pathogens include the bacteria *Aeromonas hydrophila* (see *PROBLEM 45*) and flexibacteria (see *PROBLEM 36*), water molds (see *PROBLEM 33*), and the parasites *Trichodina* (see *PROBLEM 21*) and ectocommensal protozoa (see *PROBLEMS 31* and *32*). When such pathogens or other opportunists are encountered, look closely for a primary environmental cause.

Inability to acclimate explains why fish often become sick after being handled or transported. The stress created by handling, combined with exposure to new environmental conditions (see *PROBLEM 86*), can cause severe stress against which fish cannot compensate.

CHAPTER 7

How to Use the Problem List

It is important that you fully understand the organization of the problem list because this will greatly facilitate your ability to diagnose cases.

PROBLEMS ARE LISTED IN THE ORDER THAT THEY ARE ENCOUNTERED IN THE CLINICAL WORK-UP

Starting on p. 55, *PROBLEMS 1* through *92* are listed in the order that they are encountered in the clinical work-up. This listing is summarized in Fig. I-1. Thus, as tests are performed or as tissues are examined, you should record the problems that are identified. This arrangement of problems also allows you to follow along in the diagnostic guide as various clinical techniques are performed.

Thus, problems that are identified from the history are listed first, followed by those that are made from the core water quality examination, followed by those that are made from the external (skin and gill) examinations, followed by those that are made from the postmortem examination.

It is critical to realize that a fish may have more than one problem, and thus it is important to determine which is the most serious (i.e., which requires treatment first) and which is the primary cause of the disease (see Chapter 9, *PRIORITIZING PROBLEMS*). In general, water quality problems can often incite the development of many infectious diseases, so water quality should often be improved as part of treating an infectious disease. Some infectious diseases are especially notorious as opportunistic pathogens.

CHAPTER **8**

Clinical Decision-Making: Have the Major Problems Been Identified?

When core water quality parameters have been measured and fish have been examined for infectious agents and lesions, using biopsy, culture, and necropsy exam, a decision must be made about which problems are most important and whether those identified are sufficient to explain the morbidity and mortality patterns and the clinical signs. For example, a heavy monogenean infestation on the gills, combined with clinical hypoxia, low (~1% per week) mortality, and moderately elevated unionized ammonia (0.03 mg/l UIA), would be consistent with a diagnosis of monogenean-induced mortality. The monogenean infestation could be explained by the sublethal, but stressful, ammonia concentration.

Conversely, a mild trichodinosis infestation on the gills, absence of any other infectious agents in the clinical work-up, and normal core water quality readings would not be sufficient to explain a high, acute (~5% per day) mortality rate in a population. If no other problems are identified in the clinical work-up (i.e., if all these problems are ruled out as the major cause of the fish mortalities), look to a rule-out diagnosis(es) to explain the mortalities (see Fig. I-1).

It is important to realize that rule-out diagnoses are considered **after** the clinically identifiable problems (i.e., see *PROBLEMS 1* through *72*) have been eliminated from consideration as the major cause of the disease. Rule-out diagnoses can sometimes be presumptively identified from the history (e.g., use of outdated feed in combination with clinical signs of nutritional deficiency are strongly suggestive of a nutritional imbalance; see *PROBLEM 79*). However, definitive confirmation of a rule-out diagnosis requires specialized tests that are not routinely performed in most clinics (e.g., chemical analysis of feed composition, viral isolation). Thus definitive diagnosis of rule-out diagnoses requires referral to a specialized laboratory (see Chapter 11, *WHEN TO REFER CASES*). Note that it may be impossible or economically unfeasible to obtain a definitive diagnosis. Instead, it may be better to correct the presumed problem (e.g., replace old feed with fresh feed if nutritional imbalance is suspected) and monitor for a favorable clinical response, rather than try to identify a specific problem (e.g., test for vitamin C deficiency in suspect feed).

CHAPTER 9

Prioritizing Problems

More than one problem is usually identified in a clinical work-up. Thus, the clinician must prioritize the problems using the following criteria:

1. Which problem is primarily responsible for the morbidity and/or mortality?
2. Which problem is most life-threatening?
3. Which problem is safest to treat first?

All three questions are closely interrelated; consider which problem is best addressed first. For example, gill parasites are generally considered more dangerous than skin parasites, so it would be advisable to treat gill pathogens first, especially if the fish had to be moved or otherwise stressed to treat the skin disease. In another case, if a bacterial infection and a skin parasite were both present but the fish is not eating, it would be best to treat for the skin parasite, which may stimulate the fish to begin eating, even though the bacterial infection may be more life-threatening. An antibiotic-medicated feed might then be used to effectively treat the bacterial infection. Details on treatments are given in the *PHARMACOPOEIA*.

CHAPTER 10

Treatment Plans

The clinician should provide the following two types of plans to the client:

1. **Short-term plan** — This plan should include the means to control the immediate problem that is usually the cause of the presenting complaint; this typically involves various types of medications to control infectious disease and large-scale water treatments to reduce environmental stress and toxins.

2. **Long-term plan** — This plan is often the most important and involves recommendations for improving management that will prevent the recurrence of similar problems in the future.

CHAPTER 11

When to Refer Cases

Most fish disease cases can be diagnosed by the clinician using the relatively simple techniques described in this book. However, some cases may require additional tests that are not routinely performed in most clinics (Anderson & Barney, 1991). Many rule-out diagnoses (see *PROBLEMS 73* through *85*) can be definitively diagnosed by using specialized tests. Specific details for proper referral of such cases to appropriate referral laboratories are described under individual problems. Most states have at least one government agency that can provide assistance in fish disease diagnosis. These are often affiliated with universities (veterinary colleges, fisheries departments) or state agricultural or fisheries agencies. Some federal laboratories (United States Fish and Wildlife Service, National Marine Fisheries Service in the United States) also perform fish disease diagnosis. Also an increasing number of private laboratories provide fish disease diagnostic services. A listing of fish disease diagnostic laboratories is provided annually in *Aquaculture Magazine*, Box 2329, Asheville, North Carolina 28802.

CHAPTER 12

Sample Problem Data Sheet (Key to the Headings in Part II)

PROBLEM X

Prevalence Index

This is a subjective comparison of the prevalence of the stated problem for various fish groups. The absence of a rating means that the disease does not occur in that group. Ratings are as follows: (1) very common; (2) common; (3) uncommon; and (4) rare.

The index is based only on prevalence in **cultured** fish. Prevalence of a disease in wild fish of the same species may differ considerably from individuals in culture.

The prevalence index is **subjective**, since little published quantitative data exists that documents the prevalence of diseases in cultured fish worldwide. Note that certain diseases may be much more or much less common in some geographic areas. Also, when not dealing with the species groups in the prevalence index, the prevalence may not be accurate.

Literally hundreds of fish species are cultured. However, despite this great diversity, many fish species are susceptible to the same diseases. The two most important factors that influence the types of diseases that may affect a particular fish species are salinity and temperature. These two environmental factors play an important role in limiting the distribution of infectious agents and are also an important influence on noninfectious diseases. To help you gain a better understanding of the chance of encountering certain diseases in various fish, prevalence rates are given for the following four ecological categories:

Warm Freshwater (WF) — These include fish that are submitted from freshwater environments that are warmer than approximately 20° C (68° F). Prevalence data is mainly based on diseases in tropical freshwater aquarium fish, but most diseases have a similar prevalence in ictalurids, cyprinids, and many warm water sport fish, such as centrarchids and striped bass.

Warm Marine (WM) — These include fish that are submitted from brackish (>~0.5 ppt salinity) or marine environments that are warmer than about 20° C (68° F). Prevalence data is mainly based on diseases in tropical marine aquarium fishes, but most diseases have a similar prevalence in many estuarine species, such as red drum and striped bass.

Cold Freshwater (CF) — These include fish that are submitted from freshwater environments that are colder than approximately 20° C (68° F). Prevalence data is mainly based on diseases in salmonids cultured in freshwater, but most diseases have a similar prevalence in channel catfish and many cold water game fish, such as largemouth bass, yellow perch, walleye, and pike.

Cold Marine (CM) — These include fish that are submitted from brackish or marine environments that are colder than approximately 20° C (68° F). Prevalence data is mainly based on diseases in salmonids cultured in brackish water or seawater, but most diseases have a similar prevalence in many other cold water marine species, such as flounder and cod, as well as many brackish water species, such as striped bass and sciaenids.

Note that these classifications are intended as general guidelines; many species overlap into more than one category. For example, channel catfish are normally cultured in climates where water temperatures may range from 10° C (50° F) to 30° C (86° F). The pathogens and other problems that this species encounters depend on the ecological conditions prevailing at that time. Thus, salinity and temperature should be used as the primary guides for assessing probable prevalence. Note also that the prevalence categories are primarily intended to describe problems of tropical freshwater aquarium fish (WF), tropical marine aquarium fish (WM), channel catfish (WF, CF), and salmonids (CF, CM). Thus, while other fish species are affected with similar problems, their prevalence rates may differ considerably from these given estimates.

Method of Diagnosis

This gives the data or procedure needed for the diagnosis. In some cases a definitive diagnosis cannot be obtained under typical clinical conditions. In any case the method of diagnosis that provides the most reliable result under typical clinical conditions is listed first, followed by other, usually less definitive, methods.

History

Self-explanatory. Note that **rarely** will all of the features listed be present in any single case. **None** may be present.

Physical Exam

Self-explanatory. Note that **rarely** will all of the clinical signs listed be present in any single case. **None** may be present.

Treatment

Different treatments are listed numerically (1, 2, 3, etc.). Some treatments require multiple steps; these are indicated as alphabetical subheadings of that treatment (e.g., 1a, 1b, 1c, etc.). Detailed treatment procedures are given in the *PHARMACOPOEIA*. See the *PHARMACOPOEIA* for legal considerations in treating fish.

PART II

PROBLEM LIST

Problems 1 through 9

Diagnoses made with commercially available water quality test kits or equipment that should be present in the clinician's clinic

1. Environmental hypoxia
2. Temperature stress
3. Temperature stratification
4. Ammonia poisoning
5. Nitrite poisoning
6. Too low (acidic) pH
7. Too high (alkaline) pH
8. Improper hardness
9. Improper salinity

PROBLEM 1
Environmental Hypoxia (Low Dissolved Oxygen [DO])

Prevalence Index
WF - 1, WM - 1, CF - 1, CM - 1
Method of Diagnosis
1. Measurement of oxygen concentration
2. History
History
General: Overcrowding; low water flow in raceway; algae *crash* in pond; several overcast days over pond
Acute environmental hypoxia: Acute shutdown of aeration caused by power failure; acute mortality of all but air-breathing fish; fish *piping* for air; gathering at water inflow; depression; death with opercula flared and mouth agape; acute stress response; large fish die (small fish may survive)
Chronic environmental hypoxia: Chronic stress response
Physical Examination
See *History*
Treatment
1. Acute hypoxia
    a. Restore oxygen levels immediately
    b. Monitor ammonia (see *PROBLEM 4*) and nitrite (see *PROBLEM 5*) daily for 1 week to be sure that biological filtration is functioning properly (aquaria only)

2. Chronic hypoxia
    a. Increase aeration
    b. Reduce feeding
    c. Reduce fish density

COMMENTS
Definition of Environmental Hypoxia
Environmental hypoxia means that a low concentration of dissolved oxygen (DO) exists in the water. Oxygen is the most important water quality factor for proper fish health, but it is poorly soluble in water. For example, the *maximum* amount of oxygen that can dissolve in freshwater at 28° C (82° F) is 7.84 mg/l (Table II-1; Fig. II-1, *C*) (Murray & Riley, 1969). This compares with over 150 mg O_2 per liter of air at sea level; there may be less oxygen if the culture system is crowded or has inadequate aeration.

Sources and Users of Oxygen
Oxygen can enter water from photosynthesis or by diffusion of atmospheric oxygen. In a pond without mechanical aerators, photosynthesis is the most important source of oxygen (and is also the cause of many diurnal changes in pond water quality; see Fig. II-1, *D*) (Noga & Francis-Floyd, 1991). A certain amount of algae in a pond is desirable, since it increases oxygen production and thus allows a greater number of fish to be stocked. High fish stocking densities also result in large algae populations because of the plant nutrients that are released from fish excrement.

The effect of algal metabolism on oxygen levels is dramatically illustrated by the marked diurnal variation in oxygen concentration in a pond with a large algae population (see Fig. II-1, *D*). Oxygen concentration is highest near sunset because net oxygen production occurs during the day. At night, oxygen levels decline because of the cessation of photosynthesis. Since plant and animal respiration occurs continuously, a net loss of oxygen occurs at night. Thus, oxygen levels are at their lowest level just before sunrise.

In aquaria, raceways, and other high-density culture systems, algal photosynthesis is not sufficient to support the high fish biomass. Thus, oxygen levels must be supplemented by either constant mechanical aeration

Table II-I   Dissolved oxygen (mg O$_2$ per liter) at saturation in freshwater, brackish water, and seawater at different temperatures. calculated from data in Murray and Riley (1969).

Temperature (°C)	Chlorinity (%)*										
	0	2	4	6	8	10	12	14	16	18	20
1	14.24	13.87	13.54	13.22	12.91	12.59	12.29	11.99	11.70	11.42	11.15
2	13.84	13.50	13.18	12.88	12.56	12.26	11.98	11.69	11.40	11.13	10.86
3	13.45	13.14	12.84	12.55	12.25	11.96	11.68	11.39	11.12	10.85	10.59
4	13.09	12.79	12.51	12.22	11.93	11.65	11.38	11.10	10.83	10.59	10.34
5	12.75	12.45	12.18	11.91	11.63	11.36	11.09	10.83	10.57	10.33	10.10
6	12.44	12.15	11.86	11.60	11.33	11.07	10.82	10.56	10.32	10.09	9.86
7	12.13	11.85	11.58	11.32	11.06	10.82	10.56	10.32	10.07	9.84	9.63
8	11.85	11.56	11.29	11.05	10.80	10.56	10.32	10.07	9.84	9.61	9.40
9	11.56	11.29	11.02	10.77	10.54	10.30	10.07	9.84	9.61	9.40	9.20
10	11.29	11.03	10.77	10.53	10.30	10.07	9.84	9.61	9.40	9.20	9.00
11	11.05	10.77	10.53	10.29	10.07	9.84	9.63	9.41	9.20	9.00	8.80
12	10.80	10.53	10.29	10.06	9.84	9.63	9.41	9.21	9.00	8.80	8.61
13	10.56	10.30	10.07	9.84	9.63	9.41	9.21	9.01	8.81	8.61	8.42
14	10.33	10.07	9.86	9.63	9.41	9.21	9.01	8.81	8.62	8.44	8.25
15	10.10	9.86	9.64	9.43	9.23	9.03	8.83	8.64	8.44	8.27	8.09
16	9.89	9.66	9.44	9.24	9.03	8.84	8.64	8.47	8.28	8.11	7.94
17	9.67	9.46	9.26	9.05	8.85	8.65	8.47	8.30	8.11	7.94	7.78
18	9.47	9.27	9.07	8.87	8.67	8.48	8.31	8.14	7.97	7.79	7.64
19	9.28	9.08	8.88	8.68	8.50	8.31	8.15	7.98	7.08	7.65	7.49
20	9.11	8.90	8.70	8.51	8.32	8.15	7.99	7.84	7.66	7.51	7.36
21	8.93	8.72	8.54	8.35	8.17	7.99	7.84	7.69	7.52	7.38	7.23
22	8.75	8.55	8.38	8.19	8.02	7.85	7.69	7.54	7.39	7.25	7.11
23	8.60	8.40	8.22	8.04	7.87	7.71	7.55	7.41	7.26	7.12	6.99
24	8.44	8.25	8.07	7.89	7.72	7.56	7.42	7.28	7.13	6.99	6.86
25	8.27	8.09	7.92	7.75	7.58	7.44	7.29	7.15	7.01	6.88	6.75
26	8.12	7.94	7.78	7.62	7.45	7.31	7.16	7.03	6.89	6.76	6.63
27	7.98	7.79	7.64	7.49	7.32	7.18	7.03	6.91	6.78	6.65	6.52
28	7.84	7.65	7.51	7.36	7.19	7.06	6.92	6.79	6.66	6.53	6.40
29	7.69	7.52	7.38	7.23	7.08	6.95	6.82	6.68	6.55	6.42	6.29
30	7.56	7.39	7.25	7.12	6.96	6.83	6.70	6.58	6.45	6.32	6.19

From *Fish and invertebrate culture* (p.142) by S. Spotte, 1979a, New York, John Wiley and Sons. Reprinted by permission.
*Chlorinity is a very close approximation of salinity.

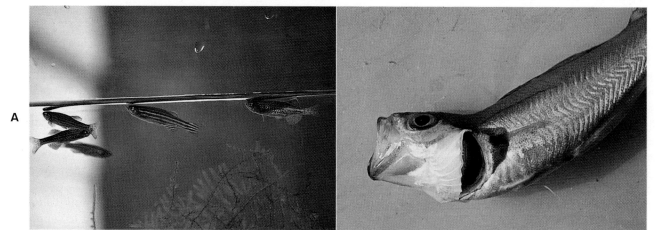

Fig. II-I   **A,** Fish *piping* for air near the surface of the water because of low dissolved oxygen (DO). The air-water interface has the highest concentration of oxygen. **B,** Fish that died because of acute environmental hypoxia.

(*A* photograph courtesy of T. Wenzel; *B* photograph from H. Moller. *C* from Piper et al., 1982; *D* from Noga & Francis-Floyd, 1991; *E* from Boyd et al., 1978.)

Continued.

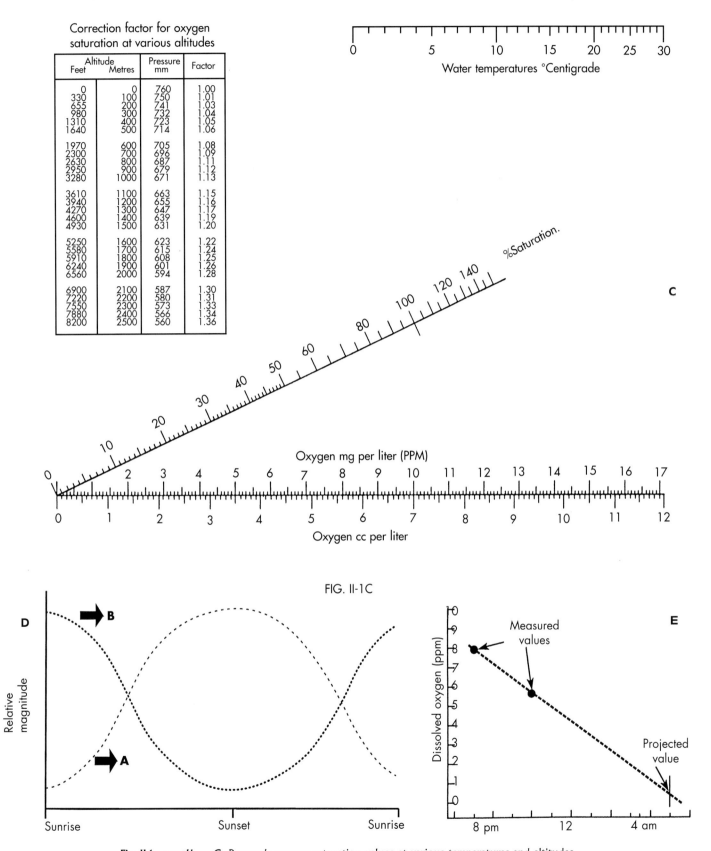

Fig. II-I—cont'd.   **C,** Rawson's oxygen saturation values at various temperatures and altitudes. **D,** Diurnal fluctuations in water quality variables in a pond. Dissolved oxygen, temperature, pH, and percentage of unionized ammonia usually increase during the day (*curve A*); dissolved carbon dioxide levels usually increase overnight (*curve B*). **E,** Extrapolation method for estimating nighttime decline in dissolved oxygen in a pond.

(aquaria) or by constantly running oxygenated water through the system (raceways). Raceways most commonly use surface water from a natural stream or lake; the latter are usually nearly saturated with oxygen.

Causes of Environmental Hypoxia

PONDS

Low oxygen is common in ponds, especially in summer, when warm temperatures both decrease oxygen's solubility (Table II-1; Fig. II-1, C) and increase the pond organisms' metabolism and subsequent oxygen demand. An intimate relationship exists between oxygen levels and pond metabolism. While it is desirable to have algae in a pond to increase oxygen production, too much algae can cause wide fluctuations in DO, because algae are both the major producers *and* consumers of oxygen in most ponds. Consequently, the large nocturnal oxygen demand can cause a low DO by sunrise.

Other circumstances can also lead to environmental hypoxia in ponds. Cloudy weather decreases photosynthesis and thus reduces net oxygen production (Tucker, 1985). Overcast weather may cause severe hypoxia by steadily decreasing oxygen production from lower light intensity. A *crash* or massive death of algae, a common but usually unpredictable event, can cause severe oxygen depletion (Boyd, 1979). Decreased oxygen production is exacerbated by the great oxygen demand of the decaying algae. Many chemicals that are commonly used to treat fish diseases (e.g., copper sulfate, potassium permanganate, or formalin) are algicidal (Schnick et al., 1989). These agents must be used with extreme caution in ponds having large algae populations.

If ice forms on a pond in winter, the oxygen can become progressively depleted, leading to anoxia (Barica & Mathias, 1979). This most commonly occurs in late winter and early spring in ponds that have a permanent winter ice cover. The ice and snow prevent oxygen diffusion into the pond and block photosynthesis, while respiration of pond organisms continues, albeit at a low metabolic rate. Many factors determine whether a kill will occur, including how long the ice cover persists and the amount of decaying matter in the pond. Shallow ponds are more susceptible, because of the smaller total amount of oxygen. Other metabolic processes, such as increased CO_2 (see *PROBLEM 80*) and hydrogen sulfide (see *PROBLEM 81*), probably contribute to mortalities. This type of winter kill should not be confused with idiopathic *winter kill* (see *PROBLEM 33*).

AQUARIA AND OTHER HIGH-DENSITY SYSTEMS

The most obvious cause of environmental hypoxia in high-density, closed-culture systems is due to failure of aerators, which leads to an acutely low oxygen level. This is a common sequela to an electrical power failure and can cause acute mortality in a home aquarium or other system. Because the oxygen may be off for only a short time and since the power often returns to normal after the fish have died without the aquarist observing the power failure, such events must be diagnosed from the history. Survival of only air-breathing fish (e.g., anabantids, clariid catfishes) is one clue that acute hypoxia may be responsible. Heavily planted aquaria could become hypoxic at night because of the plants' respiration. However, this is rare, since mechanical aeration prevents this problem.

While surface water from streams or lakes is usually well-oxygenated, ground (well or spring) water is typically low in dissolved oxygen and high in other gases; both conditions can cause hypoxia (see *PROBLEMS 10* and *80*). Nets used to confine fish in cages or pens can become fouled, impeding water flow and reducing oxygen supply.

Clinical Signs of Environmental Hypoxia

Acute environmental hypoxia is defined as a rapid (within minutes to hours) drop in DO to lethal or near-lethal levels. It is often accompanied by acute and frequently catastrophic mortalities. Common behavioral signs include lethargy (Scott & Rogers, 1980) and the congregating of fish near the air-water interface (*piping*; Fig. II-1, A), where oxygen levels are highest (Francis-Floyd, 1988). Hypoxic fish are often anorexic. A classical sign of asphyxiation is an agonal response, with the mouth open and the opercula flared (Fig. II-1, B), although this is not pathognomonic for environmental hypoxia.

Chronic environmental hypoxia is defined as a long-term (days or longer) suboptimal dissolved oxygen level in a culture system. Chronic hypoxia does not kill fish outright but causes considerable stress. At least 5 mg/l of dissolved oxygen is needed for optimal growth and reproduction of most fish (Tucker, 1985). Below this level, food consumption decreases and becomes less efficient (Hollerman & Boyd, 1980) and growth slows (Andrews et al., 1973). A DO of less than 2 mg/l is very stressful and may predispose fish to opportunistic infections (Scott & Rogers, 1980). If DO remains below 1 mg/l for any period of time, most fish die (Tucker, 1985). Many warm water fish can survive for long periods in 2 to 3 mg/l oxygen, while many cold water species (e.g., salmonids) only tolerate 4 to 5 mg/l oxygen for long periods.

Channel catfish that recover from acute environmental hypoxia may develop deep, necrotic ulcers (see *PROBLEM 92, Red Fillet Syndrome*) (Plumb & Walters, 1982).

Diagnosis of Environmental Hypoxia

Definitive diagnosis of low DO can only be done by measuring the DO in water at the site or by immediately preserving the water sample. Once the sample is removed from the aquarium or pond, its oxygen concentration changes immediately because it is mixed with air. Oxygen measurements made on unpreserved water samples submitted to the clinic are not valid. Thus, a diagnosis of environmental hypoxia is based upon the history, unless an electronic meter is used to measure oxygen on site or unless the sample is immediately preserved, using a commercial test kit.

In flow-through systems, DO is highest at the inflow and lowest at the outflow. In ponds, clinical signs are most commonly evident in early morning; hypoxic conditions often dissipate rapidly after sunrise, masking the event. The largest fish are usually most susceptible to oxygen depletion. In aquaria, survival of only air-breathing fish is strongly suggestive of acute environmental hypoxia. Although not airbreathers, goldfish can also withstand low DO for a long time.

Environmental hypoxia must be differentiated from other causes of hypoxia, including nitrite toxicity (see *PROBLEM 5*) and gill parasitosis.

Treatment of Environmental Hypoxia

Acute environmental hypoxia is an emergency situation, and immediate steps must be taken to provide fish with oxygenated water. The catastrophic nature of acute environmental hypoxia dictates that all possible measures be taken to prevent the development of this situation. For large culture systems holding high fish densities, this means having adequate emergency aerators and power sources to handle hypoxic events. Chronic environmental hypoxia is less of an emergency but is still a serious problem that should be addressed expeditiously. Reducing feeding will reduce fish and algal oxygen consumption (Andrews & Matsuda, 1975).

PONDS

Supplemental aeration should begin if DO drops below 3 to 4 mg/l (Tucker, 1985) in channel catfish ponds and 4 to 5 mg/l in salmonid culture. Aeration equipment includes both pneumatic (i.e., air pumps) and mechanical (i.e., paddlewheels) devices. Water may also be transferred from an adjacent pond to the hypoxic pond. Oxygenated well water may also be used. Aeration usually does not increase the DO throughout the entire pond but provides local areas of oxygen-rich water (Tucker, 1985), where fish remain until the dissolved oxygen level in the entire pond returns to acceptable levels. Thus, circulation is just as important as aeration because circulation increases the volume of oxygenated water in the pond. Dissolved oxygen concentrations may vary significantly at different ends of a pond because of differences in algal densities, wind direction, and related factors. Aerators should be placed where the DO is highest and thus where fish are congregating. While tractors may be used to operate aerators, electrical power is much more convenient and economical. Principles of aeration and management of dissolved oxygen problems are reviewed by Tucker (1985).

If pond fish are raised at high densities (e.g., catfish at greater than 1900 kg/ha = 2000 lb/ac), keep constant vigilance for environmental hypoxia. An oxygen meter is essential for a commercial aquaculture enterprise. Measuring DO in a pond both at dusk and 2 or 3 hours later allows the clinician to draw a straight line that can reliably predict the DO concentration at dawn (Fig. II-1, *E*).

Algae concentrations should be routinely monitored by the farmer. Algal density can be estimated by placing a Secchi disc (Tucker, 1985) or some other object (e.g., yardstick) into the water to measure turbidity. In general, pond water visibility should be no less than 0.5 m from the water's surface (Noga & Floyd, 1991). Be aware that turbidity may also result from suspended clay or other particles.

AQUARIA

Chronic environmental hypoxia is rarely a problem in aquaria because of the considerable amount of mechanical aeration. However, acute environmental hypoxia does occur because of electrical or mechanical failure of aeration equipment. Some evidence exists that adding hydrogen peroxide can provide a short-term increase in DO concentration (Maranthe et al, 1975). Ammonia and nitrite levels should be closely monitored in aquaria that have experienced an acute drop in DO because the bacteria that remove these toxins require oxygen and thus may be harmed (see *PROBLEMS 4* and *5*).

FLOW-THROUGH SYSTEMS

Water used for culture should be at close to 100% saturation. When well water is used for flow-through culture, it must usually be aerated or at least allowed to equilibrate with the atmosphere before fish are exposed to it (see *PROBLEMS 10* and *80*). In flow-through systems that are without supplemental aeration, stocking density is usually limited by oxygen concentration, especially at high ($>10°$ C [or 50° F]) temperatures (Piper et al., 1982). In trout culture, low oxygen is usually a problem in summer when low water flow, high metabolism, high organic decay, and large amounts of algae occur. The maximum stocking density recommended for salmonids in raceways can be calculated using the following Flow Index:

$$F = \frac{W}{L \times I}$$

F = Flow Index
W = the permissible weight (pounds) of fish at a given inflow
I = gallons per minute for a given fish size
L = inches

Flow Index will vary with different hatcheries, depending upon water saturation and water chemistry. Piper et al. (1982) discuss how to calculate the Flow Index for various species. Other factors will also influence stocking density (see *PROBLEMS 4* and *87*). For salmonids, oxygen levels should ideally not be less than 6 mg/l or 80% saturation and should never drop below 5 mg/l at the end of the raceway.

CAGES AND NET-PENS

Cage and net-pen systems rely on tidal currents or other water movement to supply oxygen. Fouling organisms must be removed from netting regularly to prevent blockage of water flow.

PROBLEM 2
Temperature Stress

Prevalence Index

Hypothermia: WF - 2, WM - 2, CF - 4, CM - 4
Hyperthermia: WF - 4, WM - 4, CF - 2, CM - 2

Method of Diagnosis

1. Measurement of abnormal temperature
2. History

History

General: Acute to chronic stress response

Hypothermia: Temperature at or near lower lethal limit of that particular species; shutdown of aquarium heater because of power failure or broken thermostat; thermometer not working properly; heater wattage too small for aquarium; aquarium next to window or draft; *shimmies,* lethargy; mortality of all but most cold-tolerant aquarium fishes (e.g., goldfish and koi); water mold infection

Hyperthermia: Temperature near the upper lethal limit of that particular species; dyspnea; heater thermostat improperly set; heater not adequately submerged or thermostat broken; heater wattage too large for aquarium; aquarium next to heat source or window; summer

Physical Examination

See *HISTORY*

Treatment

1. Restore proper temperature immediately
2. Move fish to environment with proper temperature

COMMENTS

Effects of Temperature on Fish Physiology

Fish are poikilothermic; therefore temperature dramatically affects their metabolism, including immunity (Avtalion et al., 1973; Finn & Nieslen, 1971). Decrease in water temperature suppresses the immune response (Clem et al., 1984). Perturbations in immune function may partly explain why many pond fish diseases are most common in the spring and fall (MacMillan, 1985), when temperature fluctuation is greatest.

Definition of Temperature Stress

Absolute temperature ranges for fish species do not exist because temperature tolerance depends on several factors, including the temperature to which the individual has been acclimated, salinity (for estuarine species), life stage, and reproductive status. The speed of temperature change is also important (see *ACCLIMATION,* p. 44). Thus, it is difficult to generalize about temperature tolerance because it is influenced by so many factors. However, it is important to be aware of the general temperature ranges (Table II-2) for the species being examined and the conditions that may influence it.

Temperate species, such as channel catfish, striped bass, and largemouth bass, often tolerate a wider temperature range than tropical fishes or cold water species (e.g., salmonids). All fish are susceptible to rapid temperature changes.

Most fish seem to tolerate a rapid drop in temperature better than an equivalent rise in temperature. This is probably due to the physiological changes that occur with increasing temperatures: metabolic rate (and thus oxygen consumption) increases with temperature. However, oxygen is less soluble at higher temperatures (see Table II-1). Thus, hypoxia may exacerbate hyperthermia. Also, stress hormone release increases with temperature. Immune function may also take time to equilibrate to the higher temperature, while pathogens can adjust much more quickly; this may explain why many bacterial and parasitic diseases are more common in spring (Meyer, 1978).

Diagnosis

As with dissolved oxygen, water temperature can only be accurately measured at the site, so a diagnosis of temperature stress at the clinic is based on the history. A history of temperature stress will vary, depending on the variables discussed above—how low or high the temperature becomes and how quickly it takes to arrive at the stressful temperature. For example, many tropical aquarium fishes can withstand a relatively low temperature as long as the change occurs slowly; this might occur during fall in an unheated aquarium. Conversely, if the heater stopped working in an aquarium in the middle of winter, dropping the temperature 10° C in 1 day, it might cause many fish to die immediately.

It is important to realize that in ponds, water temperatures may normally fluctuate as much as 10° C daily without any apparent harm to the fish (Boyd, 1990). This emphasizes the importance that acclimation plays in determining the effect of a temperature change.

HYPOTHERMIA

Because fish are cold-blooded animals, their activity depends on temperature. Thus, at low temperatures, fish become inactive and depressed. Fish exposed to subop-

Table II-2 Optimal and tolerable temperature ranges for representative fishes.

Group	Optimal	Upper tolerance	Lower tolerance
Freshwater tropicals	22 to 27	30 to 40	8 to 18
Marine tropicals	22 to 27	30 to 40	8 to 18
Goldfish; koi	15 to 22	30	2 to 4
Sunfishes	26 to 30		
American eel	30		
Striped bass juvenile	18 to 28		
Striped bass adult	18 to 25		
Channel catfish	28 to 30	35	0 to 2
Red drum	22 to 25		
Atlantic salmon	17	19	
Rainbow trout	15	19	
Brook trout	15	18	
Pacific salmon	12	18	

Note: These are general guidelines that vary considerably, depending on prior acclimation and on the prevailing environmental conditions.

timal temperatures are especially susceptible to water mold infections (see *PROBLEM 33*).

Fish that are stocked outside their normal geographic range may exhibit *winter kill*. For example, tilapia, a hardy cichlid, is often stocked in summer in subtropical or temperate areas of the United States but tilapia usually die when temperatures reach less than approximately 12° C. Low pond temperatures have been associated with an idiopathic syndrome also known as *winter kill* (see *PROBLEM 33*). Do not confuse this problem with winter kill that is caused by oxygen depletion (see *PROBLEM 1*).

HYPERTHERMIA

Hyperthermia can be a serious problem in salmonids, when temperatures in some culture systems may approach their upper lethal limit, such as during summer with trout cultured in the southern Appalachian region of the United States; this often increases susceptibility to opportunistic infections.

Treatment and Prevention

Temperature control is feasible in small, closed systems (e.g., aquaria). But, in ponds or other culture systems with large volumes of water, temperature stress is usually economically unfeasible to control. Some tropical fish farmers use plastic sheeting to insulate ponds during cold snaps, but this is not practical for food fish ponds. In flow-through systems, temperature control is only feasible when either recycling most of the water or when egg incubation systems that use very little water are employed.

It is difficult to give exact recommendations for allowable temperature change because it varies with species, environment, and prior acclimation conditions. For example, fish acclimated to a higher temperature often can withstand hyperthermia better than the same species maintained at a lower temperature. When acclimating fish to a certain temperature, a rule of thumb is that water temperature should not be changed more than about 1° C (or 1° F) per hour. While some fish may be stressed by this change, many others tolerate even more rapid changes. Fish that are normally exposed to wide temperature fluctuations (e.g., in ponds) are probably more tolerant of rapid temperature change than fish that are kept under more stable conditions (e.g., thermostatically controlled temperature in an aquarium).

HYPOTHERMIA

Tropical aquarium fish that are shipped to temperate regions in winter may be exposed to large temperature drops. If the fish are exhibiting clinical signs of hypothermia and the temperature is well outside their normal range, it should be returned to at least near their normal temperature range as quickly as possible. One way this can be done is by filling plastic aquarium bags with warm water and floating them in the shipment water.

Note that temperate species (e.g., channel catfish, salmonids) are often deliberately cooled quickly before shipping to reduce transport stress (Piper et al., 1982).

HYPERTHERMIA

As it is with hypothermia, the ability of a fish to tolerate hyperthermia depends not only on how high the temperature becomes, but also on how quickly it rises. Slow increases in temperature are tolerated much better. When acclimating aquarium-kept fish to a high temperature (such as for breeding) it is best not to raise the temperature more than approximately 3° C (or 3° F) per day. In some cases, such as when transporting fish, the temperature may be unavoidably raised above this maximum. When temperature increases, oxygen should be as close to saturation as possible because low oxygen inhibits the ability of fish to acclimate to temperature change (Weatherly, 1970). During transport, it is advisable to lower the temperature to the low end of the physiological range for that species (see *HYPOTHERMIA*).

When the temperature is near a species' upper lethal limit, it is often wise to reduce or stop feeding, since the amount of oxygen needed for both homeostasis and digestion of food may exceed the amount of oxygen that can be extracted from the water (Stevenson, 1987).

PROBLEM 3
Temperature Stratification

Prevalence Index
WF - 1, CF - 1
Method of Diagnosis
Detection of a significant thermocline
History
Deep pond (>1.5 m [5 feet]); spring/summer/fall of year; eutrophic pond
Physical Examination
Varies with sequela
Treatment
1. Provide emergency aeration
2. Prevent future stratification events

COMMENTS
Definition

Temperature stratification is not a problem in itself, but instead it causes changes in pond water quality, which can be lethal. Temperature stratification refers to the development of two distinct temperature zones in a pond (Fig. II-3); it occurs when the surface water of a pond warms up, while the bottom water remains cooler. Temperature stratification is a common problem in *farm* and *watershed-type* ponds that are often over 1.5 m deep, but it is rarely a problem in commercial catfish ponds, which are usually less than 1.5 m (5 feet) deep.

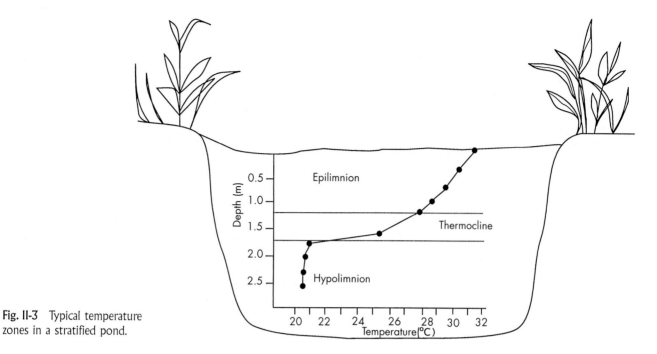

Fig. II-3 Typical temperature zones in a stratified pond.

Causes

Stratification is most likely to develop during hot, calm summer days when little water mixing occurs by wind action. As the temperature difference between the surface water (epilimnion) and bottom water (hypolimnion) increases, the pond stratifies into two layers of water that are separated by the metalimnion, or thermocline, where water temperature changes rapidly from the warm surface temperatures to the cool bottom temperatures. Warm water is lighter, and thus the thermocline acts as a physical barrier between the epilimnion and hypolimnion, and a considerable amount of energy is required to mix, or "turn over," the pond. The DO in the hypolimnion is rapidly depleted by pond metabolism and an oxygen demand builds up as anaerobic reactions are not sufficient to form final degradation products of pond metabolites. Toxic substances, such as hydrogen sulfide and methane, may accumulate under these reducing conditions.

Consequences

The longer the stratified state persists, the greater the danger of a lethal oxygen depletion and toxin release when the pond finally mixes. Inclement weather (heavy winds or cold rain), harvesting (seining), or aeration can mix a stratified pond. In addition, a stratified pond will eventually *turn over* in fall, when surface water temperatures cool. Stratification can be prevented by having the farmer run weekly *oxygen profiles* on each pond in at least two places (Noga & Francis-Floyd, 1991). The DO and temperature are measured at 0.3 m (1 foot) intervals from surface to bottom. If stratification is present, both temperature and DO will rapidly change at the thermocline, and there may be little oxygen below that depth. Any evidence of stratification should be corrected immediately by aeration. Early detection is essential to preventing a catastrophe.

PROBLEM 4
Ammonia Poisoning (New Tank Syndrome)

Prevalence Index
WF - 1, WM - 1, CF - 1, CM - 1

Method of Diagnosis
Chemical measurement of high unionized ammonia
Lethal poisoning: > ~1.00 mg UIA/l
Sublethal poisoning: > ~0.05 mg UIA/l

History
Overcrowding; recent medication or other chemicals added; newly established aquarium; aquarium gravel recently washed or other filters recently cleaned; failure of biological filters; recent algal *crash* in pond; reduced water flow in raceway; hyperexcitability, possibly other neurological signs if acute (UIA > 0.20 mg/l); acute to chronic stress response

Physical Examination
See *HISTORY*

Treatment
AQUARIA
1. 25 to 50% water change (daily to weekly, depending on ammonia concentration)
2. Add zeolite
3. Add buffer to reduce pH (freshwater only)
4. Add nitrifying bacteria
5. Add biological filtration

Major Sources of Nitrogen Input and Removal in a Culture System

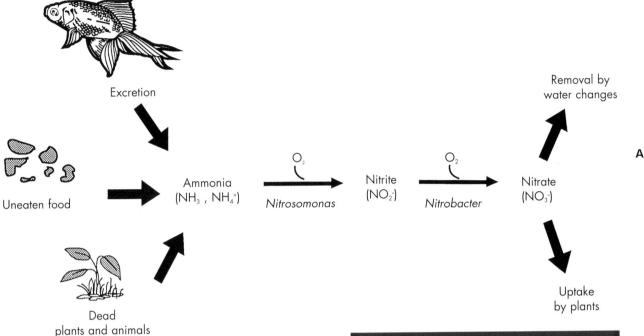

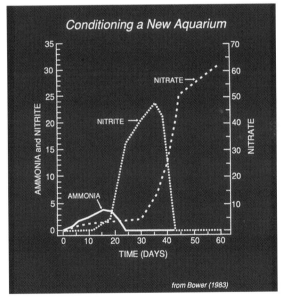

Fig. II-4 **A,** Major sources of nitrogen input and removal in a culture system. **B,** Typical ammonia and nitrite concentrations present during new tank syndrome if fish are added on day 0. Time required to establish an active filter and reduce ammonia and nitrite to nontoxic levels are ~3 weeks in freshwater aquaria (Carmignani & Bennett, 1977) and ~2 months in marine aquaria at ~20° to 22° C (Bower & Turner, 1981). Time required to establish the filter increases considerably at lower temperatures.

(B from Bower, 1983.)

6. Decrease density
7. Temporarily reduce or stop feeding

Monitor closely for possible nitrite increase

PONDS, FLOW-THROUGH SYSTEMS

1. Stop or reduce feeding
2. Decrease density
3. Add water or increase water flow

COMMENTS

Ammonia poisoning is one of the most common water quality problems diagnosed in aquaculture (Meade, 1985). Ammonia is the primary nitrogenous waste product of fish and also originates from the decay of complex nitrogenous compounds (e.g., protein). Ammonia can cause acute mortality, but most often it presents as a sublethal stress.

Aquaria

In an aquarium, ammonia accumulation is due to an inadequate number of bacteria (*Nitrosomonas* sp.) that convert ammonia to nitrite (Fig. II-4, *A*). In a new aquarium setup these bacteria are scarce. So, when fish are added to the new tank, the ammonia rapidly rises

(Fig. II-4, *B*), killing the fish; this is often referred to as *new tank syndrome.*

Ammonia poisoning can also occur in long-established aquaria. If fish are added to a tank that has many fish already present or if fish are overfed, causing an accumulation of decaying food in the tank, ammonia can rise. The total amount of ammonia that can be converted to nitrite depends entirely on the amount of biological filtration in the tank. Biological filtration (more appropriately termed *microbiological filtration,* since it refers to the filtration of water over microbes) occurs when the aquarium water passes over a surface that has *Nitrosomonas* bacteria. Thus, biological filtration (and ammonia removal) is greatest where there is a high water flow over a large surface area. This occurs in the aquarium's filters (undergravel, box, power filters). If the biological filtration capacity is too low to remove all the ammonia produced by the fish, ammonia will rise. If filters are cleaned too vigorously (e.g., gravel stirred excessively), it will cause an ammonia spike, since the bacteria are easily dislodged from the substrate and are susceptible to changes in environmental conditions.

Ponds

Ammonia is usually not a problem unless supplemental aeration is used, preventing environmental hypoxia and thus allowing higher fish densities (Boyd, 1990). As in other systems, feeding (uneaten, decaying food and ammonia generated from food consumption) is the largest source of ammonia in a commercial pond. Ammonia toxicity is most likely to occur near sunset, when pH, temperature, and thus unionized ammonia are at their peak (Fig. II-1, *D*) (see *Diagnosis of Ammonia Poisoning*). In most ponds, algae, as well as *Nitrosomonas* bacteria, are major consumers of ammonia. Most ponds, especially commercial aquaculture ponds, have large algae populations. Ammonia also tends to increase during fall and winter, possibly because of a decrease in algal and bacterial metabolism at low temperatures.

Table II-4, A   Percentage of the total ammonia nitrogen (TAN) that is present as unionized ammonia (UIA) at various temperature-pH combinations in freshwater.

Temperature (°C)	pH								
	6.0	6.5	7.0	7.5	8.0	8.5	9.0	8.5	10.0
0	0.00827	0.0261	0.0826	0.261	0.820	2.55	7.64	20.7	45.3
1	0.00899	0.0284	0.0898	0.284	0.891	2.77	8.25	22.1	47.3
2	0.00977	0.0309	0.0977	0.308	0.968	3.00	8.90	23.6	49.4
3	0.0106	0.0336	0.106	0.335	1.05	3.25	9.60	25.1	51.5
4	0.0115	0.0364	0.115	0.353	1.14	3.52	10.3	26.7	53.5
5	0.0125	0.0395	0.125	0.394	1.23	3.80	11.1	28.3	55.6
6	0.0136	0.0429	0.135	0.427	1.34	4.11	11.9	30.0	57.6
7	0.0147	0.0464	0.147	0.462	1.45	4.44	12.8	31.7	59.5
8	0.0159	0.0503	0.159	0.501	1.57	4.79	13.7	33.5	61.4
9	0.0172	0.0544	0.172	0.542	1.69	5.16	14.7	35.3	63.3
10	0.0186	0.0589	0.186	0.586	1.83	5.56	15.7	37.1	65.1
11	0.0201	0.0637	0.201	0.633	1.97	5.99	16.8	38.9	66.8
12	0.0218	0.0688	0.217	0.684	2.13	6.44	17.9	40.8	68.5
13	0.0235	0.0743	0.235	0.738	2.30	6.92	19.0	42.6	70.2
14	0.0254	0.0802	0.253	0.796	2.48	7.43	20.2	44.5	71.7
15	0.0274	0.0865	0.273	0.859	2.67	7.97	21.5	46.4	73.3
16	0.0295	0.0933	0.294	0.925	2.87	8.54	22.8	48.3	74.7
17	0.0318	0.101	0.317	0.996	3.08	9.14	24.1	50.2	76.1
18	0.0343	0.108	0.342	1.07	3.31	9.78	25.5	52.0	77.4
19	0.0369	0.117	0.368	1.15	3.56	10.5	27.0	53.9	78.7
20	0.0397	0.125	0.396	1.24	3.82	11.2	28.4	55.7	79.9
21	0.0427	0.135	0.425	1.33	4.10	11.9	29.9	57.5	81.0
22	0.0459	0.145	0.457	1.43	4.39	12.7	31.5	59.2	82.1
23	0.0493	0.156	0.491	1.54	4.70	13.5	33.0	60.9	83.2
24	0.0530	0.167	0.527	1.65	5.03	14.4	34.6	62.6	84.1
25	0.0569	0.180	0.566	1.77	5.38	15.3	36.3	64.3	85.1
26	0.0610	0.193	0.607	1.89	5.75	16.2	37.9	65.9	85.9
27	0.0654	0.207	0.651	2.03	6.15	17.2	39.6	67.4	86.8
28	0.0701	0.221	0.697	2.17	6.56	18.2	41.2	68.9	87.5
29	0.0752	0.237	0.747	2.32	7.00	19.2	42.9	70.4	88.3
30	0.0805	0.254	0.799	2.48	7.46	20.3	44.6	71.8	89.0

From Emerson et al., 1975, *Journal of the Fisheries Research Board of Canada, 32,* p. 2382. Reprinted by permission.

Ammonia may also rise after an algae *crash* or massive die-off; this not only reduces ammonia assimilation, but also adds to ammonia buildup caused by the decaying algae. Algae die-offs can occur spontaneously or may be caused by algicidal chemicals (see *PROBLEM 1*).

Flow-Through Systems

Oxygen is usually the most limiting factor in flow-through systems. However, ammonia levels can become toxic if supplemental aeration increases the maximum fish densities that can be held. Ammonia is lowest at the inflow and highest at the outflow.

Clinical Signs of Ammonia Poisoning

Acute ammonia toxicity can cause behavioral abnormalities, such as those that occur in mammals, including hyperexcitability (Daoust & Ferguson, 1984). Fish often stop feeding. Chronic ammonia poisoning has been associated with hyperplasia and hypertrophy of gill tissue, although it is unclear as to whether this nonspecific pathology is due directly to ammonia poisoning or rather to other aspects of poor water quality that frequently accompany chronically high ammonia (Daoust & Ferguson, 1984). The precise mechanism of ammonia poisoning in fish is unknown, but high aqueous ammonia increases blood and tissue ammonia levels, causing elevated blood pH, osmoregulatory disturbance, increased tissue oxygen consumption, and decreased blood oxygen transport (Schwedler et al., 1985). Chronic ammonia poisoning decreases growth (Colt & Armstrong, 1979) and disease resistance (Walters & Plumb, 1980).

Diagnosis of Ammonia Poisoning

Ammonia levels are easily determined, using commercially available kits. These kits measure the nitrogen present as ammonia, also known as total ammonia nitrogen (TAN). An ion-specific electrode can also be used to measure ammonia (e.g., Hach Chemical).

Ammonia is present in two forms: unionized (NH_3) and ionized (NH_4^+). Unionized ammonia (UIA) is toxic to fish, while ammonium (NH_4^+) is much less toxic (Russo, 1985; Meade, 1985). The amount of UIA in water depends mainly upon the pH, and also on temperature and salinity. High pH and temperature and low salinity favor the presence of UIA (Emerson et al., 1975; Meade, 1985).

The concentration of toxic UIA is determined from a standard chart. For example, if the TAN of a freshwater sample that was measured with the water quality test kit was 1.0 mg/l, the pH of the water was 8.5, and the water temperature was 25° C, 15.3% of the total ammonia would be present as UIA (NH_3) (Table II-4, *A*). Thus, the amount of UIA in the water would be 1.0 mg TAN/l × 0.153 = 0.153 mg of UIA/l. In low salinities, the fraction of total ammonia nitrogen that is present as UIA is virtually the same as for freshwater. In full-strength seawater (32 to 40 ppt), there is as much as 20%

less UIA at the same temperature and pH as in freshwater. This variation is usually not important in making a clinical diagnosis of ammonia poisoning. Bower & Bidwell (1978) provide tables for highly accurate determination of UIA in seawater.

Ammonia toxicity varies with environmental conditions (e.g., pH, temperature, salinity, water hardness) and other stresses present. Exposure to sublethal ammonia levels also increases tolerance to ammonia toxicity (Thurston et al., 1981). Sublethal levels that influence growth are especially difficult to determine, so keeping ammonia levels as low as possible is advisable. Unionized ammonia levels greater than ~1.00 to 2.00 mg/l are usually lethal within 1 to 4 days (Meade, 1985). Below this level, fish might not die, but they will be stressed. If UIA is greater than 0.05 mg/l, it should be reduced as quickly as possible.

Treatment of Ammonia Poisoning: Aquaria

Ammonia levels can be reduced with frequent water changes. But, in a long-established tank, the clinician must be careful not to cause environmental shock (see *PROBLEM 86*). Adding zeolite is a safe and effective way of reducing ammonia quickly. However, zeolite's efficacy decreases with increased salinity (see *PHARMACOPOEIA*). Reducing the pH will reduce the percentage of ammonia that is present as NH_3. For every 1 unit decrease in pH, there is a ten-fold decrease in UIA (Table II-4, *A*); this should be done with caution because a rapid drop in pH can cause other problems

Table II-4, B   Effect of various drugs on ammonia detoxification when used as prolonged immersions at recommended therapeutic levels.

Agent	Effect	Reference*
Chloramphenicol	FW: None;	A
	SW: Slight increase, accompanied by clouding of the water	B
Copper sulfate	FW: None;	C
	SW: Slight to moderate increase	B, D
Erythromycin	FW: Substantial increase	A
Formalin	FW: None	C
Gentamicin sulfate	SW: None	B
Malachite green	FW: None	C
Methylene blue	FW: Substantial increase;	C
	SW: Slight to moderate increase	B
Neomycin sulfate	SW: Slight to moderate increase	B
Nifurpirinol	FW: None;	A
	SW: None	B
Oxytetracycline	FW: None	A
Potassium permanganate	FW: None	C
Quinacrine hydrochloride	SW: None	B
Sulfamerazine	SW: None	A
Chloroquine diphosphate	SW: None	E

Compiled by Bower, 1983.
*A=Collins et al., 1976; B=Bower and Turner, 1982b; C=Collins et al., 1975; D=Kabasawa and Yamada, 1972; E=C.E. Bower (unpublished data). FW=freshwater; SW=seawater.

(see *PROBLEM 6*). Note also that reducing ammonia levels during the early stages of establishing a biological filter prolongs the time required for the biological filter to reach peak efficiency.

Water changes and zeolite or pH treatment are useful but must be part of a plan to increase biological filtration capacity of the aquarium. In a new tank, adding a commercial preparation of nitrifying bacteria can speed up the process of establishing an effective filter but usually will not instantly result in a well-established biofilter. Biofilter establishment is often quicker when filter material (gravel, filter floss) from a healthy established tank is used; however, there is the risk of introducing pathogens with such material.

In an established tank, ammonia poisoning arises when more fish are in the tank than the biological filtration can handle. In this case, either some fish must be removed or more filtration (e.g., power filter) must be added.

Many medications can be toxic to the nitrifying bacteria (Table II-4, *B*). Use of such medications can cause new tank syndrome in an established tank. If chemical damage to the biological filter occurs, a box filter with activated carbon should be added to the tank to remove all traces of the drug. The tank should then be treated as a new tank and appropriate measures taken as described above.

Treatment of Ammonia Poisoning: Ponds, Cages, Flow-Through Systems

In ponds, prevention of ammonia toxicity is preferable to therapy, since ammonia cannot be rapidly removed from most ponds. Over the short term, adding fresh water will dilute the ammonia. Ponds over 0.5 ha (1 ac) cannot be rapidly flushed, but adding fresh water will create a haven where fish can avoid the toxin.

It is advisable to feed no more than 110 kg of feed/ha/day (100 lb of feed/acre/day) to avoid ammonia accumulation in catfish ponds (Noga & Floyd, 1991). However, many producers resist this recommendation, because fish grow more slowly, lengthening the production cycle. The TAN concentration in ponds usually increases slowly; therefore, biweekly monitoring is usually adequate for commercial producers. If TAN exceeds 0.50 mg/l, it should be monitored daily until it returns to zero. Using a high-quality feed that is high in digestible protein will also reduce ammonia production.

In flow-through systems, reducing stocking densities or feeding rates or increasing water flows are the most common treatments for ammonia buildup. Treating water with zeolite is another option. Since the majority of ammonia in a flow-through system comes from fish metabolism (relatively little from the water source or from uneaten feed), an *ammonia factor* (AF) can be calculated as follows (Piper et al., 1982):

$$AF = \frac{TAN \ (mg/l) \times flow \ (gallons/minute)}{Pounds \ of \ food \ fed/day}$$

The AF is determined by measuring the TAN in a system several times during 1 day. When the AF is determined, the total amount of ammonia present at the outlet of that particular flow-through system under various feeding rates and water flows can be predicted from:

$$TAN = \frac{Pounds \ of \ food \ fed/day \times AF}{Flow \ (gallons/min)}$$

PROBLEM 5
Nitrite Poisoning (Brown Blood Disease, New Tank Syndrome)

Prevalence Index
WF - 1, WM - 4, CF - 1, CM - 4

Method of Diagnosis
1. Chemical measurement of high nitrite in water
2. Measurement of high metHb in blood

History
Overcrowding; recent medication or other chemicals added; newly established aquarium; aquarium gravel recently washed or other filters recently cleaned; failure of biological filters; fall season in pond; low $Cl^-:NO_2^-$ ratio; acute to chronic stress response

Physical Examination
Dyspnea; light tan to brown gills; tan to brown blood; acute to chronic stress response

Treatment
AQUARIA
1. Twenty-five percent to 50% water change (daily to weekly, depending on nitrite concentration)
2. Add nitrifying bacteria
3. Add chloride
4. Add biological filtration
5. Decrease density
6. Reduce temperature
7. Reduce feeding

PONDS
1. Add chloride
2. Maintain highest DO possible

COMMENTS
Epidemiology of Nitrite Poisoning
Most circumstances causing ammonia poisoning can also lead to nitrite poisoning (see *PROBLEM 4:* AQUARIA). In a newly established aquarium, nitrite buildup usually occurs after ammonia has peaked (see Fig. II-4, *B*). This is because the *Nitrobacter* bacteria that convert nitrite (NO_2^-) to nitrate (NO_3^-) require time to become active, just like the bacteria that convert ammonia to nitrite.

Table II-5 Effect of various drugs on nitrite detoxification when used as prolonged immersions at recommended therapeutic levels.

Agent	Effect on nitrite concentration	Reference*
Chloramphenicol	FW:None	A
	SW: None	B
Chloroquine diphosphate	SW: None	E
Copper sulfate	FW: None	C
	SW: Slight to moderate increase	B, D
Erythromycin	FW: Substantial increase	A
Formalin	FW: None	C
Gentamicin sulfate	SW: None	B
Malachite green	FW: None	C
Methylene blue	FW:None	C
	SW: None	B
Neomycin sulfate	SW: Substantial increase	B
Nifurpirinol	FW: None	A
	SW: None	B
Oxytetracycline	FW: None	A
Potassium permanganate	FW: None	C
Quinacrine hydrochloride	SW: None	B
Sulfamerazine	SW: None	A

Compiled by Bower, 1983.
*A=Collins et al., 1976; B=Bower & Turner, 1982b; C=Collins et al., 1975; D=Kabasawa & Yamada, 1972; E=CE Bower (unpublished data). FW=freshwater; SW=seawater.

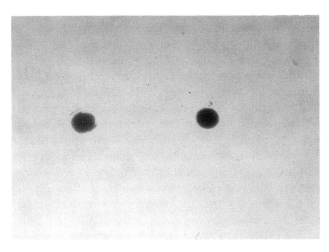

Fig. II-5 Normal drop of blood (*left*) and blood with high concentration of methemoglobin or brown blood (*right*).

Nitrite nitrifyers are also inhibited by ammonia (Moe, 1992a). Some chemicals selectively inhibit *Nitrobacter* (Table II-5), causing a nitrite spike.

In ponds, nitrite poisoning is common in fall because the temperature optima of *Nitrosomonas* and *Nitrobacter* are different, resulting in nitrite accumulation. Nitrite can rise quickly (< 24 hours) in catfish ponds (Johnson, 1993). Nitrite is not a problem in flow-through systems because there is no significant conversion of ammonia to nitrite during the short time that water is present in the system.

Clinical Signs of Nitrite Poisoning
Nitrite is actively transported across the gill, where it enters the bloodstream (Lewis & Morrios, 1986) and oxidizes hemoglobin (Hb) to methemoglobin (MetHb). Methemoglobin cannot transport oxygen efficiently, so tissues are deprived of oxygen. While oxygenated Hb is red, MetHb is brown. So fish with nitrite poisoning often have pale tan or brown gills. Methemoglobin concentrations of 25% to 30% usually give the blood a slightly brown color, but MetHb concentrations must usually be around 40% to cause grossly visible chocolate brown blood and pale tan-to-brown gills. Fish with anemia may also have pale gills but with a red tinge. Fish with severe (i.e., 80% or greater) methemoglobinemia are dyspneic even with adequate oxygen.

Behavioral changes noted with nitrite poisoning are characteristic of hypoxia, including lethargy and congre-gating near the water surface. Fish with nitrite poisoning should be disturbed as little as possible, since even minor exertion may cause acute mortality.

Diagnosis of Nitrite Poisoning
Definitive diagnosis of nitrite poisoning requires measuring the MetHb concentration in the blood (resting MetHb levels vary considerably, but > 25% is considered abnormal), combined with measuring the nitrite concentration in water. However, routine clinical diagnosis of nitrite toxicosis relies solely on measuring nitrite levels. This has its limitations, since fish vary greatly in susceptibility to nitrite poisoning. At least gross evidence of methemoglobinemia (Fig. II-5) should be sought to strengthen the diagnosis.

Colorimetic kits can be used for nitrite measurement. Analyses measure nitrite-nitrogen, which can be converted to total nitrite, using a conversion factor of 3.3. For example, if the nitrite-nitrogen (NO_2-N) measurement of the kit is 0.10 mg/l, the amount of nitrite present is 0.33 mg/l.

Nitrite poisoning has been most extensively studied in channel catfish, where firm recommendations can be made regarding toxic levels. Data also exists for other species, especially salmonids, but for most species there is no data on toxicity. Susceptibility to nitrite poisoning varies tremendously among species and some fish are resistant (Tomasso, 1986). For channel catfish in pure freshwater, nitrite should be undetectable by commercial test kits (< 0.10 mg/l of nitrite nitrogen). In contrast, sunfish tolerate high levels (96-hour LC50 often > 50 mg/l) because they do not actively take up nitrite from water. The recommended level for salmonids is < 0.50 mg/l. The 96-hour LC50 values for freshwater fish range from 0.60 to 200 mg/l. While marine fish are susceptible to nitrite poisoning, extremely high levels are required. For example, the 24-hour LC50 for spotted sea trout at 14 ppt salinity is 980 mg/l NO_2-N (Daniels & Boyd, 1987). For European sea bass at 36 ppt salinity, the 96-hour LC50 is 90 to 100 mg/l NO_2-N, and induction of methemoglobinemia requires exposure to over 25 mg/l NO_2-N for 96 hours (Scarano et al., 1984). Studies in other fish have failed to demonstrate acute toxicity at as high as 1750 mg/l (Brownell, 1981). Such high nitrite levels would never be encountered in aquaculture systems. The susceptibility of tropical aquarium fish to nitrite is unknown; however, it is best to keep levels low (< 0.10 mg/l) to avoid any possible toxicity. Long-term (over 6 months) exposure to even very low nitrite levels (0.015 to 0.060 mg/l NO_2-N) can result in mild methemoglobinemia in some fish (Wedemeyer & Yasutake, 1978).

If the water is naturally high in chloride (e.g., coastal aquifers) or chloride has been added, diagnosis of nitrite poisoning also requires measurement of Cl^-. Colorimetric tests and electronic probes are available. Nitrite toxicity is affected by many other factors, including pH, fish size, previous exposure, nutritional status, and dissolved oxygen level. Thus, it is best to keep levels as low as possible, especially for species with unknown susceptibility.

Exposure of fish to very high nitrite concentrations is also associated with the accumulation in the spleen of foci of iron-containing (Prussian blue positive staining) macrophages caused by increased erythrocyte destruction (Scarano et al., 1984).

Treatment of Nitrite Poisoning
Nitrite is much less toxic when chloride is present, possibly since Cl^- competitively inhibits nitrite uptake across the gills (Bowser, 1983). In channel catfish, chloride ion prevents mortality caused by methemoglobin-associated nitrite toxicity when present in a ratio (wt:wt) of at least 3 mg chloride to 1 mg nitrite (Bowser, 1983). Thus, a water sample with 1.2 mg/l chloride and 0.30 mg/l nitrite (= 4 mg Cl:1 mg NO_2 ratio) would not be acutely lethal to channel catfish. However, this ratio does not prevent chronic erythrocyte damage that can lead to anemia. This adverse effect is not seen when the chloride:nitrite ratio is 6:1 (Tucker et al., 1989). Similar guidelines may be satisfactory for treating nitrite toxicosis in other fish, although, as mentioned previously, most fish species have not been examined.

Sodium chloride is the least expensive and most readily available form of chloride, but calcium chloride is equally effective (Tomasso et al., 1980). The low level of salt needed to treat nitrite toxicosis (usually < 50 mg/l) is not toxic to freshwater fishes.

Once treatment is instituted, reduced hemoglobin levels usually return to normal within 12 to 24 hours and fish will begin eating. However, secondary infections may be a sequela of sublethal nitrite exposure (Hanson & Grizzle, 1985) and anemia caused by low hemoglobin can take days to return to normal (Scarano & Saroglia, 1984).

Prevention of Nitrite Poisoning
Prevention is preferable to treatment. In catfish ponds at least 20 mg/l chloride should always be present to prevent nitrite toxicity. Many natural waters have this chloride level, often obviating the need for prophylactic chloride addition. Even dilute brackish water probably has enough chloride to prevent nitrite toxicosis in most euryhaline species. For example, 1 ppt seawater contains over 500 mg/l chloride. Clinically encountered nitrite levels have never been shown to be toxic to fish in seawater, probably because of seawater's high chloride content. However, there are few studies on nitrite's effect on tropical marine reef fish, so it is advisable to keep nitrite levels in marine aquaria low.

Bicarbonate is also somewhat protective against nitrite but considerably less than chloride. High dietary ascorbate levels also protect against nitrite-induced MetHb formation (Wise et al., 1988).

PROBLEM 6
Too Low (Too Acidic) pH

Prevalence Index
WF - 2, WM - 3, CF - 2, CM - 4
Method of Diagnosis
Chemical measurement of low pH
History
Acutely low pH: Acute mortality with tremors and hyperactivity; dyspnea; acute stress response
Chronically low pH: Increased mucus production; chronic stress response
Physical Examination
See HISTORY
Treatment
AQUARIA
1. Change water
2. Add buffer
3. **Adjust pH only if ammonia levels are safe**
PONDS
1. Add buffer
2. Reduce density
FLOW-THROUGH SYSTEMS
1. Pretreat incoming water with buffer
2. Add base

COMMENTS
Fish species differ in their optimal pH range. A pH range of 6.5 to 9.0 is generally recommended for freshwater fish (Swingle, 1969). Values outside this range are stressful (Swingle, 1961). A pH of < 4.0 or > 11.0 is lethal (Swingle, 1961; Tucker, 1985). However, this is a wide range. This range is generally considered satisfactory for salmonids and channel catfish and most other freshwater

food fish. While some freshwater aquarium fish (generally, the "hardy" species most commonly sold in pet shops) can do well within this entire range, most do considerably better if maintained within a narrower range.

Many freshwater aquarium fish come from poorly buffered waters that are high in tannins or other organic acids (e.g., Amazon River basin) and thus do best in neutral-to-slightly-acidic (pH ~6.5 to 6.8) conditions (see *PROBLEM 7*). Notable exceptions include the following: African rift lake cichlids and brackish water fish (e.g., mollies, guppies, platies, swordtails) do best in hard (> 100 mg/l), alkaline (pH 7.6 to 8.0) water. Marine aquarium fish require a stable, alkaline pH. The tolerable pH for marine aquaria is generally 7.8 to 8.4 (Moe, 1992a). Optimal limits are much narrower and the pH is best kept between 8.1 to 8.3 (Bower, 1983). Fromm (1980), Schwedler et al. (1985), and Leivestad (1982) review the physiological effects and pathology of suboptimal pH.

Fish acclimated to a relatively low pH can survive a drop in pH better than the same species maintained at a higher pH. Fish routinely exposed to wide pH fluctuations (e.g., in ponds) are probably more tolerant of rapid pH change than fish kept under more stable conditions (e.g., typical aquarium).

Primary Sources of Low-pH Water
Most ground (well or spring) water has dissolved carbonates and carbon dioxide and a pH somewhere between 5 to 8 (Boyd, 1990). Ground water in contact with silicate minerals is poorly buffered and typically has a low pH and a large amount of CO_2 compared to ground water taken from carbonate substrate (e.g., limestone) that is thus well buffered. In a pond, pH is highly influenced by the soil type. Acid sulfate soils may have a pH less than 4 because of the oxidation of sulfide to sulfuric acid (Boyd, 1990), making them unsuitable for fish culture unless neutralized (see *TREATMENT*). Waters impacted by acid rain or that drain acidic soils may have low pH. This can be a problem in a raceway culture after a rain, when large amounts of acids are washed into a stream water supply. The latter is a problem in trout farms in the eastern United States. Inadequately cured silicone aquarium sealants release acetic acid.

Secondary Sources of Low-pH Water
The metabolic activity of fish and other aquatic organisms produces acids. In a closed system, such as an aquarium or pond, these acids tend to gradually reduce pH. If water changes are not regularly performed or if the pH is not otherwise adjusted, it can drop low (e.g., to pH 5 in a freshwater aquarium). A pH below 5.5 is very stressful; if too low, it is lethal. Acute exposure of fish to such a low pH (such as by adding a new fish to such a tank) can be fatal (see *PROBLEM 86*).

Buffering Capacity and pH
The bicarbonate/carbonate buffer system (Fig. II-6) is the major moderator of pH in aquatic ecosystems. Alkalinity is the buffering capacity in water, as measured by the amount of bicarbonate (HCO_3^-) and/or carbonate ($CO_3^=$) present (see *PROBLEM 8*). Alkalinity is usually expressed as mg/l of calcium carbonate equivalents. Thus, water with high alkalinity resists pH change from acids produced by the aquatic organism's respiration (i.e., CO_2) and other metabolites.

Low pH is most common in waters with low alkalinity (i.e., less than 50 mg/l as $CaCO_3$) because the lower the alkalinity, the less the buffering capacity of the water and its ability to buffer acid production. However, given enough time, the pH can drop in even highly buffered waters, such as seawater.

Pond pH is influenced not only by the amount of bicarbonate present, but also by photosynthesis. Plant photosynthesis uses CO_2, raising the pH and causing it to peak near sunset (see Fig. II-1, *D*). At night, cessation of photosynthesis results in a net accumulation of CO_2, causing a drop in pH. It is not unusual for pH to vary diurnally from 6.5 to 9.0 within a commercial aquaculture pond (Boyd, 1979). Diurnal pH variation can also occur in a heavily planted freshwater aquarium.

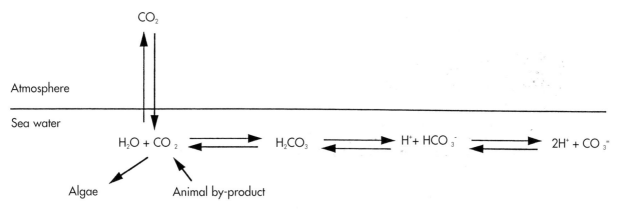

Fig. II-6 The carbonate-bicarbonate buffer equilibrium.
(From Oestmann, 1985.)

In low-alkalinity waters, the pH may fall considerably as water passes through a flow-through system, caused primarily by fish metabolism. Thus, the pH is highest at the inflow and lowest at the outflow.

Diagnosis

A good colorimetric test is adequate for routine clinical measurements of pH, but low-cost, portable pH meters (e.g., Aquatic Ecosystems; Fisher) are more convenient.

Diagnosis of acute or chronic acid stress must take into consideration the optimal pH of the species, the rate of pH change observed, and the magnitude of the change. Acclimation is also an important consideration: the pH of catfish ponds often fluctuates diurnally from 6.5 to 9.0 (Swingle, 1969). However, if this large a pH change were to occur in a typically pH-stable marine aquarium, it would cause major stress.

The toxicity of low pH is also complicated by its influence on so many water quality variables, especially ammonia (see *PROBLEM 4*) and other toxins (see *PROBLEMS 81, 83,* and *84*). Many toxins are highly affected by pH, especially metals, which become more toxic at low pH. Aluminum is one of the most common metals in soil. Aluminum ion is solubilized and is more toxic in acid pH and thus aluminum toxicity can occur concurrently (see *PROBLEM 83*) and may be the primary cause of death during acid runoff into streams. Low pH also increases the proportion of the bicarbonate buffer system that is present as free CO_2 (see *PROBLEM 80*). Thus, rapid acidification of high alkalinity water can increase the free CO_2 concentration, causing hypercarbia rather than acidosis (EIFAC, 1969).

Pure water saturated with carbon dioxide has a pH of 5.6. If the pH is < 5.6, the water must have other acids that are stronger than carbonic acid (e.g., nonmetallic oxides, hydrides of halogens, organic acids). This may suggest the possible source of the low pH.

Acute acid poisoning, characterized by tremors and hyperactivity (Schwedler et al., 1985), is much less common than chronic acid stress. Gill tissue is the primary target of acid stress (Leivestad, 1982). Low pH stimulates increased mucus production, which interferes with gas and ion exchange. Failure in acid-base balance (causing respiratory stress) and low sodium and chloride (causing osmotic stress) are the primary clinical signs. Chronic low pH stress is associated with poor growth, reproductive failure, and increased accumulation of heavy metals (Haines, 1981). Fish recovering from acute acid stress are more susceptible to infections (Jones et al., 1987).

Treatment

It is difficult to give exact recommendations for allowable pH change because it varies with species, environment, and prior acclimation conditions. When acclimating fish to a specific pH, a rule of thumb is that pH should not be changed more than about 0.2 to 0.5 pH units/day, unless the level is life-threatening. Fish are rarely stressed by this change and many tolerate even more rapid changes. For example, rainbow trout tolerate immediate transfer from pH 7.2 to pH 8.5 (Witschi & Ziebel, 1979).

Note that ammonia toxicity increases greatly with pH, so ammonia levels should be low enough to prevent possible toxic side effects before the pH is adjusted (see *PROBLEM 4*). High calcium increases the tolerance to low pH, presumably by reducing the ionic permeability of the gills (Haines, 1981).

AQUARIA

Many commercial preparations are available for adjusting the pH of aquaria. These consist of carbonate, bicarbonate, and/or phosphate buffers. Carbonate-bicarbonate buffers are preferable; they are the major source of buffer in natural waters. Frequent routine water changes (10% to 25% every 2 to 4 weeks) will prevent the drop in pH and can be used to adjust improper pH. Note that carbonate filtrants (i.e., limestone) will buffer acids but will not maintain pH over 7.5, which is outside the range required for tropical marine fish (Bower et al., 1981). Total alkalinity in marine aquaria should be 200 mg/l (4 mEq/l) and should not exceed a range of 100 to 300 mg/l (2 to 6 mEq/l) (Moe, 1992a).

PONDS

In ponds, increasing the alkalinity with buffer will also solve the pH problem. In warm water fish ponds, if pond alkalinity is less than ~50 mg/l as $CaCO_3$, buffer should be added. Some acid-sulfate soils need extremely large amounts of buffer to be neutralized. They are best managed by using buffer in combination with other management techniques (Boyd, 1990). Boyd (1990) provides detailed techniques for adding buffer to ponds.

FLOW-THROUGH SYSTEMS

Trout farms susceptible to low-pH runoff may need to lime the water supply during low-pH episodes. Agricultural lime and slaked lime do not react quickly enough to raise the pH in flow-through systems. Thus, some farms add sodium hydroxide (NaOH) solutions, using a metering device to instantaneously neutralize acidity (Boyd, 1990).

PROBLEM 7
Too High (Too Alkaline) pH

Prevalence Index

WF - 3, WM - 4, CF - 4, CM - 4

Method of Diagnosis

Chemical measurement of too high pH

History

Acutely high pH: Cloudiness of skin and gills; improper lime treatment of pond; acute stress response

Chronically high pH: Chronic stress response

Physical Examination

See *HISTORY*

Table II-7 Some tropical, freshwater aquarium fish that do best in soft, slightly acid water (pH ~6.5 to 6.8; hardness ~20 to 40 mg/l).

KILLIFISHES	TETRAS
Aphyosemion	*Cheirodon*
Aplocheilus	*Crenuchus*
Nothobranchius	*Hemigrammus*
Cynolebias	*Hyphessobrycon*
Epiplatys	*Megalamphodus*
Pterolebias	*Moenkhausia*
Rivulus	*Paracheirodon*
SOUTH AMERICAN	**LOACHES**
CICHLIDS	*Botia*
Apistogramma	
Symphysodon	**BARBS**
	Barbodes
GOURAMIES	*Capoeta*
Trichogaster	*Puntius*

Treatment

AQUARIA

1. Add buffer
2. Add deionized water
3. Add peat
4. Mechanically remove excess plants

PONDS

1. Add buffer (low-alkalinity ponds)
2. Add calcium (high-alkalinity ponds)
3. Add alum (high-alkalinity ponds)
4. Treat algae with herbicide

COMMENTS

Alkaline pH stress is much less common than acid stress because first, most closed culture systems tend to decrease in pH over time; and second, acids are much more common environmental contaminants than alkalis.

Acutely high pH may be caused by high levels of alkalis leaching out of inadequately cured concrete (Hine, 1982). Concrete containers should be allowed to leach all alkali before using for fish culture. Concrete can be *cured* with muriatic (hydrochloric) acid to speed up the process. Improper use of slaked or hydrated lime will rapidly raise the pH to 11, killing all fish (see *PHARMACOPOEIA*). The owner must then wait several weeks for the pH to return to normal before restocking.

Many fish do poorly in even moderately alkaline water and should be kept in soft, moderately acid conditions (Table II-7). Alkaline pH can also increase the mortality of incubating eggs of some species, possibly because acid waters are somewhat bacteriostatic.

Chronically high diurnal pH in ponds is almost always caused by excessive phytoplankton or vascular plant photosynthesis, which drives up the pH during the day as CO_2 is consumed (see Fig. II-1, *D*). This occurs in ponds with either low alkalinity or low calcium levels (relative to the amount of alkalinity) (Table II-8, *A*). Wide pH swings occur in low-alkalinity waters because there is not enough buffering capacity to moderate the plant-associated metabolic alkalosis. In ponds with high alkalinity and low calcium hardness, the pH can rise high during the day, sometimes over 10. This episodically high pH can be lethal to fry (Wu & Boyd, 1990). High pH can occur because the precipitation of calcium carbonate normally inhibits the rise in pH, since carbonate hydrolysis is the source of the high pH (Swingle, 1961) (see Fig. II-6).

Because most natural waters have the proper amounts and proportions of hardness and alkalinity, rising pH is an uncommon stress in pond fish. High pH in ponds is mostly important because it increases the amount of toxic, unionized ammonia (see *PROBLEM 4*).

Diagnosis

Diagnosis of alkaline pH stress should take into consideration the same factors used in diagnosing acid stress (see *PROBLEM 6*). At high pH, gill mucus cells and epithelial cells are hypertrophic (Daye & Garside, 1976). Corneal damage may also occur. These clinical signs are nonspecific. Note that alkalinity and alkaline pH are not the same (see *PROBLEMS 6* and *8* for a general discussion of acid-base balance in water).

Treatment

To correct alkaline pH stress, the clinician should take into consideration the same factors used to correct acid stress (see *PROBLEM 6*). Note especially that heavy metals are mobilized and more toxic as pH is lowered. Rapid pH decrease can also cause shock (see *PROBLEM 86*). As a general rule it is better not to lower the pH more than ~0.20 to 0.50 pH unit per day, although fish often tolerate much larger changes.

AQUARIA

Many commercial preparations are available for adjusting the pH of aquaria. Phosphate buffers are typically used to lower pH. Filtering water through peat will also reduce the pH, as well as the hardness, and is commonly used by aquarists to condition water for certain species (see Table II-7). Adding deionized water will also reduce the pH by diluting out carbonate buffers that maintain neutrality.

PONDS

In ponds with low alkalinity, adding buffer will reduce the high diurnal pH peak. Well-buffered, calcium-poor ponds can be treated with calcium; alum has also been used successfully (Boyd, 1990). Killing some of the plants with an appropriate herbicide will also dampen the daily pH spike, but this is not usually recommended because of adverse side effects (low oxygen from an algae *crash* [see *PROBLEM 1*] and possible herbicide toxicity to the fish).

PROBLEM 8
Improper Hardness
Prevalence Index
WF - 2, WM - 2, CF - 3, CM - 3
Method of Diagnosis
Chemical measurement of improper hardness
History
Acute to chronic stress response
Physical Examination
See *HISTORY*
Treatment
HARDNESS TOO LOW
Add calcium
HARDNESS TOO HIGH (AQUARIA)
1. Do water change with deionized water or other low-hardness water
2. Filter water through peat

COMMENTS
Hardness vs Alkalinity
Hardness is a measure of the divalent metal cation (e.g., calcium, iron, zinc, magnesium) concentration in water. In most waters, it is composed almost entirely of Ca++ and Mg++.

Hardness and alkalinity usually are closely related but measure different activities. Total hardness values (in mg/l as $CaCO_3$) usually will be similar to alkalinity values (in mg/l as $CaCO_3$) because the alkalinity of most natural waters comes primarily from the carbonate salts of calcium and magnesium. Other divalent or trivalent metal ions are relatively uncommon in natural waters. The hardness derived from carbonate salts is termed temporary hardness, since it is precipitated by boiling. Noncarbonate metal salts—sulfate (SO_4^{-2}); nitrate (NO_3^{-2}); chloride (Cl^-); and silicate (SiO_3^{-2})—comprise the permanent hardness, which is a less common component of total hardness. Waters where the hardness is mainly a permanent hardness are very hard but are low in alkalinity. In some waters, alkalinity is due primarily to sodium or potassium carbonate and thus may have low hardness with high alkalinity (Table II-8). The total hardness of seawater is very high (Boyd, 1990). Thus, even dilute estuarine water has considerable hardness.

Table II-8, A   Primary contributors to hardness and alkalinity in various natural waters.

		Hardness	
		Low	High
Alkalinity	Low	Low in both heavy metal salts and carbonate	Ca and Mg salts of sulfate, nitrate chloride, silicate
	High	Na_2CO_3, K_2CO_3	$CaCO_3$, $MgCO_3$

Table II-8, B   Ranges of hardness using the carbonate and °dH scales.

Water	Calcium carbonate equivalents (mg/l)*	German hardness (°dH)
Soft	0 to 75	0° to 4°
Moderately hard	75 to 150	4° to 8°
Hard	150 to 300	8° to 16°
Very hard	> 300	> 16°

*Calcium carbonate equivalents (mg/l) = °dH × 17.9 (Moe, 1992a).

Hardness Requirements
Hardness requirements vary greatly among species and somewhat with environmental conditions. Once acclimated, many fish do well over a wide range of hardness. For example, while at least 100 mg/l total hardness is considered optimal for freshwater salmonid culture, rainbow trout are successfully cultured in southern Appalachian mountain waters that have less than 10 mg/l total hardness. A total hardness of at least 50 mg/l is recommended for most warm water, freshwater, food fish (e.g., channel catfish, hybrid striped bass) (Wedemeyer et al., 1976; Piper et al., 1982).

Many freshwater aquarium fish do poorly in even moderately soft water and should be kept in waters with a high calcium content (see *PROBLEM 6* for aquarium fish that do best in hard, alkaline water). Conversely, some fish do poorly in even moderately alkaline water and should be kept in soft, moderately acid conditions (see Table II-7 for aquarium fish that do best in soft, acid water). The hardness of full strength seawater is about 6600 mg/l as $CaCO_3$, with ~1000 mg/l as $CaCO_3$ coming from calcium (~400 mg Ca/l) and ~5500 mg/l as $CaCO_3$ coming from magnesium (~1350 mg Mg/l). Calcium levels in tropical marine aquaria should be ~400 mg/l and should not exceed 200 to 450 mg/l (Moe, 1992a).

It is often easier for fish to adapt to hard water from soft water rather than vice versa. Fish that are transferred from hard to soft water also appear to be more prone to environmental shock (Grizzle et al., 1985; see *PROBLEM 86*). Calcium and magnesium are needed for osmoregulation. Calcium reduces the permeability of the gills to water, thus reducing water and electrolyte flux.

It is important to realize that hardness includes all divalent cations. For example, a hardness of at least 20 mg/l as $CaCO_3$ is needed for channel catfish health (Tucker, 1987). However, catfish in the yolk sac stage need water with at least 20 mg/l calcium, since the primary source of calcium is the water, not the diet, at this life stage. Thus, since hardness readings do not measure which metals actually constitute the hardness, it is often important to determine which minerals are contributing to the hardness.

Diagnosis of Improper Hardness

Hardness is usually expressed as mg/l equivalents of calcium carbonate, although the German hardness scale (degrees of hardness or °dH) is used extensively in the aquarium hobby (Sterba, 1983) (see Table II-8, *B*). Commercial kits are available for both measurements (e.g., Hoch Chemical; Tetra). A °dH of 3° to 10° is considered appropriate for most aquarium fish, while °dH > 10° is best for African rift lake cichlids.

In marine or brackish water pond systems, calcium levels increase with increasing salinity; thus, if the salinity is optimal for growth, calcium levels usually will be satisfactory. However, hardness reportedly can significantly decrease in marine aquaria that contain corals, crustaceans, or other invertebrates that use large amounts of calcium during growth (Moe, 1992a).

Treatment of Improper Hardness

Lime (see *BUFFERS-PONDS* in *PHARMACOPOEIA*) or other calcium salts are excellent sources of supplemental calcium for pond fish. Salt mixtures are commercially available for increasing hardness in aquaria. If aquarium hardness must be reduced, this can be done by adding distilled water available at groceries or pharmacies. Small reverse osmosis or ion exchange deionization units are available for the home aquarist (see *DEIONIZED WATER* in *PHARMACOPOEIA*). Filtering water over peat will also soften it (Sterba, 1983). Sedimentary rocks (e.g., schist, sandstone) may increase hardness because of the release of calcium and magnesium salts. Limestone substrates (e.g., coral, oyster shell) can be used in marine aquaria but are not advisable for aquaria where fish that need soft, acid waters are maintained. Metamorphic or volcanic rocks (e.g., basalt, granite, gneiss), as well as quartz, do not release divalent cations.

PROBLEM 9
Improper Salinity

Prevalence Index
WM - 3, CM - 4

Method of Diagnosis
MEASUREMENT OF SALINITY
In marine aquaria, < 30 or > 35 ppt salinity (< ~1.020 or > ~1.026 specific gravity at 25° C)

History
Maintaining salt-requiring fish in freshwater; incorrect calculation of seawater mixture; replacing seawater with freshwater during water changes; failure to replace evaporative loss of freshwater; acute to chronic stress response

Physical Examination
See *HISTORY*

Treatment
Add salt or freshwater to correct salinity

COMMENTS
Definition
Salinity is the amount (mass) of all ions in water and is most commonly expressed as parts of ions per thousand parts water (abbreviated as ppt or ‰). Freshwater has less than 0.5 ppt salinity, while natural, full-strength seawater ranges from 30 to 40 ppt salinity. Between these two extremes are various concentrations of brackish (estuarine) water, including oligohaline, mesohaline, and polyhaline. As with other water quality variables, salinity tolerance of fish varies (i.e., with age, environment).

Salinity Requirements/Tolerance
Marine aquarium fish are adapted to a narrow salinity range, and this should be maintained in the aquarium. Aquarium salinity can rapidly increase because of evaporative loss of freshwater. Salinity in a 35 ppt aquarium will often increase about 2 ppt (0.0005 to 0.001 specific gravity units) per week; it will rise more rapidly if the tank is not covered (Bower, 1983). Thus, it is best to keep the salinity of the tank at the low end of the optimal range (30 ppt).

Some *freshwater* aquarium fish are native to either estuarine environments or other waters that have a high concentration of dissolved minerals (Table II-9). It is best to keep these fish in a dilute salt solution; this can be simple table salt (NaCl), a dilute seawater mixture, or a specialized formulation for certain species groups (e.g., Malawi® salt mix for African cichlids). It is best to use a balanced salt mixture rather than pure sodium chloride because the latter lacks valuable divalent cations that are also important for osmoregulation and other physiological functions.

Many fish from freshwater environments can tolerate salinities up to 7 ppt but may not do well (McKee & Wolf, 1963). As much as 2 ppt salinity is probably safe for the great majority of freshwater fish (McKee & Wolf, 1963) (see *PHARMACOPOEIA*), but some (e.g., tetras, many catfishes) are sensitive to salt. Even the latter species seem to tolerate 1 ppt salinity indefinitely (G Lewbart, Personal Communication).

Salinity stress may occur if young freshwater salmonids (parr) are prematurely transferred to saltwater before they are ready to undergo transformation into marine-adapted fish (smolts). The parr-to-smolt trans-

Table II-9 Tropical *freshwater* aquarium fish that do best with a small amount of salt (~1 to 5 ppt salinity).

Brachygobius (bumblebee goby)
Chonerinus (puffer)
Fundulus (topminnow)
Monodactylus (mono)
Periopthalmus (mudskipper)
Poecilia (molly)—many species
Scatophagus (scat)
Toxotes spp. (archerfish)
African rift lake cichlids

formation is a stressful time during the salmonid life cycle and a transfer to seawater can often be accompanied by infectious disease outbreaks (e.g., see *PROBLEMS 49* and *52*).

Diagnosis

Salinity is difficult to measure directly but can be measured indirectly in several ways, including conductivity, chlorinity, refractive index, or specific gravity. Salinity can be measured least expensively by using a hydrometer, which measures specific gravity. However, this method is cumbersome when compared with refractometry and needs a relatively large volume of water (usually at least 50 ml). If salinity is to be measured frequently, it is easiest to use a handheld refractometer or electronic meter. A meter is the most accurate means of rapidly measuring salinity but is an expensive instrument and subject to mechanical breakdown.

Treatment

Abnormally high or low salinity places an osmotic stress on the fish and should be corrected as soon as possible with appropriate addition of salt or freshwater. It is generally recommended that the salinity be changed not more than 1 ppt/hour. For estuarine fish, salinity should not be adjusted more than 10 ppt in a few hours. As with other water quality variables, rapid changes are less tolerated.

Salt is also a useful prophylactic and can be added to freshwater aquaria to reduce prevalence of many infectious diseases, many of which are inhibited by even low salt concentrations (see *PHARMACOPOEIA*).

CHAPTER 14

Problems 10 through 42

Diagnoses made by either gross external examination of fish, wet mounts of skin/gills, or histopathology of skin/gills

10. Gas supersaturation
11. Lamprey infestation
12. Leech infestation
13. Copepod infestation/infection
14. Branchiuran infestation
15. Isopod infestation
16. Monogenean infestation
17. Turbellarian infection
18. Protozoan ectoparasites: general features
19. Ich infection
20. Marine white spot disease
21. Trichodinosis
22. *Chilodonella* infestation
23. *Brooklynella* infestation
24. Uronemosis
25. Tetrahymenosis
26. Marine velvet disease
27. Freshwater velvet disease
28. Ichthyobodosis
29. Gill *Cryptobia* infestations
30. Gill amoebic infestations
31. Sessile, solitary, ectocommensal ciliate infestations
32. Sessile, colonial, ectocommensal ciliate infestations
33. Typical water mold infection
34. Atypical water mold infection
35. Branchiomycosis
36. Columnaris infection
37. Bacterial cold water disease
38. Bacterial gill disease
39. Lymphocystis
40. Epitheliocystis
41. Miscellaneous skin and gill diseases
42. Incidental findings

PROBLEM 10
Gas Supersaturation (Gas Bubble Disease)

Prevalence Index
WF - 4, WM - 4, CF - 3
Method of Diagnosis
1. Clinical signs
2. Measurement of percentage of total gas pressure in water
History
Rapid increase of water temperature from water source to fish culture system; water intake pipe sucking in air; rapid decrease in pressure from water source to fish culture system; water falling over a deep spillway; ground water source; heavy macrophyte growth in clear pond; behavioral abnormalities; fish floating to surface
Physical Examination
Gas emboli in blood vessels of virtually any organ, including skin, gills, eyes, viscera, and peritoneal cavity; exophthalmos caused by retrobulbar gas emboli; emphysema in dermis
Treatment
Eliminate excess gas; do not stress affected fish during recovery

COMMENTS
Causes of Gas Supersaturation
Gas supersaturation (ΔP) occurs when the total pressure of gases dissolved in water is higher than the ambient atmospheric pressure. This may occur when water is pumped up from a deep (> 90-meter [300-foot]) well, since such water is often supersaturated with nitrogen and/or carbon dioxide (Colt et al., 1986). Spring water may be supersaturated with nitrogen after the spring thaw because of the overwinter accumulation of nitrogen gas (N_2) produced by natural breakdown of nitrates and nitrites (Warren, 1981). When the water is exposed to the atmosphere, the excess gas begins to equilibrate with air and thus leaves solution. If this occurs in the fish's blood vessels or other tissue, gas bubble disease results.

Gas supersaturation can also result from any other condition which leads to a higher than atmospheric concen-

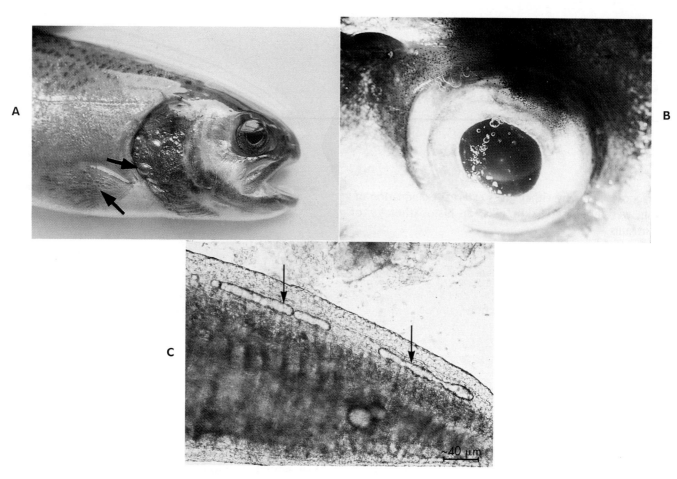

Fig. II-IO   A, Gas emboli in the fins and opercula of a trout (*arrows*). **B,** Gas emboli (*arrow*) in the eye (anterior chamber) of a European sea bass. **C,** Gas emboli (*arrows*) in the gills of a European sea bass.

(*A* photograph courtesy of H. Moller; *B* and *C* photographs courtesy of A. Colorni.)

tration of gas in water (Colt, 1986), including a leaky water pipe which can suck air under pressure, to be released at the outlet; a cavitating pump; Venturi injectors; water that is rapidly heated, such as when it is entering a heated tank or building; or water that enters a plunge pool where air is forced into solution under pressure (e.g., hydropower generating systems). Fish transported by air have also developed gas bubble disease (Hauck, 1986), but this is apparently a rare event in air-shipped fish.

In deep culture systems, fish near the surface succumb more quickly because of the difference in hydrostatic pressure (Heggberget, 1984). For example, ΔP decreases by 74 mmHg for every meter depth in freshwater at 20° C (68° F) (Colt, 1984). Thus, fish in hatcheries are especially susceptible to gas bubble disease because they cannot escape to lower depths.

Most gas emboli are produced by excess nitrogen (Marking, 1987) because oxygen is assimilated metabolically and thus less likely to form persistent bubbles. However, very high oxygen concentrations are dangerous.

In ponds that have heavy macrophyte growth (i.e., submerged aquatic weeds, such as *Hydrilla*), photosynthesis may be so great as to produce more oxygen than can diffuse into the water; this is most likely to occur in clear, shallow ponds with aquatic macrophytes. Such conditions allow oxygen to supersaturate the entire pond, not just the surface as would typically occur in a turbid pond where light penetrates less; thus, fish cannot escape the supersaturated conditions. Also, intensive culture systems using liquid oxygen to increase fish carrying capacity may accidentally *overdose* the fish.

In ponds, oxygen levels > 125% are probably not advisable, and 300% saturation is lethal (McKee & Wolf, 1963). Dissolved oxygen levels > 20 mg/l have caused mortality. Note that ponds with high photosynthetic activity often have $\Delta P > 300$ mmHg without problems if fish can escape to deeper, less saturated water (Boyd, 1990). In such cases, eggs or fry at the surface with limited mobility would be most at risk.

Sequelae of Gas Supersaturation

If fish breathe supersaturated water before it equilibrates, the excess gas may leave solution in the bloodstream, forming emboli in various tissues (*gas bubble disease*) (Fig. II-10, *A*, *B*, and *C*). Histopathology of gas bubble disease (Pauley & Nakatani, 1967) has been reported to include edema of the gill secondary lamellae, with accompanying degeneration of the overlying epithelium. Other lesions include edema and embolic disruption of buccal and intestinal mucosa, as well as vacuolar degeneration of the renal tubular epithelium. Lesions may also occur in liver and muscle.

Tissue hemorrhage and brain damage have been postulated to cause death (Ferguson, 1988), but the mechanism of tissue damage is uncertain. The severity of the damage depends on the number of emboli formed and on which tissues are affected. Behavioral abnormalities that are related to the target organs (e.g., hyperactivity, loss of equilibrium) may be present.

Clinical Signs

ACUTE GAS SUPERSATURATION

Acute gas supersaturation ($\Delta P > 50$ to 200 mmHg) can cause mortalities in as little as minutes; however, most cases present less acutely, with high mortalities after a few days' exposure. Eggs float to the surface, and larvae or fry may have hyperinflation of the swim bladder, cranial swelling, exophthalmos, swollen gill lamellae, pneumoperitoneum, or gas bubbles in the yolk sac. Up to 100% mortality can occur (Colt, 1986).

CHRONIC GAS SUPERSATURATION

Low supersaturation levels ($\Delta P < 76$ mmHg or $< 110\%$ saturation at sea level) are associated with chronic low (typically $< 5\%$) mortalities, hyperinflation of the swim bladder, and extravascular emboli in the gastrointestinal tract and mouth. Low-level supersaturation rarely produces highly visible lesions; fish must be closely examined. Secondary effects (unusually high mortalities, skeletal deformities, opportunistic infections) are most evident.

Diagnosis

The presence of gas emboli is pathognomonic for gas bubble disease. Holding fish up to a light source (*candling*) can help to visualize emboli (Ferguson, 1988). Bubbles can be squeezed from fin or gill clips while the fish is held under water, confirming the diagnosis. Do not confuse putrefaction in dead fish with gas bubble disease.

The supersaturation of just one gas may not cause gas supersaturation; for gas bubbles to form, the total gas pressure must exceed the barometric pressure. Determination of gas supersaturation is based on the measurement of the **total** concentration of dissolved gas in the water source. It is thus important to realize that some gases may be present in harmful concentrations in the absence of gas bubble disease (see *PROBLEMS 80* and *81*). Measurement of excess gases requires a saturometer (Fickeisen et al., 1975), which is commercially available (e.g., Weiss saturometer, Northwest Distribution Company).

Gas saturation can be expressed as a percentage of the total barometric pressure:

$$\text{Percentage total gas pressure} = \frac{BP + \Delta P}{BP} \times 100$$

For example, if the local barometric pressure (BP) is 760 mmHg and the ΔP measured with the saturometer is 76 mmHg, the total gas pressure is 110% saturation of water with atmospheric gases.

In general, levels of about 110% saturation are considered dangerous for fish. However, this varies with the species and with the age of the fish. For example, even low levels (101% to 105%) affect salmonid sac fry, while adult salmonids often tolerate over 125% saturation (Wood, 1976). Eggs are usually tolerant. Warm water fish are generally more tolerant of supersaturation than cold water fish.

Treatment

Treatment of gas bubble disease requires eliminating the excess gas in the water source. This can involve first aerating the water source in a reservoir to allow it to equilibrate with air, but in many cases, this is not practical. In flow-through systems that use large volumes of water, the water can be stripped of excess gas by using a packed column degasser. Packed columns are commercially available (Aquatic Ecosystems, Inc.). Construction of degassers is described by Colt (1986). Passive degassers can be used to return the gas concentration to 100%, but vacuum degassing provides a greater margin of safety.

PROBLEM 11
Lamprey Infestation

Prevalence Index
Not seen in cultured fish
Method of Diagnosis
1. Presence of lamprey on host fish
2. Lamprey lesions on host fish
History
Wild-caught fish from lamprey-endemic area
Physical Examination
Anemia; circular skin ulcers
Treatment
TFM + Bayluscide

COMMENTS
Lampreys are eel-like, jawless fish in the Class Agnatha. They are important parasites of freshwater and marine commercial fish (Fig. II-11, *A*). They feed by using a circular suctorial mouth that has sharp, horny teeth (Fig. II-11, *B*), which rasp the skin and form a characteristic, circular ulcer. In spring, lampreys spawn in freshwater; eggs hatch into small, worm-like, ammocoete larvae,

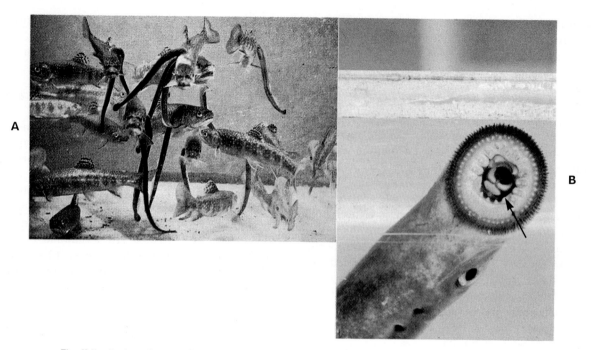

Fig. II-11 A, American sea lamprey attached to brook trout. **B,** River lamprey, showing key diagnostic features, including eel-like shape and circular, rasping mouth, with chitinized teeth (*arrow*).

(*B* courtesy of Wydoski RS and Whitney RR: *Inland fish of Washington,* Seattle, 1980, University of Washington Press.)

which filter-feed in the mud. After several years the larvae metamorphose into adult lampreys, which, depending on species, may migrate into the ocean or remain in freshwater. The American sea lamprey has become a serious problem in the Great Lakes, where it causes hemorrhagic anemia and mortality in lake trout (Wooten, 1989). Lampreys are controlled with TFM, a lampricide that is selective for the ammocoete larva. Bayluscide potentiates the effectiveness of TFM.

PROBLEM 12
Leech Infestation

Prevalence Index
WF - 4, WM - 4, CF - 4, CM - 4
Method of Diagnosis
1. Parasite on skin, gills, or in oral cavity
2. Histology of skin, gills, or oral cavity with parasite
History
Wild-caught or pond-raised fish
Physical Examination
Anemia; small red or white lesions on skin
Treatment
Organophosphate prolonged immersion

COMMENTS
Epidemiology/Pathogenesis
Leeches are rare in cultured fish but are occasionally seen in wild or pond-raised fish. They have a direct life cycle, with juveniles hatching from cocoons laid by the hermaphroditic adults. Some species have a relatively wide host range, while others are restricted to only a few fish species. Both mature and immature leeches are hematophagous, with pathology depending on the amount of blood taken (i.e., number and size of worms and the duration of feeding). Heavily infested fish (Fig. II-12, *A*) often have a chronic anemia. Leeches can also transmit microbes and hemoparasites (see *PROBLEMS 43* and *76*) during feeding. Some can cause large ulcers on the skin or in the mouth (Noga et al., 1990a).
Diagnosis
Leech infestation can be diagnosed by histopathology (Fig. II-12, *C*). Leeches should preferably be removed from the fish and then fixed, especially if species identification is desired. Leeches can be differentiated from monogeneans (see *PROBLEM 16*) by the presence of body segmentation. They are also much larger than the great majority of monogeneans. Leeches are annelids. They differ from typical free-living annelids in having anterior and posterior suckers (Fig. II-12, *B* and *D*). However, some aquatic leeches are free-living (i.e., do not feed on fish). They require examination by an expert to distinguish them from parasitic species. Leeches resemble large digenean trematodes but have a complete digestive tract, with a mouth in the anterior sucker and an anus in the posterior sucker.
Treatment
Leeches are usually easily treated with a single dose of organophosphate, although fish should be watched closely for 3 weeks to monitor for possible reinfestation.

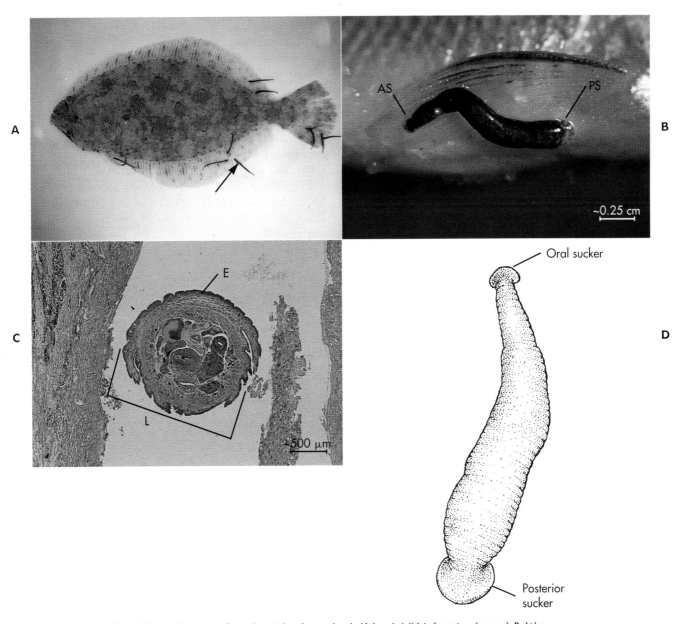

Fig. II-I2 **A,** Southern flounder with a heavy leech (*Myzobdella*) infestation (*arrow*). **B,** Wet mount of a leech (*Piscicola*) on a smelt. *AS* = anterior sucker; *PS* = posterior sucker. **C,** Histological cross-section of a leech (*L*), *Myzobdella lugubris,* in the mouth of a largemouth bass. Key diagnostic features are epithelium (*E*) on the surface of the body, circular shape, and various organs (e.g., digestive, reproductive) suspended in a true coelomic space. Hematoxylin and eosin. **D,** Diagram of a leech showing diagnostic characteristics, including suckers and segmentation.

(*B* photograph courtesy of H. Moller; *C* photograph by L. Khoo and E. Noga.)

PROBLEM 13
Copepod Infestation/Infection (Sea Louse, Fish Maggot, Anchor Worm)

Prevalence Index
WF - 2, WM - 4, CF - 3, CM - 2

Method of Diagnosis
1. Wet mount of gills, skin, or mouth with parasite
2. Histopathology of gills, skin, or mouth with parasite

History
Wild-caught, pond-raised, or cage-cultured fish; skin sores

Physical Examination
Various-sized (barely visible to 10 mm) copepods attached to gill arches, oral cavity, or skin; erosion and/or ulceration; red areas on skin, may be raised up to 5 mm in height

Treatment
1. Organophosphate prolonged immersion
2. Organophosphate bath

3. Difluorobenzuron prolonged immersion
4. Freshwater bath (*C. elongatus* only)
5. Salt prolonged immersion (freshwater copepods only)

Order Copepoda

Suborders of parasitic copepods follow, including selected families (after Kabata, 1984):

Suborder Siphonostomatoida: almost all are marine species—includes > 75% of all fish-parasitic copepod infestations/infections

Families

Grasp and anchor to gill and skin surfaces:
Cecropidae
Caligidae (*Caligus, Pseudocaligus, Lepeophtheirus*)

Hatschekiidae
Lernanthropidae
Penetrate skin and burrow deeply into tissues:
Pennellidae (*Lernaeenicus*)
Sphyriidae
Lernaeopodidae (*Salmincola, Achtheres*)
Chondracanthidae

Suborder Poecilostomatoida: almost all are marine species

Grasp and anchor to gill and skin surfaces:
Ergasilidae (*Ergasilus*)—both freshwater and marine

Suborder Cyclopoida: all but one are freshwater species

Penetrate skin and burrow deeply into tissues
Lernaeidae (*Lernaea*)

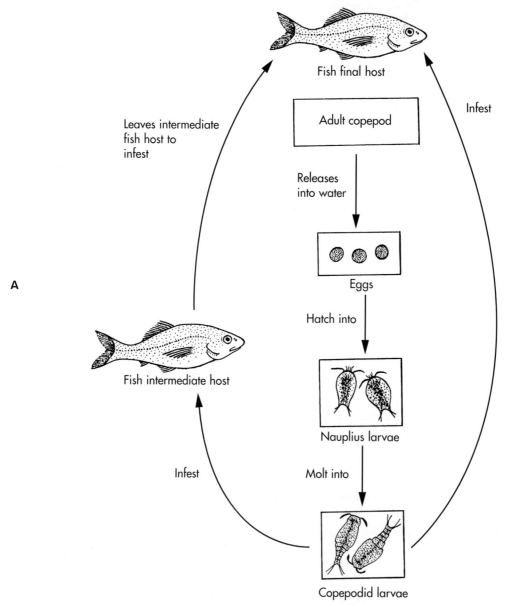

Fig. II-I3   A, Life cycles of fish-parasitic copepods. Diagrams of major types of parasitic copepods affecting cultured fish, including key diagnostic features. Egg sacs (*E*) are only present in mature females. If the adult has only recently attached to the fish, it may not be visible grossly.

Continued.

B

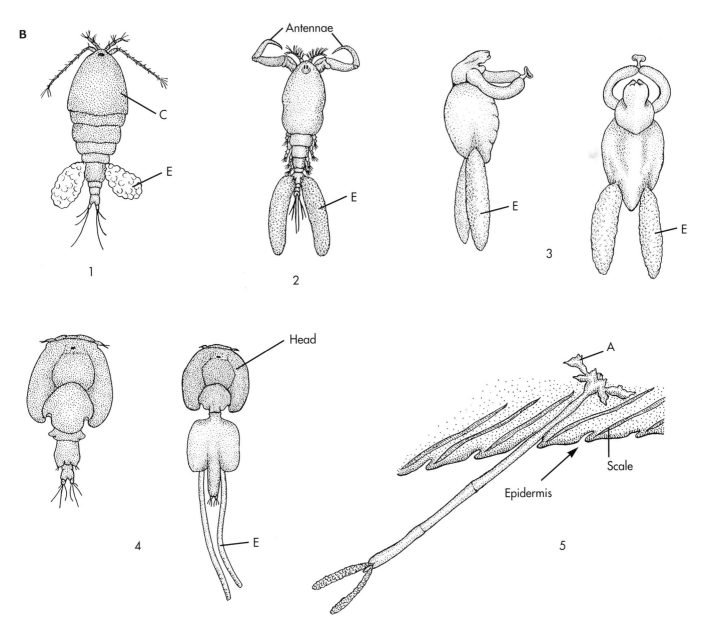

Fig. II-13—cont'd. B_1, Typical free-living copepod (*Cyclops* sp.) C=cephalothorax. B_2, Ergasiliform Type: Body divided into head, thorax, and abdomen and has a shape similar to that of free-living copepods, grasping antennae (A). Egg sacs (E) are only present in mature females. B_3, Lernaeopodid Type (lateral and dorsal views): Body more grub-like than ergasilids. B_4, Caligiform Type (male on left; female on right): Adult sea louse (5 to 10 mm), flat, broad head. Egg sacs (E) are only present in mature females. B_5, Lernaeid Type: Mature female (~5 to 25 mm), long thin body, vestigal appendages, head with anchors (A). C, Severe gill maggot (*Ergasilus*) infestation of a striped bass. The parasites are attached to the primary lamellae of the gills by their modified antennae. Note that the egg sacs (E) vary from white to grey, depending on the developmental stage of the larvae in the egg sacs. D, Sea louse infestation of wahoo. Note parasite (P) with egg sacs (E) trailing from the flat, scale-like body. E, Sea lice (*Lepeophtheirus salmonis*). F, Anchor worm (*Lernaea cruciata*) infection of a largemouth bass. The head of the parasite is embedded under the skin while the body (P) with egg sacs protrudes. Note the hemorrhage (*arrow*) where the parasite enters the fish. PF = pectoral fin. G, Close-up view of two anchor worms (*Lernaea cyprinacea*), which enter the fish at the *arrow*. E = egg sacs. H, Wet mount of a skin scraping with an immature *Lernaea cruciata* female. A = anchors. E = host epithelium. I, Histological section through an immature *Lernaea cruciata* female. Only anchors (A) are visible in this plane of section. The parasite penetrates between two scales (S), inciting inflammation. E = epithelium. Hematoxylin and eosin. J, Copepodid infestation (*Lernaea cyprinacea*) (*arrows*) on the fin of a goldfish.

(*D* photograph courtesy of T. Wenzel; *E* photograph by H. Moller; *G* photograph by G Hoffman.)

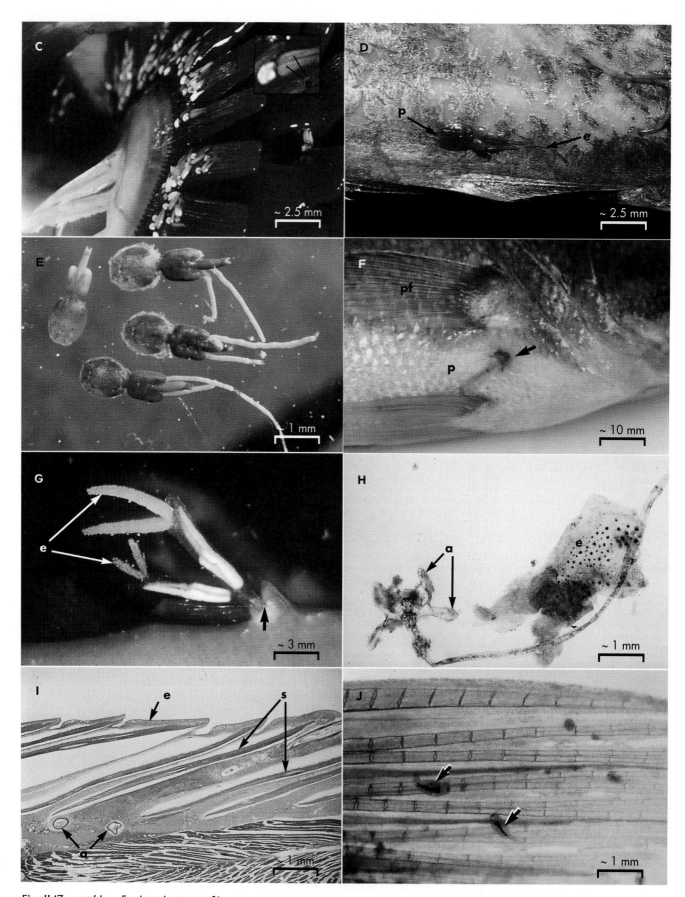

Fig. II-I3, cont'd.   *For legend see page 81.*

COMMENTS

General

Parasitic copepods are increasingly serious problems in cultured fish and can also impact wild populations. Most of the approximately 10,000 copepods are free-living, but about 1700 species are parasites. Most parasites affect marine fish, but there are some important freshwater pathogens. Parasites vary from organisms that morphologically resemble free-living copepods to others that are highly modified for parasitism (Fig. II-13, B). Most are skin or gill parasites. A few penetrate deep into host tissues, such as heart; endoparasites are not a problem in cultured fish.

The life cycle of clinically important parasitic copepods (Fig. II-13, A) typically comprises 1 to 5 free-living nauplius stages, 1 to 5 free-living or parasitic copepodid stages (Fig. II-13, J), 1 pre-adult, and finally the adult. Parasitic copepods attached to the host by a frontal filament are known as *chalimus* larvae. The life cycle is typically faster with higher temperature.

Classification of parasitic copepods is based on the structure of the buccal region (Kabata, 1981). Yamaguti (1963) provides comprehensive but outdated keys to all parasitic copepods. Kabata (1979, 1988) provides keys to northeast Atlantic and northwest Pacific species. Three major types are most commonly found on cultured fish: ergasiliform, caligiform, and lernaeiform types.

Ergasiliform Types

Ergasilids (Family Ergasilidae) appear similar to free-living copepods in having division of the body into distinct cephalothorax and abdomen and presence of paired locomotory appendages (Fig. II-13, B_2 and C). However, they are also modified for parasitism as indicated by the presence of antennae modified for grasping the host and a large trunk for reproductive products (Kabata, 1988). They are often incidental findings on wild or pond-raised fish and probably cause few problems in small numbers. However, their feeding activity does severe focal damage and heavy infestations can be damaging. Some can move around while on the host.

Ergasilus species are usually < 2 mm long, with a conical, segmented body (Fig. II-13, B_2 and C). Mostly infesting the gills of freshwater fish (Kabata, 1979), they are usually an incidental finding on feral fish in summer (Wooten, 1989).

Lernaeopodids

Lernaeopodids (Family *Lernaeopodidae*) still retain some of the typical copepod shape (Fig. II-13, B_3) but are more grub-like compared with ergasilids. *Salminicola* infests the gills of older salmonids in freshwater. Fish that return to the sea after spawning may retain the parasite; thus, individuals returing to freshwater to spawn for a second time may have severe gill damage (Hoffman, 1967).

Caligiform Types (Sea Lice)

The sea lice *Lepeophtheirus* and *Caligus* (Family Caligidae) (Fig. II-13, B_4, D, and E) infest the skin.

Species are usually restricted to certain groups (e.g., salmonids) (Table II-13). Some species are the most important parasites affecting cage-cultured salmonids in Europe (Pike, 1989). Once established in a cultured population, parasite numbers slowly increase over time, eventually causing an epidemic. Sea lice problems are most serious where salmon farming has been established for many years. Cultured fish become infested by wild fish, which usually carry low parasite burdens, although epidemics have rarely occurred in wild populations (Panasenko et al., 1986).

Grossly resembling the fish louse, *Argulus* (see *PROBLEM 14*), sea lice are dorsoventrally flattened copepods that adhere to fish; they scrape the epithelium while feeding, causing erosions and at times deep ulcers extending to bone. They attach to the host by pressing their shield-like cephalothorax onto the skin like a sucker. The second antennae and maxillipeds are used as clamps.

The life cycle of sea lice includes: nauplius (free-swimming) → copepodid (~1 mm, infective) → chalimus (~1 to 3 mm, parasitic, sessile) → pre-adult (mobile) → adult (to 10 mm, mobile) (Kabata, 1988). The life cycle is temperature-dependent, generally taking 6 to 8 weeks at optimal temperatures for salmonid parasites (Kent, 1992). Infestations can be established by copepodids, pre-adults, or adults. The pre-adult is active, scurrying on the fish's skin, where it may cause small petechial hemorrhages at feeding sites. Heavy feeding of sea lice causes deep ulcers, even exposing the cranium (Roth et al., 1993). Sea lice can survive at least 1 week in freshwater if attached to the fish.

Lernaeid Types (Anchor Worms)

Anchor worm is a general term for species of highly modified copepods that possess anchor-like processes for securing themselves to the host (Fig. II-13, B_5 and F through I). Anchor worms may be introduced into an aquarium from wild or pond-raised fish. Goldfish, koi, or wild native fish are most commonly affected. Marine aquarium fish may rarely be infected with morphologically similar but taxonomically unrelated species; such individuals are usually culled before shipment to wholesalers.

Lernaea is the most important genus of lernaeid copepods, but other genera (e.g., *Opistolernaea*, *Lernaeagiraffa*) are important in tropical environments (Paperna, 1991). *Lernaea* and related genera infect freshwater fish. *Lernaea* is most likely to be seen in summer, when reproduction usually occurs. For example, *Lernaea cyprinacea*, a cosmopolitan species that infects a wide range of fishes and even tadpoles, does not reproduce at less than 14° C (57° F). A single female may produce several hundred larvae about every 2 weeks for up to 16 weeks at optimal temperatures (> 25° C = 77° F). After several nonparasitic stages, the terminal copepodid stage (Fig. II-13, J) attaches to a fish, mates, and the male dies. The female then penetrates under the skin of the fish and differentiates into an adult.

Table II-13   Geographic and taxonomic distribution of parasitic copepods in marine fish farming (with reference to the genera *Caligus*, *Lepeoptheirius*, and *Pseudocaligus*).

Country	Species present	Host	Reference
EUROPE			
Norway	*C. elongatus, L. salmonis*	Salmonids	Johannessen, 1974; Hastein & Bergsjo, 1976; Brandal & Egidus, 1977, 1979; Hoy & Horsberg, 1991
Sweden	*Caligus* sp.	Salmonids	Lundbjorg & Ljungberg, 1977
Scotland	*C. elongatus, L. salmonis*	Salmonids	Rae, 1979; Wootten et al., 1982
Ireland	*C. elongatus, L. salmonis*	Salmonids	Tully and Morrissey, 1989
France	*C. minimus*	European sea bass	Paperna, 1980
Israel	*C. pageti, E. lizae, P. apodus*	Grey mullet	Paperna, 1975
NORTH AMERICA			
Eastern North America	*C. curtus, C. elongatus*	Salmonids	Hogans & Trudeau, 1989a, b;
	E. labracis, L. salmonis	Red drum	Landsberg et al., 1991; Richard, 1991
Western North America	*C. clemensi*	Salmonids	Johnson & Albright, 1991a, b; Richard, 1991
	L. cuneifer, L. salmonis		
SOUTH AMERICA			
Chile	*C. teres*	Salmonids	Reyes & Bravo, 1983
ASIA			
New Zealand	*C. longicaudatus*	Salmonids	Jones, 1988
Malaysia	*Caligus* sp., *E. borneoensis*	Malabaricus grouper	Leong & Wong, 1988
Philippines	*C. patulus*	Milkfish	Jones, 1980
Japan	*C. orientalis, C. spinosus*	Yellowtail	Fujita et al., 1968;
		Salmonids	Izawa, 1969; Urawa & Kato, 1991

Reprinted with permission from Roth et al., 1993.

Single lernaeid parasites are usually not life-threatening, unless they are infecting a small fish or when they penetrate near vital organs. Heavy infections can lead to debilitation and secondary bacterial or fungal infection (Noga, 1986b). Hemorrhage at the site of attachment is common (Fig. II-13, *F*), and in some cases, considerable hyperplasia or fibrosis may develop at the attachment site, which may remain even after the parasite has died. Consumers may reject disfigured fish.

Diagnosis
Diagnosis of copepod infestation/infection is based on identification of typical parasitic life stages on fish. Large, mature females are often pathognomonic (Fig. II-13, *C* through *G*). Small immature stages, such as copepodids (Fig. II-13, *J*) or even immature adults (Fig. II-13, *H*), may not be grossly visible (Noga, 1986), so microscopic examination of skin scrapings is advisable. When the skin is scraped for lernaeids, the parasite's head may remain embedded in the fish, leaving only the thin vestigal body. Histopathology may also be used to identify permanently attached forms (Fig. II-13, *I*).

Treatment
SEA LICE
Sea lice are difficult to control in caged fish. Trichlorphon or dichlorvos baths are most commonly used at present but carry potential risks to both the handler and the environment. Also, resistance has developed at some geographic sites (Roth et al., 1993).

Many other chemicals have been examined as sea lice controls, including other organophosphates, ivermectin, pyrethrum, hydrogen peroxide, formalin, carbaryl, diflubenzuron, and natural remedies (onions and garlic) (Roth et al., 1993). None of these remedies are satisfactory, either because of a narrow margin of safety or problems with potential damage to marine life. Evidence exists that parasite-eating wrasses can control infestations on salmonids (Bjordal, 1991). Freshwater controls *Caligus elongatus* infestations on red drum (Landsberg et al., 1991). Vaccines are also presently under study.

ANCHOR WORMS
For lernaeid infestations in aquarium fish, some advocate removing individual parasites with forceps (even if the head remains embedded, the parasite will die). Wounds should be watched closely for secondary infections but usually heal uneventfully within 48 hours, which is faster than if the dead parasite is expelled (G. Lewbart, Personal Communication). Note that larval stages may still remain on the fish or in the water.

Organophosphate is usually effective; prolonged immersion treatment should be repeated every 7 days for 28 days. Resistant strains have been detected on some commercial farms (Goven et al., 1980). Diflubenzuron is less toxic to fish and is highly effective (Hoffmann, 1985). It is also not inactivated at high temperatures, as are organophosphates. However, difluorobenzuron can be damaging to nontarget arthropods and is not legally approved for this use. Convalescent fish are often more resistant to lernaeid reinfection (Shields & Goode, 1978). *Lernaea cyprinacea* is inhibited by salt (Shields & Sperber, 1974).

OTHER COPEPODS

Most other parasitic copepods are probably susceptible to organophosphate treatment.

PROBLEM 14
Branchiuran Infestation (*Argulus* Infestation, Fish Louse)
Prevalence Index
WF - 3, WM - 4, CF - 3, CM - 3

Method of Diagnosis
Wet mount of skin or buccal cavity with parasite
History
Pruritus; red sores; wild-caught or pond-raised fish
Physical Examination
Focal red lesions on skin; focal color change (especially darkening) on skin
Treatment
1. Organophosphate prolonged immersion
2. Formalin bath
3. Potassium permanganate bath

COMMENTS
Epidemiology
There are about 140 species of branchiuran crustaceans. Virtually the only genus encountered is

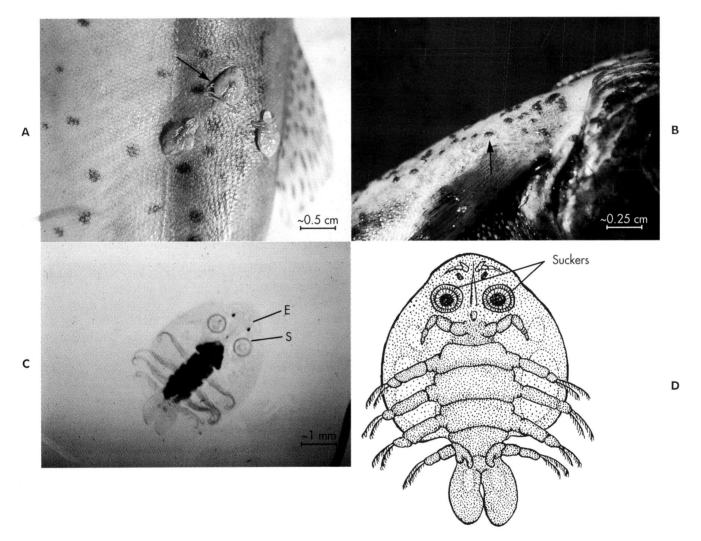

Fig. II-14 **A** and **B,** Branchiuran (*Argulus*) infestations (*arrows*). A key identifying feature is the flattened, saucer shape. **C,** Branchiuran (*Argulus*) infestation wet mount. Key diagnostic features include flattened shape, shell-like carapace covering the body, two suckers (*S*) that look like large eyes, eyespots (*E*), and jointed appendages. **D,** Diagram of a typical branchiuran (*ventral view*). Key diagnostic features include size (5 to 20 mm), oval body that looks like a scale, and suckers that look like large eyes.

(*A* photograph courtesy of D. Mitchum; *B* photograph courtesy of P. Ghittino.)

Argulus, also called the fish louse (do not confuse with sea lice; see *PROBLEM 13*). *Argulus* is uncommon in freshwater aquarium fish but may occur if wild or pond-raised fish are introduced into the tank. *Argulus* is especially common on goldfish and koi. *Argulus* is prevalent on many wild freshwater fish (e.g., centrarchids, striped bass, and other *Morone* spp., among others). Many fish lice have a wide host range.

Pathogenesis
Argulus feeds by inserting a pre-oral sting (stylet) into the host and sucking body fluids with the proboscis-like mouth (Fig. II-14, *D*). Fish can display violent erratic swimming or other behavioral abnormalities because of the irritation caused by the stylet. Fish are damaged by the repeated piercing of the skin by the stylet, which injects toxic enzymes, causing irritation. Also hooks and spines are on the appendages, which may cause mechanical damage (Kabata, 1988). This irritation may cause focal hyperpigmentation in some fish species (e.g., tilapia). *Argulus* can also transmit bacterial or viral infections (Shimura et al., 1983; Pfeil-Putzien, 1978). One or two parasites usually cause no clinical signs in large fish, but *Argulus* has a high reproductive rate.

Life Cycle
Speed of the life cycle depends upon parasite species and temperature. The entire life cycle is typically 30 days or more. Eggs laid on vegetation or other objects (which act as fomites) usually hatch into juveniles within 10 to 50 days (Paperna, 1991). Juveniles (1 to 3 mm) look like adults without suckers. Adults can survive without a host for several days.

Diagnosis
Diagnosis is easily made by morphological identification of the parasite. Branchiurans are differentiated from caligoid copepods (see *PROBLEM 13*) by having suckers and large, compound eyes (Fig. II-14, *C* and *D*). Fish lice frequently move on a host and may be seen swimming when they are in an aquarium. They often remain attached when the host is removed from the water (Fig. II-14, *A* and *B*) but can be coaxed to move by gentle nudging with a blunt probe. *Argulus* looks like a moving scale.

Treatment
As with other crustacean parasites, organophosphates are usually an effective treatment (Paperna & Overstreet, 1981). The time needed to complete the life cycle varies; therefore, it is useful to rid tanks of egg contamination by using disinfectant or by allowing the tanks to dry thoroughly for several days. Otherwise, multiple chemical treatments may be needed. Individual parasites can be removed from fish by using forceps, but this does not eliminate parasites in the environment. Mosquitofish can reportedly be used as a biological control in ponds (Langdon, 1992a).

PROBLEM 15
Isopod Infestation
Prevalence Index
WM - 4, CM - 4
Method of Diagnosis
Gross observation of parasite in gill chamber or mouth, or on skin
History/Physical Examination
Isopod grossly visible on body, in mouth, or in gill chamber
Treatment
1. Remove parasite with forceps
2. Organophosphate bath

COMMENTS
Life Cycle
Parasitic isopods (~450 species) are fairly common crustacean infestations of wild tropical marine fish. They are less common in cold marine waters and rarely found on freshwater fish. They are rare in cultured fish, although infestations have caused problems in sea-caged salmonids in Australia (Langdon, 1992a). The life cycle is simple. Most are parasitic as both juveniles and adults, although some are only parasitic as juveniles (praniza) (e.g, gnathiids) or adults (e.g., cymothids).

The are two categories with prominent differences in morphology and ecology (Kabata, 1984). The Suborder Flabellifera (Families Anilocridae, Aegidae, Corallanidae, and Cymothidae) have a typical isopod shape (Fig. II-15, *A, B,* and *C₁*) and are up to 6 cm in length. Nearly all fish groups are represented.

The much less common Suborder Gnathiidea (Family Gnathiidae) includes ~50 spp. that have larvae, and male and female adults, which differ in shape and behavior. Only the larva (Fig. II-15, *C₂*) is parasitic, living in the gastric cavity of sea anemones and tunicates, or on the skin or gills of fish. Adults are nonfeeding, live in mud tubes, and produce infective larvae.

Pathogenesis
Because of their large size, single isopods can cause considerable damage with their biting and sucking mouthparts. This may include pressure necrosis of gill tissue and growth retardation. Heavy infestations of parasitic juveniles can kill small fish when they first attach.

Diagnosis
Diagnosis of parasitic isopods is easily made from morphological characteristics. Note that free-living isopods may occasionally be seen in marine aquaria.

Treatment
There are no published studies of treatments for parasitic isopods. They are probably susceptible to organophosphates. Individuals can also be removed from fish by using forceps. Placing fish in aquaria (without mud) breaks the life cycle of gnathiid isopods (Langdon, 1992a).

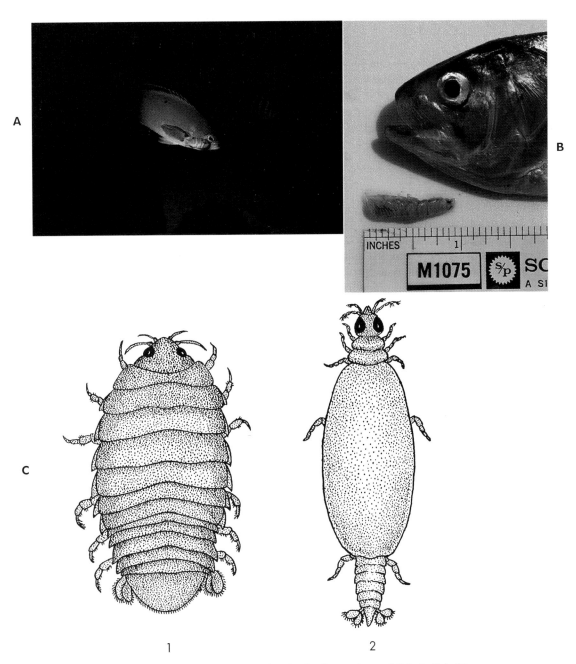

Fig. II-I5 **A,** Flabelliferan isopod attached to the cheek of a marine reef fish. **B,** Flabelliferan isopod (*Olencira* sp.) that resides in the oral cavity of Atlantic menhaden. Head with eyes on the right. **C,** Diagram of fish-parasitic isopods showing the following diagnostic features: (1) Flabelliferans—size (several mm to 6 cm), body segmentation, chitinous plates over body segments, and paired, segmented appendages; (2) Gnathiid—insect-like body; lack of segmentation because of engorgement on blood.

(*A* photograph courtesy of S. Spotte.)

PROBLEM 16
Monogenean Infestation (Skin Fluke, Gill Fluke, Eye Fluke)
Prevalence Index
WF - 1, WM - 1, CF - 1, CM - 1
Method of Diagnosis
1. Wet mount of skin or gills with parasite
2. Histology of skin or gills with parasite
History/Physical Examination
Cloudiness to skin; grey-white cast or irregular areas on skin; eroded fins; focal hemorrhages on skin; pruritus; dyspnea
Treatment
1. Formalin bath
2. Formalin prolonged immersion
3. Organophosphate bath (marine capsalids only)
4. Organophosphate prolonged immersion
5. Acetic acid bath (freshwater monogeneans only)
6. Freshwater bath (marine monogeneans only)
7. Saltwater bath (freshwater monogeneans only)
8. Potassium permanganate prolonged immersion (freshwater monogeneans only)
9. Copper prolonged immersion
10. Praziquantel bath (marine monogeneans only)
11. Praziquantel prolonged immersion
12. Mebendazole bath
13. Mebendazole prolonged immersion
14. Chloramine-T bath

COMMENTS
Epidemiology
Monogeneans are common parasites of the skin and gills of both marine and freshwater fish (Rohde, 1984; Hoffman, 1967; Bychowsky, 1957). There are many different species (~1500), most of which have a narrow host range in nature (i.e., restricted to one species, genus, or family). However, this host specificity is often lost in aquaculture (Nigrelli, 1940; Thoney & Hargis, 1991).

Heavy monogenean infestations are usually indicators of poor sanitation and deteriorating water quality (e.g., overcrowding, high ammonia or nitrite, organic pollution, or low oxygen). They can rapidly reproduce under such conditions. The doubling time for viviparous monogeneans can be as little as 24 hours. Reproductive rate is also controlled by temperature, which, although not variable in a tropical aquarium (which should have a narrow range of temperature), is important in less controlled environments (e.g., ponds, raceways). Monogeneans often *bloom* in spring.

Pathogenesis
Monogeneans feed mainly on the superficial layers of the skin and gills. This feeding activity is irritating and thus often causes skin cloudiness (see Fig. I-8) or focal reddening resulting from excess mucus production,

epithelial hyperplasia, or hemorrhage (Kabata, 1985). Some species can cause deep skin wounds. Monogeneans can probably also transmit bacteria and other agents (Cusack & Cone, 1986). Individual worms cause proportionately greater damage. In large enough numbers, monogeneans can kill, especially small fish. Even small numbers of parasites can incite excess mucus production or pruritus. There is some evidence for development of partial resistance to reinfection (Nigrelli, 1937; Evans & Gratzek, 1989).

Exotic Monogeneans
Many monogeneans have been accidentally introduced with infested fish to various parts of the world. For example, *Pseudodactylogyrus anguillae* and *P. bini* were introduced into European eel stocks from Asia (Buchmann et al., 1987), *Gyrodactylus cyprini* was introduced into the United States with European carp, and *Cleidodiscus pricei* was introduced into Europe on U.S. brown bullheads (Thoney & Hargis, 1991). The introduction of *Gyrodactylus salaris* into native Norwegian Atlantic salmon stocks caused massive damage to wild populations, presumably because native stocks were much less resistant to these exotic parasites (Johnsen & Jensen, 1986).

Types of Monogeneans
Taxonomic identification of mongeneans is based upon the morphology of the posterior attachment organ (opisthohaptor), mode of reproduction, and presence of eyespots, among other features. There are two types of monogeneans, based upon opisthohaptor morphology: in the more common Monopisthocotylea (e.g., dactylogyrids, gyrodactylids, capsalids), there is a single unit comprising several, large, centrally located, sclerotized anchors (hooks or hamuli) and often small marginal hooklets (Fig. II-16, A_1, A_2, A_3, C, D, E, F, G, and I); in the Polyopisthocotylea, the opisthohaptor consists of a battery of small, muscular, adhesive suckers or clamps that are supported by cuticular sclerites (Fig. II-16, A_4) (Egusa, 1983). The monopisthocotyleans' use of anchors or hooks for attachment tends to pierce tissue, while the polyopisthocotyleans' clamps have opposing sections that grasp host tissue between them.

Reproduction
Two major modes of reproduction are important considerations in medical management of monogeneans. Oviparous monogeneans (Fig. II-16, B) lay eggs that usually settle to the bottom to develop (Kearn, 1986). A few capsalids attach egg bundles to gill filaments (Fig. II-16, H) (Whittington, 1990). After hatching, the free-swimming infective stage (oncomiracidium) seeks out and attaches to a new host and crawls to its final site, where it usually stays for the rest of its life. In contrast, viviparous monogeneans give birth to living young (Fig. II-16, A_1, C, and D).

Important Pathogens
GYRODACTYLOIDEA

The most economically important monogeneans in cultured fish are in the monopisthocotylean Superfamilies Gyrodactyloidea and Dactylogyroidea (Wooten, 1989). The viviparous gyrodactylids (Fig. II-16, *C* and *D*) are skin and gill parasites of both freshwater and marine fish (Yamaguti, 1968). Various species of *Gyrodactylus* are pathogenic to eels, salmonids, cyprinids, ictalurids, clariids, fundulids, poeciliids, gasterosteids, cyclopterids, cichlids, and pleuronectids (Thoney & Hargis, 1991).

DACTYLOGYROIDEA

The oviparous dactylodyrids are primarily gill parasites of freshwater fish (Yamaguti, 1968). There are many species in various genera, especially *Dactylogyrus*, *Pseudodactylogyrus*, and *Cleidodiscus* (Fig. II-16, *E* and *F*).

CAPSALOIDEA

Some capsalids (Fig. II-16, *G*) can be important pathogens of marine fish. They are large, monopisthocotylean worms (up to ~3 to 10 mm) that concomitantly can cause large wounds on the skin or eyes (erosion, ulceration). Feeding activity of the capsalids can induce hyperplasia, which may partly enclose the flukes. Skin

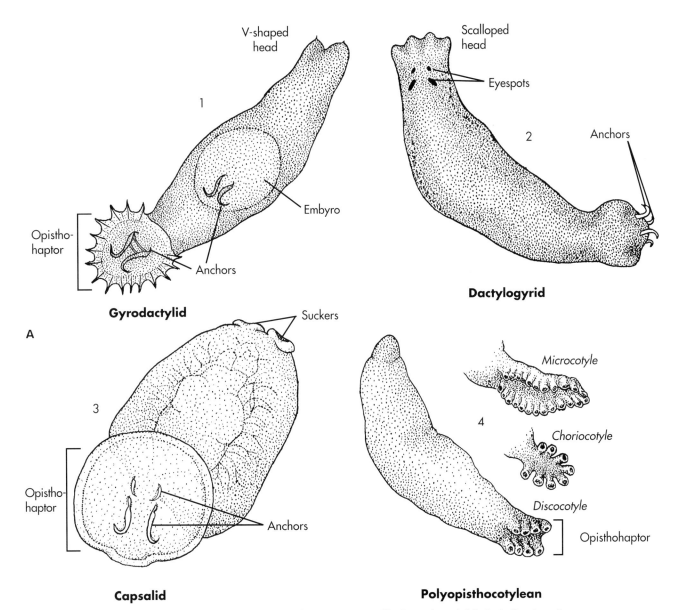

Fig. II-16 Diagrams of major types of monogeneans affecting cultured fish, including key diagnostic features. A_1, Gyrodactylid Type. Note size (0.3 to 1 mm), V-shaped head, lack of eyespots, developing embryo with anchors, single pair of anchors. A_2, Dactylogyrid Type. Note size (to 2 mm), scalloped head, one or more pairs of eyespots, ovary without embryo, 1 to 2 pair of anchors; primarily on gills. A_3, Capsalid Type. Note size (often > 4 mm), anchors; some also have anterior suckers. A_4, Polyopisthocotylean Type. Note clamps and lack of anchors on various opisthohaptors.

Continued.

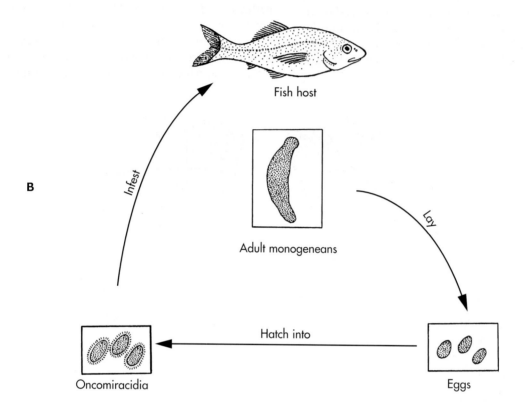

Life cycle of oviparous monogeneans

Fig. II-16—cont'd.   **B,** Life cycle of oviparous monogeneans. **C,** Wet mount of a gyrodactylid monogenean attached to goldfish fin (*F*). *O* = opisthohaptor; *A* = anchors of embryo's opisthohaptor. **D,** Wet mount of a typical monopisthocotylean monogene (*Gyrodactylus*). Key identifying features include size, worm-like appearance, and anchors (*A*). Note the embryo (*arrows*), which differentiates it from oviparous monopisthocotyleans. *O* = opisthohaptor. **E,** Wet mount of a heavy dactylogyrid (*Cleidodiscus*) infestation (*arrows*) of channel catfish gills. *P* = primary lamella. **F,** Wet mount of a typical dactylogyrid monogenean (*Cleidodiscus*) attached to gill. *E* = eyespots. **G,** Wet mount of capsalid monogenean (*Benedenia*). Note the two pairs of tightly apposed, curved anchors (*A*), which differentiate it from *Neobenedenia*, which has three pairs of tightly apposed, curved anchors. Both genera have two anterior suckers (*S*). *O* = opisthohaptor. **H,** Wet mount of *Benedinia* eggs, with threads used for attachment to fish or other objects. **I,** Histological section through a monopisthocotylean monogenean infesting the skin (*S*) (detachment is an artifact). Note the refractile anchors (*A*). Hematoxylin and eosin.

(*D* photograph courtesy of G. Hoffman; *F* photograph courtesy of A. Mitchell; *G* and *H* photographs courtesy of A. Colorni.)

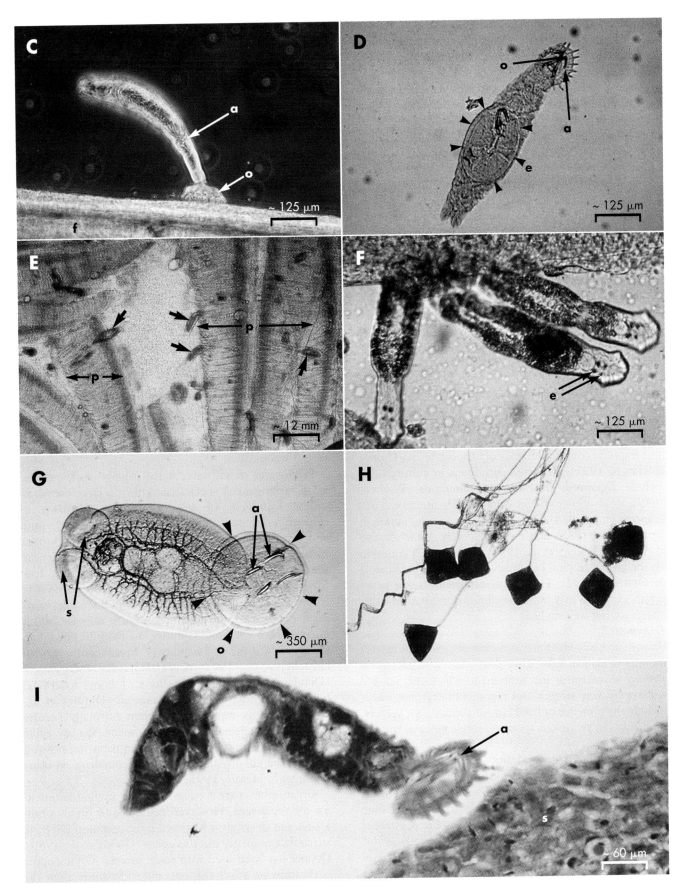

Fig. II-16—cont'd. *For legend see opposite page.*

infestations induce flashing and resultant long scratches on lightly scaled fish (e.g., pompano, kingfish, dolphin). Capsalids can produce large numbers of eggs (over 80/day in some species) (Thoney, 1990).

Neobenedenia melleni causes serious skin damage and has a predilection for the eye (i.e., eye fluke; don't confuse with digenean eye flukes; see *PROBLEM 55*); its large hooks cause ophthalmic lesions leading to blindness (Nigrelli, 1940). It infests numerous species, including various tropical reef fish, including members of the Acanthuridae, Ariidae, Balistidae, Diodontidae, Carangidae, Chaetodontidae, Holocentridae, Labridae, Lutjanidae, Malacanthidae, Ostraciidae, Pomadasyidae, Percichthyidae, Pomatomidae, Psettidae, Scatophagidae, Sciaenidae, Serranidae, Sparidae, and Triglidae (Thoney & Hargis, 1991).

Other pathogens in cultured fish include *Entobdella solea* on dover sole (Anderson & Conroy, 1968), *Benedenia seriolae* on yellowtail (Egusa, 1983), *Benedenia* sp. on pompano (Lawler, 1977b), and *Dermophthirius* or *Dermophthioides* spp. on various elasmobranchs (Thoney & Hargis, 1991).

POLYOPISTHOCOTYLEA

Relatively few polyopisthocotyleans are problems in cultured fish; most that affect cultured fish have a wide host range. They feed on blood and do not browse like monopisthocotyleans. Thus, they usually elicit a less severe host response compared to monopisthocotyleans (Thoney & Hargis, 1991). Reported pathogens in cultured fish include *Discocotyle* in European salmonids (Wooten, 1989), *Allobivagina* on *Siganus* in the Mediterranean Sea (Paperna et al., 1984), *Axine* or *Heteraxine* on *Siganus* in Japan (Egusa, 1983), and *Polylabroides* on *Acanthopagrus* in Australia (Diggles et al., 1993). *Microcotyle* is common on the gills of tropical butterflyfish and angelfish (Blasiola & Gratzek, 1992). Heavy infestations of some polyopisthocotyleans may cause few clinical signs, but sublethal effects are not well studied.

Diagnosis

Worms are easily identified as monogeneans by using wet mounts of skin or gills. They often have a characteristic *jerking* or caterpillar-like motion, in which the parasite will repetitively stretch and recoil. Other key features include the presence of hooks (most commonly), suckers, or clamps. In viviparous species, a single embryo is easily seen developing within the adult worm (Fig. II-16, *C* and *D*). Capsalids are large but transparent flukes. Fixation in formalin or alcohol causes them to turn white, rendering them more visible. The great majority of monogeneans do not exceed 4 mm, although species from large marine fish (e.g., sailfish) may be up to 3 cm (Moller & Anders, 1986). Identification to species or even genus is not essential for successful treatment but can be useful, since species vary considerably in pathogenicity (Cone & Odense, 1984) and in response to treatment. Live or pre-

served samples (p. 31) are best sent to a reference laboratory for specific taxonomic identification.

Monogeneans may be present in low numbers without causing disease; for example, the presence of a single parasite in a skin scraping or gill clip of a 10 cm–long fish would not be compatible with a history of mortalities in a fish population, and thus, other causes should be sought under those circumstances.

Treatment

GENERAL CONSIDERATIONS

Several therapies have been successfully used to control monogenean infestations, but it is important to realize that monogenean species and even populations differ in their sensitivity to treatments, so the clinician must often try different therapies to determine which works best in a particular situation. For example, toltrazuril has shown experimental effectiveness against pseudogyrodactylosis in some cases (Schmahl et al., 1988) but not others (Buchmann et al., 1990).

One important consideration in designing an effective treatment is whether the monogenean is viviparous or oviparous because the eggs of some monogeneans are resistant to treatment and thus several drug applications may be required for control. In capsalids, resistant eggs take 10 to 21 days to hatch; visible reinfestation occurs about 2 weeks after treatment at 20° to 25° C (68° to 77° F). Thus, control requires weekly treatments for at least 3 weeks.

Freshwater or saltwater baths usually work only on small monogenean species (i.e., not on large capsalids, unless followed 48 hours later by formalin or organophosphate treatment [Langdon, 1992a]). Adult and juvenile polyopisthocotyleans were only removed by high-dose formalin treatment (400 ppm for 25 minutes). This dose is not tolerated by many fish. Monogeneans on estuarine species are also resistant to freshwater or saltwater baths. However, if feasible, long-term exposure to suboptimal salinity may be highly effective. For example, salinities less than 20 ppt significantly reduce the egg viability of *Neobenedenia melleni* (Mueller et al., 1992) or *Polylabroides multispinosus* (Diggles et al., 1993). Only long (1 hour) freshwater baths cured fish of *P. multispinosus* (Diggles et al., 1993). This is much longer than normally recommended for marine fish. Gill monogeneans are often more resistant to treatment than skin parasites, possibly because the gill provides protection from drug exposure (Thoney & Hargis, 1991).

Organophosphate is one of the most useful treatments for monogeneans. However, resistance to organophosphates can develop; it has been most commonly seen in farms that regularly use this agent (Goven et al., 1980). Copper has been used with some success. While copper is thought to affect the oncomiracidia more than the adults, this is not always true (Thoney, 1990).

Interestingly a bath of 80 mg/l benzocaine has successfully treated some monogenean infestations (Svendsen & Haug, 1991). Mebendazole and praziquantel have both been recently used with success against several marine or freshwater monogeneans (Szekely & Molnar, 1987; Thoney & Hargis, 1991), but whether they will supplant other more traditional treatments (e.g., formalin) remains to be seen.

Biological control may be feasible in tropical marine aquaria, since *cleaner fish*, such as French angelfish, neon gobies, and Pacific cleaner wrasse, reportedly pick monogeneans off other fish (Moe, 1992a).

ENVIRONMENTAL CONSIDERATIONS

Chemical treatments often only control and do not eradicate monogeneans, emphasizing the need for environmental management. Monogeneans cannot survive for more than 2 weeks off a host (unless present as overwintering eggs); many will die much more quickly (some within minutes). Because of their reproductive cycle, the offspring of viviparous monogeneans remain on the same host; thus, transmission can occur via fish-to-fish contact. Reducing crowding may be more significant in reducing such transmission than in oviparous monogeneans, where a free-swimming larva may attach to any host.

PROBLEM 17
Turbellarian Infection (Tang Turbellarian, Black Ich)

Prevalence Index
WM - 3
Method of Diagnosis
1. Wet mount of skin or gills with parasite
2. Histopathology of skin or gills with parasite
History/Physical Examination
Black (rarely white) skin lesions up to ~1 mm; white lesions may interconnect into larger foci
Treatment
1. Freshwater bath
2. Formalin bath
3. Organophosphate prolonged immersion

COMMENTS
Epidemiology/Pathogenesis

Turbellarians are a phylum of mainly free-living worms related to trematodes. *Ichthyophaga*, *Paravortex*, and several other genera have been reported from free-ranging marine fish (Cannon & Lester, 1988).

Most of what is known about these parasites is based on studies of the *tang turbellarian* (tentatively identified as a *Paravortex* sp.) (Kent & Olson, 1986) (Fig. II-17, *A* through *C*). The tang turbellarian has been most commonly observed on yellow tangs but also infects at least 16 tropical marine species in 5 families,

including butterflyfish, angelfish, gobies, opisthognathids, and other tangs. Less well described turbellarian infections on other marine species have also been suspected to be caused by this organism. The tang turbellarian induces a hypermelanization reaction, resulting in dark foci on the skin, which are best seen on light-colored fish; there may be acute, focal dermatitis and hemorrhage. Parasites less commonly infect gill epithelium.

The life cycle is direct and is analogous in many ways to marine white spot disease (see *PROBLEM 19*), with a proliferative stage off the host. After feeding for about 6 days on the fish (growing from 77 μm to 450 μm), the parasite leaves the host and falls to the sediment, where it continues to increase in size (to ~750 μm) over the next 3 to 4 days. During this time, progeny form and the young are brooded internally. An adult can produce as many as 160 juveniles at once. The adult's body wall ruptures, releasing juveniles that can immediately infect a host. The life cycle takes ~10 days at 24.5° C (76° F) (Kent & Olson, 1986).

Because of the high reproductive rate, fish can harbor up to 4500 parasites in as little as 20 days. Death can ensue in 10 to 23 days. Infestations can also spread from fish to fish when worms in the parasitic phase change hosts. Fish-to-fish transmission takes less than 24 hours.

Another turbellarian, tentatively identified as an *Ichthyophaga* sp. (Julian Smith, Personal Communication), has caused epidemics in lookdowns and other cultured carangids in North Carolina (Noga, Camper, & Smith, Unpublished Data). This organism induces a proliferative epithelial response (Fig. II-17, *D* and *E*).

Diagnosis

Lesions produced by the tang turbellarian look grossly similar to those caused by digenean metacercariae (see *PROBLEM 55*) and lesions caused by the lookdown turbellarian look grossly similar to cryptocaryonosis (see *PROBLEM 20*). Both are easily identified using wet mounts or histopathology. Note that the lookdown turbellarian is easily crushed when covered with a coverslip (E. Noga, Unpublished Data). Thus, wet mounts should be examined without coverslips when suspect skin lesions are seen but no parasites are detected. Brooding adults of the tang turbellarian can also be detected in detritus samples from the tank bottom. Do not mistake the parasite for free-living turbellarians, which are common, nonpathogenic pests in freshwater and marine aquaria.

Treatment

Formalin or organophosphate controls the tang turbellarian. Two to three treatments are usually advisable (Kent & Olson, 1986). The lookdown turbellarian is resistant to both copper and formalin but responds well to a freshwater bath (John Camper, Personal Communication).

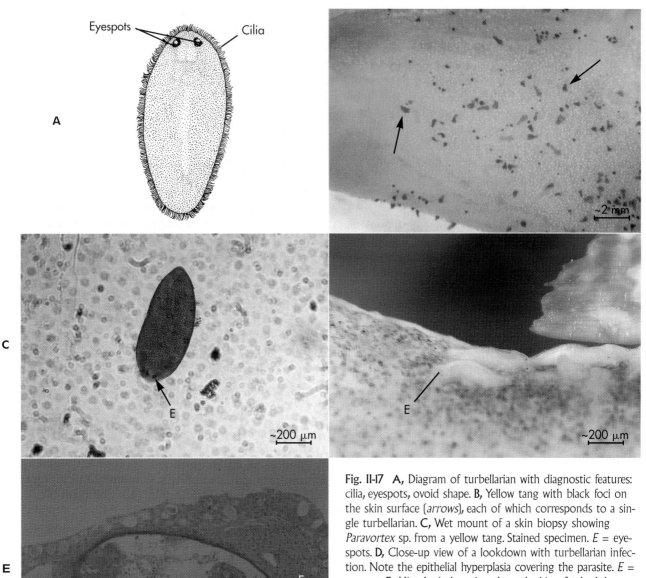

Fig. II-17 **A,** Diagram of turbellarian with diagnostic features: cilia, eyespots, ovoid shape. **B,** Yellow tang with black foci on the skin surface (*arrows*), each of which corresponds to a single turbellarian. **C,** Wet mount of a skin biopsy showing *Paravortex* sp. from a yellow tang. Stained specimen. *E* = eyespots. **D,** Close-up view of a lookdown with turbellarian infection. Note the epithelial hyperplasia covering the parasite. *E* = eyespot. **E,** Histological section through skin of a lookdown showing turbellarian. Key diagnostic features include complete ciliation, two eyespots, size (~100 to 500 μm), and ovoid shape.

(*A* from Cannon & Lester, 1988; *B* and *C* photographs courtesy of G. Blasiola.)

PROBLEM 18
Protozoan Ectoparasites: General Features

Prevalence Index
WF - 1, CF - 1, WM - 1, CM - 1

Method of Diagnosis
1. Wet mount of skin or gills with parasite
2. Histopathology of skin or gills with parasite

History/Physical Examination
All caused by feeding activity of the parasite; typical signs include pruritus ("flashing"), dyspnea, "cloudy" skin, secondary microbial infections

Treatment
Usually antiseptic-type treatment

COMMENTS
Protozoan ectoparasites are the most common parasites encountered in cultured fish (MacMillan, 1991); they are also frequently found on wild fish. This group is a diverse array of mainly ciliates and flagellates that feed on the most superficial skin layer (i.e., epithelium). Most feed only on the epithelium's surface, but a few (e.g., *Ichthyophthirius*) penetrate into the epithelium.

Clinical signs are due to damage caused by parasite feeding activity. Parasites are irritating, which often causes a reactive hyperplasia of the epithelium and/or increased mucus production. When the hyperplasia is severe, this response appears as a *cloudiness* to the skin (see Fig. I-8). The same response can occur on the gills and leads to hypoxia.

All protozoan ectoparasites have a direct life cycle, which is faster at higher temperature. Generation time of some species may be as little as 24 hours under optimal conditions. Thus, these parasites can quickly overwhelm a host population. All are easily diagnosed via wet mount of live material or from histopathology.

Effective treatment of protozoan ectoparasites depends on an understanding of the two major types of life styles: nonencysting and encysting. Nonencysting protozoans (e.g., *Trichodina*, *Ichthyobodo*) complete their life cycle on the host and are easily treated, usually with a single, short-term drug application. Encysting protozoans (e.g., *Ichthyophthirius*, *Amyloodinium*) produce a reproductive cyst off the host. Both the fish-feeding stage and the reproductive cyst are resistant to treatment, so therapy must be directed at the free-swimming, infective stage (see Fig. II-19, *A*). This requires that chemicals be present for a long time or that several treatments be applied to ensure that all infective stages are killed.

PROBLEM 19

Ich Infection (Freshwater White Spot Disease, *Ichthyophthirius Multifiliis* Infection, Ichthyophthiriosis)

Prevalence Index
WF - 1, CF - 2
Method of Diagnosis
1. Wet mount of skin or gills with parasite
2. Histopathology of skin or gills with parasite
History/Physical Examination
Typical signs of protozoan ectoparasite; also white nodules up to 1 mm on skin or gills that may interconnect into larger foci
Treatment
1. Formalin prolonged immersion
2. Formalin/malachite green prolonged immersion
3. Salt prolonged immersion
4. Raise temperature to > 30° C (86° F) for 10 days
5. Formalin bath weekly until cured
6. Transfer fish to new aquarium daily for 7 days at 25° C (77° F)

COMMENTS

Life Cycle
Ich is one of the most common diseases of freshwater fish. Virtually all freshwater fish are susceptible to infec-

tion, although scaleless fish, such as catfish and loaches, are especially vulnerable. Up to 100% mortality may occur (Meyer, 1974).

The ich trophozoite (feeding stage) feeds in a nodule formed in the skin or gill epithelium (Ewing & Kocan, 1986) (Fig. II-19, *A*). After it feeds within the skin or gills, ich breaks through the epithelium, falls off the host, and forms an encapsulated dividing stage (tomont). The tomont secretes a capsule, which is sticky and adheres to plants, ornaments, nets, or other objects. It divides up to 10 times by binary fission, producing tomites that break through the nodule wall to form motile, infective, ~20 × 50 μm theronts (Fig. II-19, *A*). A single trophont may produce over 1000 theronts. Thus, ich can overwhelm a population quickly.

Epidemiology
A common temperature for ich outbreaks is 15° to 25° C (59° to 77° F). However, outbreaks often develop at low (< 10° C [50° F]) temperatures in spring, when fish are stressed from overwintering (J. Lom, Personal Communication). Parasites complete their life cycle in 3 to 6 days at 25° C (77° F), 10 days at 15° C (59° F), and a month or more at 10° C (50° F), when the disease is rarely serious (Meyer, 1974). While ich is typically a warm water disease, it can also infect salmonids or other cold water fish at as low as 4° C (39° F). Many epidemics in salmonids are during summer, when fish are heat-stressed (>17° to 19° C [63° to 66° F]). Considerable acquired immunity is present in fish that recover from infection (Dickerson et al., 1986).

Pathogenesis
Ich cysts appear grossly as small white nodules that produce a salt-like dusting (Fig. II-19, *B*). The nodules protrude slightly from the surface (Fig. II-19, *B*), being from ~0.10 to 1.0 mm in size. In advanced, heavy infections, individual cysts may appear to coalesce, forming mucoid masses on the skin (Fig. II-19, *C*). Fish having such heavy infections are not likely to survive, even if they are treated.

The epithelial erosion and ulceration that result from the parasite's entrance into and exit from the host are probably at least as damaging as its feeding activity while it is on the host. Lesions produced by the parasites may also lead to secondary microbial infections.

Diagnosis
The presence of a ciliate encysted **within** the host's epithelium (Fig. II-19, *D*) is pathognomonic. The cilia move constantly while the trophont is within the cyst. *Ichthyophthirius* is a holotrich ciliate; thus, cilia are evenly distributed over the entire body surface. Other diagnostic features of the trophont include a C-shaped macronucleus (may not be easily visible on small trophonts) (Figs. II-19, *E* and *F*), large size variation of trophonts (Fig. II-19, *E*), and pleomorphic shape.

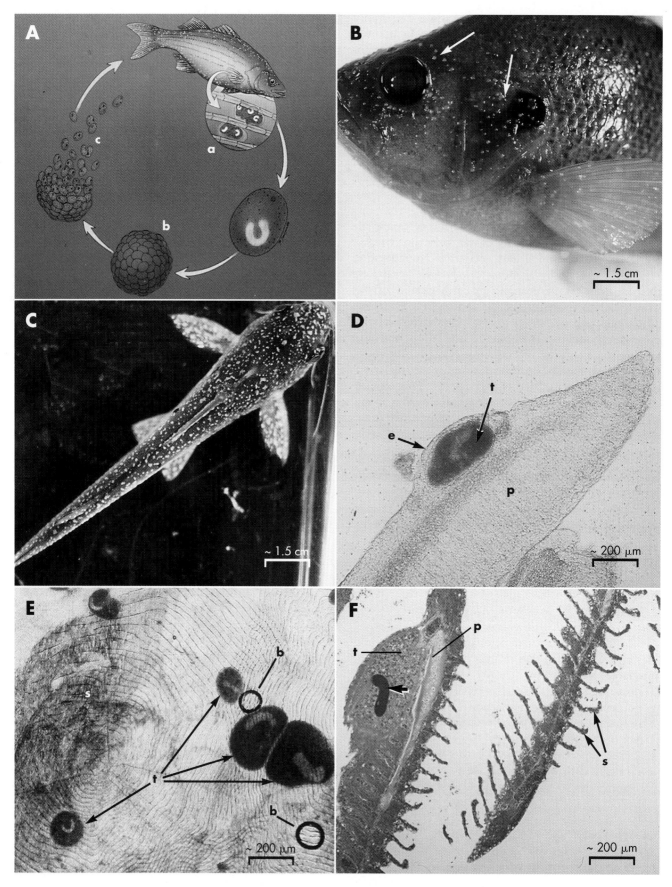

Fig. II-19   *For legend see opposite page.*

Treatment

AQUARIA

Detection of even a single ich trophont warrants immediate treatment. Fish with extensive lesions (see Fig. II-19, *B* and *C*) have a guarded prognosis. The theront stage is most susceptible to therapy and thus drugs must remain at therapeutic levels for a sufficient time to ensure that all parasites have passed through this stage. At optimum temperatures (24° to 26° C), treatment must be maintained for 1 week, since the life cycle is completed in 3 to 7 days (Parker, 1965). Formalin prolonged immersion is effective; three treatments on alternate days are recommended to ensure that all emerging theronts are killed. In advanced cases, formalin/malachite green may be preferable, because these two agents are synergistic (Gilbert et al., 1979). Watch closely for recurrence and extend treatment if parasites are still seen.

At lower temperatures, the cycle takes longer. Thus, if a client has goldfish in an unheated tank at 7° C, it may take 6 weeks or longer for all parasites to form theronts. Instead of treating for a longer time, it is best, if possible, to temporarily raise the temperature of the system and treat accordingly. This may not be possible in large culture systems. Ich cannot complete its life cycle at > 30° C (86° F) (Parker, 1965), but many fish cannot tolerate such high temperatures (see *PROBLEM 2*).

Ichthyophthirius multifiliis cannot tolerate over 1 ppt salinity (Allen & Avault, 1970), and thus salt can be used both as a cure and as a preventative. It is especially useful for euryhaline fish such as poeciliids, which are prone to develop ich when kept in freshwater; most fish tolerate low salt levels (see *PHARMACOPOEIA*). Salt also helps to alleviate the osmotic stress caused by the epithelial damage.

Transferring fish to a new aquarium daily for 7 days will cure fish by preventing reinfection. This treatment is stressful to the fish and cumbersome. Daily vacuuming of the bottom of the aquarium has also been reported to control the infection by removing developing cysts (Brown & Gratzek, 1980). At 25° C (77° F), theronts only remain infective for 30 hours after excystment, but delayed emergence of some theronts requires that aquaria be left without fish for 7 days to be rid of the infection. All stages are also killed by drying.

PONDS

For pond fish, the treatment of choice for ich is copper sulfate. At 20° to 25° C (68° to 77° F), treatments must be applied every other day at least thrice. At 15° C (59° F), this should be extended to every 3 to 4 days. At cooler temperatures, ich causes more chronic outbreaks. Its prolonged life cycle at low temperatures necessitates extended treatment (Post, 1987).

During outbreaks, quarantine of infected fish and disinfection of equipment (e.g., nets, aerators) are essential. Adjacent ponds should be closely monitored, since birds feeding on diseased fish or carcasses can spread the infection.

FLOW-THROUGH SYSTEMS

Fish in flow-through systems require repeated bath treatments, until no parasites are detected (usually at least three treatments). Increasing the flow in a raceway has also been reported to cure fish by sweeping away infective theronts (Brown & Gratzek, 1980).

PROBLEM 20
Marine White Spot Disease (Cryptocaryonosis, Marine Ich)

Prevalence Index

WM - 1

Method of Diagnosis

1. Wet mount of skin or gills with parasite
2. Histopathology of skin or gills with parasite

History/Physical Examination

Typical signs of protozoan ectoparasite; also, white foci up to ~0.5 mm on skin that may interconnect into larger masses; white "tags" on skin; acute mortality

Treatment

1. Hyposalinity (16 ppt or less) for 14 days
2. Hyposalinity (10 ppt) for 3 hours q 3 days × 4
3. Transfer fish to new aquarium q 3 days × 4
4. Lower temperature to < 19° C (66° F)
5. Copper prolonged immersion

Fig. II-19 **A,** *Ichthyophthirius multifiliis* life cycle. *a* = trophonts; *b* = dividing tomont; *c* = tomites/theronts. **B,** Close-up view of a bluegill with ich. Note that the parasite nodules (*arrows*) protrude slightly above the skin surface. **C,** Channel catfish with a heavy ich infection. **D,** Wet mount of a gill biopsy showing *I. multifiliis* trophont (*t*) encysted within the epithelium (*e*) of the primary lamella (*p*). **E,** Wet mount of a skin scraping showing *I. multifiliis* trophonts (*t*). Key features include the size variation of the pleomorphic parasites and the C-shaped macronucleus. *s* = fish scale. *b* = air bubble. **F,** Histological section through trophont (*t*). Note the macronucleus (*arrow*). The C-shape is not apparent in every section through a parasite. *p* = primary gill lamella; *s* = secondary gill lamellae.

[*A* figure by B. Davison-DeGraves and E. Noga; *C* photograph by R. Bullis and E. Noga; *F* photograph courtesy of L. Khoo.]

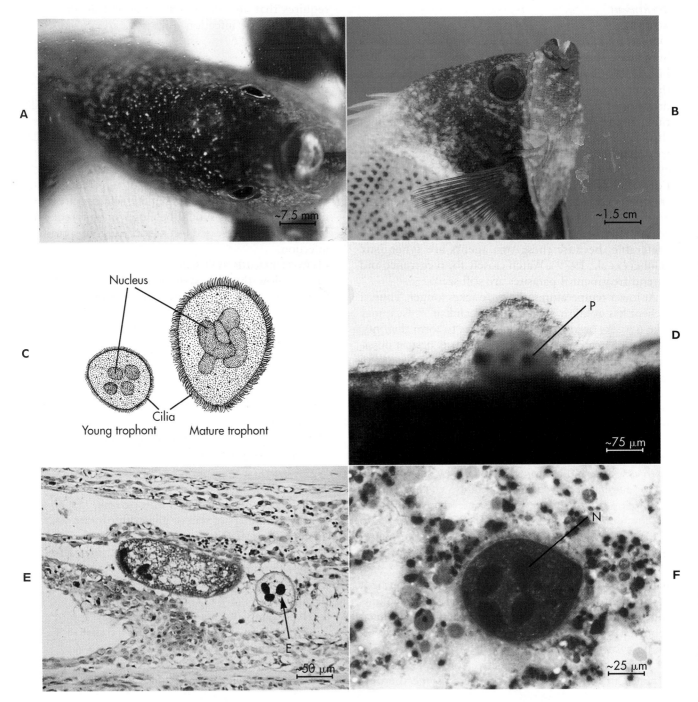

Fig. II-20 **A,** Red sea damselfish with a heavy *C. irritans* skin infection. The infection looks like a dusting of salt on the body. **B,** Queen angelfish with multifocal depigmented skin erosions affecting the entire head, caused by a prior *C. irritans* skin infection. **C,** *Cryptocaryon irritans.* Diagram with key characteristics of trophont: size (up to 450 μm), cilia evenly distributed over body, spherical-to-oval shape, multilobed nucleus. See ich (see *PROBLEM 19*) for life cycle. **D,** Fin clip with *C. irritans.* The parasite (*P*) is within the epithelium. **E,** Histological section of a fish infected with *Cryptocaryon irritans* (Mediterranean Sea strain). Note the presence of the two parasites <u>under</u> the epithelium, which is pathognomonic, and the lobated macronucleus (*arrow*). **F,** Stained smear of a *Cryptocaryon* trophont. *N* = nucleus. Modified Wright's.

[*A, D,* and *E* photographs courtesy of A. Colorni; *B* photograph by B. Brglz and E. Noga; *F* photograph by L. Khoo, C. Harms, and E. Noga.]

COMMENTS
Epidemiology/Pathogenesis
Traditionally a problem in aquarium fish, *Cryptocaryon irritans* has recently become a serious disease in cultured warm water marine fish (Tookwinas, 1990). It plays the same role in the marine environment that *Ichthyophthirius multifiliis* does in freshwater. While these two ciliates have a similar life cycle and pathology, recent studies have shown this to be due to convergent evolution rather than phylogenetic relatedness (Colorni et al., 1993). *Cryptocaryon irritans* has the same life cycle (see Fig. II-19, *A*) and also produces *white spots* on the skin (Fig. II-20, *A*) (Brown, 1951). The parasites are somewhat smaller than ich and thus produce slightly smaller nodules. Affected skin often appears to have a fine dusting of salt. Skin lesions may appear less like discrete white spots and more like multifocal white patches (Fig. II-20, *B*). More than one species of *Cryptocaryon* may exist (Diamant et al., 1991).

Cryptocaryon is pathogenic at 20° to 30° C (68° to 86° F), with optimal reproduction at 30° C (86° F). At 21° to 24° C (70° to 75° F), the life cycle is completed in as little as 6 days, with most parasites completing their life cycle in 11 to 15 days (Nigrelli & Ruggieri, 1966; Colorni, 1985). Up to 200 theronts may be produced by one tomont.

Diagnosis
Even fairly heavy infections may require close examination to be grossly detectable. Shining a light on top of the fish in a darkened room can be helpful. *Cryptocaryon* is most readily diagnosed when seen under the skin or gills (Fig. II-20, *D*). The presence of a ciliated protozoan **within** the host's epithelium (Fig. II-20, *D*) is pathognomonic. Unlike ich, it does not have a C-shaped macronucleus. A moniliform macronucleus, consisting of four linked, bead-like segments, may be seen in histological sections or stained smears of trophonts (Kaige & Miyazaki, 1985; Colorni & Diamant, 1993) (Fig. II-20, *C*, *E*, and *F*) but not at all stages of development. The macronucleus is obscured in wet mounts by the granular cytoplasm. Trophonts range from 48 to 450 μm × 27 to 350 μm (Nigrelli & Ruggieri, 1966).

Treatment
Treatment should be prompt because the parasite reproduces quickly. Tomonts can be lysed by hyposalinity (Colorni, 1985). Thus, euryhaline fish are easily treated if the salinity can be lowered. The least stressful procedure is probably to lower the salinity for short time intervals (see *HYPOSALINITY* in *PHARMACO-POEIA*). Alternatively, the salinity can be lowered indefinitely to 16 ppt or less (Cheung et al., 1979); even many stenohaline reef fish tolerate this well, although some fish become hyperactive or aggressive during treatment. Hypersalinity in combination with drug treatment has also been used (Huff & Burns, 1981). Cryptocaryonosis also responds well to copper therapy.

Lowering the temperature below 19° C (66° F) will stop reproduction (Wilkie & Gordin, 1969) but is impractical in most instances and probably not advisable for most tropical reef fish. Transferring fish to a clean aquarium every 3 days will also effect a cure but is stressful. Evidence exists that suggests recovered fish are more resistant to reinfection (Colorni, 1985).

At 25° C (77° F), theronts remain infective for only 24 hours after excystment, but the long time for emergence of some theronts requires that aquaria be left without fish for at least 3 months to be rid of the parasite. Tomonts have been observed to survive and release theronts as long as 72 days after leaving the fish (A. Colorni, Personal Communication). All stages are also killed by drying.

PROBLEM 21
Trichodinosis

Prevalence Index
WF - 1, WM - 4, CF - 1, CM - 1
Method of Diagnosis
1. Wet mount of skin or gills with parasite
2. Histopathology of skin or gills with parasite
History/Physical Examination
Typical signs of protozoan ectoparasite; chronic mortality
Treatment
1. Formalin bath
2. Formalin prolonged immersion
3. Potassium permanganate prolonged immersion
4. Acetic acid bath (freshwater only)
5. Salt bath (freshwater only)
6. Freshwater bath (marine only)
7. Copper prolonged immersion

COMMENTS
Epidemiology/Pathogenesis
Many trichodinid species infest marine or freshwater fish, including *Trichodina*, *Trichodinella*, *Tripartiella*, *Paratrichodina*, *Hemitrichodina*, and *Vauchomia* species. All have a similar morphology (Fig. II-21, *A* through *C*). Almost all clinically important species infest the skin and/or gills. Some species infect the urinary bladder, oviducts, or gastrointestinal tract, but they are not proven pathogens. In general, the larger (> 90 μm), skin-dwelling trichodinids have a broad host range, while smaller (< 30 μm), gill-dwelling parasites tend to infest one or a few fish species (Van As & Basson, 1987). There are important exceptions (e.g., *Trichodinella epizootica* infests at least 19 fish species). Many species infest both skin and gills. Other aquatic animals (e.g., amphibian larvae) can be reservoirs for some fish trichodinids (Lom & Dykova, 1992).

Trichodinosis is usually a relatively mild disease that presents as chronic morbidity or mortality (Hoffmann,

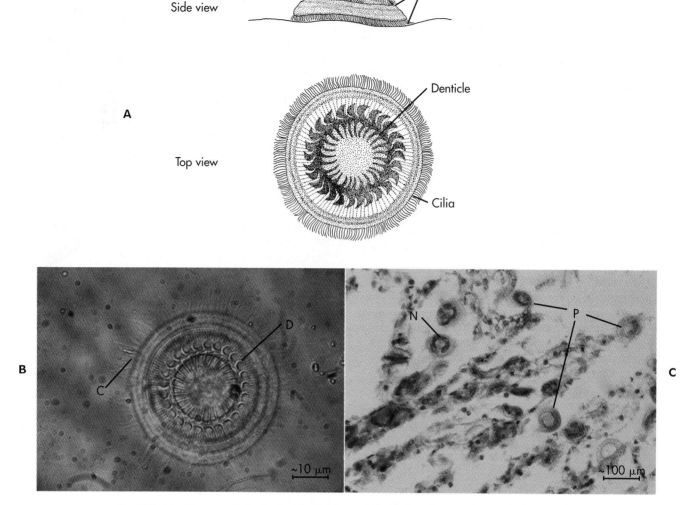

Side view

Cilia

A

Denticle

Top view

Cilia

B

D

C

~10 μm

N

P

C

~100 μm

Fig. II-2l   A, Diagram of a typical trichodinid parasite with key characteristics: size (l5 to l20 μm, usually 40 to 60 μm in diameter), cilia for locomotion, round shape when seen from top of parasite (dorsally), and ring with hook-like denticles. **B,** Wet mount of a typical trichodinid parasite. *C* = cilia; *D* = denticle. **C,** Histological section through the gill of a goldfish with a heavy trichodinid infestation. Parasites (*P*) can be recognized by their round shape from above. *N* = nucleus.

(*B* photograph courtesy of F. Meyer.)

1978). While trichodinids only inhabit the surface of the fish, adherence to and suction on the epithelium may cause damage (Lom, 1973a). Heavily infested fish are anorexic, lose condition, and usually experience low-level (1% per week) mortality. Mortalities can be much higher, especially in young fish. Secondary bacterial infections can greatly escalate mortalities. Trichodinid infestations are seen mainly in fish that are debilitated because of some other condition (e.g., poor nutrition, overcrowding, another disease). At least some trichodinids can survive off the host for 1 to 2 days (J. Lom, Personal Communication).

Diagnosis

Trichodinids are easily recognized (Fig. II-2l, *A* through *C*). They often exhibit a characteristic scooting motion on tissue surfaces. All trichodinids are treated similarly, so there is no need for identification to genus (which requires silver staining of fixed samples). The observation of low numbers (e.g., 1 per 100X field of view) of trichodinids on a skin or gill biopsy is inconsequential; other problems should be sought in the clinical work-up. However, because of their tenuous attachment to the tissues, they are easily lost during fixation.

Treatment

Trichodinids are easily killed with one application of appropriate treatment. Fish will often recover spontaneously if water quality is improved. Some trichodinid species can infest both freshwater and marine fish (Lom & Dykova, 1992), but virtually all common pathogens are restricted to either fresh or salt water environments.

PROBLEM 22
Chilodonella Infestation (Chilodonellosis)

Prevalence Index
WF - 1, CF - 1

Method of Diagnosis
1. Wet mount of skin or gills with parasite
2. Histopathology of skin or gills with parasite

History/Physical Examination
Typical signs of protozoan ectoparasite, especially whitish or bluish sheen on body, "tattered" appearance to skin; also, a drop in temperature or previous injury

Treatment
1. Formalin bath
2. Formalin prolonged immersion
3. Potassium permanganate prolonged immersion
4. Acetic acid bath
5. Salt bath
6. Copper prolonged immersion

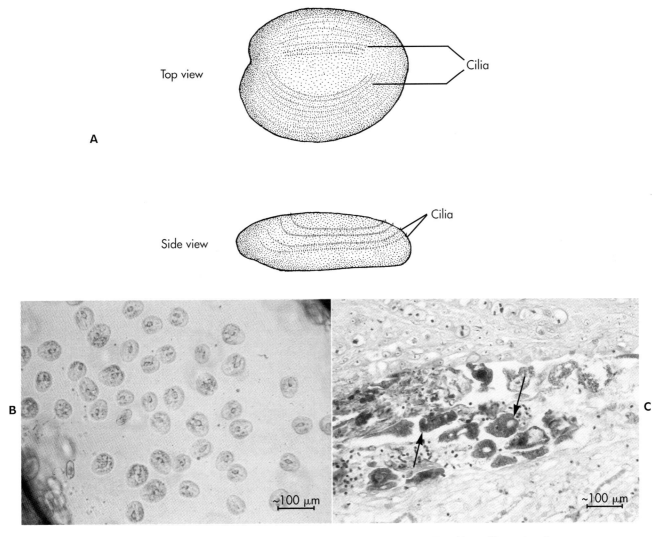

Fig. II-22 A, *Chilodonella.* Diagram of key characteristics: size (usually ~40 to 60 μm long); bands of cilia; when viewed from above (*top view*), oval-to-heart-shape, with notched anterior end; parasites are flattened shape when viewed from the side (*side view*). **B,** Wet mount of *Chilodonella piscicola.* **C,** Histological section of gill with *Chilodonella* (*arrows*). Giemsa.

(*B* photograph courtesy of G. Hoffman.)

COMMENTS

Epidemiology/Pathogenesis

Most *Chilodonella* species are free-living, but two species (*C. piscicola* and *C. hexasticha*) are pathogenic for fish. *Chilodonella piscicola* (formerly *C. cyprini*) infests virtually all freshwater fish, mainly fingerlings (Shulman & Jankovski, 1984). It can also infest fish in brackish water. *Chilodonella hexasticha* is less widely distributed but produces similar lesions, mainly in older fish.

Chilodonellosis is more insidious than ich, since severe damage can occur before gross pathology is evident. *Chilodonella* elicits a strong cellular response, which suggests that it may feed directly on epithelium (Paperna & Van As, 1983). It appears to feed by penetrating the host cells with its cytostome and sucking out the contents (Wiles et al., 1985). Advanced *Chilodonella* infestations are sometimes associated with skin ulcers, which may have a *tattered* appearance (see Fig. II-23, *A*). High numbers can cause secondary bacterial infections and substantial mortality (10% per week).

Chilodonellosis has a wide temperature tolerance. For example, outbreaks in cold water species often occur at 5° to 10° C (41° to 50° F), while tropical fish are affected when temperature drops to 20° C (68° F). Outbreaks can also occur at higher temperatures. Mass mortalities have occurred in wild populations (Langdon et al., 1985).

Some free-living *Chilodonella* species (e.g., *C. cucullulus*, *C. uncinata*) can damage weakened fish in polluted waters (Lom & Dykova, 1992). They are apparently not as widespread as the two more pathogenic *Chilodonella* species.

Diagnosis

Chilodonella is easily recognized in wet mounts or histological sections (Figs. II-22, *A* through *C*). Because of their tenuous attachment to the tissues, they are easily lost during fixation. In wet mounts, *Chilodonella* glides slowly over gill lamellae, sometimes turning in wide circles (Brown & Gratzek, 1980). It is differentiated from the holotrichs ich (see *PROBLEM 19*) and *Tetrahymena*

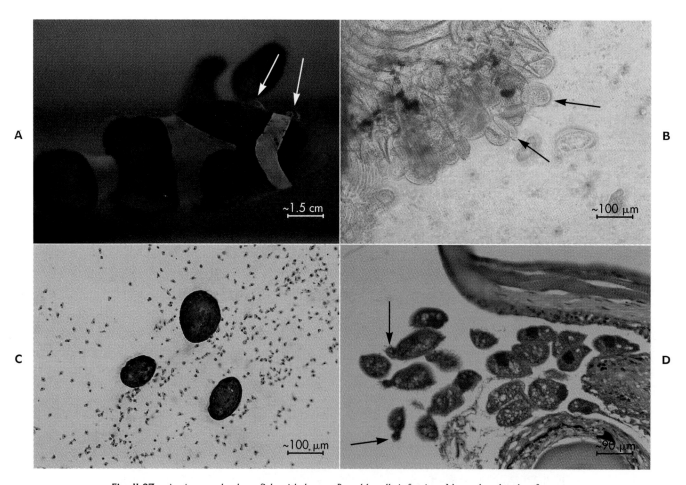

Fig. II-23   A, A percula clownfish with heavy *Brooklynella* infection. Note the shreds of detaching skin (*arrows*). **B,** Wet mount of skin from a percula clownfish with brooklynellosis. Note ovoid shape on top view and flat shape on side view (*arrows*). **C,** Modified Wright's stained smear of the skin lesion in Fig. II-23, *A*, with three *Brooklynella* trophozoites. **D,** Histological section of the skin lesion in Fig. II-23, *A*, with many parasites. Key features include size, shape, and notched anterior end (*arrows*).

(*C* and *D* photographs by L. Khoo and E. Noga.)

(see *PROBLEM 25*) by its flattened shape. Also characteristic are its bands of cilia on the ventral surface, which require high magnification to see and are best visualized with silver staining. *Chilodonella piscicola* is 30 to 80 × 20 to 60 μm, with 8 to 11 bands of cilia, while *C. hexasticha* is smaller (30 to 65 × 20 to 50 μm), with 5 to 9 cilia bands (Fig. II-22, *A*). Identification to species is not needed for proper treatment.

Treatment

One application of an appropriate treatment usually controls chilodonellosis. *Chilodonella piscicola* produces long-lasting cysts (Bauer & Nikolskaya, 1957), but whether these are resistant to treatment is not known.

PROBLEM 23
Brooklynella Infestation (Brooklynellosis)

Prevalence Index
WM - 2

Method of Diagnosis
1. Wet mount of skin or gills with parasite
2. Histopathology of skin or gills with parasite

History/Physical Examination
Typical signs of protozoan ectoparasite

Treatment
1. Formalin bath

COMMENTS
Brooklynellosis (Fig. II-23, *A* through *D*) is the marine analogue of chilodonellosis. It has been associated with acute mortalities of tropical marine fish. *Brooklynella hostilis* is morphologically similar to *Chilodonella*, having an oval shape with more numerous ciliary rows. Its most easily recognized diagnostic features are dorsoventral flattening, notched anterior end, size, and slow, *Chilodonella*-like movement. Its size range is 56 to 86 × 32 to 50 μm.

Unlike most marine fish ectoparasites, it is often not susceptible to copper, but formalin baths are effective (C.E. Bower, Personal Communication). While reported to be only a gill pathogen (Lom & Nigrelli, 1970), it can also cause serious skin lesions (Fig. II-23, *A*). It commonly occurs after transport stress.

PROBLEM 24
Uronemosis *(Uronema* Infestation / Infection)

Prevalence Index
WM - 4

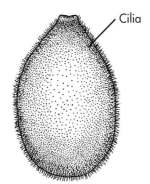

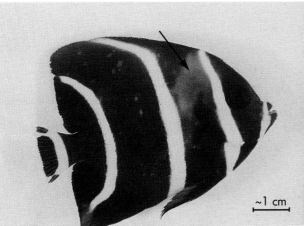

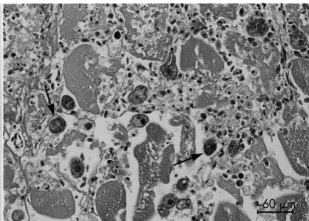

Fig. II-24   **A,** *Uronema marinum.* Diagram with key characteristics: size (~13 to 20 × 32 to 38 μm), tear-drop shape (narrow anteriorly), cilia (*C*) evenly distributed over body (after Lom & Dykova, 1992; from Kahl). **B,** Immature French angelfish with large area of depigmentation (*arrow*) caused by uronemosis. **C,** Histological section of lesion in Fig. II-24, *B,* necrotic muscle with trophozoites, some with ingested erythrocytes (*arrows*). Hematoxylin and eosin.

Method of Diagnosis:
1. Histopathology of skin, gills, or internal organs with parasite
2. Wet mount of skin, gills, or internal organs with parasite

History/Physical Examination

Focal depigmentation, pitting, ulceration of skin; dyspnea; hyperactivity, then lethargy

Treatment

Freshwater bath followed after 24 hours by formalin prolonged immersion (useful only in early stages)

COMMENTS
Epidemiology/Pathogenesis

Uronema marinum (Fig. II-24, *A*) seems to be the marine counterpart of *Tetrahymena* (see *PROBLEM 25*). Both are holotrich ciliates that cause skin/gill lesions and systemic infections. *Uronema* appears to have a wide host range and can infect fish over a wide range of temperature (8° to 28° C [46° to 82° F]) and salinity (20 to 31 ppt) (Cheung et al., 1980). Unlike other ectoparasitic protozoa, *Uronema* often invades internal organs and causes deep ulcers (Fig. II-24, *B*). Muscle (Fig. II-24, *C*), kidney, liver, spinal cord, and urinary bladder may be affected (Cheung et al., 1980). There is typically little inflammatory response (Fig. II-24, *C*). Fish usually develop white skin foci, which progress to areas of depigmentation and ulceration (Bassler, 1983). Some fish may show no external signs, except lethargy. There may be skin hemorrhage/necrosis and gill aneurysms. Once established in a host, death is swift.

The closely related and morphologically similar *Miamiensis avidus* has only been reported once from nodular lesions on seahorse (Thompson & Moewus, 1964). Both *Uronema* and *Miamiensis* are free-living protozoa and thus may exist in an aquarium without fish. A *Uronema*-like ciliate has caused disease in cultured Japanese flounder and red sea bream in Japan (Yoshinaga & Nakazoe, 1993). Pathology is similar.

Diagnosis

Even if skin lesions are present, skin scrapings may not detect the organisms in wet mounts if they are deep in the tissues. Thus, scraping deep into the muscle or examining tissues histologically may be needed for diagnosis. Unlike *Brooklynella*, *Uronema* is smaller, ellipsoid, and holotrichous (Thompson, 1963). It is also smaller than *Cryptocaryon* and does not incite the typical proliferative nodule present in cryptocaryonosis (see *PROBLEM 20*).

Treatment

Early stages of uronemosis can reportedly be controlled by a freshwater bath followed by prolonged immersion in formalin (Blasiola & Gratzek, 1992). Advanced lesions have reportedly responded to methylene blue or nitrofurazone (Cheung et al., 1980; Bassler, 1983). However, systemic or deep muscle infections probably have a poor prognosis.

PROBLEM 25
Tetrahymenosis *(Tetrahymena* Infestation/Infection, TET Disease, Guppy Disease)

Prevalence Index

WF - 3, CF - 4

Method of Diagnosis

1. Wet mount of skin, gills, or internal organs with parasite
2. Histopathology of skin, gills, or internal organs with parasite

History/Physical Examination

Typical signs of protozoan ectoparasite; also, areas of muscle swelling

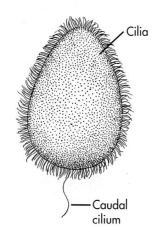

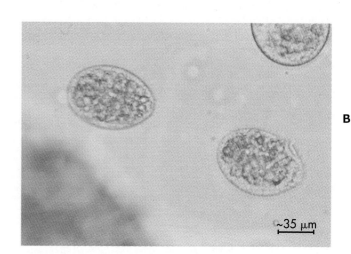

Fig. II-25   A, *Tetrahymena.* Diagram with key characteristics: size (~30 to 60 × 50 to 100 μm); pyriform or radially symmetrical, ovoid body; evenly distributed cilia; long caudal cilium (present only in some species [e.g., *T. corlissi*]). **B,** Wet mount of *Tetrahymena.* Note long cilia covering body. Formalin-fixed specimen.

(B photograph courtesy of G. Hoffman.)

Treatment
1. Formalin bath

COMMENTS
Epidemiology/Pathogenesis
Tetrahymenids (Fig. II-25, *A* and *B*) are typically free-living ciliates, but some species can be highly lethal fish pathogens. In advanced cases, *Tetrahymena* may invade various internal organs, with parasite foci in muscle, kidney, or brain. Reproduction is typically by binary fission; some species (e.g., *T. corlissi*) can produce small reproductive cysts (2 to 8 tomites).

The species most commonly causing disease is *Tetrahymena corlissi*, which can infest/infect fish and amphibians. Called *guppy disease* because of its predilection for guppies, the disorder also affects other livebearers, cichlids, and tetras (Hoffman et al., 1975). Clinical signs are nonspecific, but muscle swelling may be evident grossly (Ferguson, 1988). Guppies can appear normal one day and be dead the next; a mass of ciliates may form a rim around the orbit (*spectacle eye*). In black mollies, *T. corlissi* induces white patches caused by massive numbers of ciliates in copious amounts of mucus (Johnson, 1978).

Tetrahymena pyriformis-like ciliates can damage the skin and invade the internal organs of common carp, catfish (*Ameiurus* sp.), and rainbow trout (Shulman & Jankovski, 1984). Other *Tetrahymena* isolates cause deep ulcerative dermatitis in Atlantic salmon in freshwater (Ferguson et al., 1987).

Diagnosis
The mucus production and epithelial damage caused by *Tetrahymena* may appear grossly similar to ich (see *PROBLEM 19*) but are easily differentiated by identifying the parasite. *Tetrahymena* may be confused with free-living, nonpathogenic ciliates, such as *Paramecium*, which may occasionally be found in low numbers on the skin or gills. Shape, size, movement (like a spiraling football), and presence of typical invasive lesions should be used for differentiation. Penetration of ciliates into muscle and deep tissues is highly diagnostic for *Tetrahymena*.

Treatment
Only cases without systemic disease are treatable and may require several treatments. The environment should also be improved.

PROBLEM 26
Marine Velvet Disease (Amyloodiniosis, Marine Velvet Disease, Marine *Oodinium* Disease, Oodiniosis)
Prevalence Index
WM - 1
Method of Diagnosis
1. Wet mount of skin or gills with parasite
2. Histopathology of skin or gills with parasite

History/Physical Examination
Typical signs of protozoan ectoparasite; also, golden, dust-like sheen ("velvet") on skin
Treatment
1. Copper prolonged immersion
2. Chloroquine diphosphate prolonged immersion
3. Freshwater prolonged immersion

COMMENTS
Epidemiology
Amyloodiniosis is one of the most important diseases of warm water marine fish (Paperna et al., 1981), infesting both food fish and aquarium fish worldwide (Lawler, 1977a). *Amyloodinium ocellatum* is one of the few fish parasites that can infest both elasmobranchs (sharks, rays) and teleosts (Lawler, 1980), and most fish that live within its ecological range are susceptible to infestations. Even freshwater fish, such as centrarchids or tilapia, are susceptible to infestation when they are in brackish water (Lawler, 1980). Species most resistant to infestations tend to produce thick mucus or tolerate low oxygen levels (Lawler, 1977a).
Life Cycle
Amyloodinium is a dinoflagellate that is highly adapted to parasitism; the trophont bears little resemblance to free-living dinoflagellates. Typical dinoflagellate morphology is apparent only during the disseminative (dinospore) stage (Fig. II-26, *A*).

The life cycle is virtually identical to that of *I. multifiliis* (see *PROBLEM 19*). The trophont (Fig. II-26, *A* through *D*) attaches to and feeds on the host's epithelium. After the trophont feeds for several days, it detaches from the host, retracts its rhizoids (root-like structures used to attach to the epithelium), and becomes a tomont. The tomont divides, producing up to 256 (usually 64 or less) motile, infective dinospores (Brown, 1934; Nigrelli, 1936). Dinospores are 8 to 13.5 μm long by 10 to 12.5 μm wide. The dinospores attach to a host, differentiate into a trophont, and continue the cycle.

Environmental Requirements
Optimal temperature for most isolates is 23° to 27° C (73° to 81° F). Tomont division is limited to 16° to 30° C (61° to 86° F) (Paperna, 1984). Infestations do not occur at less than 17° C (63° F) (A. Colorni, Personal Communication). Tomonts stop dividing at low temperatures, but some isolates can produce dinospores when returned to 25° C (77° F), even after 4 months at 15° C (59° F) (C.E. Bower, Personal Communication).

Amyloodiniosis has caused disease in salinities ranging from 3 to 45 ppt. Isolates vary in salinity tolerance. For example, Red Sea isolates do not divide below 12 ppt salinity (Paperna, 1984), while epidemics commonly occur at 3 ppt salinity in the Gulf of Mexico (Lawler, 1977a). Salinity tolerance decreases at suboptimal temperatures.

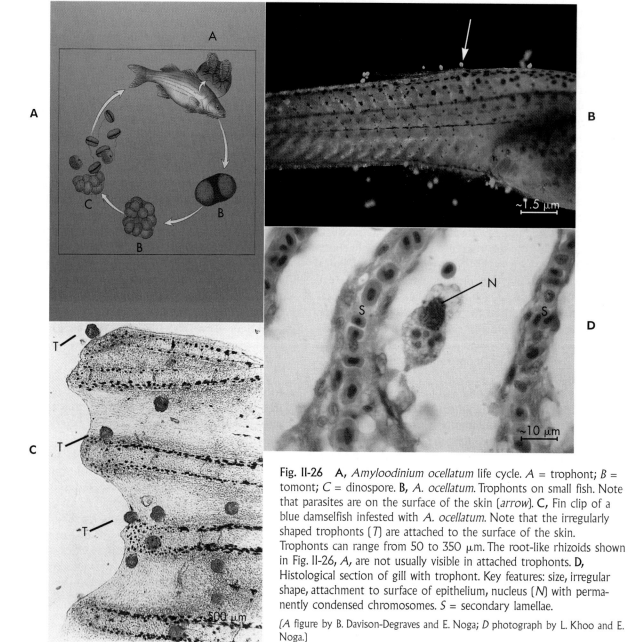

Fig. II-26 **A,** *Amyloodinium ocellatum* life cycle. *A* = trophont; *B* = tomont; *C* = dinospore. **B,** *A. ocellatum.* Trophonts on small fish. Note that parasites are on the surface of the skin (*arrow*). **C,** Fin clip of a blue damselfish infested with *A. ocellatum.* Note that the irregularly shaped trophonts (*T*) are attached to the surface of the skin. Trophonts can range from 50 to 350 μm. The root-like rhizoids shown in Fig. II-26, *A,* are not usually visible in attached trophonts. **D,** Histological section of gill with trophont. Key features: size, irregular shape, attachment to surface of epithelium, nucleus (*N*) with permanently condensed chromosomes. *S* = secondary lamellae.

(*A* figure by B. Davison-Degraves and E. Noga; *D* photograph by L. Khoo and E. Noga.)

Pathogenesis

The gills are usually the primary site of infestation. Heavy infestations may also involve the skin and eyes. Tomonts that are occasionally seen in the gastrointestinal tract (Hojgard, 1962; Brown, 1934) were probably swallowed by the host.

Rhizoids (Fig. II-26, *A*) anchor the parasite to the host cells (Lom & Lawler, 1973). A single trophont can damage and kill several host cells (Lom & Lawler, 1973; Noga, 1987), which probably accounts for the severe injury inflicted on the host by trophonts.

Mild infestations (e.g., 1 to 2 trophonts per gill filament) cause little pathology. However, heavy infesta-tions can cause serious gill hyperplasia, inflammation, hemorrhage, and necrosis. Death can occur within 12 hours (Lawler, 1980). Some acute mortalities are associated with apparently mild infestations, suggesting that hypoxia may not always be the cause of death in all primary gill infestations. Osmoregulatory impairment and secondary microbial infections caused by severe epithelial damage may also be important.

Diagnosis

Gross skin infestation by *Amyloodinium* is most easily seen on dark-colored fish as is also true for freshwater velvet (Fig. II-27, *A*), using indirect illumination, such as by shining a flashlight on top of the fish in a darkened room. Observing fish against a dark background also helps. Heavily infested skin may have a dusty appearance (*velvet disease*); however, this is not a common finding, and fish often die without obvious gross skin lesions.

Definitive diagnosis is easily made by identification of trophonts in biopsies (see Fig. II-26, *C*) or histological sections (see Fig. II-26, *D*). Parasites can also be *brushed* off the surface of heavily infested skin. Trophonts can be dislodged by placing fish in a small (as small as possible) container of freshwater for 1 to 3 minutes (Bower et al., 1987). Trophonts settle to the bottom of the container after 15 to 20 minutes. The parasites can be aspirated from the sediment and identified microscopically. Note that tomonts will also be present, since dislodgement stimulates the trophonts to form tomonts.

RELATED NONPATHOGENIC DINOFLAGELLATES

The closely related *Crepidoodinium* only infests estuarine topminnows (*Fundulus*, *Lucania*, and *Cyprinodon*) in the Gulf of Mexico and the Atlantic Ocean near Virginia, U.S.A. *Crepidoodinium* is not pathogenic but only uses the fish as an attachment site. Trophonts are 670 × 130 μm and green because of the presence of chloroplasts (Lom & Lawler, 1973).

Treatment

Amyloodinium ocellatum is highly virulent and must be treated as soon as it is detected to prevent a catastrophe. The free-swimming dinospore is susceptible to chemotherapy (Paperna, 1984; Lawler, 1980), but trophonts and tomonts are resistant, making eradication difficult. For example, tomonts tolerate copper concentrations that are over 10 times the levels that are toxic to dinospores (Paperna, 1984). Even tomonts inhibited from dividing can often resume dividing when returned to untreated water (Paperna et al., 1981). Treatment with 100 to 200 mg/l formalin for 6 to 9 hours detaches trophonts from fish, but they resume division after removal of formalin (Paperna, 1984). Thus, treatments must be long enough to allow all trophonts and tomonts to form dinospores. Periodic examination for reinfestation after treatment is advisable.

The most widely used treatment is copper (Bower, 1983; Cardeilhac & Whitaker, 1988), which will control outbreaks, but some parasites may remain latent on the fish (C.E. Bower, Unpublished Data). Bower (Personal Communication) discovered that the antimalarial chloroquine diphosphate is safe and effective. It is less toxic than copper and may also eliminate latent infestations, but it is expensive. Many other agents have been tested with little success against amyloodiniosis (Noga & Levy, In Press).

Lowering the temperature to 15° C (59° F) arrests the disease (Paperna, 1984), but this is almost never feasible. Lowering salinity delays but does not prevent infestations (Barbaro & Francescon, 1985), unless fish are

placed in freshwater. A 5-minute freshwater bath dislodges most but not all trophonts (Lawler, 1977a; Kingsford, 1975).

Dinospores can be killed with ultraviolet radiation (Lawler, 1977a). Quarantine of new fish for at least 20 days may reduce but not eliminate the risk of parasite introduction. Dinospores remain infective for at least 6 days at 26° C (79° F) (Bower et al., 1987). There is some evidence that fish may produce an immune response after natural challenge (Smith et al., 1994). Vaccines are being explored (Smith et al., 1993).

PROBLEM 27

Freshwater Velvet Disease (Freshwater Velvet, Rust Disease, Gold Dust Disease, Pillularis Disease, Freshwater *Oodinium*)

Prevalence Index

WF - 2

Method of Diagnosis

1. Wet mount of skin or gills with parasite
2. Histopathology of skin or gills with parasite

History/Physical Examination

Typical signs of protozoan ectoparasite; also, golden, dust-like sheen (*velvet*) on skin

Treatment

1. Salt prolonged immersion

COMMENTS

Epidemiology

Piscinoodinium is the freshwater analogue of *Amyloodinium* (see *PROBLEM 26*). Most reports of the parasite have been on aquarium fish in North America (*P. limneticum*) and Europe (*P. pillulare*), as well as food fish in Malaysia (Shaharom-Harrison et al., 1990; Lom & Schubert, 1983).

Many tropical fish are susceptible to *Piscinoodinium*, with anabantids, cyprinids, and cyprinodontids frequently affected. Temperate species (e.g., common carp, tench) and larval amphibians (*Amblystoma mexicanum*, *Rana temporaria*, and *R. arvalis*) are also susceptible (Geus, 1960).

Life Cycle

The life cycle is the same as for *Amyloodinium* (see Fig. II-26, *A*). Trophonts are yellow-green, pyriform or sac-like, up to 12 × 96 μm. They are almost round when mature (Lom & Schubert, 1983) and somewhat less irregular in texture, compared with *Amyloodinium*. Up to 256 dinospores (10 to 19 μm long × 8 to 15 μm wide in *P. limneticum*) are produced from each tomont. The life cycle may be completed in 10 to 14 days under optimal condition. Optimal temperature for *P. pillulare* is 23° to 25° C (73° to 77° F), with sporulation requiring 50 to 70 hours for an average-sized tomont. At 15° to 17° C (59° to 63° F), sporulation requires 11 days (van Duijn, 1973). Optimal conditions are probably similar for *P. limneticum*.

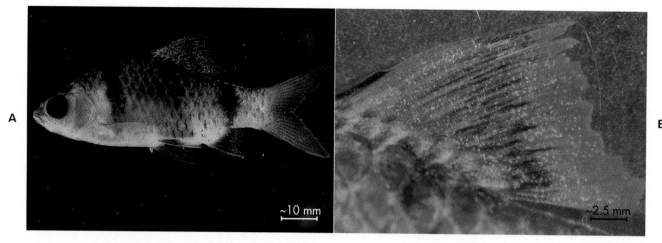

Fig. II-27 A, Infestation of a tiger barb with *P. pillulare*. Note the fine dust-like covering of parasites. B, Close-up of Fig. II-27, A.

Under crowded conditions or in stagnant water, sporulation is inhibited and smaller dinospores are produced. Lower temperature slows the life cycle (Jacobs, 1946).

Pathogenesis

Clinical signs are similar to amyloodiniosis, except that fish can withstand much heavier infestations. The parasite is most pathogenic in young fish that may die within 1 to 2 weeks; older fish may live for months. Heavy infestations (Fig. II-27, A and B) produce a yellow or rusty sheen to the skin when viewed under direct light. There may also be excess mucus, darkening of the skin, dyspnea, anorexia, and/or depression (Shaharom-Harrison et al., 1990). Skin ulcers (Shaharom-Harrison, 1990) and tattered, sloughing epithelium (Schaperclaus, 1951) have been seen in some cases.

Histopathology ranges from separation of the respiratory epithelium to severe hyperplasia of the entire gill filament. Filament degeneration and necrosis may occur. Some parasites may become almost entirely covered by hyperplastic epithelium (Shaharom-Harrison et al., 1990; van Duijn, 1973), probably because of the chronic irritation caused by infestation. Some of these parasites may even sporulate (Geus, 1960).

Diagnosis

Definitive diagnosis is easily made by identification of trophonts in biopsies. Trophonts look almost identical to *Amyloodinium* (see Fig. II-26, A through C).

Treatment

Both species of *Piscinoodinium* are treated the same. The relatively mild pathogenicity of *Piscinoodinium* usually allows ample time to control outbreaks. It is often advisable to raise the temperature to 24° to 27° C (75° to 81° F) to speed up the life cycle during treatment. Leaving aquaria without fish for 2 weeks at this temperature will eliminate the parasites. Dinospores remain infective for only up to 48 hours (Jacobs, 1946; van Duijn, 1973), but ample time must be allowed for

delayed emergence of dinospores from tomonts. Reducing lighting to inhibit autotrophy has also been advocated during treatment (van Duijn, 1973).

The safest and most effective treatment for piscinoodiniosis is prolonged immersion salt (about 1 teaspoon per 5 gallons of water). This is also an effective prophylactic (R. Goldstein, Personal Communication). For heavy, life-threatening infestations, a 35 ppt, 1- to 3-minute salt bath dislodges trophonts.

Copper has been advocated as a treatment (van Duijn, 1973), but its unpredictable toxicity in soft, acid water often makes it dangerous to use, especially since many commonly affected aquarium fish are maintained under those conditions. Heating water to 33° to 34° C (91° to 93° F) reportedly controls infestations (Untergasser, 1989), but some aquarium fish cannot tolerate such high temperatures (see *PROBLEM 2*). Chloroquine diphosphate has not been tested against piscinoodiniosis, but its success with amyloodiniosis suggests that it may be useful.

PROBLEM 28

Ichthyobodosis (Costiosis)

Prevalence Index

WF - 2, CF - 1, CM - 4

Method of Diagnosis

1. Wet mount of skin or gills with parasite
2. Histopathology of skin or gills with parasite

History/Physical Examination

Typical signs of protozoan ectoparasite; especially, drop in temperature; bluish or whitish film on body

Treatment

1. Formalin bath
2. Formalin prolonged immersion
3. Potassium permanganate prolonged immersion
4. Raise temperature > 30° C (86° F)
5. Salt bath (freshwater only)

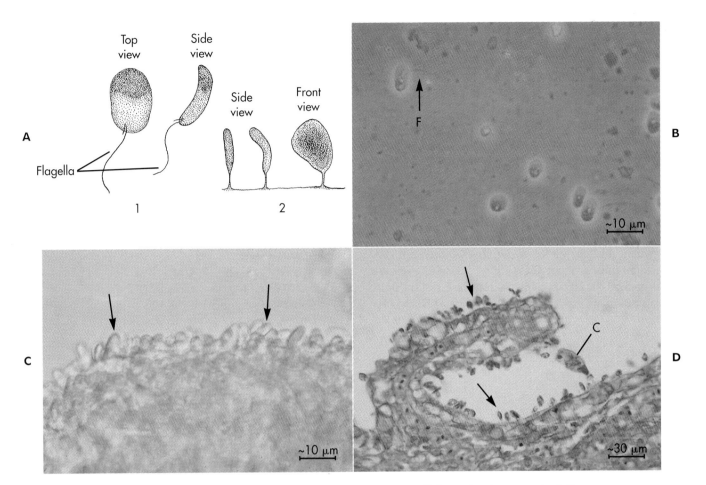

Fig. II-28 **A,** *Ichthyobodo.* Diagrams with key characteristics: (*1*) Free-swimming stage: size (~5 to 8 × 10 to 15 μm), slightly asymmetrical, oval body on top view; flattened, crescent shape on side view; single or paired flagella directed posterolaterally. (*2*) Attached stage: pyriform shape; flagella are not easily seen when attached. **B,** Wet mount of the free-swimming stage of *I. necator.* F = flagellum. **C,** Wet mount of many *Ichthyobodo* (*arrows*) attached to the gill epithelium. **D,** Histological section of gill with a heavy *I. necator* infestation (*arrows*). Note the pyriform, dorsoventrally flattened shape. A larger, unrelated ciliate (*C*) is also present. Giemsa.

(*B* and *C* photographs courtesy of G. Hoffman.)

COMMENTS

Epidemiology

Ichthyobodo necator (previously known as *Costia necatrix*) is one of the smallest ectoparasites that infest fish (about the size of a red blood cell). *Ichthyobodo* is especially dangerous to young fish and can attack healthy fry and even eggs. In older fish it is associated with some type of predisposing stress.

Ichthyobodo necator causes disease over a wide temperature range (2° to 30° C [36° to 86° F]). In warm water fish it is usually a problem in cooler temperatures (< 25° C [77° F]) and is reported to die above 30° C (86° F) (Langdon, 1990). Parasites from cold water fish (e.g., salmonids) have concomitantly lower temperature optima.

While classically a disease of freshwater fish, *I. necator* can survive transfer to saltwater and cause mortality in marine-adapted salmonids (Urawa & Kusakari, 1990). *Ichthyobodo*-like parasites also occur in purely marine fish (Cone & Wiles, 1984; Diamant, 1987; Bokeny et al., 1994; Morrison & Cone, 1986), and there is evidence that marine isolates from flatfish may be a different species of *Ichthyobodo* (Urawa & Kusakari, 1990). *Ichthyobodo*-like flagellates also occur on octopus (Forsythe et al., 1991); it is not known if these can infest fish.

Pathogenesis

Ichthyobodo necator exists in two forms (Joyon & Lom, 1969). The **detached**, mobile form (Fig. II-28, A_1 and B) has two or, if predivisional, four flagella, all of which are difficult to see in actively moving parasites. While the parasite feeds on the fish, it is curled into a pyriform shape and is **attached** to and penetrates the epithelium (Fig. II-28, A_2, C, and D). The transition between forms occurs within a few minutes.

Ichthyobodo can cause considerable mortalities—sometimes with little obvious pathology (Fig. II-28, *D*) but other times with spongiosis and epithelial sloughing. Tissue irritation also leads to epithelial hyperplasia and increased mucus production, giving fish a bluish cast (*slime*).

Diagnosis

Diagnosis is easily made from skin or gill biopsies (Fig. II-28, *B* and *C*). The free-swimming form exhibits a characteristic *flickering* motion when it moves, which is caused by the change of refractility when it turns its crescent-shaped body. Attached parasites are more difficult to detect, but, in heavy infestations, they can be located by focusing up and down at 400X magnification on the edge of the gill epithelium, where they form palisades. They may also be seen slowly swaying while attached.

Small numbers of parasites (e.g., < ~2 per high power field on a gill biopsy) usually do not cause clinical signs. *Ichthyobodo* may quickly leave a dead host, making estimations of parasite numbers in histological sections dif-

ficult. Note that cryptobids (see *PROBLEM 29*) and nonpathogenic, ectocommensal bodonid flagellates may also be found on fish skin and gills; these should not be confused with *Ichthyobodo*.

Treatment

One application of an appropriate treatment usually controls ichthyobodosis, but infestations on euryhaline species may be resistant to salt treatment. *Ichthyobodo* appears to be an obligate parasite.

PROBLEM 29
Gill *Cryptobia* Infestation (Cryptobiosis)

Prevalence Index
WF - 3, WM - 3, CF - 3, CM - 4

Method of Diagnosis
1. Wet mount of gills with parasite
2. Histopathology of gills with parasite

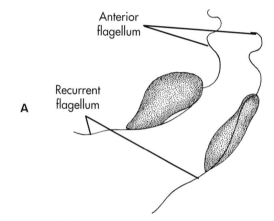

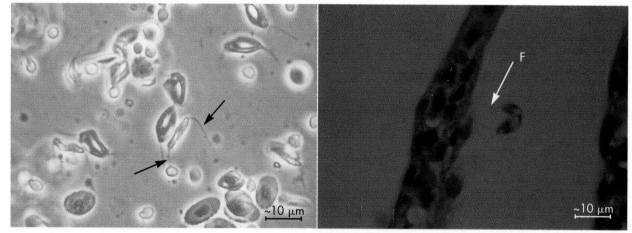

Fig. II-29 **A,** *Cryptobia.* Diagram with key characteristics: size (~10 to 20 × ~3 to 6 μm), pleomorphic shape; two flagella (one directed anteriorly and the other [recurrent flagellum] directed posteriorly). The recurrent flagellum sometimes forms a short, undulating membrane (see *Trypanoplasma*). **B,** Wet mount of *Cryptobia eilatica* from the gills of European sea bass. Note the two flagella (*arrows*), directed anteriorly and posteriorly. **C,** Histological section of two cryptobids from striped bass attached to a gill secondary lamella by their recurrent flagellum (*F*). Hematoxylin and eosin.

[*B* photograph courtesy of A. Diamant; *C* photograph by L. Khoo and E. Noga.]

History/Physical Examination

Typical signs of protozoan gill ectoparasite; especially emaciation, anorexia

Treatment

1. Formalin bath
2. Formalin prolonged immersion

COMMENTS

Epidemiology/Pathogenesis

Cryptobia is a widely distributed group of 10 species of kinetoplastid flagellates that can colonize many freshwater or marine fish. They are weak pathogens. One of the most common species is *Cryptobia branchialis*, a drop-shaped (12 to 22 × 3.5 to 4.5 μm) bacteriovore common in polluted fresh or marine waters.

Diagnosis

Cryptobia is distinguished from the morphologically similar *Trypanoplasma* (see *PROBLEM 43*) by its less developed undulating membrane and its tissue predilection (gill or gastrointestinal tract; see *PROB-* *LEMS 43* and *71*). Taxonomically related nonpathogenic, ectocommensal, bodonid flagellates occasionally inhabit the gills. *Cryptobia* is differentiated from *Ichthyobodo* (see *PROBLEM 28*) by its morphology, flowing, amoeboid motility; and relatively superficial attachment to gill tissue via its recurrent flagellum (Fig. II-29, *A*, *B*, and *C*).

Treatment

Gill cryptobids are easily treated with formalin, but eliminating the culpable stress will often allow spontaneous recovery.

PROBLEM 30
Gill Amoebic Infestations

Prevalence Index
CF - 4, CM - 4

Method of Diagnosis
1. Wet mount of gills with parasite
2. Histopathology of gills with parasite

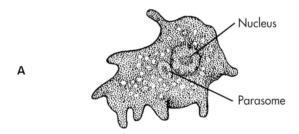

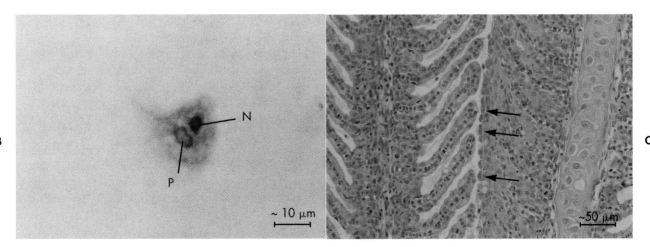

Fig. II-30 **A,** *Paramoeba pemaquidensis.* Diagram with key characteristics: size (~25 μm), nucleus, parasome. **B,** Stained smear of *Paramoeba.* Note the nucleus (*N*) and parasome (*P*). Feulgen stain. **C,** Histological section of cochliopodid amoeba (*arrows*) on the gills of a rainbow trout. Hematoxylin and eosin.

[*B* photograph courtesy of M. Kent; *C* photograph by L. Khoo and E. Noga.]

History/Physical Examination
Typical signs of protozoan gill ectoparasite
Treatment
1. Transfer to < 10 ppt seawater (*Paramoeba* only)
2. Freshwater bath for 3 hours (*Paramoeba* only)
3. Formalin bath (cochliopodid only)

COMMENTS
Epidemiology/Pathogenesis
Amoebae have been rarely reported as infestations of the gills of salmonids.

PARAMOEBA
Paramoeba pemaquidensis has caused chronic mortality (up to 2% per day) in sea cages in the western United States, Canada, and Tasmania, Australia (Kent, 1992). Severity increases with temperature, with disease occurring above 15° C (59° F).

Paramoeba (Fig. II-30, *A* and *B*) causes proliferative gill lesions. Crowding, poor water exchange, cage fouling, and previous gill damage appear to be risk factors (Kent et al., 1988b). Outbreaks typically occur in the first summer after transfer of fish from freshwater to sea cages. Clinically affected fish develop elevated serum sodium levels before the onset of behavioral signs, which may allow early detection of the disease (Munday, 1988).

Histopathologically, there is focal lamellar hypertrophy with epithelial hyperplasia and metaplasia. There is a primary focal neutrophilic, then mononuclear infiltrate. Recovery, especially in rainbow trout, is characterized by focal lymphoid nodules at the base of the secondary lamellae.

COCHLIOPODID AMOEBA
Cochliopodid amoebae (Fig. II-30, *C*) have incited proliferative responses in rainbow trout that may appear as grossly visible nodular gill masses (*nodular gill disease*) in the United States, Canada, and Germany (Daoust & Ferguson, 1985; J. Lom, Personal Communication); in some cases, cochliopodid infestations have developed after fish were treated for bacterial gill disease (A. Noble, Personal Communication; Bullock et al., 1994).

Diagnosis
All amoebae are best diagnosed by examining them in wet mounts. In many cases, this is mandatory for identification.

PARAMOEBA
Wet mounts reveal free-floating amoebae with digitiform pseudopodia. Amoebae will attach to the slide within an hour, allowing observation of the parasome. Fixation and Fuelgen-staining also reveals the parasome (Fig. II-30, *B*). Amoebae remain best attached with Bouin's or Davidson's fixative and have a hyaline ectoplasm fringing the granuloplasm.

COCHLIOPODID AMOEBA
Presumptive identification is based on the presence of amoebae forming palisades on gill lamellae (Fig. II-30,

C). On Bouin's fixed smears, the nucleus has an unusual heterochromatin pattern that resembles *Schizamoeba*, which was previously identified from rainbow trout stomach (T. Sawyer, Personal Communication). Definitive identification awaits further studies.

Treatment
Paramoeba seems somewhat resistant to formalin (and other common ectoparasiticides) and effective formalin treatment requires high concentrations for long periods. The best treatment is to transfer fish to brackish water, which probably not only kills the amoebae, but also reduces the osmotic stress from gill damage. Some fish, especially rainbow trout, appear to develop resistance to reinfection after a single exposure.

The amoebae associated with nodular gill disease are susceptible to a formalin bath (A. Noble, Personal Communication).

PROBLEM 31
Sessile, Solitary, Ectocommensal Ciliate Infestations
Prevalence Index
WF - 1, CF - 2
Method of Diagnosis
1. Wet mount of skin or gills with parasite
2. Histopathology of skin or gills with parasite
History/Physical Examination
Typical signs of protozoan ectoparasite; also, organically polluted water
Treatment
1. Formalin bath
2. Formalin prolonged immersion
3. Copper prolonged immersion

COMMENTS
Epidemiology/Pathogenesis
The sessile, solitary, ectocommensal ciliates *Apiosoma*, *Riboscyphidia*, and *Ambiphrya* attach to the skin or gills with a holdfast (scopula, Fig. II-31, *A₁*, *A₂*, *A₃*, *B*, and *C*) (Lom, 1973b). Attachment apparently causes only superficial damage to the epithelium (Lom & Corliss, 1968), which belies the ectocommensal nature of these organisms. Like the sessile, colonial ectommensals (see *PROBLEM 32*), they reproduce by binary fission and use the host primarily for attachment. They derive little, if any, nutrition directly from the fish. They feed on bacteria and suspended organic debris, which is prevalent in nutrient-rich (i.e., polluted) water. Thus, they are good indicators of poor water quality. Many of these ciliates can probably be free-living. They are only moderately pathogenic, but high numbers on the gills can physically impede gas exchange. They may also act as a nidus for bacterial colonization.

Capriniana piscium (formerly *Trichophrya*) is a common suctorian ciliate that commonly infests gills of channel catfish, among other species (Fig. II-31, A_4). It has no cilia when attached to fish; instead, it has characteristic tentacles that emanate from an amorphous body (Fig. II-31, *D* and *E*). Attachment probably causes little damage to the epithelium, but heavy infestations can cause mechanical blockage of respiration. *Capriniana* feeds on ciliates and suspended organic debris. *Capriniana* is not taxonomically related to *Apiosoma*, *Riboscyphidia*, or *Ambiphrya* and reproduces by budding, forming motile, ciliated stages that can colonize a new host (Lee et al., 1985).

Diagnosis
Diagnosis is easily made from wet mounts or histology. Identification to species is not needed, since all members of the same genus are treated similarly.

Treatment
Like the sessile, colonial, ectocommensal ciliates (see *PROBLEM 32*), medical treatment should always be accompanied by an improved environment. Treatment with formalin is usually effective for freshwater species of *Apiosoma*, *Riboscyphidia*, and *Ambiphrya*. Treatments for marine pathogens have not been established, but they probably respond to similar remedies. *Capriniana* can be resistant to formalin and should be treated with copper.

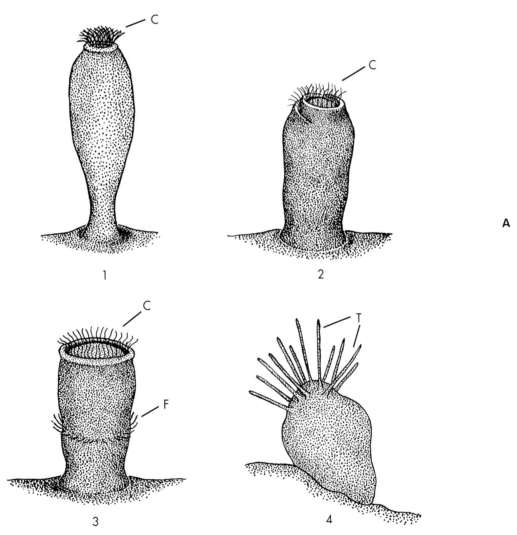

Fig. II-31   A, Sessile, solitary, ectocommensal ciliates. Diagrams with key characteristics (*C* = cilia). Most range from ~40 to 100 μm. All except *Capriniana* may occur on skin or gills:
1. *Apiosoma* (66 species); elongated body; only oral cilia; freshwater
2. *Riboscyphidia* (~18 species): cylindrical to conical body; only oral cilia; freshwater or marine
3. *Ambiphrya* (4 species): cylindrical to conical body; oral cilia; permanent, motionless, equatorial, ciliary fringe (F); freshwater
4. *Capriniana piscium*: variable size (usually 40 to 110 × 25 to 70 μm); pleomorphic shape; feeding tubes (T); body adhered to secondary lamella of gill

Continued.

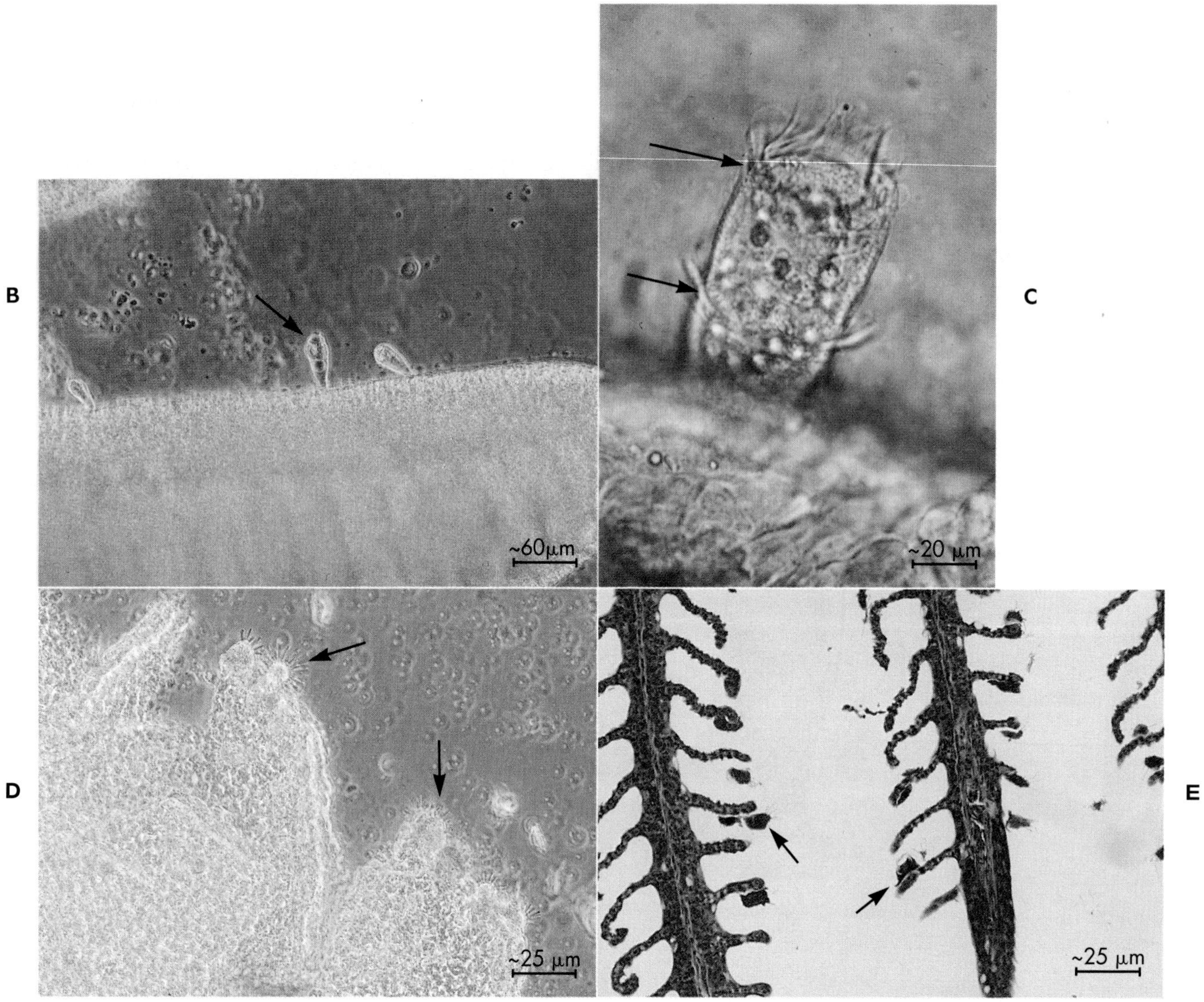

Fig. II-31—cont'd. **B,** Wet mount of *Apiosoma* (formerly *Glossatella*) infestation (*arrow*). Note the vase shape. **C,** Wet mount of *Ambiphrya* (formerly *Scyphidia*). Note the oral and aboral cilia (*arrows*). **D,** Wet mount of *Capriniana piscium* (*arrows*). Note the feeding tubes. **E,** Histological section of *Capriniana piscium* (*arrows*). Note the feeding tubes protruding from parasites that have adhered to base of secondary lamella. Hematoxylin and eosin.

(*B* photograph courtesy of A. Colorni.)

PROBLEM 32
Sessile, Colonial, Ectocommensal Ciliate Infestations (Red-Sore Disease)

Prevalence Index
WF - 1, CF - 4
Method of Diagnosis
1. Wet mount of skin or gills with parasite
2. Histopathology of skin or gills with parasite
History/Physical Examination
Typical signs of protozoan ectoparasite; also, various-sized amorphous masses on the skin, in mouth, or on gill arches; organically polluted water

Treatment
1. Formalin bath
2. Formalin prolonged immersion
3. Potassium permanganate prolonged immersion
4. Salt bath weekly × 3
5. Salt prolonged immersion

COMMENTS
Epidemiology/Life Cycle
Epistylis is the most common and pathogenic type of sessile, colonial ectocommensal ciliate. It is commonly associated with a mixed infection of gram-negative bacteria known as red-sore disease (Esch et al., 1978). This bac-

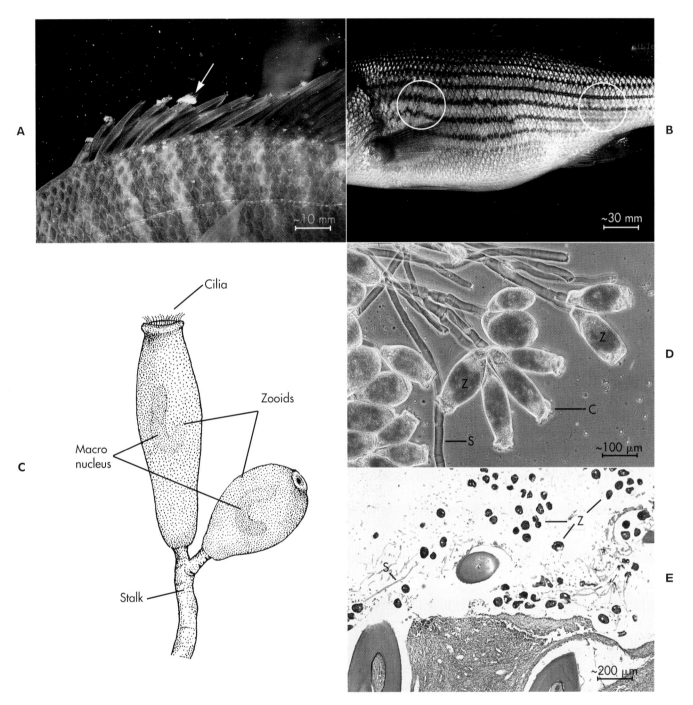

Fig. II-32 **A,** *Epistylis* infestation on the dorsal fin of a bluegill (*arrow*). **B,** *Epistylis* infestation on the skin of a striped bass (*circles*). **C,** *Epistylis*. Diagram with the following key characteristics: size of individual zooids (150 to 300 × 40 to 60 μm or 50 to 80 × 20 to 30 μm), cilia surrounding the mouth; stalk connecting zooids. **D,** *Epistylis*. Wet mount of a skin scraping: *Z* = zooids; *C* = cilia; *S* = stalk. **E,** *Epistylis*. Skin lesion with zooids (*Z*). *S* = stalk. Hematoxylin and eosin.

(*A* photograph by S. Smith and E. Noga.)

teria-parasite complex is common in pond-raised fish in the southern United States and elsewhere, especially during warmer months. Centrarchids, ictalurids, *Morone* spp., and many other fish are susceptible.

Stalked ectocommensal ciliates reproduce by binary fission along the longitudinal axis. To move to another site, the zooid in the colony transforms into a disc-shaped telotroch with equatorial cilia for locomotion. Like other ectocommensal protozoa (see *PROBLEM 31*), these organisms feed on bacteria and other small food items present in the water. They use the fish as a surface for attaching. Thus, their presence is indicative of organically polluted water that would tend to have a high concentration of bacteria. *Epistylis* can be free-living (W. Rogers, Personal Communication), but such species can only colonize severely debilitated fish (J. Lom, Personal Communication). Most *Epistylis* infestations are caused by species that are more adapted to feeding on fish. One species of *Epistylis* was transferred by some investigators into the genus *Heteropolaria* (Foissner et al., 1985).

Pathogenesis

Epistylis produces white or hemorrhagic lesions (*red-sores*) on the flanks or on the tips of bony prominences, such as the fins (Figs. II-32, *A* and *B*), jaws, or gill cover. They may also infect the oral cavity or gills. They must attach to a hard surface and thus anchor to some calcified tissue (e.g., fin ray, scale). The skin is ulcerated wherever they are attached and lesions always have bacterial infections, especially aeromonads and other gram-negative rods (Esch et al., 1976) (see *PROBLEM 45*). Red-sore lesions may become secondarily invaded by water molds. Gross lesions may also look similar to water mold infections (see *PROBLEM 33*). Lesions tend to be chronic, but acute mortalities can occur, usually caused by systemic bacterial infection.

Diagnosis

Typical stalked, noncontractile zooids are diagnostic (Fig. II-32, *C, D,* and *E*). *Epistylis* zooids have a C-shaped macronucleus and should not be mistaken for ich trophonts (see *PROBLEM 19*) or trichodinids (see *PROBLEM 21*) when they are detached from their colonies. The colony stalk without zooids should not be mistaken for fungal hyphae. Several other colonial peritrichs rarely colonize debilitated fish: the stalks of *Vorticella*, *Zoothamnium*, and *Carchesium* are contractile, and either unbranched with a single zooid or branched, bearing many zooids (Lom & Dykova, 1992).

Treatment

Epistylis infestations are occasionally resistant to formalin; salt baths (Foissner et al., 1985) or prolonged salt exposure is usually effective, if tolerated by the fish. Advanced cases may need to be treated for systemic bacterial infections. Other stalked ectocommensals from freshwater fish probably respond to the treatments listed. Marine ectocommensals are probably susceptible to formalin or a freshwater bath.

PROBLEM 33
Typical Water Mold Infection (Saprolegniosis, Oomycete Infection)

Prevalence Index
WF - 1, CF - 1

Method of Diagnosis
Wet mount of skin or gills having broad (7 to 30 μm), nonseptate hyphae

History/Physical Examination
White, brown, red, or green cottony mass on skin or gills (slimy glistening mass when fish is out of water); acute stress, especially temperature drop, recent transport, or trauma

Treatment
1. Salt prolonged immersion
2. Malachite green bath
3. Malachite green prolonged immersion
4. Malachite green flush
5. Malachite green constant flow
6. Malachite green swab
7. Formalin bath
8. Methylene blue prolonged immersion (eggs only)
9. Hydrogen peroxide bath (eggs only)

COMMENTS
Epidemiology

Water molds (Class Oomycetes) are by far the most common fungal infections of freshwater fish and are increasingly recognized as important pathogens of estuarine fish (see *PROBLEM 34*); they are distributed worldwide. Virtually every freshwater fish is probably susceptible to at least one species. The Class Oomycetes is divided into four orders, three of which have species that can infect fish (Saprolegniales, Leptomitales, and Peronosporales). The great majority of fish pathogens are in the Family Saprolegniaceae (Saprolegniales). Some Oomycetes can infect amphibians; others are important pathogens of aquatic invertebrates.

Water molds are classical opportunists that normally feed saprophytically on dead organic matter. As in other animals, there is increasing evidence that fungal infections in fish are associated with immunosuppression. Outbreaks often occur after a drop in temperature or when temperatures are near the physiological low end for a particular fish species (Roberts, 1989c). This may be due not only to lower immunity, but also because many Oomycetes are more active in the cooler months of the year (Hughes, 1962). Skin wounds caused by mechanical trauma or other pathogens provide a portal of entry for water molds (Tiffney, 1939a; Scott & O'Bier, 1962). Handling, crowding, heavy feeding rates, and high organic loads also appear to increase the risk of saprolegniosis.

Most lesions are caused by *Saprolegnia* (which is why the disease is called saprolegniosis), but other Oomycetes cause a clinically identical disease. There may be primarily parasitic strains of water molds. For example, *Saprolegnia parasitica* appears to be highly pathogenic, while *Pythium* and *Leptomitus* are only weakly pathogenic (Scott & O'Bier, 1962). Of all the Oomycetes, *Saprolegnia parasitica* and *S. diclina* are probably the two species most commonly isolated from fish; they are closely related to each other and are often referred to as the *S. diclina-S. parasitica* complex (Neish & Hughes, 1980; Noga, 1993b). Most studies of this complex have involved salmonids. More than one pathogen may occur in lesions (Pickering & Willoughby, 1977).

Transmission

Water molds are ubiquitous saprophytes in soil and freshwater. They are appropriately named, requiring water for growth and sporulation; this differentiates them from most terrestrial fungi that can produce aerial spores. Most transmission is probably by motile zoospores (Fig. II-33, *A*) produced by the vegetative hyphae, although other reproductive stages (e.g., gemma) may also be important. The zoospore allows dissemination to distant sites. It is important to realize that most fish infections are probably acquired from inanimate sources (i.e., fungi sporulating on dead organic matter).

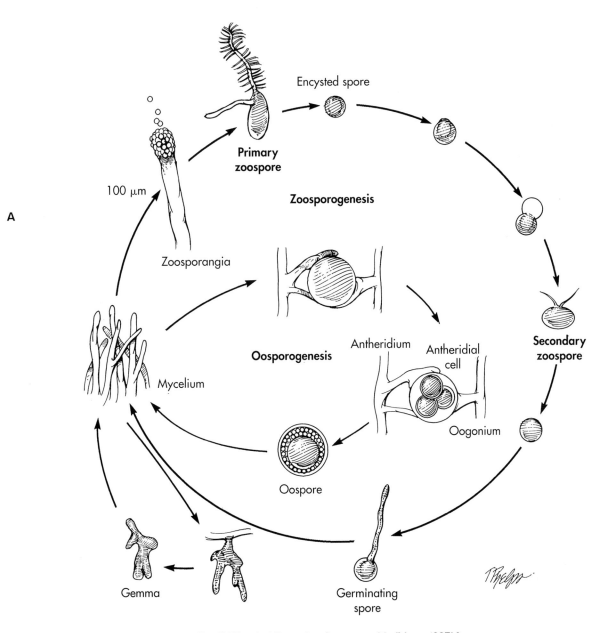

Fig. II-33   **A,** Life cycle of water molds (Noga, 1993b).

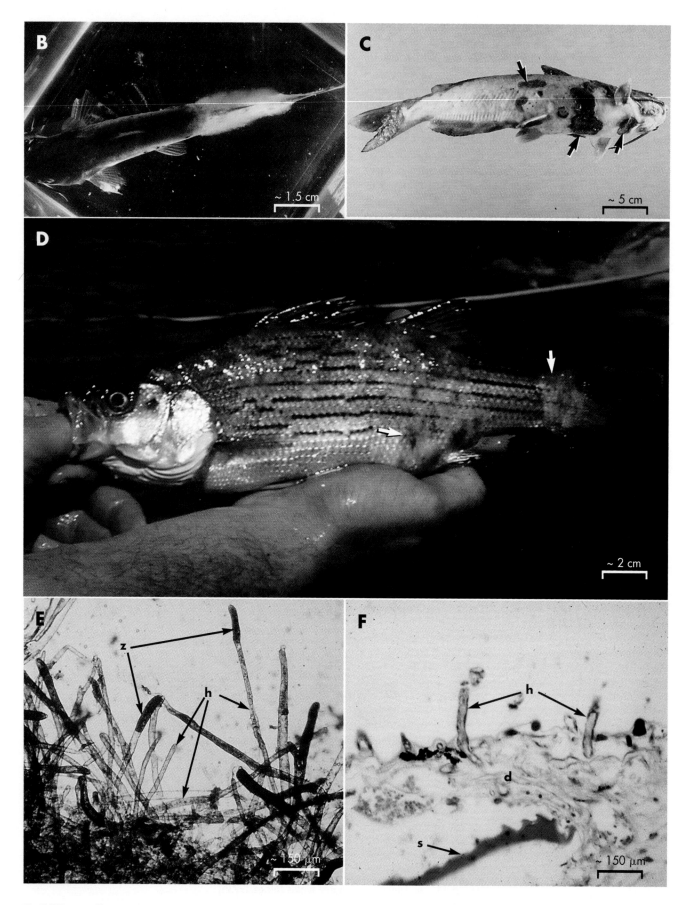

Fig II-33—cont'd. *For legend see opposite page.*

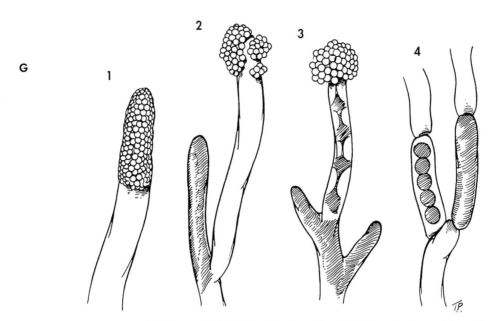

Fig. II-33—cont'd.   B, Water mold infection of a channel catfish. Note the large, white, cottony mass of fungus and the loss of normal black pigment over the infected skin. C, Water mold infection of a channel catfish with winter kill. The fungal mycelium (*arrows*) is brown because of trapping of debris. D, Water mold infection (*arrows*) of a hybrid striped bass. Note the glistening, matted appearance compared to Fig. II-33, *B*. The fungal mycelia are darker because of the trapped debris. E, Wet mount from a water mold infection. Broad, nonseptate hyphae (*H*). Zoosporangia (*Z*) are not always present in wet mounts of lesions. F, Histological section of a water mold infection of skin. Note the absence of epithelium, the superficial nature of the lesion, and the lack of inflammation. *H* = hypha; *S* = scale; *D* = dermis. Hematoxylin and eosin. G, Zoosporangia of some fish-pathogenic Oomycetes. *1, Saprolagnia. 2, Achlya. 3, Aphanomyces. 4, Leptolegnia* (Noga, 1993a).

[*B* photograph by R. Bullis and E. Noga; *E* photograph courtesy of A. Colorni.]

Pathogenesis

Typical water mold infection presents as a relatively superficial, cottony growth on the skin or gills (Fig. II-33, *B*). Such lesions usually begin as small, focal infections that can rapidly spread over the surface of the body. It is not unusual for large lesions to suddenly appear within 24 hours. Newly formed lesions are white due to the presence of the mycelia; with time, the lesions often become colored red, brown, or green because of the trapping of sediment, algae, or debris in the mycelial mat (Fig. II-33, *C*). If the water mold is observed on a fish removed from the water, the mycelium appears as a slimy, matted mass on the body (Fig. II-33, *D*).

Although they grow rapidly over the skin's surface, typical water mold infections rarely penetrate beyond the superficial muscle layers (Fig. II-33, *F*). Superficial damage to the skin or gills can be fatal. Loss of serum electrolytes and protein is proportional to the percentage of skin affected (Richards & Pickering, 1979). Thus, morbidity and mortality increase as the amount of affected skin or gill tissue increases. With acute lesions, fish usually die within several days or recover within several weeks.

Oomycetes are important pathogens of fish eggs (see *PROBLEM 93*). Infections most often begin in unfertilized or otherwise nonviable eggs. Once established, they can rapidly spread to healthy eggs, eventually resulting in complete loss of the brood. Oomycetes rarely infect the gastrointestinal tract of small fry and may penetrate into the viscera.

WINTER KILL

Winter kill is an idiopathic disease that often has a prominent fungal component (Fig. II-33, *C*). Clinical signs include endophthalmia; a *dry*, mucus-depleted skin; and focal water mold infections (Durborow & Crosby, 1988). The disease occurs when pond temperatures drop below 15° C (59° F) and often after a cold front has rapidly dropped the temperature. The disease may be caused by immunosuppression because of the rapid temperature drop, possibly in combination with chronically high ammonia levels or exposure to some environmental stress in the prior summer/fall.

Diagnosis

Observation of a cottony, proliferative growth on the skin or gills should alert the clinician to a possible diagnosis of typical water mold infection. Some other pathogens (e.g., *Flavobacterium, Epistylis*) can cause grossly similar lesions but are easily differentiated microscopically.

Clinical diagnosis of typical water mold infection is easily made from wet mounts, which have broad, aseptate, fungal hyphae of variable width (~7 to 30 μm) (Fig. II-33, *E*). Histologically, presumptive diagnosis of saprolegniosis is based upon the presence of relatively shallow lesions that have broad, aseptate hyphae. Hyphae are usually visible with hematoxylin and eosin stain (H&E) and stain strongly with silver (e.g., Gomori methenamine silver, Fig. II-34, *D*). There is little inflammation, and the fungi usually do not extend past the superficial muscle layers.

Diagnosis requires that affected fish be alive when examined, because water molds are ubiquitous saprophytes in soil, freshwater and, to some extent, estuarine environments; dead fish are fertile substrates for colonization. Oomycetes are also common secondary invaders of wounds initiated by other pathogens (e.g., bacteria, parasites). In summary, the clinician should always look for other initiating causes when water molds are identified in a lesion.

IDENTIFICATION OF SPECIFIC WATER MOLDS
Presumptive diagnosis (i.e., identification of broad, aseptate, fungal hyphae in skin or gill lesions) is sufficient for clinical treatment decisions. Oomycetes vary in drug susceptibility in vitro, but the lack of similar data on clinical response to various drugs has made these differences academic. However, determining the type of oomycete involved will become a more important consideration as various therapies are compared in clinical situations.

Determining that a fungal organism is an oomycete requires the observation of asexual sporangia. Asexual sporangia also allow classification to genus (Fig. II-33, *G*). While sporangia are seen occasionally on infected fish (Fig. II-33, *E*), a culture is usually required to elicit these structures. Identification to species is based on sexual stages (Figs. II-33, *A*). Many isolates will not produce sexual stages in culture. See p. 35 for details about isolation of water molds from lesions. Details of culture methodology and induction of reproductive stages are provided in Fuller and Jaworski (1987). Immunological methods also hold promise as future diagnostic tools (Bullis et al., 1990).

IMPORTANCE OF WATER MOLDS IN THE CASE
A diagnosis of saprolegniosis should always include a thorough search for underlying predisposing factors.

Treatment
PROGNOSIS
The chance of recovery from saprolegniosis is directly related to the amount of skin or gill infected by fungus. While mildly infected fish have a good chance of recovery with proper management, fish with large areas covered by fungus (e.g., Fig. II-33, *B* through *D*) usually die. Prophylactic antibiotics may be needed to combat secondary bacterial infections.

TREATMENT OPTIONS
Water molds are among the most difficult diseases to treat. Except for salt, agents legally approved for food fish (Schnick et al., 1986) are of limited effectiveness. Malachite green is the most effective agent for treating water mold infections in fish, but it is not approved for food fish use in many countries because of its teratogenic and mutagenic properties.

None of the hundreds of other agents that have been tested against Oomycetes are as efficacious as malachite green (Bailey, 1984; Alderman & Polglase, 1984; Scott & Warren, 1964; Olah & Farkas, 1978; Bailey & Jeffrey, 1989). While there are species differences in the tolerance to antifungal agents (e.g., *Saprolegnia* is usually more resistant than *Aphanomyces*), whether these are clinically relevant differences is unknown.

Most fish-pathogenic water molds are inhibited by even low prolonged immersion salt concentrations (> 3 ppt), which is probably why they do not affect marine fish in high salinities (see *PROBLEM 34*). Prolonged immersion salt also helps to counteract osmotic stress caused by skin damage and subsequent ion loss. Unfortunately, prolonged immersion salt is impractical in most commercial production situations.

PROPHYLAXIS
Because of the acute, fulminating nature of many oomycete infections and their resistance to chemotherapy, prophylaxis is the best strategy. Avoid skin damage and predisposing stresses. Prolonged immersion salt is an effective prophylactic when transporting fish or acclimating them to a new environment. Water molds cannot be eliminated from any culture systems.

PROBLEM 34
Atypical Water Mold Infection (Ulcerative Mycosis, UM, Red-Spot Disease, RSD, Epizootic Ulcerative Syndrome, EUS)
Prevalence Index
WF - 3
Method of Diagnosis
1. Culture of water mold from typical ulcers
2. Histology of skin or gills having broad (7 to 20 μm), nonseptate hyphae with typical ulcers
3. Wet mount of skin or gills having broad (7 to 20 μm), nonseptate hyphae with typical ulcers
History/Physical Examination
Shallow to deep skin ulcers
Treatment
None proven

COMMENTS
Epidemiology

Atypical water mold infection differs from typical water mold infection (see *PROBLEM 33*) in being an extremely deep, penetrating lesion (Fig. II-34, *A* and *B*; compare with Fig. II-33, *B*). While atypical water mold infection is less common than typical water mold infection, it is a serious disease in some areas (Frerichs et al., 1986).

Atypical water mold infection occurs in numerous estuarine and freshwater fish populations worldwide (Table II-34). The disease is a problem in wild, estuarine fish populations of the western Atlantic Ocean (Noga, 1990). In the Australo-Pacific and in southern Asia, it is considered by some to be the most important disease affecting cultured fish (Frerichs et al., 1986). Atypical water mold infections have also been rarely seen in some freshwater aquarium fish (Wada et al., 1994).

Morbidity and mortality can be high, and epidemics can develop rapidly. Interestingly, once an epidemic has occurred in an area, the prevalence and severity of future outbreaks often subside (Roberts, 1989b).

Clinical Signs/Pathogenesis

The two most characteristic features of atypical water mold infections are first, the frequently deep, extremely aggressive ulcers that often penetrate into the body cavity (Fig. II-34, *A* and *B*) and second, the severe chronic inflammation that is largely directed at the fungal component (Fig. II-34, *C*). Neither of these features is characteristic of typical water mold infections (see *PROBLEM 33*).

Some lesions are small (~5 mm) foci of reddening on the skin, but many are large, deep, necrotic ulcers up to 25 mm in diameter. When the lesions are examined early in an epidemic, they often contain white, friable material that usually has numerous hyphae interspersed within necrotic muscle. Eventually, the necrotic, fungus-infected tissue sloughs, leaving a crater-shaped cavity that is surrounded by dark red-to-white colored muscle. *Aphanomyces* is the water mold most commonly isolated

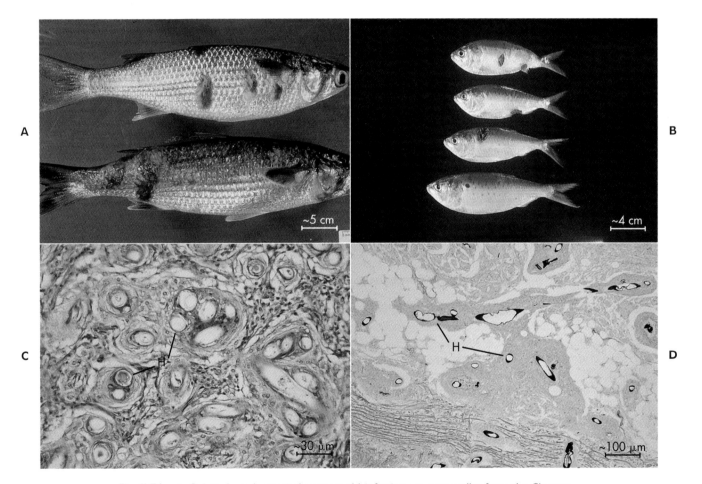

Fig. II-34   A, Relatively early, atypical water mold infection on grey mullet from the Clarence River, Australia. **B,** Advanced atypical water mold infection on Atlantic menhaden from Pamlico River, U.S.A. **C,** Histological section of an atypical water mold infection showing chronic inflammatory response to broad, aseptate hyphae (*H*). Hematoxylin and eosin. **D,** Silver stain of atypical water mold lesion. *H* = hyphae. Gomori methenamine silver.

Table II-34 Fish species most commonly affected by atypical water mold infections.

Disease	Geographic range	Primary host range	References
Red spot (Bundaberg disease; Australian epizootic ulcerative syndrome)	Australia, New Guinea	Barramundi; grey mullet; yellowfin bream; luderick; grunters (Teraponidae); rainbowfish (Melanotaenidae)	McKenzie & Hall, 1972 Callinan, 1988 Pearce (undated) Fraser et al., 1992
Asian epizootic ulcerative syndrome (EUS)	Malaysia, Indonesia, Thailand, Burma, Laos, Sri Lanka, India	Snakeheads; clariid catfishes; gouramies	Roberts et al., 1986 Chinabut & Limsuan, 1983 Roberts et al., 1993
Ulcerative mycosis (UM)	Western Atlantic (United States)	Atlantic menhaden; southern flounder; striped bass; sciaenids (sea trout, silver perch, spot, others); gizzard shad	Noga, 1993b
Mycotic granulomatosis (MG)	Japan	Goldfish; ayu; bluegill	Miyazaki & Egusa, 1972 Hatai et al., 1984 Grier & Quintero, 1987 Dykstra et al., 1989

From Noga, 1993b.

from lesions, but other water molds have also been cultured (Noga, 1993). Numerous bacteria are also usually present, especially aeromonads or vibrios (Noga & Dykstra, 1986; Roberts et al., 1986).

Diagnosis

PRESUMPTIVE DIAGNOSIS

A presumptive diagnosis of atypical water mold infection is based on the presence of deep skin ulcers that contain broad (at least 7 μm in diameter), aseptate hyphae that usually incite severe, chronic inflammation (Fig. II-34, C). Inflammatory cells are often seen surrounding the hyphae in wet mounts. In histological sections, hyphae may be difficult to see with hematoxylin and eosin but can be seen easily with silver stains (e.g., Gomori's methenamine silver) (Fig. II-34, D).

Other fungi can also cause chronic ulcers in fish, and this type of response is common in other deep mycoses (see *PROBLEM 68*). Other fungal infections can be differentiated from atypical water mold infection on the basis of hyphal size and color and on the presence of septa. *Ichthyophonus* hyphae (see *PROBLEM 67*) have similar morphology, but other developmental stages (e.g., cysts) are usually also present. Oomycetes can also be identified ultrastructurally because their tubular mitochondrial cristae differentiate them from all other broad, aseptate fungi, which have plate-like cristae (Dykstra et al., 1986).

DEFINITIVE DIAGNOSIS

Definitive diagnosis is based on culture of water mold fungi from lesions. Culture is best accomplished by using a nutrient-poor medium, such as corn meal agar or YpSs agar (Seymour & Fuller, 1987), which tends to reduce the growth of bacterial contaminants. Culturing Oomycetes from atypical water mold lesions is especially difficult because of the many bacteria also present in lesions. In heavily contaminated lesions, adding penicillin (about 500 U/ml) and/or streptomycin (about 0.2 μg/ml) may improve yields; however, *Aphanomyces*, which is the most common oomycete in atypical water mold lesions, is inhibited by antibiotics.

CAUSES OF INFECTION

While atypical water mold infection can be diagnosed as a *disease* by confirming that a water mold is present, the primary *cause* of the ulcers is unknown in many cases. While the fungi and bacteria present in lesions probably play an important role in killing fish, they are probably not responsible for initiating many of the lesions. There is strong evidence that skin damage caused by a toxic dinoflagellate, *Pfeisteria piscicida* (see *PROBLEM 85*), has been linked to atypical water mold infection in Atlantic coast estuarine fish (Noga et al., In Press). The cause(s) of the clinically similar red-spot and EUS is unknown, although there is evidence for some agent being spread; this disease complex appears to have spread from the Australo-Pacific region to now encompass most of southern Asia (Noga, 1993b).

Treatment

There is no known treatment for atypical water mold infection. While various medications (antibiotics to antiseptics) have been used, there is no evidence for their efficacy. In Thailand, EUS is empirically treated by "improving water quality" by either: (1) adding 60 to 100 kg of lime/1600 m² and repeating this treatment after 3 weeks; or (2) adding 200 to 300 kg of salt/1600 m² (K. Tonguthai, Personal Communication). Avoiding exposure to *Pfeisteria piscicida* is advisable for fish that are at risk of exposure to this organism in Atlantic coast estuaries.

PROBLEM 35
Branchiomycosis (*Branchiomyces* Infection, Gill Rot)

Prevalence Index
Not reported in species listed
Method of Diagnosis
1. Histology of gills with *Branchiomyces*
2. Wet mount of gills with *Branchiomyces*
History/Physical Examination
Necrotic gill lesions
Treatment
No known treatment

COMMENTS
Epidemiology
Branchiomycosis is a fungal disease that has caused acute, often high, mortality in several freshwater fish, including American eel, European eel, boyeri atherinid, largemouth bass, smallmouth bass, pumpkinseed, bluegill, northern pike, three-spined stickleback, and European perch (Neish & Hughes, 1980). It has been reported primarily from Europe and Taiwan, but isolated cases have also occurred in the United States (Arkansas) (Meyer & Robinson, 1973).

There are two species. *Branchiomyces sanguinis* affects common carp, tench, and three-spined stickleback in Europe, while *Branchiomyces demigrans* infects largemouth bass, northern pike, tench, and striped bass in Europe, Taiwan, or the United States (Neish & Hughes, 1980). Some have speculated that branchiomycosis is a type of water mold infection (Alderman, 1982), but there is too little published morphological data to assign a classification to *Branchiomyces*.

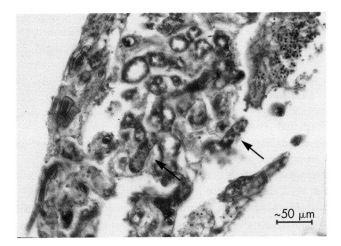

Fig. II-35 Histological section through *Branchiomyces*-infected gills. Key diagnostic feature is sporulating hyphae (*arrows*). Giemsa.

Clinical Signs/Pathogenesis
Gills may be *mottled* in appearance because of areas of thrombosis and ischemia, which cause alternating areas of light and dark regions in the tissue. Histologically, there are branched, aseptate hyphae with intrahyphal, eosinophilic (by hematoxylin and eosin), round bodies ("aplanospores") (Fig. II-35), which look similar to *Saprolegnia* sporangia (see Fig. II-33, *A*). Both *Branchiomyces* species cause similar pathology, except that *B. demigrans* affects the entire gill, with hyphae penetrating though blood vessel walls into the lumen, while *B. sanguinis* is restricted to gill blood vessels (Wolke, 1975).
Diagnosis
Diagnosis of branchiomycosis can be made by examining wet mounts or histopathology of lesions. Characteristic hyphae (Fig. II-35), causing deep branchial infection, are diagnostic.
Treatment
There is no known treatment. Reducing organic loading and reducing the temperature below 20° C (68° F) have been suggested.

PROBLEM 36
Columnaris Infection (Myxobacterial Disease, Peduncle Disease, Saddleback, Fin Rot, Cotton Wool Disease, Black Patch Necrosis)

Prevalence Index
WF - 1, CF - 1, CM - 4
Method of Diagnosis
1. Culture of bacteria from lesions
2. Wet mount of skin or gills with typical bacteria
3. Histopathology of skin or gills with typical bacteria
History
High temperatures; dyspnea; recent acute stress; late spring to early fall; acute morbidity/mortality
Physical Examination
Ulcers (usually shallow), reddening, erosion, and necrosis of skin; gill necrosis; yellow mucoid material on skin or gills
Treatment
Surface infection only:
1. Potassium permanganate prolonged immersion
2. Copper sulfate prolonged immersion
3. Quaternary ammonium bath
Systemic infection:
Appropriate antibiotic

COMMENTS: FRESHWATER PATHOGENS
Epidemiology
Columnaris, mistakenly referred to as *myxobacterial* infection, is a common bacterial disease that affects the skin or gills of freshwater fish. *Flexibacter columnaris* is the most prevalent member of this group, which has a worldwide

distribution and can probably infect most freshwater fish. *Flexibacter columnaris* is an important fish pathogen. It can rapidly infect a population and cause large mortalities (Becker & Fujihara, 1978; Fijan, 1968; Chen et al., 1982). Water temperature and strain virulence are the most important factors determining disease severity.

RISK FACTORS/VIRULENCE MECHANISMS
Flexibacter columnaris is usually pathogenic at higher than ~15° C (59° F). Both mortality and acuteness of disease increase with temperature. For example, experimental infections can kill oriental weatherfish within ~7 days at 15° C (59° F) and in only 1 day at 35° C (95° F) (Wakabayashi, 1993). While disease may occur at less than 15° C (59° F), it is less severe. Virulence mechanisms are unclear, but mineral content of the water is important. *F. columnaris* is less pathogenic in soft water (Fijan, 1968). In one study, optimum hardness was ~70 mg/l and some isolates were virtually nonpathogenic in distilled water (Chowdhury & Wakabayashi, 1988b). Pathogenicity paralleled bacterial survival in various media (Chowdhury & Wakabayashi, 1988a). There is no apparent relationship between serotype and virulence.

Other risk factors include physical injury (e.g., net damage), low oxygen (Chen et al., 1982), organic pollution (Fijan, 1968), and high nitrite (Hansen and Grizzle, 1985). Exposure to high arsenic levels increased the susceptibility of striped bass to columnaris (MacFarlane et al., 1986). Uneaten feed supports growth of *Flexibacter columnaris* and thus is a source of infection (Sugimoto et al., 1981).

SOURCE OF INOCULUM
It is likely that many of the flexibacteria and related bacteria infecting fish may occur naturally on healthy fish and in aquatic ecosystems, since many can be routinely isolated from such sources (Austin & Austin, 1987).

Clinical Signs/Pathogenesis
Columnaris is primarily an epithelial disease (Fig. II-36, A and B). It causes erosive/necrotic skin and gill lesions that may become systemic. It often presents as whitish plaques that may have a red periphery on the head, back (saddleback lesion), and/or fins (*fin rot*), especially the caudal fin. Fragments of the fin rays may remain after the epithelium has sloughed, leaving a ragged appearance. Lesions rapidly (often within 24 hours) progress to ulcers, which may be yellow or orange due to masses of pigmented bacteria. Ulcerations spread by radial expansion and may penetrate into deeper tissues, producing a bacteremia.

Channel catfish may have systemic *F. columnaris* infections without external lesions; internally, there may be swelling of the posterior kidney (Hawke & Thune, 1992). The clinical significance of the latter infections is unknown.

Gill infections are less common but more serious. Columnaris begins at the tips of the lamellae and causes a progressive necrosis that may extend to the base of the gill arch. A less common peracute syndrome presents as sudden death with systemic infection.

Diagnosis
Rapid, presumptive identification of *Flexibacter columnaris* can be made by examining wet mounts of lesions, which have long, thin rods (~0.50 to 1.0 × 4 to 10 μm) (Fig. II-36, C) with a characteristic flexing or gliding motion. If wet mounts are allowed to stand for a few minutes, the bacteria often aggregate into a writhing mass that appears like a column or haystack (Fig. II-36, D). Other shorter rods (mostly nonmotile *Flavobacterium* spp.) that do not have a flexing motility have also been associated with similar gross lesions. Lesions may be secondarily infected by water molds (see *PROBLEM 33*) or other opportunists. Related bacteria cause epithelial lesions at low temperatures (see *PROBLEM 37*). These diseases are often proliferative, as well as necrotic.

Presumptive diagosis is sufficient in routine clinical cases. Culture is not usually warranted because most columnaris infections are predictably susceptible to either antiseptics or certain antibiotics. *Flexibacter* does not grow well on standard bacteriological media; it requires specialized media for both isolation and antibiotic sensitivity testing.

If culture and sensitivity is desired (such information may be useful in case of treatment failure), one must use medium with a low nutritional content and high moisture content (e.g., *Cytophaga* agar [Anaker & Ordal, 1959]; a 1:10 dilution of nutrient broth in 1% agar has also been used). Media should be fresh so that there is enough moisture. Selective media containing antibiotics greatly enhance isolation, especially from mixed bacterial infections (Bullock et al. 1986; Hawke & Thune, 1992).

TAXONOMY
Flexibacter columnaris is usually the cause of columnaris disease in freshwater fish. However, Pyle and Shotts (1980, 1981) and Starliper et al. (1988) provided phenotypic and genotypic evidence, suggesting that not all flexibacteria associated with fish disease were actually *F. columnaris* but that as many as several different species may be involved.

In addition, a large number of other similar, gram-negative bacterial rods have been isolated from fish epithelial lesions, including *Cytophaga*, *Flavobacterium*, *Sporocytophaga*, and *Myxobacterium*. Most notable among these are *Flexibacter psychrophila* (*Cytophaga psychrophila* = *Flexibacter aurianticus*), the cause of bacterial cold water disease in salmonids (see *PROBLEM 37*) and *Flavobacterium branchiophila*, a cause of proliferative gill disease (see *PROBLEM 38*). All these gram-negative bacteria form colonies that are orange or yellow pigmented, rhizoid, and spreading.

Both *Flexibacter* and *Cytophaga* spp. exhibit gliding motility, while flavobacteria are nonmotile. Key differen-

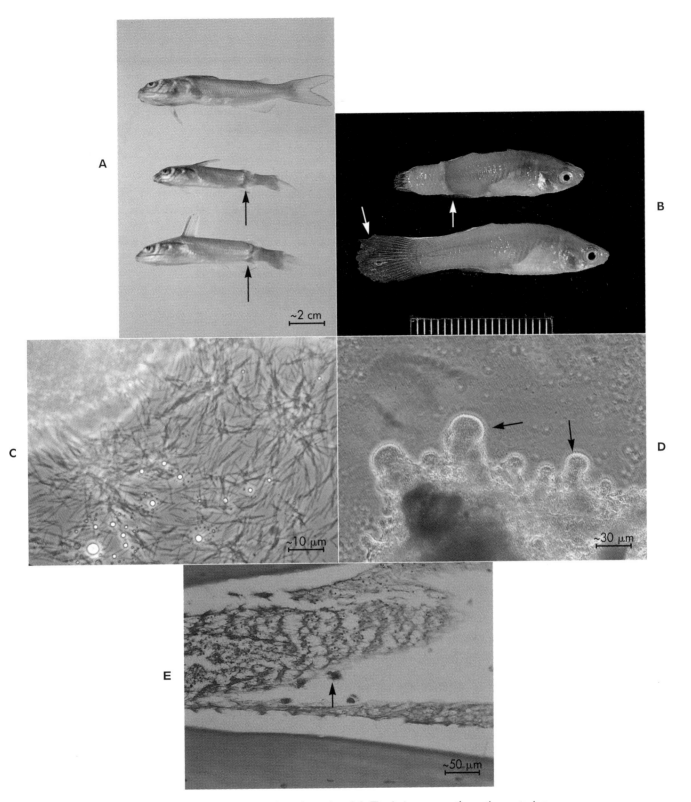

Fig. II-36 **A,** Columnaris in fingerling channel catfish. The lesion covers the entire posterior portion of the body of the bottom two fish. The leading (anterior) edge of the lesion is much deeper; this area (*arrow*) was secondarily invaded by water molds and other bacteria. **B,** Severe columnaris in a guppy (*top*). The entire tail has sloughed, and the infection extends halfway up the flank (*arrow*). There is little chance that this fish will survive, even if it is treated. The lower fish has a mild infection on the tail (*arrow*); bar = 2 cm. **C,** Wet mount of a columnaris lesion showing the characteristic long, thin rods. **D,** Wet mount of a columnaris lesion showing the typical haystack appearance (*arrows*) produced by aggregations of bacteria. Phase contrast. **E,** Histological section through a columnaris lesion of the caudal fin that is entirely infected with long, thin rods (*arrow*) associated with tissue necrosis (*N*). Hematoxylin and eosin.

tiating features of the presently known pathogens are summarized by Austin and Austin (1987). Reichenbach (1989) places all the above fish-pathogenic bacteria into the genus *Cytophaga*. Whether this will withstand challenge is uncertain.

Definitive diagnosis of *Flexibacter columnaris* is based upon biochemical tests or agglutination. *F. columnaris* is a homogeneous species, although potential cross-reactivity with related organisms has not been fully determined.

Treatment

Early cases of columnaris may be successfully treated with surfactant baths or prolonged immersion in potassium permanganate or copper sulfate. However, advanced cases (i.e., lesions with exposed muscle or over 5% of body surface area being affected) warrant systemic antibiotics. Isolates are usually susceptible to oxytetracycline and/or nifurpirinol, but many are resistant to ormetoprim-sulfadimethoxine (Anonymous, 1986; Hawke & Thune, 1992).

If fish with advanced lesions are anorexic, a potassium permanganate treatment may stimulate enough appetite to begin oral medication. Medical therapy must always be accompanied by an improvement in environment. Avoid exposing cultured salmonids to feral fish, which often carry the infection. Lowering the temperature (e.g., adding cold water) will reduce disease severity (Wood, 1974). Vaccination has shown some promise experimentally (Moore et al., 1990), but no vaccines are commercially available.

COMMENTS: MARINE PATHOGENS

Columnaris-type infections caused by *Flexibacter maritimus* or related bacteria have recently been reported in young marine fish. Juvenile (> 6 cm) black sea bream and red sea bream usually develop lesions in spring after being transported to sea cages (Wakabayashi et al., 1986). Dover sole (black patch necrosis, Campbell & Buswell, 1982), Japanese flounder (Baxa et al., 1987), Atlantic salmon smolts (Kent et al., 1988a), and turbot (Pazos et al., 1993) develop similar superficial skin lesions. Stomatitis lesions have also been seen in Atlantic salmon.

Much less is known about marine columnaris, but the bacteria are microscopically similar to freshwater columnaris lesions. Isolation methods are similar to that for *F. columnaris*, except that salt or seawater should be added to media. *Flexibacter maritimus* requires medium having at least 15 ppt and some require 30 ppt seawater (not NaCl only) for isolation. Oxytetracycline has been used to treat infections in bream, but this treatment has not always been effective (Wakabayashi, 1993). Black patch necrosis is resistant to many antibiotics but responds to placing sole on a sand substrate to reduce abrasions.

PROBLEM 37
Bacterial Cold Water Disease (Peduncle Disease, *Flexibacter Psychrophilus* Infection, BCWD)

Prevalence Index
CF - 1, CM - 3

Method of Diagnosis
1. Culture of bacteria from lesions
2. Wet mount of skin with typical bacteria
3. Histopathology of skin with typical bacteria

History
Cold temperatures; early spring; acute to chronic morbidity/mortality

Physical Examination
Erosion and ulceration (usually shallow) of skin

Treatment
1. Quaternary ammonium bath
2. Potassium permanganate flush
3. Appropriate antibiotic
4. Diquat bath

COMMENTS
Epidemiology

Bacterial cold water disease, caused by *Flexibacter psychrophilus*, is common in freshwater salmonids and is a serious problem in salmonid hatcheries. It is probably endemic in salmonid culture. Coho salmon are especially vulnerable, but all salmonids are probably susceptible. As with columnaris (see *PROBLEM 36*), water temperature and strain virulence are the most important factors determining disease severity. BCWD is often associated with erythrocytic inclusion body syndrome (EIBS) (see *PROBLEM 43*). EIBS anemia may predispose fish to BCWD (Holt et al., 1993).

RISK FACTORS/VIRULENCE MECHANISMS

Flexibacter psychrophilus is usually pathogenic at less than ~10° C (50° F). The disease usually appears in spring, when temperatures are 4° to 10° C (39° to 50° F) (Holt et al., 1993). Mortality is most acute at 15° C (59° F); mortality decreases at higher temperature (Holt et al., 1993). Like *F. columnaris*, strains vary widely in pathogenicity (Holt et al., 1993). Extracellular products may be the major cause of clinical signs (Otis, 1984).

SOURCE OF INOCULUM

The natural reservoir has not been identified. It can be isolated from the surface of clinically normal fish (Holt et al., 1993); skin damage may be needed to initiate infections. Vertical transmission is likely because the bacterium is commonly found on eggs and can be isolated from reproductive tissues of a high percentage of fish (up to 76%) (Holt et al., 1993).

Clinical Signs/Pathogenesis

Bacterial cold water disease causes epithelial erosions and necrotic skin lesions but often becomes systemic (Wood

& Yasutake, 1956). In young fish (yolk sac fry = alevins), erosions damage the skin covering the yolk.

In older fish, typical signs of peduncle disease appear, which are similar to columnaris infections (Fig. II-37). Internally, there may be hemorrhage (Otis, 1984). Bacteria are most common in highly vascularized tissues, including secondary lamellar capillaries, kidney, heart, and spleen (Wood & Yasutake, 1956). Inflammation is typically mild or absent. Moribund fish with no external lesions and dark color are seen late in epidemics.

Recovered coho salmon often develop spinal deformities (lordosis, scoliosis, vertebral compression) at 3 to 4 months of age (Wood, 1974). Fish that recover from typical BCWD disease may also develop neurological disease, presumably from the localization of bacteria in the cranium. Unilateral hyperpigmentation also suggests nervous tissue damage. The bacterium is readily isolated from brain (Kent et al., 1989).

Diagnosis
Rapid, presumptive identification of *Flexibacter psychrophila* can be made by examining wet mounts of lesions, which have long, thin rods (~0.50 to 1.0 × 4 to 10 µm) with a characteristic flexing or gliding motion, like *F. columnaris* (see Fig. II-36, *C*). Histopathology can also be used for presumptive diagnosis; some bacteria may be lost during processing.

Presumptive diagnosis is sufficient in routine clinical cases. Culture is not usually warranted because *Flexibacter* does not grow well on standard bacteriological media, requiring specialized media for both isolation and antibiotic sensitivity testing. Fortunately, most BCWD infections are predictably susceptible to either antiseptics or certain antibiotics.

Treatment
Early cases of BCWD may be successfully treated with quaternary ammonium or oxytetracycline baths.

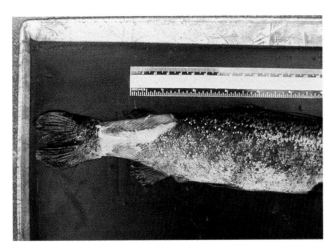

Fig. II-37 Rainbow trout with typical bacterial cold water disease (peduncle disease).

(Photograph courtesy of National Fish Health Research Laboratory.)

However, systemic infections are common, requiring systemic antibiotics. Sulfas are not effective compared with oxytetracycline (Wood, 1974). Treating alevins is difficult because at this life stage they do not eat until the yolk sac is absorbed. In fish with advanced lesions, treatment with potassium permanganate flush followed by antibiotic has been effective (Schachte, 1983). Keeping alevins in shallow rather than deep troughs, keeping water flows in incubators low (Wood, 1974), and inhibiting excessive movement of alevins to prevent abrasions (Leon & Bonney, 1979) can reduce infections. Avoid exposing cultured salmonids to feral fish, which often carry the infection.

PROBLEM 38
Bacterial Gill Disease (BGD, Proliferative Gill Disease, PGD, *Flavobacterium Branchiophila* Infection, Pigmented Bacteria Gill Disease)

Prevalence Index
CF - 1
Method of Diagnosis
1. Culture of bacteria from lesions
2. Wet mount of gills with typical bacteria
3. Histopathology of gills with typical bacteria
History
Overcrowding; low DO; high ammonia; high turbidity
Physical Examination
Lethargy; flared opercula; coughing; dyspnea; mucus strands trailing from gills
Treatment
1. Salt bath
2. Quaternary ammonium bath
3. Chloramine-T bath
4. Diquat bath

COMMENTS
Epidemiology
Bacterial gill disease is an important disease in cultured freshwater salmonids (Wakabayashi et al., 1989). *Flavobacterium branchiophila* causes a chronic, proliferative response in gill. No studies have examined the pathophysiological effects of BGD, but it probably causes respiratory and osmoregulatory impairment, which depends on normal epithelium function. Up to 25% mortality can occur (Speare et al., 1991).
RISK FACTORS/VIRULENCE MECHANISMS
While there appear to be differences in pathogenicity among BGD bacteria isolates, bacterial gill disease is mainly a production management disease. Risk factors include low oxygen, high turbidity, high ammonia, and overcrowding. Water temperature does not appear to affect pathogenicity. Outbreaks have occurred at 5° C (41° F) in cyprinids and almost 20° C (68° F) in

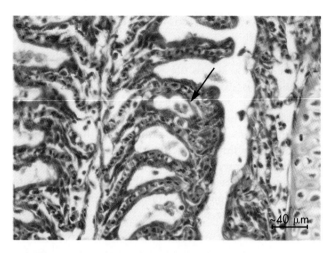

Fig. II-38 Bacterial gill disease. Hyperplasia and fusion of adjacent secondary lamellae. The hyperplastic lesions surround bacteria and cell debris (*arrow*). Hematoxylin and eosin.

salmonids (Turnbull, 1993a). Transmission is via water (Ferguson et al., 1991).

Clinical Signs/Pathogenesis

GROSS LESIONS

The gill is the only target organ. There are clinical signs of respiratory impairment, including lethargy, dyspnea, coughing, and flared opercula. Strands of mucus may trail from the gills. In early stages, the gills may be hyperemic, with swollen primary lamellae. Increased mucus may trap debris. Later, secondary water mold infections (see *PROBLEM 33*) or opercular damage may occur (Ostland et al., 1990).

HISTOPATHOLOGY

Bacterial gill disease is primarily an epithelial disease. Bacteria may initially colonize the tips of the secondary lamellae and then spread inward, inducing a proliferative branchitis (Fig. II-38) that causes epithelial hyperplasia. Fusion of secondary lamellae may occur distally, forming a partially enclosed space with bacteria, sloughed epithelial cells, and mucus (Fig. II-38). Hyperplasia may also cause obliteration of the entire interlamellar space and in severe cases may cause fusion of adjacent primary lamellae.

Diagnosis

Rapid, presumptive identification of *Flavobacterium branchiophila* can be made by examining wet mounts or histopathology of lesions, which have long, thin rods (~0.50 to 1.0 × 4 to 10 μm), similar to *F. columnaris* (see Fig. II-36, *C*). Flexibacteria have also been implicated in some cases of bacterial gill disease. Flavobacteria are nonmotile, while *Flexibacter* exhibits gliding motility (see *PROBLEM 36* for a taxonomic summary of this group). Early lesions of BGD can be hard to detect with histopathology because bacteria are often lost during processing (Turnbull, 1993).

The susceptibility of bacterial gill disease to antiseptic-type therapies makes presumptive diagnosis sufficient for clinical cases. If desired, culture may be performed as described for columnaris (see *PROBLEM 36*). *Flavobacterium branchiophila* can be difficult to isolate in the absence of clinical disease (Heo et al., 1990).

Treatment

Bacterial gill disease usually responds to antiseptic baths. Providing adequate oxygen is useful supportive therapy. Reducing stressors is important. It is likely that this organism may occur naturally on healthy fish and possibly in aquatic ecosystems.

PROBLEM 39
Lymphocystis

Prevalence Index
WF - 1, WM - 1

Method of Diagnosis
1. Histology of skin or gills showing massively enlarged dermal fibroblasts.
2. Wet mount of skin or gills showing massively enlarged dermal fibroblasts

History/Physical Examination
Recent stress; various-sized, white to pink, pinpoint to mulberry-size masses, especially on skin, but also in the buccal cavity and on the gills; rarely present on serosal surfaces of internal organs

Treatment
1. Isolate affected individual(s)
2. Prophylactic antibiotics

COMMENTS
Epidemiology
Lymphocystis is a chronic (usually many weeks), self-limiting disease affecting many cultured and wild marine and freshwater fish (Lawler et al., 1977). It has been reported from over 125 species in 34 families (Wolf, 1988). Lymphocystis is a disease of higher (i.e., evolutionarily advanced) teleosts and does not affect salmonids, catfish, or cyprinids. An iridovirus, it is the most common viral infection of aquarium fish. While it causes only low mortality, lymphocystis is disfiguring and can render affected fish unsalable.

It probably consists of several closely related viruses; specific isolates may only be able to infect related fish in the same family or genus. Transmission probably occurs by rupture or sloughing of lesions followed most often by infection of abraded integument (Lawler et al., 1977). Virus is viable in water for about 1 week. The incubation period may be long (weeks to months). Many fish probably carry a latent infection, which may appear after shipping or other stress. Tropical aquarium fish often *break* with lymphocystis after arrival at a retailer's facility.

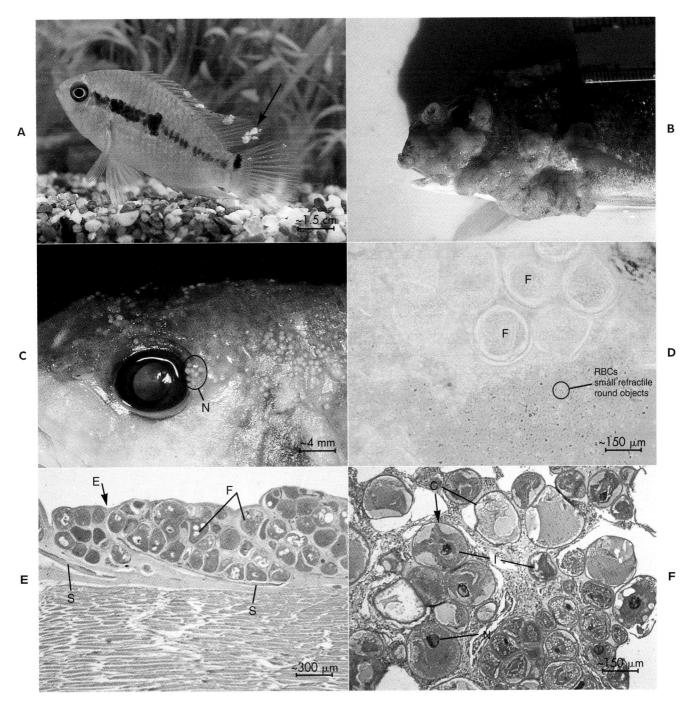

Fig. II-39 A, Severum cichlid infected by lymphocystis on the dorsal fin (*arrow*). **B,** Atlantic croaker with a severe lymphocystis infection. The reddening (hemorrhage) suggests that this lesion may be secondarily infected by bacteria. **C,** Atlantic croaker with extensive lymphocystis nodules (*N*). Note the granular, sand grain–like appearance. Preserved specimen. **D,** Wet mount of lymphocystis lesions showing massively enlarged, virus-infected dermal fibroblasts (*F*) that are over 500 times the size of red blood cells (*RBCs*). Photographed with green filter. **E,** Histological section through a lymphocystis lesion. Note massively enlarged dermal fibroblasts (*F*) or lymphocysts (*E* = epithelium; *S* = scale). Hematoxylin and eosin. **F,** Close-up of a lymphocystis lesion that shows diagnostic features, including infected fibroblasts with irregular inclusions (*I*), capsule (*C*), and enlarged, undisplaced nucleus (*N*). Hematoxylin and eosin.

(*A* photograph courtesy of T. Wenzel; *C* photograph by M. Jansen and E. Noga; *F* photograph courtesy of L. Khoo.)

Clinical Signs/Pathogenesis

GROSS LESIONS

The lymphocystis virus infects the dermal fibroblasts, producing tremendously hypertrophied cells that are often just visible to the naked eye. Early or mild stages of the disease appear as a salt-like dusting of the body (Fig. II-39, *C*), which may later coalesce into large neoplastic-like masses of hypertrophied cells (Fig. II-39, *A* and *B*). Lesions less commonly affect internal organs or gill (Russell, 1974).

HISTOPATHOLOGY

Histopathology of infected tissue shows hypertrophied fibroblasts with basophilic, intracytoplasmic inclusions (Pritchard & Malsberger, 1968) (Fig. II-39, *E* and *F*). Viral inclusion material may be lacy with scattered, small condensations of chromatin (plaice type) or large and cord-like, with blebs (mullet type) (Ferguson, 1989). These *lymphocysts* are surrounded by a hyaline *capsule*, which may be responsible for the initially mild inflammatory response. In later stages, as the lymphocysts rupture, numerous inflammatory cells surround the lesions.

Diagnosis

Wet mounts of skin lesions that have typical pathology (Fig. II-39, *D*) provide strong presumptive evidence for lymphocystis infection and are usually sufficient for clinical diagnoses. Epitheliocystis (see *PROBLEM 40*) can also produce grossly hypertrophied cells but appears to be less common than lymphocystis. Epitheliocystis also primarily affects the gills.

If a definitive diagnosis is required, epitheliocystis can be readily distinguished from lymphocystis histopathologically by its presence in epithelial cells that have a hypertrophic host nucleus that is peripheral to a granular basophilic inclusion containing many coccoid or coccobacillary bodies (see Fig. II-40, *B*) (Herman & Wolf, 1987). Lymphocysts are dermal fibroblasts, have irregular inclusions, and have an undisplaced nucleus (Fig. II-39, *F*). Mild gross lesions may be confused with ich (see *PROBLEM 19*) but are easily differentiated via wet mount.

Lymphocystis may also be confused grossly with some forms of idiopathic epidermal hyperplasia (see *PROBLEM 72*), but the latter lesions are rare compared with lymphocystis. Lesions such as walleye dermal sarcoma can be differentiated with histopathology.

Treatment

There is no treatment for lymphocystis. Fish should be watched closely for secondary infections and medicated accordingly. Affected fish should be quarantined, preferably for at least 1 month after recovery. Lesions will often regress spontaneously. Stress reduction and avoidance of skin trauma are essential to control. Recovered fish that are stressed will often recrudesce, although some recovered fish appear immune to reinfection.

PROBLEM 40
Epitheliocystis (Mucophilosis)

Prevalence Index

WF - 4, WM - 4, CF - 4, CM - 4

Method of Diagnosis

1. Histology of gills or skin with massively enlarged epithelial cells
2. Wet mount of gills or skin with massively enlarged epithelial cells

History/Physical Examination

Small pinpoint masses, mainly on gills but rarely on the skin

Treatment

1. Isolate affected individual(s)
2. Prophylactic antibiotics

COMMENTS

Epidemiology

Epitheliocystis has been reported from over 25 species of freshwater and marine fish worldwide. It has been associated with mortalities in common grey mullet, grey liza mullet, striped bass, gilthead sea bream, red sea bream, common carp, rainbow trout, lake trout, and amberjack (Turnbull, 1993b; Herman & Wolf, 1987; Paperna et al., 1981). Some evidence exists that epitheliocystis *strains* may only infect fish within the same family (Hoffman et al., 1969).

When present in small numbers, epitheliocystis may be an incidental finding, but in high concentrations it has been associated with considerable mortalities. Details of its life cycle and pathogenesis are largely unknown. The disease has never been experimentally reproduced.

Clinical Signs/Pathogenesis

While not yet proven to be a cause of disease, epitheliocystis has been associated with varying degrees of morbidity and mortality. Gills and rarely skin and pseudobranch are the primary target organs (Turnbull, 1993b). Lesions present as white miliary nodules up to ~1 mm in diameter on the skin or gills. Host response varies from no reaction to severe epithelial hyperplasia. Host response is usually most severe with heavy infections, but light infections will occasionally incite inflammation.

Diagnosis

Lesions may grossly resemble *Ichthyophthirius multifiliis* (see *PROBLEM 19*), lymphocystis (see *PROBLEM 39*), or other nodular skin lesions but are easily distinguished with histopathology. Epitheliocystis infects skin and gill epithelial cells, resulting in the cells enlarging to 20 to 400 μm in diameter. Presumptive diagnosis can be made from wet mounts, showing nodular masses in the tissue (Fig. II-40, *A*).

All major types of epithelial cells can be infected, including chloride and goblet cells (Ferguson, 1989).

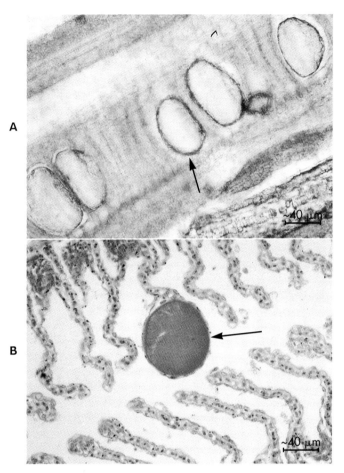

A

B

Fig. II-40 A, Wet mount of gill from gilthead sea bream infected by epitheliocystis. Infected host epithelial cells are massively enlarged, each having a smooth, homogeneous inclusion (*arrow*). B, Histological section through epitheliocystis-infected gill cell (*arrow*). Key diagnostic feature is a large, granular, basophilic inclusion, filled with coccoid bodies, which occupies virtually the entire cell. Hematoxylin and eosin.

(*A* photograph courtesy of A. Colorni.)

The hypertrophic cytoplasm is peripheral to a granular basophilic inclusion, containing large numbers of coccoid or coccobacillary bodies (Fig. II-40, *B*). When the nucleus is seen in sections, it is on the periphery of the cell. Histologically, the major differential is lymphocystis virus infection (see *PROBLEM 39*), which can be distinguished based on its infection of dermal fibroblasts, presence of irregular inclusions, and undisplaced nucleus. Unlike lymphocystis, epitheliocystis can also infect salmonids, catfish, or cyprinids.

Epitheliocystis is tentatively considered a chlamydia-like organism, although it has never been successfully cultured to confirm this hypothesis.

Treatment

There is no known treatment, except disinfection and quarantine.

PROBLEM 41
Miscellaneous Skin and Gill Diseases

The following agents are primarily systemic pathogens but may occasionally cause skin or gill lesions:

Myxozoans: Diagnostic spores or developmental stages are easily identified via wet mounts or histopathology (see *PROBLEM 59*).

Microsporidians: Diagnostic spores are easily identified via wet mounts or histopathology (see *PROBLEM 66*).

Helminths: Digeneans (see *PROBLEM 55*) and nematodes (see *PROBLEM 56*) are easily identified via wet mounts or histopathology.

Trypanoplasms: These are mainly hemoparasites but may occur on the gills as well; they are easily identified in wet mounts or smears (see *PROBLEM 43*).

Bacterial infections: Some bacterial infections mainly affect the skin or gills, but skin lesions are often a manifestation of systemic disease (see *PROBLEM 44*).

Ichthyophonus: *Ichthyophonus* (see *PROBLEM 67*) may cause skin lesions.

Fungal infections: Some systemic fungal infections (see *PROBLEM 68*) may cause skin lesions.

The following are mainly skin diseases but are diagnosed by rule-out of other problems:

Idiopathic epidermal hyperplasia: (see *PROBLEM 72*)

The following agents are uncommon to rare diseases that infest/infect the skin or gills:

Dermocystidium: This is a poorly studied group of organisms that typically produces various-sized (usually 0.1 to 4.0 mm), white, macroscopic nodules on the skin or gills of many fish species (Hatai, 1989) (Fig. II-41, *A*). The cysts contain spherical, 3 to 10 μm spores. Often an incidental finding, some species have caused mortality in salmonids and other fish. *Dermocystidium* is probably related to the protozoa or to the fungi, but its classification is unclear (Perkins, 1974). The most diagnostic feature is the presence of a spherical stage (*spores*), having a large central vacuole or refractile body (Fig. II-41, *B*). Hyphal-like structures are produced by some species (Dykova & Lom, 1992). Various species have been reported from Europe, Japan, China, Russia, and the United States.

X-cells: X-cells are amoeba-like cells that produce masses in the gills pseudobranchs and skin of some marine fish, especially Atlantic cod and dab in the North and Baltic Seas (Waterman & Dethlefsen, 1982; Diamant & McVicar, 1989). They have been speculated to be aberrant host cells (i.e., neoplasia), but others believe that they are protozoan parasites. X-cells often form "cysts," which are subivided into compartments (Fig. II-72, *D*).

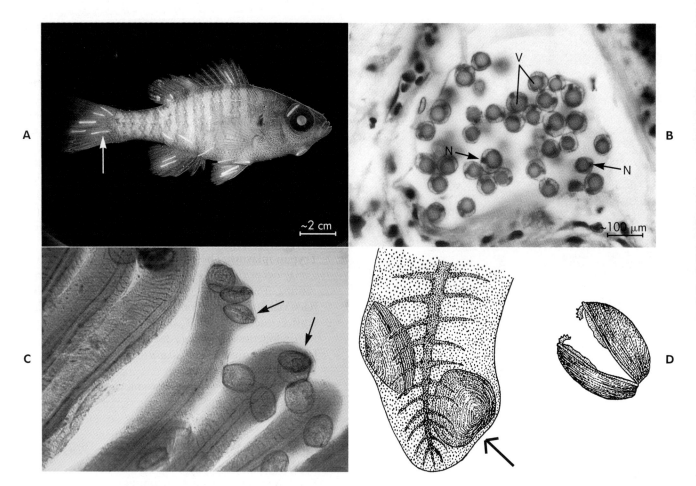

Fig. II-41   **A,** *Dermocystidium* gross lesion (*arrow*) in the fin of a sunfish. **B,** *Dermocystidium* spores. The mature spore has a large, PAS (periodic acid–Schiff stain) positive vacuole (V) surrounded by a thin rim of host cytoplasm, except where it thickens to make room for the nucleus (*N*). The inclusion is PAS (+) and hematoxylin and eosin (-) (Hatal, 1989). **C** and **D,** Glochidia infestation (*arrows*) of the gills of a fish.

(*A* photograph courtesy of D. Demont; *B* photograph courtesy of J. Lom; *C* photograph courtesy of A. Mitchell.)

Algal infections: Algal infections have been reported from a few fish (Edwards, 1978), especially centrarchids. Bony prominences are common infection sites (Vinyard, 1953; E.J. Noga, Unpublished Data). Infections of the eye (Hoffman et al., 1965), intestinal mucosa (Langdon, 1986), and skin (Blasiola & Turnier, 1979) have also been reported. No treatments have been reported.

Glochidia-producing freshwater bivalve molluscs: Primarily members of the Family Unioidae, this group of freshwater bivalves has an obligatory parasitic stage. The infective larvae (*glochidia*) are released by the adult clams and are passively dispersed via water currents. They attach to the gills and/or skin of fish, using sharp hooks on each shell valve. This incites a hyperplastic response in the fish's epithelium (Fig. II-41, *C*). Eventually, the parasites are shed when they metamorphose into adult clams. Infestations are usually innocuous unless heavy. No treatments have been reported.

Mycoplasma: *Mycoplasma mobile* is the only mycoplasma that has been isolated from fish. It was cultured from the gills of tench (Stadtlander & Kirchoff, 1989). While extensively studied, it has not yet been proven to be pathogenic to fish, although it can damage gill tissues cultured in vitro.

Miscellaneous pathogens: Various other invertebrates have been rarely reported to infest mainly marine fish, including *cnidarians, amphipods, cirripeds* (*barnacles*), and *ostracods* (Kinne, 1984). Candiru are small, pencil-thin, South American catish that infest the gill chamber of larger fish (Axelrod et al., 1980).

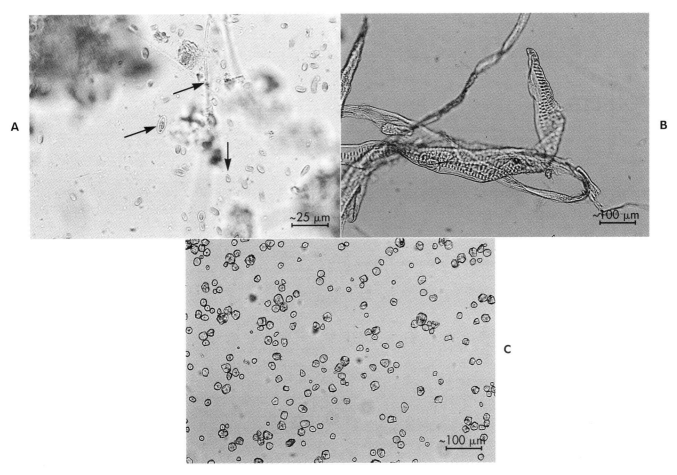

Fig. II-42   **A,** Various unicellular and filamentous algae (*arrows*). **B,** Fiber from paper separating plastic coverslips. Do not confuse with fungal hyphae (see Fig. II-33). **C,** Talcum crystals from powdered gloves.

PROBLEM 42
Incidental Findings

Prevalence Index
WF - 1, WM - 1, CF - 1, CM - 1
Method of Diagnosis
Wet mount of skin or gills with organism/foreign body

COMMENTS

Nonpathogenic protozoans and other organisms are commonly seen in wet mounts from the skin or gills of fish. It is important to recognize these as incidental findings, so that the true cause of the problem is pursued. Fish possess an endogenous skin and gill flora, which probably includes protozoa. It is not unusual to see an occasional ciliate or flagellate on a wet mount of normal skin or gill. Gills commonly trap debris in proportion to the amount of suspended matter in the water and may have various types of algae (Fig. II-42, *A*), protozoa, and nonpathogenic bacteria. Inanimate objects (Fig. II-42, *B* and *C*) may also be seen occasionally.

Gill and especially skin wounds are often secondarily colonized by a wide array of organisms that are simply taking advantage of the nutrient soup provided by this damaged tissue. Some may be present in high numbers. For example, a wound having a large number of bacteria often also has a large complement of phagotrophic protozoa. While these organisms may make some contribution to disease, there is no documented proof of their pathogenicity.

CHAPTER 15

Problem 43

Diagnoses made by examination of a gill clip or a blood smear

Primary Hemopathies

Prevalence Index
WF - 4, WM - 4, CF - 4, CM - 4

Method of Diagnosis
1. Wet mount of blood or tissue with pathogen
2. Blood or tissue smear with pathogen
3. Histopathology of tissue with pathogen

History
Lethargy, weight loss, chronic mortality; leech infestation; may be no clinical signs; wild-caught or pond-raised fish

Physical Examination
May be anemia, cachexia, or other clinical signs but is often an incidental finding

Treatment
See specific pathogen; usually best to increase oxygen content of water

COMMENTS

Primary hemopathies are diseases that primarily affect the peripheral blood. Other organs may be affected secondarily. Note that other diseases not mentioned in this chapter may secondarily cause hemopathies (e.g., many viral and bacterial infections, some parasites, toxins).

Blood Flukes
Blood flukes are digenean trematodes that infect the circulatory system. *Sanguinicola* and *Cardicola* infect salmonids and can cause mild-to-heavy mortalities in hatcheries in the western United States that use surface water (Evans & Heckmann, 1973). *Sanguinicola* also infects common carp in Europe and mullet in Australia. Sanguinicolids (*Paradeotacylix* spp.) have caused mass mortalities in cultured amberjack in Japan (Ogawa et al., 1993).

The general life cycle is similar to that of other digeneans (see Fig. II-55, *A*), with fish acting as the final host. Blood flukes need only one intermediate host.

Cercariae penetrate the fish and migrate to target organs. Interestingly, some species that infect marine fish use a polychaete as an intermediate host (They are the only digeneans known to not require a mollusk in their life cycle [Lester, 1988].)

Adults reside in blood vessels and in heart or peritoneal cavity. They release fertilized eggs, which lodge in gill blood vessels (intestinal blood vessels in mullet), causing thrombosis, lethargy, and gill irritation, as indicated by flashing. Lamellae are swollen and ischemic. Eggs may incite an inflammatory response. Eggs gradually make their way to the outside. They often embryonate while undergoing the migration and may have fully developed miracidia (Fig. II-43, *C*).

Infections are usually diagnosed by identifying the ova or miracidia in the gills (or intestine in mullet) (Fig. II-43, *D*). Avoidance of surface water that contains the intermediate host is the only proven control, although praziquantel might be effective.

Trypanosomes
Trypanosomes (Fig. II-43, A_1) are uncommon blood infections in cultured fish but are common in wild populations, especially cold water species (e.g., European carp, tench). They may be encountered on routine examinations, such as when gill clips are examined for other pathogens. They may be found in high concentrations (reportedly up to 1,000,000 organisms/μl blood) and often localize in blood-filtering organs, such as the kidney.

PATHOGENESIS
Trypanosomes can cause anemia, hematopoietic damage, and death. Common pathogenic trypanosomes include *Trypanosoma carassii* (*T. danliewski*) (Woo, 1987) infecting goldfish, common carp, and some noncyprinids (Woo, 1987; Dykova & Lom, 1979b), *T. cobitis* infecting weatherfish (cobitids) (Letch, 1980), and *T. murmanense*, a well-known North Atlantic species that infects 13 diverse fish species (e.g., cod, plaice, eels) (Khan, 1985).

LIFE CYCLE
Fish trypanosomes are transmitted by leeches—a process that is necessary for the completion of the trypanosome species' life cycle. A single leech species can often transmit more than one trypanosome species. They develop

in the gut of the leech, producing large numbers of the fish-infective stage (trypomastigotes), which are then transferred to a fish host with the leech's blood meal.

Trypomastigotes in fish blood may be either small forms (acute infection) or large forms (chronic infection), since they increase in size the longer they remain in the blood. Some trypomastigotes of marine fish are up to 100 μm, but most freshwater species are not more than about 50 μm. There may be a mixture of forms in blood because of repetitive infections by leeches. It is not known if all fish forms can start a leech infection. When ingested by a leech, the trypomastigotes form amastigotes, which have no flagellum. The trypanosome then goes through several other developmental stages, eventually producing a trypomastigote, which is infective for fish.

DIAGNOSIS

The major differential is trypanoplasms (Fig. II-43, A_2), which have two flagella. Trypanosomes also wriggle vigorously in one place. Controlling the leech population is the only known method of treatment.

Trypanoplasms

Trypanoplasma (Fig. II-43, A_2) is morphologically similar to *Cryptobia* (see *PROBLEM 29*) and both genera have been combined by some researchers (Woo, 1987). Thirty-five fish species are infected by trypanoplasms.

LIFE CYCLE

The life cycle is similar to trypanosomes, with a prepatent period immediately after a leech infects the fish, followed by a parasitemia and then either death of the fish or eventual absence of the parasite from the peripheral blood. At this point, there is often a nonsterile immunity (i.e., no parasites in peripheral blood, but the fish is still infected). In some species, there can be several cycles of parasitemia.

PATHOGENESIS

Trypanoplasma borreli causes anemia (*sleeping sickness*) in goldfish, koi, and other cyprinids (Kruse et al., 1989). In freshwater salmonids, *T. salmositica* causes a virulent systemic disease, with progressive anemia (pale gills), exophthalmos, abdominal distension, and splenomegaly,

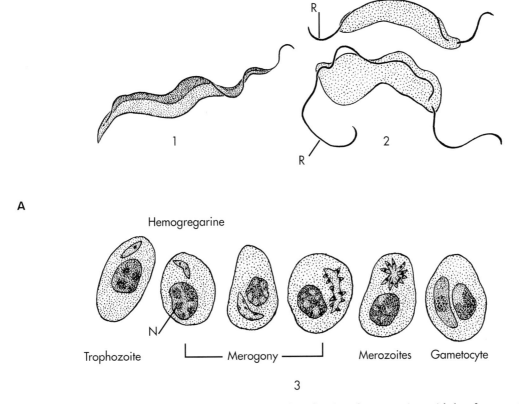

Fig. II-43 Diagram of representative examples of various hemoparasites, with key features: A_1, Trypanosomes: shape; single flagellum directed anteriorly. A_2, Trypanoplasm: pleomorphic shape; two flagella, one directed anteriorly, the other (*R* = recurrent flagellum) directed posteriorly. The recurrent flagellum forms a characteristically wide, wavy, undulating membrane; these organisms are highly similar to *Cryptobia* (see *PROBLEM 29*). A_3, Hemogregarine (typical development stages). *N* = host cell nucleus.

Continued.

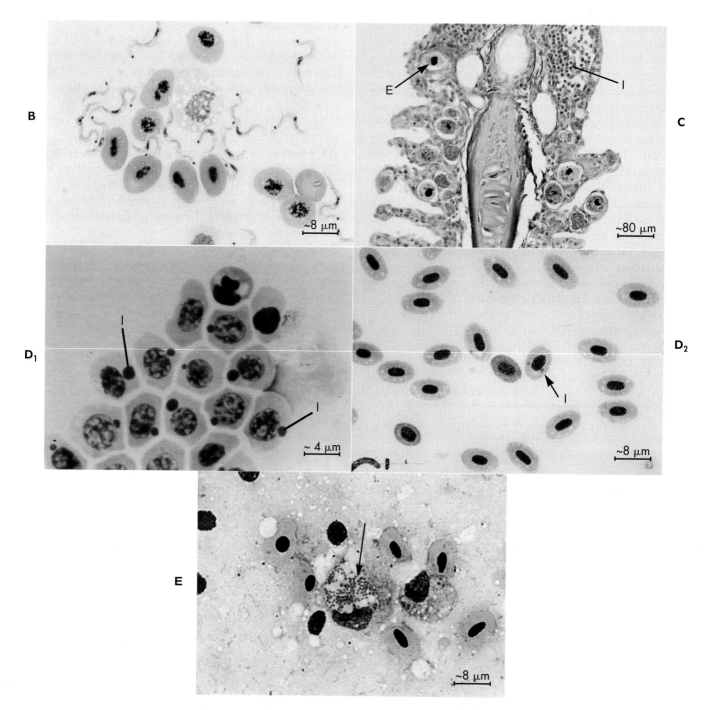

Fig. II-43—cont'd.   **B,** Blood smear with trypanosomes. Giemsa. **C,** Histological section of *Sanguinicola* miracidia lodged in gill vessels of a salmonid. Note the parasite's characteristic, darkly pigmented eyespot (*E*). There is also some branchial inflammation (*I*). Hematoxylin and eosin. **D,** Blood smears of (*1*) viral erythrocytic necrosis; (*2*) erythrocytic inclusion body syndrome (EIBS). *I* = inclusions. Giemsa. **E,** Blood smear of rickettsia-like organisms (*arrow*) in a tilapia macrophage. Giemsa.

(*A₃* modified from Khan, 1972; *B* photograph courtesy of C. Huang; *D₁* photograph courtesy of M. Kent; *D₂* photograph courtesy of C. Smith; *E* photograph courtesy of C. Tu.)

presumably caused by hypoproteinemia and vascular damage (Woo, 1991). Parasites may also cause immunosuppression. *Trypanoplasma bullocki* infects 13 diverse species of marine fish along the western Atlantic and Gulf of Mexico and may contribute to natural mortality in some flatfish (Burreson & Frizzell, 1986). Affected fish have a distended abdomen because of edema.

DIAGNOSIS/TREATMENT

Trypanoplasma is distinguished from trypanosomes by its flowing, amoeboid motility and by the presence of two flagella (Fig. II-43, A_2). It is distinguished from the morphologically similar *Cryptobia* (see *PROBLEM 29*) by its more developed undulating membrane, predilection for blood, and indirect life cycle (leech vector). Note, however, that *T. salmositica* may also occur on the gills and can also be transmitted mechanically (Woo, 1991). There is no treatment, except for eliminating the leech vector.

Apicomplexan Hemoparasites

Several types of apicomplexan hemoparasites are uncommonly encountered, mainly in wild fish: coccidia (e.g., *Haemogregarina*) and piroplasmids (e.g., *Babesiosoma, Haemohormidium, Mesnilium*) (Fig. II-43, A_3). Diagnosis is based on identification in blood smears. Little is known about their life cycles, but all probably require an intermediate host, such as a leech or parasitic crustacean. Most are incidental findings, but *Haemogregarina sachai* infection of cultured turbot in Scotland caused anemia, leucocytosis, and tumor-like granulomas in various tissues (Ferguson & Roberts, 1975).

Microsporidian Hemoparasites

Enterocytozoon salmonis has been recently associated with plasmacytoid leukemia, a serious infectious anemia of salmonids in seawater (Hedrick et al., 1990a). It primarily infects chinook salmon, but also infects rainbow trout in the Pacific Northwest of the United States and Canada and in France. It occurs mainly in the nucleus of hematopoietic cells, but also occurs in rodlet cells, renal tubule epithelium, and glomerular mesangial cells. Infected cells appear to have intranuclear inclusions via light microscopy. This organism is probably not the cause of plasmacytoid leukemia (see salmon leukemia virus, *PROBLEM 78*).

Rickettsia-Like Hemoparasites

SALMONID RICKETTSIAL SEPTICEMIA (SRS, COHO SALMON SYNDROME, *PISCIRICKETTSIA SALMONIS*)

Discovered in Chile in the late 1980s, this disease has caused serious losses in sea-reared coho salmon in that country. It also affects Atlantic salmon, chinook salmon, and rainbow trout (Turnbull, 1993b). Salmonids may be an aberrant host. Monthly mortalities average 1% to 20% on affected farms, with up to 90% cumulative losses. The most diagnostic gross signs are anemia (as low as 2% PCV), whitish-to-reddish skin ulcers, and ascites. There may be petechial visceral hemorrhages and multifocal nodules on the liver. Histologically, there is a systemic vasculitis, often necrotizing, with granulomatous inflammation. Diagnosis is made by identifying small (0.4 to 1.5 μm), basophilic, rickettsia-like organisms (RLO) both free in tissues and in macrophages (Fig. II-43, *E*). Isolates are susceptible to many antibiotics, including tetracyclines and quinolones, but not to penicillins. Gram-staining of broodstock tissues is presently used to screen for the organism (Turnbull, 1993b).

Viral Hemopathies

Viral hemopathies typically present as various types of inclusions, especially in erythrocytes. Some have been associated with disease, but others are only incidental findings. Presumptive diagnosis is usually made from stained blood smears. Definitive diagnosis of specific types of viral hemopathies requires electron microscopic examination of infected cells to identify the specific virus present. The only known treatment is to decrease stress to prevent infection by opportunistic pathogens.

VIRAL ERYTHROCYTIC NECROSIS (VEN, PISCINE ERYTHROCYTIC NECROSIS, PEN)

Viral erythrocytic necrosis (previously known as piscine erythrocytic necrosis) refers to a morphologically heterogenous group of viruses that infect members of 14 families of marine fish, including Atlantic salmon, Atlantic cod, and Atlantic herring. Affected fish include 23 genera in North America; 3 genera in the Pacific Northwest, and 4 genera in Atlantic waters of Europe (MacMillan et al., 1980, 1989a). Some populations have 100% prevalence. The infection can be experimentally transmitted with infected blood within species but not between species. This suggests that a hematophagous vector may be required for transmission. Vertical transmission is also suspected.

Clinically, VEN presents as intracytoplasmic inclusions in the erythrocytes, consisting of masses of viral particles and/or degenerative changes (e.g., karyolysis) of the nucleus (Fig. II-43, D_1). Affected erythrocytes are irregular, more osmotically fragile, with degenerative nuclear and cytoplasmic changes. There are single (rarely multiple), 0.3 to 4.0 μm inclusions that stain green with acridine orange. Anemia occurs in some infected salmonids, but this has not been experimentally documented.

ERYTHROCYTIC INCLUSION BODY SYNDROME (EIBS)

EIBS causes a progressive, severe anemia in juvenile to yearling chinook and in coho salmon in the Pacific Northwest. It can be transmitted experimentally via water, as well as orally. Recovered fish are resistant. The time-course of infection may be up to 5 months; clinical course and recovery are faster at high temperatures.

Blood smears stained with pinacyanol chloride (best) or Leishman-Giemsa reveal a single, purple-pink, 0.8 to 3.0 μm inclusion in erythrocytes (Fig. II-43, D_2). Acridine orange staining reveals a red inclusion (Holt & Piacenti, 1989). There is also splenic hemosiderosis.

COHO ANEMIA

Coho anemia affects seawater-reared coho salmon in California. By Leishman-Giemsa, there are many 1 to 2 μm (often rod-shaped) inclusions in erythrocytes. There is also macrophage hemosiderosis in kidney, spleen, and liver (Hedrick et al., 1987b).

INTRAERYTHROCYTIC VIRAL DISEASE OF RAINBOW TROUT

Only one case of this disease has been documented (in Donaldson strain of rainbow trout). It presented as exsanguinating hemorrhage, hypoxia, and sudden death. There were small, basophilic, pleomorphic inclusions in erythrocytes.

Toxicoses

NITRITE POISONING (see PROBLEM 5)

Idiopathic Hemopathies

INFECTIOUS SALMONID ANEMIA (ISA)

Infectious salmonid anemia is a recently described, serious anemia of seawater-cultured Atlantic salmon in Norway. Affected fish can also have abdominal swelling and liver damage. Losses are variable but can be high. The disease has been associated with increasing temperatures in spring and at times to decreasing temperatures in fall, as well as other stresses. A virus is strongly suspected but has not yet been identified.

NO BLOOD DISEASE (WHITE LIP DISEASE)

This is a chronic, often severe, anemia of channel catfish. Hematocrits can be as low as 1% (Plumb et al., 1986). At least some cases may be caused by folate deficiency (Plumb et al., 1991).

CHAPTER 16

Problems 44 through 54

Diagnoses made by bacterial culture of kidney or affected organs

44. Bacterial dermatopathies/systemic bacterial infections: general features
45. Motile aeromonad infection
46. *Aeromonas salmonicida* infection
47. Enteric septicemia of catfish (ESC)
48. *Edwardsiella tarda* infection
49. Vibriosis
50. Pasteurellosis
51. Enteric redmouth disease
52. Bacterial kidney disease
53. Mycobacteriosis
54. Miscellaneous systemic bacterial infections

PROBLEM 44
Bacterial Dermatopathies/Systemic Bacterial Infections: General Features

Prevalence Index
WF - 1, WM - 1, CF - 1, CM - 1
Method of Diagnosis
1. Culture of clinically relevant numbers of bacteria from skin lesions and/or internal organs
2. Clinical signs with histopathological/immunological evidence of infection
History
Varies with pathogen; acute to chronic morbidity/mortality
Physical Examination
Red areas on body; skin ulcers; depression; exophthalmos; peritonitis (swollen abdomen)
Treatment
1. Appropriate antibiotic
2. Eliminate responsible stress
3. Disinfect and quarantine if appropriate

COMMENTS
Epidemiology/Pathogenesis
Bacteria are important pathogens in both wild and cultured fish and are responsible for serious economic losses. Some may cause primarily a surface (skin/gill)

infection (see *PROBLEMS 36, 37,* and *38*); most can cause systemic disease. A wide array of bacteria cause infections in marine or freshwater fish. Few pathogens infect both freshwater and marine fish. Most pathogens are gram-negative rods.

Many pathogens can present as only skin infections, especially flexibacteria, aeromonads, and vibrios. Fish may present with *fin rot*, an imprecise general term for ulcerative, necrotic lesions that affect the fins (see Fig. I-3). Various bacteria are often present in fin rot lesions, but some stress is considered to be the primary cause. The fin rot syndrome includes several diseases and idiopathic responses. Bacterial skin infections can advance to become systemic, leading to much greater and more acute mortality. In at least one case, typical *Aeromonas salmonicida*, skin ulcers may originate from the hematogenous spread of a systemic infection.

The classical signs associated with systemic bacterial infection are indicative of a bacterial toxemia/septicemia and include diffuse hemorrhage and necrosis of internal organs, especially those involved in filtering blood (spleen, kidney). Kidney and/or spleen is often enlarged. External signs may include skin ulcers, fin necrosis, or hemorrhages on the body (petechiation, ecchymoses) and fins (Fig. II-44, *A* through *C*). Fish often have unilateral or bilateral exophthalmos (see Fig. I-3) and fluid accumulation in the abdomen (see Fig. I-3).

Not all bacteria that cause systemic disease produce the above clinical signs, but these signs are common. Bacteria are also an important cause of egg mortality (see *PROBLEM 93*).

Most fish-pathogenic bacteria can reside in the environment or on/in apparently normal fish (latent carriers). Thus, infections are often precipitated by some stress that upsets the natural defenses against these agents (e.g., overcrowding, low DO, high ammonia).
Diagnosis
Definitive diagnosis of bacterial disease requires the culture of the pathogen from skin lesions and/or internal organs, since clinical signs are rarely pathognomonic or even diagnostic for any specific pathogen. Culture is also essential to determining antibiotic sensitivity, which often varies widely between isolates.

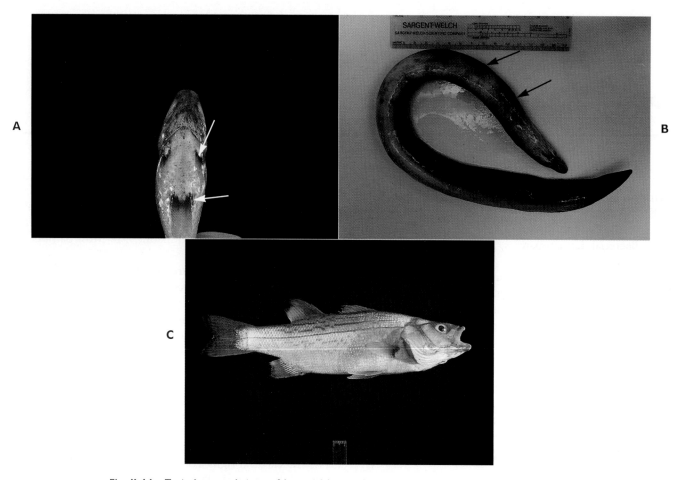

Fig. II-44 Typical external signs of bacterial hemorrhagic septicemia. **A,** Goldfish (*ventral view*). Petechial hemorrhages and congestion or hemorrhage at the base of the fins (*arrows*). **B,** American eel (*ventral view*). Ecchymotic hemorrhages (*arrows*). **C,** Striped bass. Reddening of fins. This could be caused by hemorrhage, hyperemia, or congestion.

Bacteria may often infect the skin, producing erosions or ulcers. Skin lesions are especially a diagnostic challenge, often having multiple pathogens. It is often difficult to determine the initiating (i.e., primary) pathogen. It is best to identify the predominant colony type, but this ignores the fact that unrelated organisms may have a similar colonial appearance. Also, the primary pathogen may not be the most common organism at the time of culture, especially if lesions are chronic (see *PROBLEM 46*).

Culture of internal organs is usually more straightforward, although even here, multiple bacterial species may be present. Kidney is the best tissue for routine isolation of systemic pathogens. However, other tissues may be preferable for certain pathogens or for identifying asymptomatic carriers. Multiple infections are common, and determining all the important pathogens is important. See *CULTURING FOR BACTERIA* (p. 30) for details on sampling for bacteria. For rapid identification of the pathogen involved, immunodiagnosis is frequently used (Anderson & Barney, 1991). Companies selling immunodiagnostic kits include Diagxotics and Micrologix.

Treatment

Medical management is similar for all pathogens and usually requires treatment with antibiotics, although early stages of skin/gill infections may be amenable to antiseptic baths. Treatment options are limited for food fish (see *PHARMACOPOEIA*). Treatment should be initiated as soon as possible, since outbreaks can rapidly move through a population. Removing the initiating stress(es) is also essential. Feeding antibiotics is the delivery method of choice, but sick fish will often be anorexic. If fish are not eating, treating for other complications, such as external parasites, may help. However, keep in mind that external treatments may also precipitate or enhance the severity of low-grade bacterial infections. There is an increasing prevalence of antibiotic-resistant strains. Antibiotic resistance is highly correlated with prior antibiotic use, so farms that frequently use antibiotics have the most problems. See the *ANTIBIOTICS* section of the *PHARMACOPOEIA* for discussion of this problem.

PROBLEM 45
Motile Aeromonad Infection (MAI, Motile *Aeromonas* Septicemia, MAS, Red Sore)

Prevalence Index
WF - 1, WM - 4, CF - 1
Method of Diagnosis
Culture of large numbers of motile aeromonad bacteria from typical skin and/or internal lesions
History
Acute to chronic morbidity/mortality
Physical Examination
Red areas on body; skin ulcers; depression; exophthalmos; peritonitis (swollen abdomen)
Treatment
1. Eliminate primary cause
2. Appropriate antibiotic

COMMENTS
Epidemiology
Motile aeromonad infection (MAI) is probably the most common bacterial disease of freshwater fish. All freshwater fish are probably susceptible. Motile aeromonads may also inhabit brackish water (Hazen et al., 1978) but decrease in prevalence with increasing salinity (Kaper et al., 1981). MAI has been associated with several members of the genus *Aeromonas*, which are ubiquitous in freshwater environments, including *A. hydrophila*, *A. sobria*, *A. caviae*, *A. schuberti*, and *A. veronii*. Many other *Aeromonas* species have been recently taxonomically identified, but only a few aeromonads have been strongly documented as true fish pathogens (e.g., *Aeromonas saccharophila* [Martinez-Murcia et al., 1992], *A. sobria* [Toranzo et al., 1989]). By far the most important fish pathogen is *A. hydrophila* (syn. *A. liquefaciens*, *A. formicans*), and this group is often referred to as the *A. hydrophila* complex. Motile aeromonads are also commonly isolated from the mucosal surfaces and internal organs of clinically healthy fish (MacMillan, 1985). Highest prevalence is in organically polluted waters (Hazen et al., 1978). Ingestion of contaminated feed may also be a source of infection (King & Shotts, 1988).

Motile aeromonads can infect many vertebrates, including frogs, alligators, and man. Reports of gastrointestinal and systemic infection in humans have increased, but the ubiquity of these bacteria, combined with the frequent exposure of humans to these pathogens, suggests that risk of zoonotic infection may be relatively low.

Predisposing risk factors include high temperatures, overcrowding, organic pollution, and hypoxia. Motile aeromonads often invade skin wounds, commonly with water molds (see *PROBLEM 33*), or ectoparasites (Noga, 1986b). *Aeromonas hydrophila* is often associated with the protozoan *Epistylis* in causing widespread

epidemic skin lesions known as *red-sore disease* (Esch & Hazen, 1980) (see *PROBLEM 32*).

Motile aeromonads are relatively weak pathogens, but isolates vary widely in pathogenicity (Lallier et al., 1980). An S-layer on the cell wall (Chabot & Thune, 1991) and more elastase production (Shotts et al., 1985) are present in more pathogenic strains, but there is little correlation of pathogenicity with most exotoxins (proteases, hemolysins).
Clinical Signs/Pathogenesis
GROSS LESIONS
Clinical signs of motile aeromonad infection range from superficial to deep skin lesions (Fig. II-45, *A* and *B*), to a typical, gram-negative bacterial septicemia (see Fig. II-44, *A*), with or without skin lesions.

Skin lesions include variously sized areas of hemorrhage and necrosis on the skin and the base of the fins (Fig. II-45, *A*). These may progress to reddish or gray ulcers with necrosis extending to the muscle (Fig. II-45, *B*). Ulcers may progress to hemorrhagic septicemia, with exophthalmos, a distended abdomen that has serosanguinous fluid, visceral petechiation, and a hemorrhagic and swollen lower intestine and vent (Fig. II-45, *C*). Peracute infections are not associated with skin lesions. Anorexia and dark color are most common with systemic disease.

HISTOPATHOLOGY
Skin lesions include acute-to-chronic dermatitis/myositis. In septicemias, there may be depletion and necrosis of the renal and splenic hematopoietic tissue; necrotic intestinal mucosa; and focal necrosis in the heart, liver, pancreas, and gonad (Bach et al., 1978; Huizinga et al., 1979). The presence of free melanin or lipofuscin from ruptured melanomacrophage centers is characteristic (Roberts, 1989b).
Diagnosis
Definitive diagnosis of motile aeromonad infection requires biochemical identification of *clinically significant* numbers of the suspect bacterium in target tissues, with attendant clinical signs. It is important to be certain that this is the primary infectious cause of the problem. Motile *Aeromonas* spp. are frequent secondary invaders, following channel catfish virus (see *PROBLEM 74*), rhabdovirus carpio (see *PROBLEM 78*), *Aeromonas salmonicida* (see *PROBLEM 46*), or other infections. Kidney is probably the best organ for isolation; lesions should also be sampled. Proper care should be taken when skin lesions are sampled (see *CULTURING FOR BACTERIA*, p. 30). A culture of four to six fish is advisable to confirm the diagnosis. Motile aeromonads often overgrow less fastidious bacteria (e.g., *Edwardsiella ictaluri*, *Aeromonas salmonicida*).

Isolates vary widely in antigenicity, making immunological identification difficult. They are ~0.8 to 1.0 × 1.0 to 3.5 μm and motile by a single polar flagellum.

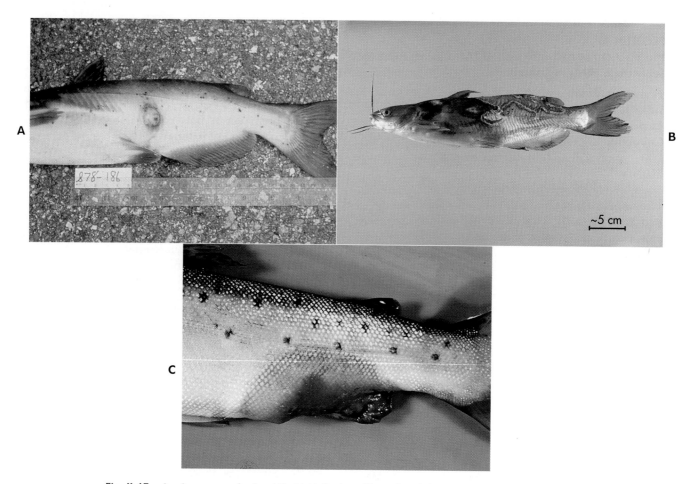

Fig. II-45 A, *Aeromonas hydrophila* skin infection. Channel catfish with shallow ulcer. **B,** Channel catfish with *Aeromonas hydrophila* infection. Note the extensive, relatively deep skin ulcer. **C,** Rainbow trout with motile *Aeromonas* infection. Note the reddened, swollen vent.

[*A* photograph courtesy of A. Mitchell; *C* photograph courtesy of R. Roberts.]

Treatment

Motile aeromonad infection is a classical example of a stress-borne disease. Losses because of MAI are highly dependent on the severity of the environmental stress that precipitated the outbreak. Outbreaks will often resolve themselves without antibiotic intervention if environmental problems are corrected. Also, antibiotic treatment may not be economically justifiable. Thus, whether to medicate should depend on the acuteness of the outbreak (mortality rate, feeding activity), severity of the stress, and how quickly the stress can be eliminated.

Oxytetracycline, chloramphenicol, and nifurpirinol have successfully controlled some outbreaks. Chloramphenicol is also used prophylactically in eastern European carp culture just before times of stress (Roberts, 1993). However, many isolates are resistant to these and many other antibiotics (Shotts et al., 1976; Dixon et al., 1990). Sulfadimethoxine-ormetoprim is often used in the United States for oxytetracycline-resistant isolates.

PROBLEM 46

Aeromonas Salmonicida Infection (Furunculosis, Ulcer Disease)

Prevalence Index

CF - 1, CM - 1

Method of Diagnosis

Identification of *Aeromonas salmonicida* from typical skin and/or internal lesions

History

Acute to chronic morbidity/mortality

Physical Examination

Skin ulcers and "furuncles"; red areas on body; depression; exophthalmos; swollen abdomen

Treatment

Appropriate antibiotic

COMMENTS

Epidemiology

Aeromonas salmonicida infection is a common bacterial disease of freshwater fish and is becoming a serious problem in marine fish, especially Atlantic salmon culture (Munro & Hastings, 1993). It is one of the most important diseases of salmonids. Atlantic salmon are most susceptible; rainbow trout are most resistant. Any age salmonid is susceptible. The organism is also an important pathogen of nonsalmonids. Goldfish, common carp, koi, and American and Japanese eels are most often affected, but bream, roach, dace, chub, tench, pike, bullhead, sculpin, catfish (McCarthy, 1978), wrasse (Treasurer & Cox, 1991), as well as smallmouth bass, northern pike, yellow perch, brook stickleback, sablefish, hybrid striped bass (*Morone saxatilis* × *M. chrysops*), and lamprey are susceptible. Disease can occur in wild fish.

TYPICAL VS ATYPICAL STRAINS

There are three subspecies of *A. salmonicida* (Austin & Austin, 1987): The *typical* subspecies *A. salmonicida* subspecies *salmonicida* is usually associated with systemic disease (furunculosis), while the *atypical* subspecies *A. salmonicida* subspecies *achromogenes* and *masoucida*, which do not conform to the typical phenotypic pattern in culture, are usually associated with infections localized to the skin (ulcer disease). However, this distinction is not perfectly demarcated; typical strains have been isolated from ulcer disease lesions (Noga & Berkhoff, 1990), and atypical isolates can cause furunculosis (Munro & Hastings, 1993).

TRANSMISSION

Skin ulcers are a major source of infection during epidemics, but the mechanism of horizontal transmission is not known. A high percentage of carriers can develop after an epidemic; shedding is via the feces. Vertical transmission via infected ova occurs rarely, if ever (Bullock & Stuckey, 1987). In salmonids, outbreaks are typically associated with stress, especially high temperatures. Isolates vary in pathogenicity.

Clinical Signs/Pathology

Clinical signs of *Aeromonas salmonicida* infection range from superficial or deep skin lesions without systemic involvement (ulcer disease) to a typical, gram-negative bacterial septicemia (furunculosis) (Fig. II-46, A through D).

FURUNCULOSIS—GROSS LESIONS

The classical form of *Aeromonas salmonicida* infection primarily affects salmonids. Clinical signs of furunculosis depend on the time-course of infection, with gross signs more apparent with increasing chronicity

Peracute disease, which is the least common presentation, has been seen in salmonid fry. Fish die rapidly, typically without any gross lesions except darkening (McCarthy & Roberts, 1980).

The acute form is the most common, especially in growing fish. It presents as a typical bacterial hemorrhagic septicemia, with bacteria disseminated in many tissues; fish often die in 2 to 3 days.

The subacute/chronic form is less common than the acute form. Mostly seen in adults, it presents as a more chronic form of bacterial hemorrhagic septicemia, which

may include exophthalmos, bloody discharge from nares and vent, and multifocal hemorrhages in the viscera and muscle (Herman, 1968; Roberts, 1989b). The gills may be pale from anemia or may have hemorrhages (Bruno et al., 1986). Fibrinous edema and serosanguinous fluid may be present. The gastrointestinal tract may have a necrotic enteritis and catarrhal exudate (Ferguson & McCarthy, 1980). The classical but inconsistently present clinical sign of chronic disease is the "furuncle," actually a dark, raised tumefaction, which ulcerates to release serosanguinous fluid (Fig. II-46, A). *Furuncles* develop from localization of hematogenous bacteria in the muscle or skin, not from an external skin infection.

FURUNCULOSIS—HISTOPATHOLOGY

Lesions are typical of a bacterial septicemia, with necrosis and hemorrhage, especially of well-vascularized organs (e.g., liver, spleen, kidney) (McCarthy & Roberts, 1980). There is often a characteristic lack of immune cell response to infection, probably because of potent leukocidin production (Ellis, 1991). Bacterial microcolonies are present in target organs (Fig. II-46, E). Leukopenia is common. Degranulation of eosinophilic granular cells of mainly the intestinal submucosa but also the gills is diagnostic (Vallejo & Ellis, 1989).

ULCER DISEASE

Ulcer disease is the most common form of *A. salmonicida* infection in nonsalmonids; salmonids can also be affected. Unlike furunculosis, ulcer disease is typically localized to the skin and only becomes systemic late in the disease.

Carp erythrodermatitis (CE), an important disease in cultured carp in Europe, is caused by a skin infection with atypical *A. salmonicida* (Bootsma et al., 1977). This disease is part of the infectious dropsy of carp (IDC) complex. Infectious dropsy of carp encompasses two types of diseases in cultured carp: the acute form of IDC is now known to be caused by *Rhabdovirus carpio* (see *PROBLEM 78*), while the chronic form of IDC is caused by atypical *Aeromonas salmonicida*.

ULCER DISEASE—GROSS LESIONS

Skin lesions range from whitish discolorations to shallow hemorrhagic ulcers to deep lesions that expose underlying muscle or bone (Shotts et al., 1980; Fig. II-46, B and C). Because of their chronicity, lesions are often secondarily infected with water molds, protozoa, and other bacteria. Fish may have hemorrhage on the body and the base of the fins.

In eels, infections begin as depigmented foci that spread to form large patches of necrotic skin up to 16 cm² in area. The depigmented patches detach at the dermoepidermal junction, forming large ulcers that expose underlying muscle. The infection commonly affects the head, producing cranial swelling and corneal edema (*swollen head disease* of Japanese eels, Fig. II-46, D) (Ohtsuka et al., 1984).

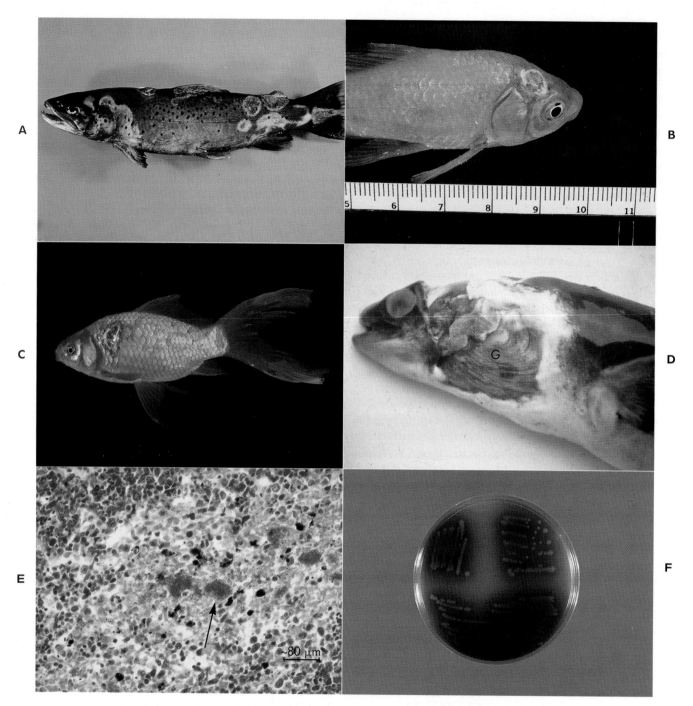

Fig. II-46 A, Salmon with furunculosis. Typical skin ulcers. B, Goldfish with relatively shallow, grey ulcer on head caused by *A. salmonicida.* C, Goldfish with deep, red ulcer caused by *A. salmonicida.* D, American eel with ulceration of head and corneal edema caused by *Aeromonas salmonicida* infection. *G* = exposed gill arches. E, Kidney of a salmonid with several focal *A. salmonicida* microcolonies (*arrow*). Eosinophilic area of necrosis surrounds the colonies. Hematoxylin and eosin. F, Brown, diffusible pigment surrounding *A. salmonicida* colonies grown on trypticase soy agar.

(*A* photograph courtesy of R. Roberts.)

ULCER DISEASE—HISTOPATHOLOGY

A mild to severe, primarily mononuclear infiltrate may be present. In eels many lesions have extensive collagen deposition, which contributes to the tissue swelling and belies the chronic nature of the disease (Noga & Berkhoff, 1990). Chronic inflammation has also been reported in Atlantic cod skin lesions (Morrison et al., 1984).

Diagnosis

CLINICAL DISEASE—PRESUMPTIVE DIAGNOSIS

Presence of furunculosis is suggested by the presence of necrotic lesions with bacterial microcolonies (Fig. II-46, E). Necrosis of cardiac atrial endothelium may be the only lesion seen in peracute mortality of fry. On tissue smears, cells are bipolar staining, small coccoid to coccobacillary (~1 μm × 2 μm) rods. Other bacteria (e.g., *A. hydrophila*, *Vibrio*) can cause similar lesions, making this a presumptive diagnosis at best. Histopathological lesions of ulcer disease are not diagnostic.

CLINICAL DISEASE—DEFINITIVE DIAGNOSIS

Definitive diagnosis of clinical *A. salmonicida* infection requires identification of the bacterium in target tissues, with attendant clinical signs.

In clinical cases of systemic disease, the bacterium is readily isolated from kidney, spleen, or internal lesions. Isolating the bacterium from ulcer disease lesions can be difficult. Ulcer disease isolates of *A. salmonicida* are often fastidious and difficult to isolate. An enriched medium, such as brain or heart infusion agar or 5% blood agar, should be used for primary isolation. Opportunists, such as *Aeromonas hydrophila*, can rapidly outcompete *A. salmonicida*, so primary cultures must be watched carefully daily. It is advisable to sample several fish, especially those with early lesions, where the primary pathogen is more likely to be isolated. Atypical *A. salmonicida* colonies are usually small, circular, grey, up to 1.5 mm in diameter after 4 to 7 days at room temperature.

COLONY CHARACTERISTICS

Presumptive identification of typical *A. salmonicida* colonies is indicated by the presence of brown, diffusible pigment around colonies after 24 hours of incubation; this is most easily seen on clear agar (Fig. II-46, F) but is also visible on blood agar. However, both false-positives (e.g., some *Aeromonas hydrophila*, *A. media*, and *Pseudomonas* isolates) and false-negatives can occur. Most atypical strains produce no pigment or take several days to produce pigment.

Characteristically, colonies of most isolates can be *pushed* along the agar surface with an inoculating loop (Shotts & Teska, 1989). The bacterium is nonmotile (differentiating it from motile aeromonads).

Definitive identification of *A. salmonicida* can be accomplished with biochemical tests. However, atypical strains do not conform to the typical biochemical profile for this species (Shotts & Teska, 1989), so definitive diagnosis should include immunological confirmation,

such as with latex bead agglutination or immunofluorescent antibody (Austin & Austin, 1987). Atypical *A. salmonicida* infecting salmonids has previously been misidentified as *Haemophilus piscium*.

CARRIERS

The kidney and lower intestine should be cultured when searching for asymptomatic carriers (Bullock et al., 1983; Rose et al., 1989). Skin and gills also can be cultured, but other bacteria commonly overgrow isolates (Munro & Hastings, 1993). False negatives are common. More asymptomatic carriers can be detected by stressing suspect fish with heat shock (raising temperature to 18° C [64° F] from 12° C [50° F]) or glucocorticoid immunosuppression (0.80 mg triamcinolone acetamide in small brook trout, 8 mg in large fish) (Bullock & Stuckey, 1975). Using both heat and corticosteroids increases recovery rate of the bacterium.

Treatment

SALMONIDS

During outbreaks, all moribund fish, especially those with skin ulcers, should be promptly removed and disposed of properly (i.e., do not allow contagion to reenter the system). Oral oxytetracycline, furazolidone, oxolinic acid, and potentiated sulfonamides have been used successfully, but many isolates are resistant. In Europe, isolates with multiple resistance are much more prevalent in sea-caged fish, compared with those in freshwater fish (Munro & Hastings, 1993). Amoxicillin is most effective against European isolates, although *Achromogenes* is often resistant (Barnes et al., 1991). Sulfadimethoxine-ormetoprim is used for oxytetracycline-resistant isolates in the United States. Fluoroquinolones are more effective than oxolinic acid (Austin & Austin, 1993) and are under study for licensing.

Disinfection and quarantine, followed by stocking specific-pathogen-free fish and eggs, can eliminate the infection from facilities, so long as stocks are not reexposed to water that has infected feral fish. Riverine waters containing wild salmonids and the presence of infected nonsalmonids around sea cages present important risks to cultured salmonids (Munro & Hastings, 1993).

Aeromonas salmonicida is probably an obligate pathogen but may survive for long periods off host fish. Bacteria can survive in water for up to about 3 weeks and may possibly survive for months in sediments (Munro & Hastings, 1993). The 6-week period used to fallow sea cages may not be long enough to eliminate the pathogen. Reducing stress is imperative for long-term management.

Furunculosis vaccines are commercially available, but they have not been as successful as bacterins for other diseases (e.g., yersiniosis, vibriosis).

NONSALMONIDS

Except for carp erythrodermatitis, treatment has not been attempted in most cases of nonsalmonid furunculosis. Similar antibiotics should be considered. It is speculated that death from ulcer disease may be due to osmoregulatory damage, rather than toxemia (Munro & Hastings, 1993). This is supported by the fact that the adding of estuarine water reduced morbidity in American eels held in freshwater impoundments in North Carolina (N. Marquardt, Personal Communication). Inhibition of some isolates by seawater cannot be ruled out.

Because isolation of atypical *A. salmonicida* is often difficult, individual pet goldfish or koi are often treated based on the presence of typical lesions. However, other diseases, such as mycobacteriosis, may cause similar lesions, so necropsy and culture is advised when possible.

PROBLEM 47
Enteric Septicemia of Catfish (ESC, *Edwardsiella Ictaluri* Infection)

Prevalence Index
WF - 1
Method of Diagnosis
Culture of *Edwardsiella ictaluri* from typical lesions
History
Usually acute, but sometimes chronic, mortality; corkscrew spiral swimming
Physical Examination
Raised open ulcer on frontal bone of skull; bloody or clear fluid in peritoneal cavity; swollen abdomen; exophthalmos; red or white areas on body; skin ulcers; depression
Treatment
Appropriate antibiotic

COMMENTS
Epidemiology/Pathogenesis
Enteric septicemia is the most important disease that affects channel catfish, causing millions of dollars in losses annually in the United States. It has a high predilection for channel catfish but has been occasionally isolated from other ictalurids (brown bullhead, blue catfish, white catfish), other catfish (walking catfish), and unrelated species, such as green knife fish and devario danio (Kent & Lyons, 1982; Blazer et al., 1985). It has also caused neurological disease in poeciliid tropical aquarium fish (R. Francis-Floyd, Personal Communication). European catfish are experimentally susceptible. Surprisingly, rainbow trout and chinook salmon are very susceptible to experimental challenge (Baxa-Antonio & Hedrick, 1992). Whether these fish can asymptomatically carry the infection is unknown. Golden shiner, bighead carp, and largemouth bass are totally resistant (Plumb & Sanchez, 1983).
TEMPERATURE-DEPENDENT PATHOGENICITY
ESC is a markedly seasonal disease, with outbreaks occurring when water temperatures hover around 24° to 28° C (75° to 82° F) during the day (Francis-Floyd et al., 1987), which is optimum for the bacterium's growth. Thus, it is most prevalent during May and June and September and October in ponds in the southeast United States. Outside this temperature range, mortalities may occur, but they are low and chronic.

The ESC bacterium can survive for over 90 days in pond mud at 25° C (77° F) (Plumb & Quinlan, 1986), which may account for recurrent epidemics in ponds. It can probably be carried in the gut of asymptomatic channel catfish.
Clinical Signs/Pathogenesis
GROSS LESIONS
There are two forms of ESC that are related to the route of exposure:

Acute form: In the gut route, bacteria are ingested, enter the bloodstream through the intestine, and apparently colonize various organs, causing necrosis and ulceration. There is typically acute mortality and in some cases few external signs.

Clinically affected fish may occasionally hang head up in the water and exhibit corkscrew spiral swimming, usually followed by death. Fish may have abdominal distension, exophthalmos, or pale gills. Blood-borne bacteria localizing in the dermis cause necrosis and hemorrhage that result in red-to-tan and slightly raised-to-depressed petechiae on the dorsum, flanks, jaw, and operculum. Petechiae on dark areas of skin appear as small (1 to 3 mm), depigmented foci (*false spots*) (Fig. II-47, *A*).

Internally, the peritoneal cavity contains bloody or clear fluid (which is especially characteristic), hemorrhage and necrosis of the liver, and splenic and renal hypertrophy. There may be petechial hemorrhages in the muscles.

Chronic form: In the nervous route, bacteria invade the olfactory organ via the nasal opening and migrate up the olfactory nerve to the brain, where the infection spreads from the meninges to the skull and finally to the skin, forming the hole-in-the-head lesion (Fig. II-47, *B*) (Shotts et al., 1986). This is a raised or open ulcer on the frontal bone of the skull. The brain can be entered without cutting the skull. Disease progression is more chronic than via the gut route.
HISTOPATHOLOGY
Histologically, enteritis, hepatitis, myositis, and interstitial nephritis begin as acute lesions and develop into chronic-active and then chronic foci. Fish with the nervous form initially develop inflammation in the olfactory sac, which progresses up the olfactory nerve, eventually reaching the olfactory lobe of the brain. The telencephalon (meningoencephalitis) and overlying bone and skin are primarily affected. Macrophages in lesions often have bacteria (Shotts et al., 1986).

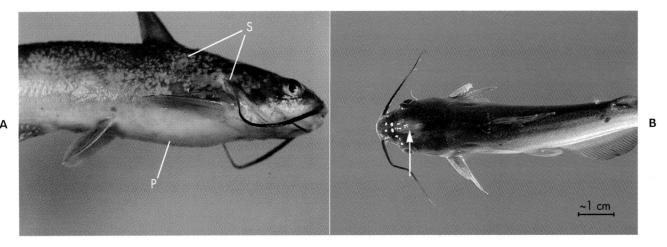

Fig. II-47   **A,** Channel catfish with ESC. Note skin erosion and ulceration, which appear as false spots (*S*) on the flank and focal petechiation (*P*) on the ventrum. **B,** Channel catfish with classical hole-in-the-head lesion caused by the erosion of the fontanelle of the skull (*arrow*).

(*A* photograph courtesy of M. Beleau.)

Diagnosis

Definitive diagnosis of clinical ESC requires identification of the gram-negative bacterium in target tissues, with attendant clinical signs. In the acute form, kidney is the organ of choice, while in the chronic form, brain is the best organ for isolation. *Edwardsiella ictaluri* is somewhat fastidious for a fish pathogen and can be overgrown by other bacteria. Colonies are typically pinpoint in size after 24 hours at 30° C (86° F). Fluorescent antibody or enzyme-linked immunosorbent assay (ELISA) can be used for rapid presumptive diagnosis in tissue smears of infected fish.

In young fish, ESC can be clinically identical to channel catfish virus disease (CCVD) (see *PROBLEM 74*). The major distinguishing feature is the *hole-in-the-head* lesion (do not confuse with *hole-in-the-head* of pet fish; see *PROBLEMS 89* and *90*), which is considered highly diagnostic for ESC.

Treatment

Losses because of ESC are highly dependent on the speed with which fish are placed on medication. Fish quickly go off feed after an ESC epidemic begins, making treatment impossible. If ESC is suspected, an attempt should be made to isolate the bacterium for identification and sensitivity testing as soon as possible. The trend is toward using rapid immunodiagnosis (e.g., ELISA) if ESC is suspected, so that fish can be placed on medication as soon as possible. Medication can later be modified if subsequent culture and sensitivity results warrant it.

Oxytetracycline and ormetoprim-sulfadimethoxine have both been used with varying success, but increasing numbers of *E. ictaluri* isolates are resistant. Also, not all isolates from the same case exhibit the same resistance pattern (Taylor & Johnson, 1991). The importance of this finding

to choice of medication is not yet known. Some isolates have also been found to be susceptible to kanamycin, streptomycin, neomycin, nitrofurantoin, and/or oxolinic acid in vitro (Waltman & Shotts, 1986). Outbreaks will often spontaneously subside when the water temperature leaves the optimal range. Experimental bacterins have shown promise (Plumb et al., 1986), and a commercial vaccine has recently been marketed (Biomed). Stress, especially crowding, increases the severity of ESC outbreaks but is not needed to initiate epidemics.

PROBLEM 48
Edwardsiella Tarda Infection (Edwardsiellosis, Emphysematous Putrefactive Disease, *Edwardsiella* Septicemia)

Prevalence Index
WF - 3
Method of Diagnosis
Culture of *Edwardsiella tarda* from typical skin and/or internal lesions
History
Low, chronic mortality; fish continue to eat
Physical Examination
Deep, malodorous ulcer on flank; red areas on body
Treatment
Appropriate antibiotic

COMMENTS
Epidemiology
Edwardsiella tarda (formerly *Edwardsiella anguillimortifera* and *Paracolobactrum anguillimortiferum*) is an economically important but relatively uncommon bacterial disease in channel catfish in the United States

(Waltman et al., 1986). While it is not reported from American eels, it causes serious losses in Japanese eels in Japan and Taiwan (Waltman et al., 1986). It has been isolated from the gastrointestinal tract of numerous cold-blooded animals, from mussels to alligators. Reptiles and amphibians are especially common carriers (Waltman et al., 1986). It can also cause disease in striped bass, goldfish, common carp, grass carp, chinook salmon, largemouth bass, nilotica tilapia, striped mullet, Japanese flounder, yellowtail, red sea bream, and crimson sea bream (Plumb, 1993). Wyatt (1979) also found that up to 100% of the crayfish, frogs, and turtles in ponds that contain infected catfish are infected.

RISK FACTORS AND TRANSMISSION

The disease is mainly a problem in older channel catfish and Japanese eels, but fingerlings and elvers are susceptible. Most disease seems to occur at high temperature. It is most prevalent in channel catfish at ~30° C (86° F) (Meyer & Bullock, 1973) and is most prevalent in Japanese eels during summer. However, it has caused disease in Taiwan-cultured eels at 10° to 18° C (50° to 64° F) (Liu & Tsai, 1980). It is also associated with organic pollution. In catfish ponds, mortalities are usually low and chronic (< 5%), but if fish are stressed, mortalities may be high. Hemolysin and chondroitin sulfate activities may be pathogenic factors.

Transmission and the source of infection during outbreaks in fish are uncertain, although the infection is known to remain dormant in fish tissues. Carrion-eating birds may also be an important source of infection (Winsor et al., 1981).

ZOONOTIC ASPECTS

Edwardsiella tarda is an important zoonotic problem and is a serious cause of enteric disease in humans. It can be isolated from the urine and feces of many mammals, including man (Clarridge et al., 1980) and marine mammals (Coles et al., 1978), although it is typically associated with freshwater environments. In humans, it has been implicated in meningitis, liver abcesses, wound infections, and most commonly gastroenteritis. It is often recovered from catfish fillets in processing plants and may spread to man via the oral route.

Clinical Signs/Pathogenesis

Clinical signs of edwardsiellosis vary with the species affected but often have masses of bacteria, both surrounded by inflammatory cells and free within lesions.

CHANNEL CATFISH

Lesions are initially seen as 3 to 5 mm red cutaneous foci on the flanks and caudal peduncle. They are caused by fistulas originating deep in the muscle that extend from malodorous fluctuant subdermal masses (Meyer & Bullock, 1973) (Fig. II-48). There is also petechiation and malodorous (hydrogen sulfide production) liquefactive necrosis of the viscera with fibrinous peritonitis. Characteristically, fish may continue to eat even if

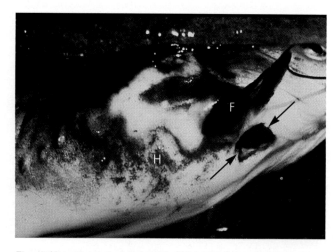

Fig. II-48 Channel catfish with *Edwardsiella tarda* infection. Note the deep fistula on the flank (*arrows*). F = pectoral fin; H = hemorrhage.

(Photograph courtesy of F. Meyer.)

severely affected. There may be posterior paresis in late stages. Larger fish (> 40 cm [16 inches]) are most commonly affected, often broodfish.

JAPANESE EELS

Japanese eels may exhibit one of two forms (Miyazaki & Egusa, 1976a, 1976b): The nephric form (*suppurative interstitial nephritis*) is more common and is associated with necrotic renal foci that spread to other organs (spleen, liver, gills, stomach, and heart). In the hepatic form (*suppurative hepatitis*), microabscesses form in the liver and spread to other organs. These lesions appear as light-colored nodules on the viscera. Abscesses may ulcerate through the body musculature.

OTHER SPECIES

In striped bass, unusual features include epithelial hyperplasia, which can give the fish a tattered appearance, and necrosis in the lateral line and on the body surface and gills (Herman & Bullock, 1986). Anemia and hypoxia also occur. In tilapia, lesions include skin depigmentation, swollen abdomen, and corneal opacity. There are white, bacteria-filled nodules in the gills, kidney, liver, spleen, or intestine (Kubota et al., 1981).

Diagnosis

Definitive diagnosis is based on standard biochemical tests and agglutination. Fluorescent antibody has also been used to identify the pathogen (Amandi et al., 1982).

The agent can be isolated from affected tissues, especially the kidney, using a simple medium, such as trypticase soy agar (Waltman et al., 1986). Isolates grow best at 37° C (98.6° F) but will appear after 2 to 4 days at 25° C (77° F) as small, grey, circular, transparent colonies composed of motile gram-negative rods (Shotts & Teska, 1989).

Treatment

As with many fish bacterial pathogens, *E. tarda* is associated with polluted environments. Thus, systemic antibiotic treatment (oxytetracycline) should be accompanied by an improvement in water quality. Some strains of *E. tarda* are resistant to oxytetracycline (Hilton & Wilson, 1980). Drug-resistant strains of *E. tarda* that carry transferable R-plasmids have appeared at high frequency in cultured Japanese eels (Aoki et al., 1987). Scarring may occur on surviving fish (Meyer & Bullock, 1973).

PROBLEM 49
Vibriosis (Salt Water Furunculosis, *Vibrio* Infection, Hitra Disease)

Prevalence Index
WM - 1, CF - 4, CM - 1
Method of Diagnosis
Culture of large numbers of vibrios from typical skin and/or internal lesions
History
Acute to chronic morbidity/mortality
Physical Examination
Red areas on body; skin ulcers; depression; exophthalmos; swollen abdomen
Treatment
Appropriate antibiotic

COMMENTS
Epidemiology/Pathogenesis
Vibriosis is caused by infection with one of several members of the primarily marine genus *Vibrio* and is one of the most important diseases affecting marine fish. All marine fish are probably susceptible to at least one species. Vibrios have been infrequently isolated from freshwater aquarium fish and freshwater salmonids that have been fed marine offal (Hacking & Budd, 1971; Kitao et al., 1983).

Vibrios are facultative pathogens that can readily survive and multiply in the environment, although the relative pathogenicity of environmental versus fish isolates is uncertain. Vibrios are commonly isolated from the mucosal surfaces and internal organs of clinically healthy fish, as well as from invertebrates, sediments, and the water column. Highest environmental prevalence is in organically polluted water and high salinity.

A major predisposing risk factor for vibriosis in salmonids and other species is high temperatures, making this a summer disease. Crowding, organic pollution, and other stressors can also precipitate outbreaks. Strains also vary considerably in virulence, and some strains can cause disease without any predisposing stress. Some vibrios produce hemolysins (which may cause anemia) and proteases (which may cause muscle damage) (Hjeltnes & Roberts, 1993).

Clinical Signs/Pathology
VIBRIO ANGUILLARUM (SALT WATER FURUNCULOSIS)
Vibrio anguillarum is the most common fish-pathogenic vibrio. Recent phylogenetic studies of ribosomal RNA (ribonucleic acid) suggest that this organism should belong in a new genus (*Listonella* [MacDonnell & Colwell, 1985]); however, the name *Vibrio* will be retained for this discussion, since this change has yet to be widely adopted.

Clinical signs of systemic *Vibrio anguillarum* infection are similar to *Aeromonas salmonicida* infection (ergo, salt water furunculosis). Both localized skin ulcers and systemic infections can occur. Systemic infections often localize in iron-rich filtering organs, such as spleen and kidney. In salmonids, three systemic forms of the disease have been described (Hjeltnes & Roberts, 1993).

The peracute form presents as anorexia, darkening, and sudden death in young fish. Histopathological features include cardiac myopathy with sarcoplasmic vacuolation (which may be the only lesion) and renal and splenic necrosis.

In the acute form, dark, fluctuant, subdermal cavitations ulcerate to release serosanguinous fluid. There is also abdominal distension, anemia, and dermal hemorrhage. Internal signs of typical septicemia include visceral petechiation, splenomegaly, and liquefactive renal necrosis. Histologically, there is necrosis of the liver, spleen, kidney, and heart, as well as depletion of hematopoietic elements. A necrotic enteritis produces a catarrhal, yellow, mucoid exudate.

The chronic form presents as organized, deep, granulomatous muscle lesions on various parts of the body, including the head. Deep muscle lesions may not be apparent until slaughter. Eye lesions are common, including corneal edema, ulceration, and exophthalmos.

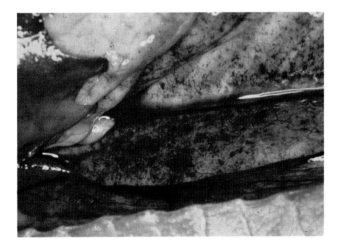

Fig. II-49 Atlantic salmon with vibriosis (Hitra disease). Massive hemorrhages in viscera.

(Photograph courtesy of H. Moller.)

There is also hemorrhage in the abdominal cavity, contributing to anemia and fibrinous adhesions. Histologically, there is heavy hemosiderin deposition in melanomacrophage centers, presumably because of hemolysins produced by the bacteria.

VIBRIO SALMONICIDA (HITRA DISEASE, COLD WATER VIBRIOSIS)

Vibrio salmonicida is a serious problem in sea-cultured Atlantic salmon in Europe (Hjeltnes & Roberts, 1993) and has been recently identified in cultured stocks in the northwest Atlantic, including Canada and the United States (O'Halloran et al., 1992). It has also recently been identified in Atlantic cod (Jorgensen et al., 1989). In salmonids, clinical signs are similar to *V. anguillarum*, ranging from peracute mortality with no clinical signs to a chronic, hemorrhagic septicemia. Outbreaks occur in winter, typically when temperatures drop below 5° C (41° F), and continue until the temperature drops below 2° C (35.6° F). Morbidity can resume when temperatures warm to 2° to 3° C (35.6° to 37.4° F) in spring and continue until temperatures exceed 8° C (46.4° F). Outbreaks begin with anorexia, depression, and disorientation, proceeding to abdominal distension, rectal prolapse, reddening of the fins and skin, and pale gills.

Internally, there may be fluid in the peritoneal cavity and hemorrhages on the swim bladder, abdominal fat, and other viscera (Fig. II-49). Histopathology is similar to *V. anguillarum* but often with severe heart and muscle damage (myonecrosis).

OTHER VIBRIOS

Other less commonly isolated vibrios cause either skin lesions or bacterial hemorrhagic septicemia in various fish species:

Vibrio ordalii (V. anguillarum biotype II): This agent is pathologically and biochemically similar to *V. anguillarum* (formerly known as *V. anguillarum* biotype I), causing a bacterial hemorrhagic septicemia in marine fish in Japan and the Pacific Northwest of the United States (Schiewe et al., 1981). Differentiating features include the tendency of *V. ordalii* to form bacterial microcolonies in muscle, gill, and gastrointestinal tract (Ransom et al., 1984). Bacteremia also typically develops later in the course of the disease.

Vibrio damsela: This agent causes skin ulcers or systemic disease in a wide range of fish, including blacksmith damselfish, yellowtail, turbot, gilthead sea bream, and brown shark (Fouz et al., 1992). It is also a zoonotic pathogen, causing skin ulcers in humans (Love et al., 1981). It is now considered a member of the genus *Photobacterium* (Austin & Austin, 1993).

Vibrio carchariae: This agent causes systemic disease and skin ulcers in sharks. It has been isolated from a sandbar shark and lemon sharks (Colwell & Grimes, 1984). Affected fish develop subdermal necrotic "cysts" and necrosis and inflammation of viscera and brain (Grimes et al., 1985).

Vibrio alginolyticus: This agent appears to cause disease only in highly stressed individuals, including gilthead sea bream, mullet, and other marine species (Colorni et al., 1981).

Vibrio vulnificus biogroup 2: This agent is pathologically similar to *V. anguillarum* and has caused bacterial hemorrhagic septicemia in Japanese eels in Japan and European eels in England, Spain, and the Netherlands (Austin & Austin, 1993).

Vibrio cholerae (non 01): This agent has been reported only once as a fish pathogen, from ayu in Japan (Muroga et al., 1979). Experimental challenges demonstrated the organism to be highly pathogenic to ayu and Japanese eels.

Vibrio fischeri: This agent was isolated from diseased turbot in Spain that exhibited skin papillomas and visceral neoplasia (Lamas et al., 1990).

Vibrio harveyi: This agent was isolated from common snook in Florida, USA, that developed corneal opacity within 24 hours of being transported (Kraxberger-Beatty et al., 1990). This agent was also isolated from deep skin ulcers in feral jack crevalle.

Vibrio splendidus: This agent has been isolated from cultured turbot in Spain, Atlantic salmon in Scotland, and turbot and European sea bass in Norway (Austin & Austin, 1993). It causes a typical bacterial hemorrhagic septicemia.

Diagnosis

Definitive diagnosis of vibriosis requires identification of the bacterium in target tissues, with attendant clinical signs. Isolation in a mixed culture from normal colonization sites (e.g., skin, gastrointestinal tract) on fish does not necessarily indicate that vibriosis is reponsible for the disease. It is important to be certain that this is the primary infectious cause of the problem. Vibrios can be secondary invaders. Kidney is probably the best organ for isolation; lesions should also be sampled. Note that *V. salmonicida* is psychrophilic and should be incubated at low temperatures (12° to 16° C [54° to 61° F]) to achieve isolation; *V. salmonicida* colonies take 3 to 5 days to appear; the small, translucent colonies may be missed without careful examination.

Vibrios are gram-negative, short (~0.5 to 2.0 μm), motile, usually curved rods. Almost all either require or have enhanced growth in the presence of sodium, but fish pathogens are usually readily isolated on a rich nutrient medium (e.g., Columbia blood agar). Tissue-invading pathogens typically have low sodium requirements, which is a factor in their ability to survive in the host.

Treatment

Vibriosis is a classical example of a stress-borne disease. Losses caused by vibriosis are highly dependent on the severity of the environmental stress that precipitated the outbreak, varying from acute to chronic. Salmonids often *break* with vibriosis after movement from freshwater to seawater. Exposure to copper (>30 μg/ml) or iron (> 10 μg/ml) also increases susceptibility to vibriosis (Hetrick et al., 1979; Austin & Austin, 1993).

Oxytetracycline, potentiated sulfonamides, and oxolinic acid have been used successfully, but there is increasing resistance to these drugs, especially in *V. anguillarum* and *V. salmonicida* (Hjeltnes & Roberts, 1993). Commercial bacterins, available for *V. anguillarum*, *V. ordalii*, and *V. salmonicida*, provide good protection for populations at risk. Reducing stress is imperative for long-term management.

PROBLEM 50
Pasteurellosis (Tuberculosis, Pseudotuberculosis, *Pasteurella Piscicida* Infection)

Prevalence Index
Does not affect listed species groups
Method of Diagnosis
Culture of *Pasteurella piscicida* from typical skin and/or internal lesions
History
Acute to chronic morbidity/mortality
Physical Examination
Multiple, raised, white nodules on spleen and kidney (chronic form only)
Treatment
Appropriate antibiotic

COMMENTS
Epidemiology
Pasteurellosis is a common disease in cultured marine fish in Japan, including ayu, black sea bream, red sea bream, red grouper, oval fish, and yellowtail (Kitao, 1993a).

Pasteurella piscicida has also caused isolated epidemics in white perch, striped bass, and gulf menhaden in coastal waters of the United States (Snieszko et al., 1964; Paperna & Zwerner, 1976; Robohm, 1983; Hawke et al., 1987; Lewis et al., 1970). It has also been isolated from snakehead in Taiwan (Tung et al., 1985). Rudd and chub isolates in England (Ajmal & Hobbs, 1967) may actually be atypical *Aeromonas salmonicida* (see *PROBLEM 48*). Most recently, it has been isolated from cultured and wild marine fish in the Mediterranean areas of Spain, France, and Italy (Margarinoz et al., 1992), as well as Israel (R. Avtalion, Personal Communication).

Mode of transmission is unknown, although fish-to-fish contact and an invertebrate vector have both been suggested. Oral transmission is likely. The reservoir of infection is uncertain, although striped bass were believed to be the major source of infection in Chesapeake Bay. Host susceptibility varies significantly, since many unrelated fish species were not clinically affected during a striped bass epidemic (Hawke et al., 1987).

In Japan, epidemics occur when salinities drop to < 30 ppt after a heavy rain and temperatures rise over 25° C (77° F) (Kitao, 1993). Epidemics do not develop if the temperature remains below 25° C (77° F). High temperature has also been associated with outbreaks in the United States (Hawke et al., 1987).

Clinical Signs /Pathogenesis
Pasteurella piscicida causes a bacteremia/septicemia that takes one of two forms.

ACUTE FORM
In the acute form, few clinical signs are present. There may be small hemorrhages around the gill covers or the bases of the fins (Snieszko et al., 1964), or there may be abnormal skin pigmentation and enlarged spleen and kidney (Hawke et al., 1987). Histologically, there is acute necrosis of spleen, liver, and pancreas with no inflammation.

CHRONIC FORM
In the chronic form, there are 1 to 2 mm miliary lesions in the kidney and spleen that are composed of bacteria that incite a chronic inflammatory response. The appearance of this latter lesion has led to its being misleadingly called tuberculosis or pseudotuberculosis.

Diagnosis
Presumptive diagnosis of *Pasteurella piscicida* is based on presence of typical gross lesions having gram-negative, nonpigmented, short (~0.5 to 0.75 × 1 to 2 μm long), nonmotile rods that stain bipolarly. Note that *Aeromonas salmonicida* (see *PROBLEM 46*) is morphologically similar and has been mistaken for *Pasteurella* (Hastein & Bullock, 1976). Confirmatory diagnosis can be performed by using slide agglutination or immunofluorescence.

The agent can be isolated from affected organs, especially kidney and spleen, by using nutrient agar at room temperature. Shiny grey-yellow, entire, convex, 1 to 2 mm colonies develop after 48 to 72 hours. Culturally, *P. piscicida* most closely resembles non-pigment-forming isolates of *Aeromonas salmonicida*.

Treatment
Infections in Japan have been treated with many different antibiotics, such as ampicillin (Kusuda & Inoue, 1977) and potentiated sulfonamides (Fujihara et al., 1984). However, there are serious problems with resistance (Kitao, 1993).

Oxytetracycline was not very effective in controlling an outbreak in striped bass; however, this was believed to be due to inadequate tissue levels attained in target organs and not to resistance of the bacterial isolate (Hawke et al., 1987). Experimental vaccines show promise (Fukuda & Kusuda, 1981; Kusuda et al., 1988).

PROBLEM 51
Enteric Redmouth Disease (ERM, Redmouth, Yersiniosis, Blood Spot, *Yersinia Ruckeri* Infection)

Prevalence Index
CF - 1
Method of Diagnosis
Culture of *Yersinia ruckeri* from typical skin and/or internal lesions
History
Dark fish that cannot find food (blind); acute to chronic mortalities
Physical Examination
Typical of hemorrhagic septicemia; especially dark coloration, exophthalmos, hemorrhage in mouth and eyes, depression, swollen abdomen
Treatment
Appropriate antibiotic

COMMENTS
Epidemiology
Yersiniosis has been reported in the United States, Canada, Australia, Africa, and Europe. *Yersinia ruckeri* is an important pathogen of salmonids. Rainbow trout are especially susceptible, but steelhead, cutthroat, brown and brook trout, and coho, sockeye, chinook, and Atlantic salmon are also affected. While any age salmonid is susceptible, ERM primarily affects market-sized fish, making it a potentially devastating disease.

The bacterium has also been less frequently isolated from diseased European sea bass, emerald shiners, fathead minnows, cisco, sturgeon, turbot, peled, whitefish, and muskum whitefish. It has also been isolated from asymptomatic goldfish, common carp, European eel, burbot, coalfish, and arctic char (Stevenson et al., 1993). The bacterium is widespread in freshwater environments.

Pathogenesis
ERM outbreaks usually begin with chronic, low mortality, which generally escalates. Severity of ERM outbreaks depend mainly on strain virulence and degree of environmental stress. There are six serovars of *Y. ruckeri*, Types I to VI. Type I (Hagerman) is the most common, widely distributed, and pathogenic. But, not all serovar I isolates are pathogenic, and other serovars can be highly lethal (Stevenson et al., 1993).

The incubation period at 15° C (59° F) is about 1 week. There is lower morbidity/mortality at low (< 10° C [50° F]) temperatures. Mortalities may occur for up to 60 days. A high percentage (> 75%) of recovered fish may become carriers (Busch & Lingg, 1975). Subclinical carriers cyclically shed bacteria from the lower intestine (Busch & Lingg, 1975). About monthly shedding has occurred in experimentally affected populations, but the periodicity of the shedding cycle probably varies with environmental conditions (Stevenson et al., 1993). Cyclic shedding helps to explain fluctuation in pathogen prevalence in fish populations (Bruno & Munro, 1989). The carrier state can be maintained indefinitely (> 100 days) with an average 10% infection (Busch & Lingg, 1975).

High (15° to 18° C [59° to 64° F]) temperature can cause carriers to begin shedding, leading to clinical disease (Rucker, 1966). Clinical signs can develop within several days of the stress. Grading (Rucker, 1966) and copper exposure (Knittel, 1981) may also initiate outbreaks. There may be up to 70% mortality initially. The mechanisms responsible for virulence are unknown.

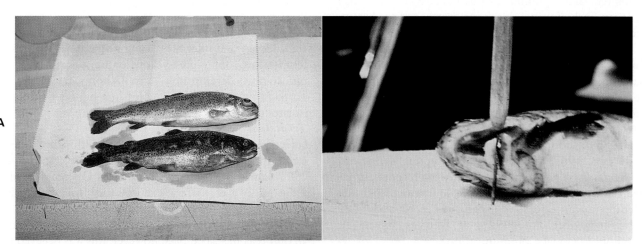

A   B

Fig. II-51   **A,** Rainbow trout with exophthalmos (*top fish*) and darkened color (*bottom fish*) exhibit common clinical findings with ERM. **B,** The lower jaw of a trout has been propped open, revealing hemorrhage in the roof of the mouth, a classical lesion of ERM.

(*A* photograph by K. Townsend and E. Noga; *B* photograph courtesy of C.L. Davis Foundation for Veterinary Pathology.)

Clinical Signs/Pathogenesis

GROSS LESIONS

The early stages of ERM resemble aeromonad and vibrio infections. There is darkening of the dorsum, anorexia, and lethargy. Internal lesions are typical of other gram-negative bacterial septicemias, including visceral petechiation, splenomegaly, and necrosis of the intestinal mucosa with a catarrhal exudate.

With chronic disease, there is also abdominal distension, unilateral or bilateral exophthalmos (Fig. II-51, *A*), and hyphema (*blood spot*). In this case, darkening is due to the ophthalmic lesions, which cause blindness, leading to lack of melanin pigment control (Fig. II-51, *A*). Fish also accumulate near the outlet screens of the raceway (see Fig. I-3).

CLINICAL PATHOLOGY/HISTOPATHOLOGY

Clinical pathological changes include leucocytosis, reticulocytosis, low hematocrit, and low total plasma protein. Histologically, there is bacterial colonization of well-vascularized tissues, causing hemorrhage and/or telangiectasis of gills, kidney, liver, spleen, and heart, as well as muscle. This leads to necrosis of the hematopoietic tissue, causing anemia. There is also necrosis and sloughing of the gastrointestinal tract.

Diagnosis

Gross lesions that differentiate ERM from other bacterial septicemias include reddened skin erosions found mainly on the head or mouth (Fig. II-51, *B*), especially the lower jaw, and *blood spot* (hyphema). The latter is characteristic of infections in Atlantic salmon. While these lesions are good presumptive evidence for ERM in salmonids, they are not always present (Frerichs et al., 1985).

Definitive diagnosis of ERM requires identification of the bacterium in target tissues, with attendant clinical signs. Kidney is the best organ for isolation during epidemics. Lower intestine appears to be better for isolating the bacterium from asymptomatic carriers (Busch & Lingg, 1975). The bacterium is sometimes difficult to isolate, and enrichment by first incubating samples in trypticase soy broth for 2 days at 18° C (64° F) has been advocated (Stevenson et al., 1993). However, this may not be successful with intestinal samples because of the large numbers of other bacteria.

Some other members of the Enterobacteriaceae (e.g., *Hafnia alvei* and *Serratia liquefaciens*) are phenotypically and even immunologically similar to *Y. ruckeri*. A selective medium based on positive Tween 80 hydrolysis and negative sucrose fermentation is useful for North American isolates (Waltman & Shotts, 1984) but is not as successful in identifying isolates from other geographic areas (Austin & Austin, 1993).

Treatment

In the United States oxytetracycline is the antibiotic of choice for food fish, but many *Y. ruckeri* isolates are resistant. Ormetoprim-sulfadimethoxine is more expensive, but less resistance is present. Many isolates are also susceptible to oxolinic acid (Rogers & Austin, 1982).

Carriers are the most important source of infection, especially when stressed (Hunter et al., 1980). Keeping the water supply free of carrier fish is the best method of control. Carriers can also be kept downstream of susceptible populations. Vertical transmission has not been demonstrated. Eggs from infected broodstock should be treated with antiseptic. Maintain good sanitation and keep stress to a minimum to reduce recrudescence of carriers. Keep fish-eating birds and mammals away from culture facilities, since many can transport the bacterium in their intestines (Stevenson et al., 1993). Natural disease does not confer complete immunity, but commercial *Y. ruckeri* bacterins offer good protection and are important in managing populations at risk for ERM.

PROBLEM 52

Bacterial Kidney Disease (BKD, Dee Disease, *Renibacterium Salmoninarum* Infection)

Prevalence Index

CF - 1, CM - 2 (salmonids only)

Method of Diagnosis

1. Culture of *Renibacterium salmoninarum* from typical skin and/or internal lesions
2. Identification of *R. salmoninarum* with immunological probe

History

Acute to chronic morbidity/mortality

Physical Examination

Focal, white nodules in spleen, kidney, other viscera; pseudodiphtheritic membrane covering viscera; cavitations in muscle

Treatment

Appropriate antibiotic

COMMENTS

Epidemiology

Renibacterium salmoninarum is an important pathogen of salmonids, especially rainbow, brown, and brook trout and coho and chinook salmon. BKD only affects salmonids. Any age fish is susceptible, but losses often do not occur until the fish are well grown (> 6 months old), which makes it a potentially devastating disease. It occurs in virtually all areas where salmonids occur, except Australia, New Zealand, and Russia (Evelyn, 1993). It is a serious problem in the northeast Pacific (United States, Canada) and in Japan.

Some nonsalmonids can be experimentally infected with *R. salmoninarum* (Traxler & Bell, 1988), but none develop BKD. It is unlikely that nonsalmonids are a significant reservoir of infection because there are no published reports of natural infections in nonsalmonids. The

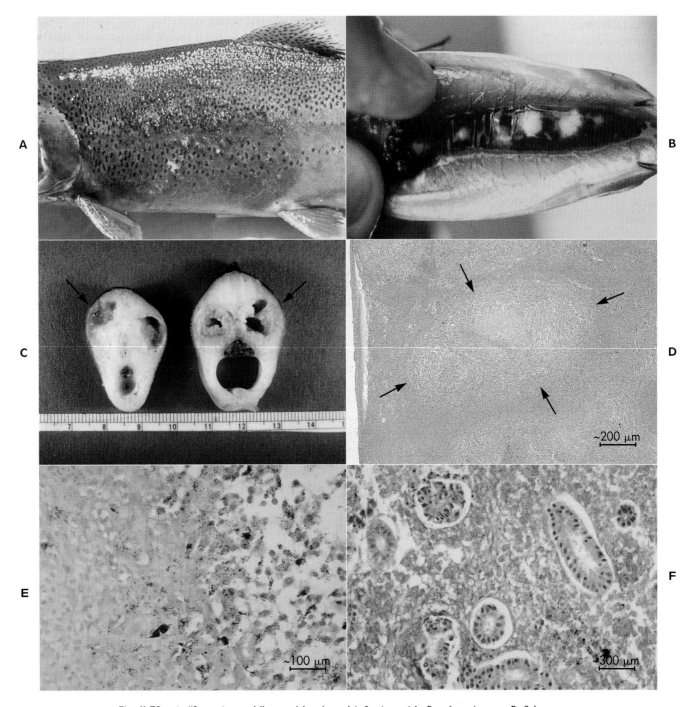

Fig. II-52 A, "Spawning rash" caused by dermal infection with *R. salmoninarum*. B, Salmon with abdominal cavity opened and viscera removed, revealing focal, white nodules in the kidney caused by BKD. C, Cross-sections through the body of a salmon, revealing large cavitations in muscle (*arrows*) caused by *R. salmoninarum* infection. D, Histological section of anterior kidney, showing a large area of focal necrosis (*arrows*) caused by *R. salmoninarum* infection. Hematoxylin and eosin. E, Gram stain of section in Fig. II-52, *D*, with numerous, gram-positive, short bacterial rods. Brown and Brenn. F, *R. salmoninarum* infection. Chronic interstitial nephritis. Kidney hematopoietic tissue has been replaced with a macrophage infiltrate. Compare with Fig. I-3, *E*. Hematoxylin and eosin.

(*A* and *B* photographs courtesy of National Fish Health Research Laboratory, USA; *C* photograph courtesy of R. Wolke.)

bacterium is an obligate pathogen and dies quickly in the environment (Evelyn, 1993).

Horizontal transmission can occur in both freshwater and seawater via cohabitation with infected fish, ingestion, skin wounds, or contact with contaminated water. Feeding of raw viscera was responsible for epidemics in the 1960s. Vertical transmission is a major problem. The bacterium is commonly within the eggs of infected females (Evelyn et al., 1984). It resides in the yolk, protected from antiseptics (Evelyn et al., 1986). Infected peritoneal fluid is a major source of egg infection, but there is evidence that intraovum infections may also occur before ovulation (Evelyn, 1993).

Clinical disease is most likely to develop during times of stress, especially during transfer of salmonids from freshwater to seawater, or during spawning (Fryer & Sanders, 1981). While BKD is typically a chronic infection, stress may precipitate acute mortalities. There can be a higher incidence of BKD in soft water, probably because of biological factors.

Clinical Signs/Pathogenesis

GROSS LESIONS

Fish with severe BKD may have no external signs. Affected fish may present with dark coloration, exophthalmos, pale gills, abdominal distension, or hemorrhages at the vent or base of the fins. Small vesicles on the flanks (Fig. II-52, A), filled with clear or turbid fluid, rupture to form small ulcers.

The major target organ is the kidney, which has white, nodular masses (Fig. II-52, B). Nodules may also occur in other viscera, especially spleen. There may be fluid in the abdomen. A pseudodiphtheritic membrane may be present over the abdominal viscera, most often at less than 10° C (50° F). A less common finding is large cavitations in skeletal muscle (Fig. II-52, C).

HISTOPATHOLOGY

Nodules are focal, often large, granulomas consisting of macrophages containing various numbers of phagocytized bacteria. In relatively resistant species (e.g., Atlantic salmon), granulomas are often encapsulated, indicating a successful host response. In more susceptible Pacific salmon, granulomas are rarely well-encapsulated (Evelyn, 1993) (Fig. II-52, D). In advanced lesions, there is often caseous necrosis with numerous free bacteria (Bruno, 1986).

Diagnosis

CLINICAL DISEASE

Tissue smears having 0.5×1 to 2 μm, coryneform-like, gram-positive rods can be used for a rapid presumptive identification of BKD but are not reliable in light infections because of the difficulty in differentiating the bacterium from melanin granules (see Fig. I-3, A). Histopathology can also provide presumptive identification (Fig. II-52, D through F) but is best accompanied by immunological confirmation.

Definitive diagnosis of clinical BKD requires identification of the bacterium in target tissues, with attendant clinical signs. The corpuscle of Stannius, a paired, white, endocrine organ in the anterior kidney, should not be mistaken for a BKD nodule. Kidney is the best organ for sampling during epidemics.

Renibacterium salmoninarum is fastidious and extremely slow-growing, typically requiring 3 to 6 weeks to appear after primary isolation (Evelyn, 1977). It grows best at 15° to 18° C (59° to 64° F) and does not grow at 25° C (77° F) (Evelyn, 1993). It also requires a specialized medium for isolation, which is not commercially available (see Shotts & Teska, 1989). Thus, clinical diagnosis of BKD is almost always based on immunological identification of R. salmoninarum antigen in tissues. The bacterium is an immunologically homogeneous taxon. Direct fluorescent antibody is presently the most widely used technique but is being supplanted by enzyme-linked immunosorbent assay (Pascho et al., 1987; Anonymous, 1991). An ELISA kit (Diagxotics), as well as antisera (Kirkegard and Perry Labs), is commercially available for diagnosis. Tissue samples can also be sent to a specialized laboratory for confirmatory diagnosis. False positives are a serious problem, especially when small numbers of fish are positive (Austin & Austin, 1987).

The only bacteria that may be mistaken for R. salmoninarum are a group of small, gram-positive rods that cause pseudokidney disease (see PROBLEM 54). They are easily differentiated from R. salmoninarum based on their rapid growth at 30° C (86° F) on trypticase soy or brain-heart infusion agar (Hiu et al., 1984). Renibacterium salmoninarum is not acid-fast, which differentiates it from Mycobacterium (see PROBLEM 53).

CARRIERS

Detection of carriers is mainly focused on identifying infected broodstock. Ovarian fluid is the best material for identifying the bacterium from asymptomatic carriers during spawning because it is a known source of infection for eggs and bacterial load is proportional to the infection status of ovary tissue (another source of inoculum). Unfortunately, fluorescent antibody is not always sensitive enough to detect all carriers (Evelyn, 1993). Newly developed ELISA methods appear to be more sensitive (Myers et al., 1993). However, membrane filtration followed by fluorescent antibody is also good for ovarian fluid (Elliott & Barila, 1987).

Treatment

There are no proven therapies that can unequivocally cure fish of BKD (Elliott et al., 1989). The intimate association of the bacterium with host defenses, coupled with its chronic, insidious nature, make it difficult to control. Macrolide antibiotics (e.g., erythromycin) are the most effective agents in treating both clinical and asymptomatic infections (Austin, 1985; Moffitt, 1991). Only erythromycin, thiocyanate, and phosphate were effective prophylactically or therapeutically against BKD; other forms tested (stearate, ethylsuccinate, or estolate) were not (Austin, 1985).

CLINICAL DISEASE

Oral erythromycin and thiocyanate appear to reduce severity of outbreaks but have not been proven to cure fish of the infection (Austin, 1985). Oral oxytetracycline has also been used to try to control infections, since it is less expensive (Kent, 1992). However, oxytetracycline was ineffective in either prophylaxis or treatment of experimental BKD (Austin, 1985).

ASYMPTOMATIC INFECTIONS

Injection of erythromycin base (as Erythro® 100 or Erythro® 200) into female broodstock before spawning significantly reduces the incidence of infected eggs (Moffitt, 1991). This occurs because it kills bacteria in the fish and because the procedure "loads" antibiotic into the eggs. Erythromycin is detectable into the alevin stage (Evelyn, 1993). There is preliminary evidence that this procedure may entirely eliminate the infection from broods (Lee & Evelyn, 1991).

Female broodstock should be injected with erythromycin between 9 and 56 days before spawning (Armstrong et al., 1989). In one preliminary study, there was no evidence of bacteria when fish were injected about 28 days before spawning (Lee & Evelyn, 1991). As an added precaution, eggs should also be treated with potentiated iodine antiseptic after spawning (Evelyn, 1993). Treating eggs only with antiseptic is ineffective because antiseptics do not penetrate the egg (Evelyn et al., 1986). Male broodstock are not treated, since they do not seem to be a significant source of vertical transmission, even when milt is heavily infected with the bacterium (Evelyn, 1993).

Exposure of eggs to erythromycin phosphate before water hardening is not effective in reducing infection incidence, since therapeutic antibiotic levels are not maintained long enough and the antibiotic does not penetrate the yolk where some bacteria occur (Elliot et al., 1989).

AVOIDANCE

Use of specific-pathogen-free stock is the best means of control, but this may be difficult to achieve with anadromous stocks that are frequently exposed to feral fish har-

boring the bacterium. Successful screening relies heavily on sensitive and specific testing for asymptomatic carriers. Clean stocks should be kept away from waters having feral salmonids. If possible, only one age group should be kept on a farm at one time.

PROBLEM 53

Mycobacteriosis (Tuberculosis)

Prevalence Index
WF - 1, WM - 3, CF - 4, CM - 3
Method of Diagnosis
1. Culture of *Mycobacterium*
2. Histology of lesions (spleen, liver, kidney, skin)
History
Chronic morbidity/mortality
Physical Examination
Nonhealing, shallow to deep skin ulcers; corneal ulcers; pale coloration; emaciation; white nodules on viscera
Treatment
Disinfect and quarantine

COMMENTS

Epidemiology

HOST RANGE

Mycobacteriosis is probably the most common chronic disease that affects aquarium fish. Virtually all freshwater and marine aquarium fish are probably susceptible, especially members of the freshwater families Anabantidae, Characidae, and Cyprinidae (Nigrelli & Vogel, 1963). Aquarium fish mycobacteriosis is caused by the mycobacteria *Mycobacterium marinum* and *M. fortuitum*.

Although disease is presently uncommon in salmonids, asymptomatic *Mycobacterium* infections are common in some populations; over 25% of some hatchery salmonids are infected with *M. chelonae* along the northeastern Pacific coast (Arakawa & Fryer, 1984). *Mycobacterium* was historically a serious problem in salmonids, when they were fed raw fish offal (Ross et al., 1959). *Mycobacterium neoaurum* was recently isolated from a mixed culture from Atlantic salmon with ocular lesions (Backman et al., 1990). Mycobacteriosis has also

---

Fig. II-53 A, Dwarf gourami with a large chronic skin ulcer caused by mycobacteriosis. **B,** Mozambique tilapia with corneal ulceration and chronic, hyperpigmented ulcerations on the flank and fins (*arrow*) caused by *Mycobacterium marinum*. **C,** Massively hypertrophied spleen (*S*) of a Mediterranean sea bass with multifocal granulomas caused by *Mycobacterium marinum*. **D,** Wet mount of the spleen of a Mozambique tilapia with mycobacterial granulomas (*G*). Note the dark, necrotic center and lighter periphery of inflammatory cells, which is diagnostic for granulomatous response. **E,** Granulomas (*G*) in the spleen of fish in Fig. II-53, *A*. Hematoxylin and eosin. **F,** Numerous acid-fast mycobacteria in a granuloma of fish in Fig. II-53, *A*. Fite-Faraco. **G,** Culture of *Mycobacterium marinum* on Lowenstein-Jensen agar. Note bright yellow (photochromogenic) colonies.

(*C* photograph courtesy of A. Colorni; *G* photograph courtesy of L. Khoo and E. Noga.)

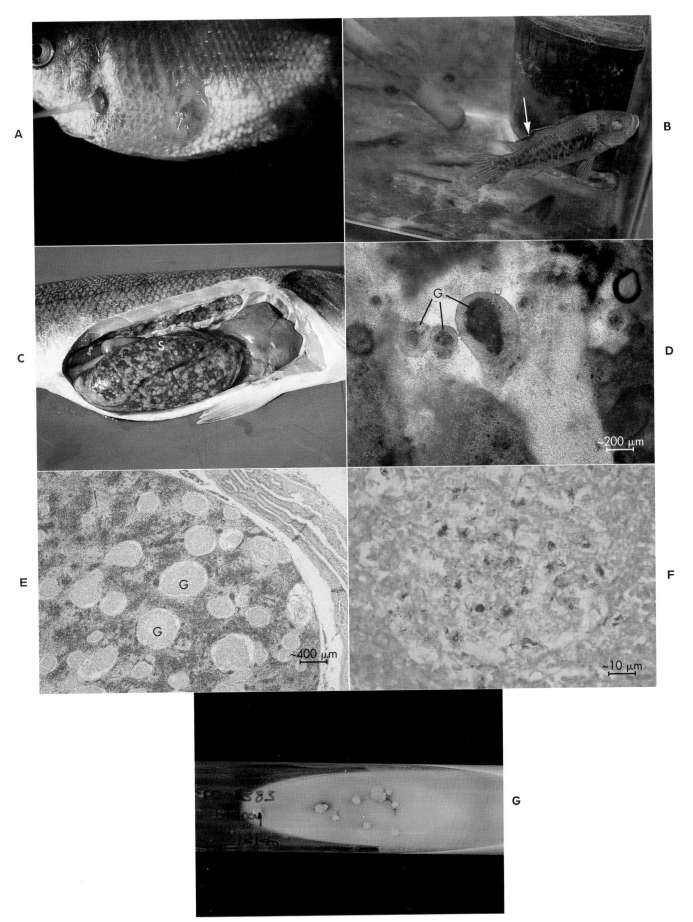

Fig. 11-53   *For legend see opposite page.*

been a serious problem in other cultured food fish, such as European sea bass (Colorni et al., 1993), tilapia, and striped bass (Hedrick et al., 1987a), especially in intensive culture systems.

TRANSMISSION

Shedding of bacteria from infected skin ulcers, as well as the intestine, is probably a major source of inoculum. Ingestion is probably the major source of infection, including fish that have recently eaten dead tankmates. The bacteria can survive for 2 years in the environment (Reichenbache-Klinke, 1972). Transovarian transmission has been demonstrated in platyfish (Conroy, 1966) but does not occur in salmonids (Ross & Johnson, 1962).

ZOONOTIC CONSIDERATIONS

Fish-pathogenic mycobacteria can infect humans, usually causing localized, nonhealing ulcers (*fish tank granuloma, swimming pool granuloma*) that may be difficult to treat because of the resistance of some isolates to most antituberculosis drugs (Noga et al., 1990). Owners should be cautioned about contacting potentially infected fish or fomites. The ubiquity of fish mycobacteriosis coupled with the apparently low numbers of human cases suggest that it fortunately appears to be a low risk for healthy humans. However, a small number of *M. marinum* infections have been reported from HIV-infected persons (Glaser et al., 1994). All acquired the infection from contact with pet fish, usually when cleaning the aquarium. Gloves should be worn by persons at risk when cleaning an aquarium or when handling fish (Angulo et al., 1994).

Clinical Signs/Pathogenesis

GROSS LESIONS

Emaciation, poor growth, or retarded sexual maturation may be the only clinical signs of mycobacteriosis. Other lesions include skeletal deformities; chronic, nonhealing, shallow to deep ulcers (Figs. II-53, *A* and *B*); or fin erosion. Internally, 1 to 4 mm white nodules may be present on the viscera, especially hypertrophic kidney or spleen (Fig. II-53, *C*).

HISTOPATHOLOGY

There is a chronic inflammatory response with epithelioid macrophages surrounding the bacteria. Lesions often have necrotic centers and may have melanomacrophages or melanocytes. Bacteria are typically located in the center of the inflammatory focus.

Diagnosis

Mycobacteriosis is strongly suggested by the typical clinical signs in combination with the presence of large numbers of granulomas in wet mounts (Fig. II-53, *D*), especially spleen and kidney. Granulomas can be caused by many other pathogens, but if large numbers are present, histological material should be stained for acid-fast bacteria (Fig. II-53, *E* and *F*). Fite-Faraco is often better than Ziehl-Neelsen for demonstrating piscine mycobacteria (Wolke & Stroud, 1978). Tissue smears can also be

stained, but this is less advisable, since fresh, infective lesion material must then be handled, risking infection of the clinician. Note that an occasional granuloma is a common incidental finding on necropsy. Granulomas also look similar to melanomacrophage centers (see Fig. I-26, *A*). When in doubt about the significance of wet mount lesions, samples should be processed for histology.

Mycobacteria are ~0.4 × 1.0 to 4.0 μm long, are acid-fast, and often stain unevenly. Mycobacteria are also gram-positive but often do not stain well (Frerichs, 1993). Other acid-fast rods (i.e., *Nocardia* [see *PROBLEM 54*]) are longer and branching. *Nocardia* is also much less common in aquarium fish and salmonids than mycobacteriosis.

Isolation on Lowenstein-Jensen (Fig. II-53, *G*) or Middlebrook LH10 agar allows definitive diagnosis by biochemical identification, as well as determination of the species involved. Isolation may take up to 30 days; sometimes organisms cannot be cultured even when large numbers are seen in lesions (Frerichs, 1993). Some isolates may grow on blood agar or trypticase soy agar, if the inoculum is heavy (Shotts & Teska, 1989). Culture is usually not necessary unless treatment is anticipated.

Treatment

As with so many fish diseases, mycobacteriosis usually gains a foothold under suboptimal environmental conditions. Once established, it can be difficult to control because there is no nonlethal means of detecting carriers, although nucleic acid probes hold promise of improved detection of carriers (Colorni et al., 1993). The apparently high prevalence of subclinical disease in feral fish also makes it difficult to exclude. Disinfection and quarantine are the best methods of control.

Many drugs have been advocated for treating this disease, but there are few rigorous clinical trials yet published. In one study, erythromycin, rifampicin, or streptomycin was effective against experimental infections (Kawakami & Kusuda, 1990). There is some clinical evidence that kanamycin may be effective in some cases (Conroy & Solaro, 1965), although some strains are resistant in vitro (Noga et al., 1990b), and we know nothing of the bioavailability of any antimycobacteriosis drugs for fish. This disease can be insidious and difficult to eradicate. Improved management is mandatory. Freezing does not kill bacteria in carcasses (Ross et al., 1959).

PROBLEM 54
Miscellaneous Systemic Bacterial Infections

The most clinically important diseases in this group include botulism, streptococcosis, nocardiosis, pseudokidney disease, and pseudomonad infections. Other agents have only been isolated sporadically or in some instances from only a single epidemic.

Table II-54 Miscellaneous bacterial infections of fish.*

Disease/pathogen	Hosts	Geographic/ ecological range	Key diagnostic features	Treatment	References
ANAEROBES					
Eubacterium meningitis [Eubacterium tarantellus = Catenabacterium sp.]	Grey mullet, snook, redfish, flounder	Southeast USA, marine	Chronic onset of neurological signs (spiral swimming); filamentous, asporogenous, gram + rods in brain smears or histological sections	None proven[†]	Udey et al, 1977 Henley & Lewis, 1976 Lewis & Udey, 1978
Botulism [Clostridium botulinum Type E]	Rainbow trout, coho salmon	Northwest USA; England; Denmark; freshwater	Chronic mortality with intermittent depression; alternatively float and sink until death; common in sediment and fish intestines; diagnosis requires presence of clinical signs, not just isolation of pathogen (bacteria are common in sediment and gastrointestinal tract)	Oxytetracycline oral; destroy infected stock; remove detritus; lime pond	Eklund et al, 1982 Cann & Taylor, 1984 Schiewe et al, 1988
GRAM-POSITIVE AEROBIC COCCI					
Streptococcosis§ [Streptococcus spp.]	Striped mullet, sea trout, pinfish, spot, Atlantic croaker, Gulf menhaden, yellowtail, ayu, striped bass, pagrus sea bream, amago salmon, rainbow trout, hardhead sea catfish, stingray, tilapia, bluefish, siganid, golden shiner, silver sea trout, Japanese flounder, jacopever	Southeast USA; Chesapeake Bay, USA; South Africa; Japan; Israel; Italy; marine and freshwater	Acute to chronic mortality with exophthlalmos; hemorrhages on body; serosanguinous fluid in peritoneal cavity and intestine; reportedly problem in aquarium fish; many different Streptococcus spp.; dull grey, 1 to 2 mm colonies at 48 hours; very important disease	Ampicillin oral; erythromycin oral; oxytetra-cycline oral; see Kitao, 1993b, for other antibiotics	Plumb at al, 1974 Austin & Austin, 1987 Baya et al, 1990a Shotts & Teska, 1989 Shiomitsu et al, 1980 Gratzek et al, 1992 Kitao, 1993b
Staphylococcus epidermidis	Red sea bream, yellowtail	Japan; marine	Exophthalmos; skin ulcers; disease only reported once	None proven	Kusuda & Sugiyama, 1981
Staphylococcus aureus	Silver carp	India; freshwater	Corneal damage progressing to phthisis bulbi; disease only reported once	None proven	Shah & Tyagi, 1986
Planococcus sp.	Atlantic salmon, rainbow trout	England; freshwater	Associated with RTFS‡ and skin lesions in trout; kidney damage in salmon; sporadic cases	None proven	Austin & Stobie, 1992a Austin & Austin, 1993
Micrococcus luteus	Rainbow trout	England; freshwater	Isolated from fish with RTFS‡; disease only reported once	None proven	Austin & Stobie, 1992a

Continued.

Table II-54 Miscellaneous bacterial infections of fish, contd.

Disease/pathogen	Hosts	Geographic/ecological range	Key diagnostic features	Treatment	References
GRAM-POSITIVE AEROBIC RODS					
Nocardiosis (*Nocardia asteroides*)	Brook trout; steelhead trout; Pacific salmon; rainbow trout; paradise fish [E]; three-spot gourami [E]; neon tetra; green sunfish [E]; bluegill [E]; blue minnow [E]; Jack mackerel [E]; Formosa snakehead [E]; largemouth bass [E]	Worldwide; freshwater and marine	Clinically resembles mycobacteriosis; short, coccobacillary to long, slender, branching rods in chronic inflammatory lesions (*Mycobacterium* not branching); usually acid-fast in histological sections; abundant bacterial filaments in routine stains; growth on Lowenstein-Jensen agar after 21 days; important disease	None proven; destroy stock	Conroy, 1964 Van Duijn, 1981 Wood & Ordal, 1958 Chen, 1992
Nocardiosis; gill tuberculosis (*Nocardia seriolae = N. kampachi*)	Yellowtail	Japan; marine	See *N. asteroides* above	None proven; destroy stock	Kusuda et al, 1974 Kudo et al, 1988
Pseudokidney disease (*Lactobacillus piscicola = Carnobacterium piscicola*); also *Lactococcus piscium* and *Vagococcus salmoninarum*)	Salmonids; common carp; striped bass; catfish	USA; Canada; Europe; freshwater	Post-spawning fish; large amount of fluid in peritoneal cavity; liver, spleen, kidney damage; clinically similar to BKD (see *PROBLEM 52*); adults affected in North America; trout fry/fingerlings and common carp in Europe; chronic, stress-related disease	None proven	Hiu et al, 1984 Michel et al, 1986 Evelyn, 1993 Baya et al, 1991a
Corynebacterium aquaticum	Striped bass	Maryland, USA; freshwater	Nervous signs because of infection of the CNS; disease only reported once	None proven	Baya et al, 1992a
Streptoverticillium salmonis	Salmonids	USA	Gram-positive mycelia; only sporadic cases	None proven	Rucker, 1949
Rhodococcus sp.	Atlantic and chinook salmon	Canada; freshwater	Corneal damage; exophthalmos; may be kidney granulomas; may confuse with BKD (see *PROBLEM 52*); only sporadic cases	None proven	Backman et al, 1990
GRAM-NEGATIVE AEROBIC RODS **Pseudomonadaceae**					
Fin rot (*Pseudomonas fluorescens*, *P. putida*, *P. putrefaciens*, *P. pseudoalkaligenes*, *Pseudomonas* sp.)	Goldfish; silver, bighead, grass and black carp; tench; hybrid striped bass; tilapia; white catfish; rainbow trout; probably many other species	Worldwide; freshwater, marine	Typical bacterial septicemia; often fin erosion, ulceration; often pathogenic at low temperatures; often resistant to antibiotics (need to test sensitivity of isolate)	Appropriate antibiotic	Bauer et al, 1973 Csaba et al, 1981 E. Noga (unpublished data) Shotts & Teska, 1989 Lio-Po & Sanvictores, 1987 Roberts & Horne, 1978 Meyer & Collar, 1964 Austin & Stobie, 1992b

Sekiten-byo (Pseudomonas anguilliseptica)	Japanese and European eels; bluegill (E); common carp (E); golfish (E); loach (E); ayu (E); crucian carp (E)	Japan; Scotland; marine	Petechiae around mouth, operculum, and ventrum; internal gross signs may not be present; 1 mm, pale grey, round, raised, shiny colonies after about 7 days; acute, often high, mortalities	Raise temperature to 27° C for 2 weeks, then drop to <20° C; nalidixic acid; oxolinic acid; piromidic acid	Muroga et al., 1977; Ellis et al., 1983a

Enterobacteriaceae

Serratia plymuthica	Rainbow trout	Spain; Scotland; freshwater	Often no external signs; may only be skin lesions; sporadic cases	None proven	Nieto et al., 1990; Austin & Stobie, 1992b
Serratia liquefaciens	Atlantic salmon; lake trout; brook trout	Scotland; (marine); Ontario, Canada; [freshwater]	Few external signs; nodules on kidney/spleen; mottled liver; only sporadic cases	Oxolinic acid, possibly oxy-tetracycline	McIntosh & Austin, 1990; Stevenson et al., 1993
Serratia marcescens	White perch	Black River, Chesapeake Bay, USA; freshwater	Isolated only from clinically normal fish during a disease survey	None proven	Baya et al., 1992b
Hafnia alvei	Rainbow trout	Bulgaria; freshwater	Typical of hemorrhagic septicemia; also see PROBLEM 5; disease only reported once	None proven	Gelev et al., 1988
Citrobacter freundii	Marine sunfish; Atlantic salmon; rainbow trout; carp	Japan; Spain; Scotland; India; marine and freshwater	Erratic swimming; eroded and hemorrhagic skin; focal nodules (granulomas) in kidney; other lesions typical of hemorrhagic septicemia	None proven	Sato et al., 1982; Austin et al., 1992b; Austin & Austin, 1993; Baya et al., 1991b
Enterobacter agglomerans	Dolphin	Florida; Bermuda; marine	Hemorrhages in eyes and muscles; disease only reported once	None proven	Hansen et al., 1990
Proteus (Providencia) rettgeri	Silver carp	Israel; freshwater	Red ulcers on body (head, fin bases, and abdomen); bacterium associated with poultry feces; disease only reported once	None proven; handle fish carefully	Bejerano et al., 1979
Salmonella arizonae	Piracuru	Japan (aquarium); freshwater	Corneal opacity; mild gross signs of hemorrhagic septicemia; disease only reported once	None proven	Kodama et al., 1987

Vibrionaceae

Plesiomonas (Proteus) shigelloides	Rainbow trout	Portugal; freshwater	Emaciation; red anus with yellow exudate; petechiation of muscle lining peritoneum; ascites in peritoneal cavity; only reported once, but may be fairly common	Sulfadiazine-trimethoprim oral	Cruz et al., 1987

Continued.

Table II-54   Miscellaneous bacterial infections of fish, cont'd.

Disease/pathogen	Hosts	Geographic/ ecological range	Key diagnostic features	Treatment	References
Alteromonas piscicida [= *Flavobacterium piscicida*]	Marine fish	Florida, USA; marine	Mass mortality associated with phytoplankton bloom (*red tide*); disease only reported once	None proven	Meyers at al., 1959
Shewanella putrefaciens [= *Pseudomonas putrefaciens*]	Rivulatus rabbitfish	Red Sea, Egypt; marine	High mortalities in caged fish; disease only reported once	Killed vaccine may protect	Saeed et al., 1987
Moraxellaceae					
Acinetobacter-like	Atlantic salmon	Norway; marine	Hemorrhage, hyperemia, ulceration, and edema of skin; hemorrhage in peritoneum and swim bladder; isolated on blood agar, with 0.5% NaCl; disease only reported once	Oxytetra- cycline, intramuscular	Roald & Hastein, 1980
Moraxella sp.	Striped bass; rainbow trout (E)	Potomac River, Maryland, USA; freshwater	Large skin hemorrhages, missing scales; hemorrhage in swim bladder; pale liver, possibly with adhesions; disease only reported once	None proven	Baya et al., 1990b
MISCELLANEOUS					
Deleya cupida [= *Alkaligenes cupidus*]	Schlegeli black sea. bream	Japan; marine	Heavy mortalities in fry; isolated from mixed bacterial culture of fry homogenate; disease only reported once	None proven	Kusuda et al., 1986
Janthinobacteriun lividum	Rainbow trout	Scotland	Associated with RTFS‡ Fry: exophthalmos; hyperpigmentation; pale gills; swollen abdomen; swollen spleen and kidney Larger fish: skin ulcers; disease only reported once; produces purple colonies	None proven	Austin et al., 1992a

*All isolated using routine procedures (blood agar or simple nutrient agar at room temperature) unless noted otherwise.
†None proven: no clinical trials have been published that determine if a particular treatment will control the disease. Most of these bacteria have been tested for suceptibility to various antibi-
otics in vitro, but in most cases in vivo trials that substantiate the usefulness of those specific antibiotics have not been published.
‡RTFS = rainbow trout fry syndrome (Austin & Austin, 1993).
§Some *Streptococcus* species from Japan are now classified as *Enterococcus seriolicida* (Kusada et al., 1991].
E = experimental host.

CHAPTER 17

Problems 55 through 72

Diagnoses made by necropsy of the viscera and examination of wet mounts or histopathology of internal organs

55. Digenean trematode infections
56. Nematode infections
57. Cestode infections
58. Acanthocephalan infections
59. Myxozoan infections: general features
60. Proliferative gill disease
61. *Ceratomyxa shasta* infection
62. *Hoferellus carassii* infection
63. Proliferative kidney disease
64. Whirling disease
65. Miscellaneous important myxozoan infections
66. Microsporidian infections
67. Ichthyophonosis
68. Miscellaneous systemic fungal infections
69. Hexamitosis
70. Tissue coccidiosis
71. Miscellaneous endoparasitic infections
72. Idiopathic epidermal proliferation/neoplasia

PROBLEM 55
Digenean Trematode Infections (Digenean Fluke Infection, Metacercarial Infection, Black Spot, White Grub, Yellow Grub)

Prevalence Index
Larvae: WF - 2, WM - 4, CF - 4, CM - 3
Adults: WF - 4, WM - 3, CF - 4, CM - 4
Method of Diagnosis
1. Wet mount of gut contents or affected tissue that has larvae or adults
2. Histological section of gut contents or affected tissue having larvae or adults
History
Wild-caught or pond-raised fish
Physical Examination
Larvae: White, yellow, or black, flat to raised, about 1 to 4 mm nodules in skin, muscle, or viscera
Adults: Worms, usually 1 to 5 mm, in gut lumen

Treatment: Larvae
1. Keep infected birds or mammals away from ponds
2. Disinfect and quarantine
3. Bayluscide (as molluscicide)
4. Copper (as molluscicide)
5. Praziquantel oral
6. Praziquantel injection
7. Praziquantel bath

COMMENTS
Epidemiology
Digeneans are common, asymptomatic infections in wild fish. About 1700 species of adult digeneans infect fish. Metacercariae are even more common than adults. Digeneans are uncommon in cultured fish, except when the other hosts needed for the life cycle are present. Freshwater aquarium fish are commonly infected because they are often collected in the wild; such infections do not progress in aquaria.
Life Cycle
Adult digeneans produce large, usually operculated eggs that pass out of the gut of the final host (fish, bird, or mammal), hatch into a miracidium, and infect a mollusc (usually a snail). Cercariae develop, are released by the mollusc host, and penetrate a fish. After reaching the host's target tissue, the cercaria differentiates into a metacercaria, which usually produces a cyst. When the fish is eaten by the final host, the metacercaria differentiates into an adult. Variations to this life cycle are shown in Fig. II-55, *A*.
Pathogenesis
Adult digeneans mostly inhabit the gastrointestinal tract, rarely infecting the swim bladder, ovary, peritoneal cavity, urinary bladder, or circulatory system. All but the hemoparasites (see *PROBLEM 43*) are usually an incidental finding.

Host damage is most likely to occur during cercarial migration, causing hemorrhage, necrosis, and inflammation along the migration path (Sommerville, 1981). Heavy, acute infections can be fatal, especially to small fish (Hoffman, 1967; Sindermann 1990).

Metacercaria (Fig. II-55, *B* through *D*) are almost always innocuous. If they displace enough host tissue, they can compromise organ function. However, fish can carry amazingly high worm burdens without any apparent ill effects (Fig. II-55, *D*), probably because of the stable host-parasite relationship. Cyst formation is probably responsible for the characteristic lack of host response to metacercariae. Metacercariae can be found in virtually any tissue, depending on the infecting digenean species.

While they are usually harmless, metacercariae are often disfiguring (Fig. II-55, *B* and *C*) and render fish unpalatable or aesthetically unpleasing. Lesions may be white or yellow (white grub, yellow grub) because of the color of the worms, or they may be black (black spot disease) because of a hyperpigmentation host reaction (Fig. II-55, *C*). In aquarium fish this pigmentation may be mistaken by the owner as the host's normal color pattern (G. Lewbart, Personal Communication).

Some metacercariae are dangerous; *Diplostomum* (eye fluke) metacercariae infect the lens of salmonids and other fish, causing blindness and a subsequent inability to find food. Heterophyid metacercariae cause severe gill damage, decreased respiratory tolerance, and mortality in pond-raised fish in the subtropics and tropics

(Paperna, 1991) (Fig. II-55, *G* and *H*). They have caused serious morbidity in Florida (United States) and Israel. Infections of eels have been damaging (Yanohara & Kagei, 1983). The severity of the host response in these heterophyid infections may be due to these fish being aberrant hosts.

Zoonotic Potential
Many heterophyids (e.g., *Heterophyes, Haplorchis, Metagonimus*) and opisthorchids (e.g., *Chlonorchis, Opisthorchis*) can infect humans that eat metacercaria-infected fish if the fish are not cooked well or are not heavily salted.

Diagnosis
Almost all metacercariae are encysted in tissues, while adults are usually free in the gut lumen. Worms are easily identified as digeneans by using wet mounts or tissue sections (Fig. II-55, *E* through *H*). Digeneans typically have anterior (oral) and ventral suckers (Fig. II-55, *I*), although the suckers may be vestigal or completely absent in adults of some species (e.g., *Sanguinicola*). Worms are typically 1 to 5 mm, although adult parasites of some large, oceanic fish may be several centimeters or more.

Life cycles of fish-parasitic digeneans

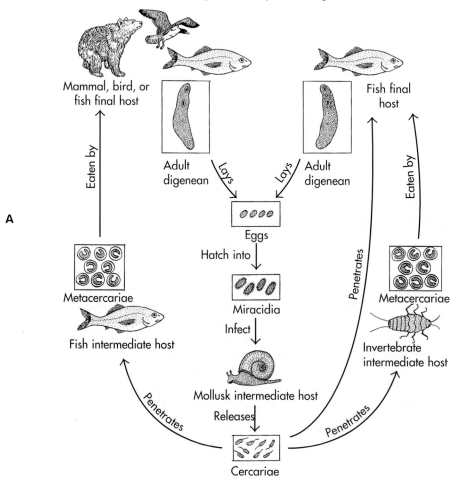

Fig. II-55 **A,** Life cycles of digeneans infecting fish.

Continued.

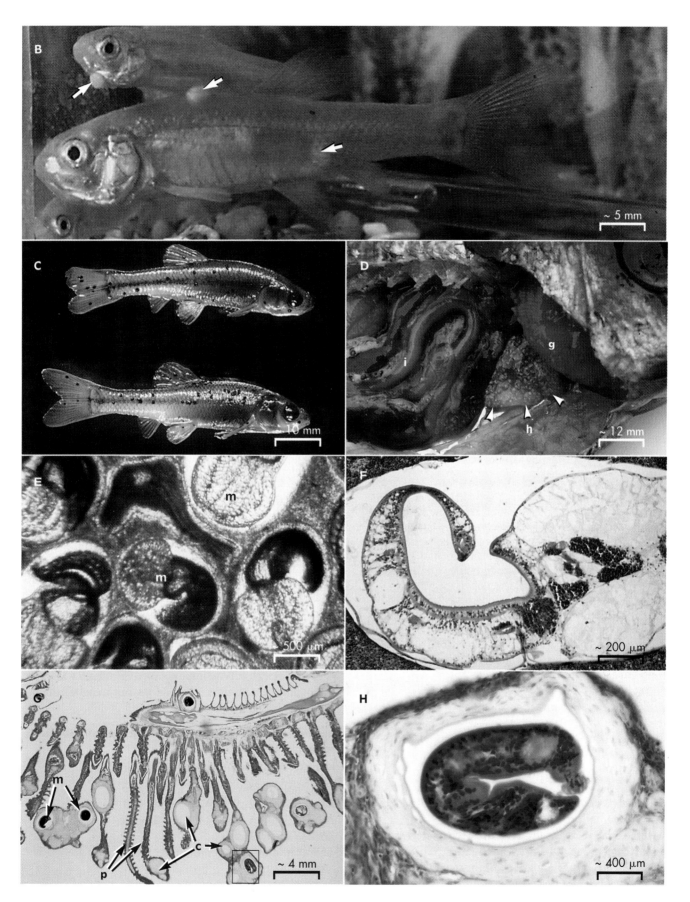

Fig. II-55—cont'd.   *For legend see page 166.*

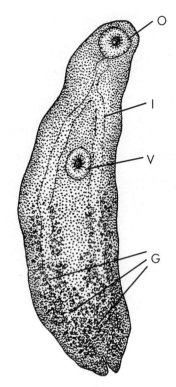

I

Fig. II-55—cont'd. **B,** Minnows with yellow grub metacercariae (*arrows*) encysted in muscle and just below the skin. Note that some cysts protrude above the skin surface. **C,** Minnows with numerous black spots caused by the host's reaction to invading metacercariae (*Neascus*). **D,** Feral bluegill with body wall dissected away. Massive metacercarial infection of heart (*H*). Each white focus is a single metacercaria. The ventral portion of the heart is white because of the massive number of white worms. This fish was clinically normal when collected. *I* = intestine; *G* = gill. **E,** Wet mount of metacercaria (*m*) of *Posthodiplostomum minimum* in a tissue squash. **F,** Histological section of a metacercaria (*Posthodiplostomum minimum*). Hematoxylin and eosin. **G,** Heterophyid metacercarial (*m*) infection of the gill of a dwarf gourami. Note the extensive chondrodysplasia (*c*) surrounding the parasites. *p* = primary lamella. Hematoxylin and eosin. **H,** Close-up of metacercaria in Fig. II-55, *G.* **I,** Diagram of typical digenean trematode. Diagnostic features: oral sucker (*O*), ventral sucker (*V*), blind gut (*I*), gonads (*G*). Metacercariae usually do not have mature gonads.

(*B* photograph courtesy of T. Wenzel; *C* photograph by L. Khoo and E. Noga; *E* photograph courtesy of G. Hoffman.)

Digeneans are distinguished from monogeneans (see *PROBLEM 16*) by the absence of chitinous hooks or polyopisthocotylean-type suckers (see Fig. II-16, *A*) and from cestodes (see *PROBLEM 56*) by the presence of a ventral sucker and a gut, as well as by the absence of body segmentation.

Metacercariae typically have most characteristics of adult digeneans but usually lack mature reproductive organs. Since the size and shape of the genital organs are used for species identification, it is usually impossible to key metacercariae to species. However, all metacercariae are managed similarly.

Treatment
MEDICAL/SURGICAL
Adult digeneans are not usually a problem in cultured fish; although Di-N-butyl tin has been tested against infections in trout (Mitchum & Moore, 1966).

Praziquantel was partially successful in eliminating yellow grub metacercariae in channel catfish. Reduction in parasite burden was not evident until 5 months after treatment (Lorio, 1989). Praziquantel has also experimentally reduced metacercaria burdens of *Diplostomum spacaceum* in trout and sculpins (Bylund & Sumari, 1981). Metacercariae close to the skin can be surgically excised by cutting down to the cyst with a sharp scalpel and then gently removing the worm with forceps. The worm should be completely removed to avoid excessive postoperative inflammation.

ENVIRONMENTAL
To acquire metacercariae, fish must be exposed to the intermediate host infected with cercariae. This typically occurs in ponds or natural waters where there is exposure to the appropriate intermediate and final hosts (usually a specific snail and fish-eating bird, respectively). Eradicating snails with molluscicides can be difficult because snails are often resistant to treatment. Even ichthyotoxic levels of copper and slaked lime can be ineffective (R. Francis-Floyd, Personal Communication). Bayluscide appears to be the most effective chemical, but fish must be removed before treating the pond (R. Francis-Floyd, Personal Communication). Treatments are best done at night, when snails are more active (Francis-Floyd, 1993). Snail-eating fish (e.g., black carp) are under investigation as a biological control (R. Hodson, Personal Communication).

Snails usually proliferate in oligotrophic or mesotrophic ponds containing solid substrates, such as earth or gravel, and having low fish density (i.e., ponds used for broodstock, spawning, or nursery). They also proliferate in extensive systems, such as impounded lakes. Snails are not a problem in intensive culture systems that have a muddy bottom and high organic loads (Paperna, 1991). Avoiding exposure of culture waters to the final host will prevent infections but may be equally difficult.

PROBLEM 56
Nematode Infections (Roundworm Infection)
Prevalence Index
Larvae: WF - 2, WM - 2, CF - 4, CM - 4
Adults: WF - 3, WM - 4, CF - 4, CM - 4
Method of Diagnosis
1. Wet mount of gut contents or viscera with adults, larvae, or eggs
2. Histology of gut contents or viscera with adults, larvae, or eggs
3. Fecal sample with eggs

History
Gradual weight loss; lethargy; pond-raised or wild fish
Physical Examination
Emaciation; worms protruding from anus
Treatment: Larvae
No proven treatment for encapsulated forms
Treatment: Adults
1. Fenbendazole oral
2. Levamisole oral
3. Piperazine oral

COMMENTS
Epidemiology
Fish are either intermediate or final hosts for nematodes. About 650 species of nematodes parasitize fish as adults and many others use fish as intermediate hosts. While nematodes are common in wild fish, neither adult nor larval nematodes are usually a problem in most cultured fish because of the absence of other hosts in the life cycle (Fig. II-56, *A*). However, pond-raised fish or those fed live and wild-caught arthropods can become infected. Also, some nematodes infecting aquarium fish have a direct life cycle (see Fig. II-56, *A*).

Freshwater fish are often infected by members of the Camallanoidea and Ascaroidea. Marine fish are usually infected by members of the Ascaridoidoiea (*Contracecum, Pseudoterranova, Anisakis*), Camallanoidea (*Camallanus, Culcullanus*), Dracunculoidea (*Philonema, Philometra*), and Spiruroidea (*Metabronema, Ascarophis*). Most of the camallanoids, dracunculoids, and spiruroids have two host life cycles where fish are the final host. *Spirocamallanus* can be pathogenic to tropical marine fish (Rychlinski & Deardorff, 1982).

Life Cycle
Sexes are separate in nematodes. Most fish-parasitic nematodes are oviparous; eggs usually hatch in the water, releasing a free-swimming larva. Some (*Camallanus, Philometra*) are viviparous, with females releasing live young. In either case, the larva is ingested by an intermediate host, often a crustacean, and then by a fish, where it either matures to an adult or encysts. Larvae encysted in fish are ingested by a bird, mammal, or another fish as final host (Rohde, 1984; Hoffman, 1967).

Some nematodes have a direct life cycle: *Capillaria pterophylli* infects freshwater angelfish and other cichlids (Moravec, 1983); at 20° to 23° C (68° to 73° F), eggs embryonate in 3 weeks, and the prepatent period is 3 months. *Capillostrongyloides ancistri* infects ancistrid catfish (Moravec et al., 1987) and probably also has a direct life cycle. Other capillarids infect cyprinids or gouramies (Moravec et al., 1987). *Camallanus*, a bright-red live bearer, affects poeciliids. They typically present as red worms protruding from the anus.

Pathogenesis
Adults are almost always found in the digestive tract (Fig. II-56, *F*), where some (e.g., *Capillaria*) can cause chronic wasting if present in high numbers. Some adult nematodes inhabit the peritoneal cavity, gonads (Fig. II-56, *B*), or swim bladder, but none are documented problems in cultured fish except the swim bladder nematode *Anguillicola* (Fig. II-56, *D*).

Anguillicola crassus (from Japan) and *Anguillicola novazelandiae* (from New Zealand) have caused serious problems in freshwater cultured European eels, apparently after introduction with exotic eels (Paperna, 1991). In Japan, infections occur during grow-out in earthen ponds but rarely occur in intensive systems, since the copepod intermediate host cannot survive (Hirose et al., 1976). Lesions are most evident in postjuvenile eels. The swim bladder has a foamy fluid that later becomes brown-red. The swim bladder wall is thickened and opaque. There is up to 20% mortality from secondary bacterial infections after swim bladder rupture. Adult worms are grossly visible (~20 to 70 mm); juveniles are ~600 to 800 μm and can be seen with a magnifying glass in the swim bladder wall, often near capillaries.

Wild or pond-raised fish are common hosts for larval nematodes, which rarely cause any problem, even in high numbers. However, migrating larvae of *Anisakis, Contracaecum, Eustrongyloides*, and *Philonema* may cause tissue damage. Larval worms may be present in virtually any organ, most commonly the skin, muscle, viscera, or peritoneal cavity (Fig. II-56, *C*).

Some larval nematodes are serious public health problems and can cause larva migrans when ingested by humans (e.g, *Anisakis, Pseudoterranova*) (Fig. II-56, *E*). Most zoonotic problems are caused by infections of feral, cold water marine fish.

Diagnosis
Fecal exam can be used to identify eggs in the digestive tract (Fig. II-56, *G*). Worms are easily identified as adult or larval nematodes by using wet mounts or tissue sections. The main criteria used to identify species are size, fine structure of the head and tail, position of the excretory pore, and structure of the transitional area between the esophagus and intestine. Most of these criteria are also valid for older larval stages. Species confirmation is best done by sending samples to a reference laboratory.

Free-living nematodes may occasionally colonize chronic skin lesions or recently dead fish. Parasites are distinguished from free-living nematodes by the lack of long sensory setae on the head (Moller & Anders, 1986).

Treatment
Anthelminthics can control adult nematodes. Fenbendazole, levamisole, and piperazine have been used with some success. Ivermectin has also been used for treatment (Heckmann, 1985) but has a low therapeutic index in fish and is thus dangerous to use. Encysted nematodes are difficult to treat. For example, levamisole kills adults of the eel swim bladder worm,

Life cycles of fish parasitic nematodes

Fig. II-56 A, Life cycles of nematodes infecting fish. **B,** Adult red worm (*Philometra* sp.) in the ovary of a croaker. **C,** Liver of Atlantic cod with encysted, anisakid, nematode larvae. Each larva (*arrows*) is curled and in a capsule. **D,** Swim bladder worms (*Anguillicola*). Dark color is due to feeding on blood. **E,** Nematodes responsible for anisakiasis: *Pseudoterranova decipiens* (*PD*) and *Anisakis simplex* (*AS*). The milky white ventricle is characteristic of *A. simplex*. **F,** Freshwater angelfish intestine with nematodes (*N*) invading the mucosa. Diagnostic features: cylindrical shape; pseudocoelom, giving appearance of a "tube-within-a-tube." Hematoxylin and eosin. **G,** Wet mount of intestinal squash from a fish with *Capillaria* sp. eggs. Note the plug on each end (*arrow*).

(*B, C, D,* and *E* photographs courtesy of H. Moller.)

Continued.

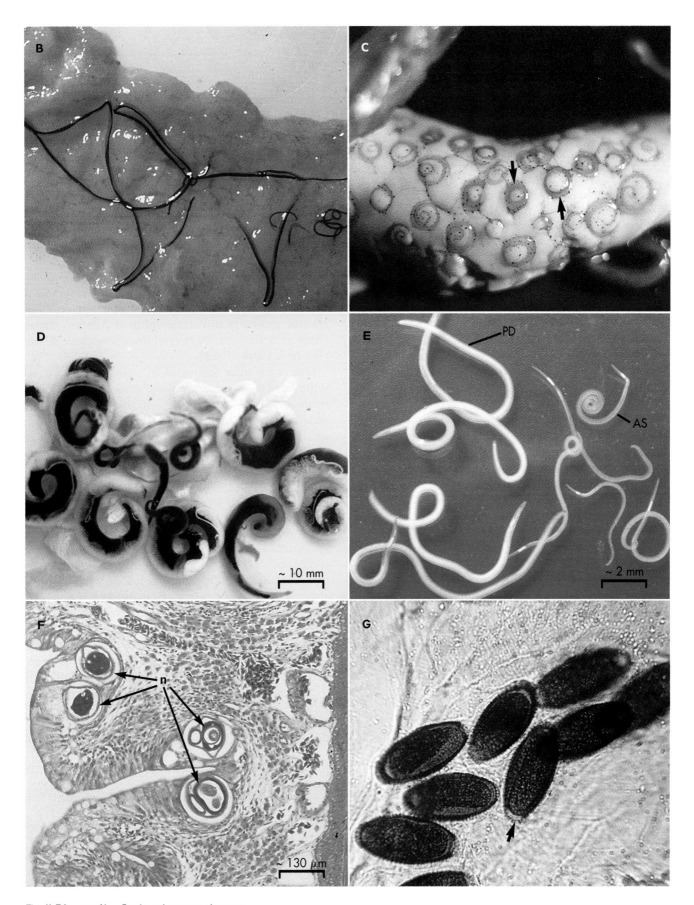

Fig. II-56—cont'd.   *For legend see opposite page.*

Anguillicola, but not the L3 larvae, which are in the swim bladder wall and are not hematophagous. The glass eel stage cannot eat the L3 because their digestive tract is still closed. Thus, the best prevention for anguillcolosis is to catch the glass eels before they begin to eat (Blanc et al., 1992).

To prevent infections having an intermediate host, avoid feeding organisms that may harbor larvae. Copepods and live fish are the most common sources. Fish can even become infected when fed frozen fish (Gaines & Rogers, 1971). Proper sanitation should help to mitigate infections with a direct life cycle.

PROBLEM 57
Cestode Infections (Tapeworm Infection)
Prevalence Index
Larvae: WF - 4, WM - 4, CF - 4, CM - 4
Adults: WF - 3, WM - 4, CF - 4, CM - 4
Method of Diagnosis
Wet mount of affected tissue having cestode larvae or adults
History
Wild-caught or pond-raised fish; worms in tissue or body cavity; feeding live copepods or other intermediate hosts
Physical Examination
Adult worms in intestine or larvae in peritoneal cavity, liver, or muscle; emaciation with heavy worm burdens; usually asymptomatic
Treatment: Larvae
No proven treatment
Treatment: Adults
1. Disinfect pond
2. Praziquantel oral
3. Praziquantel bath

COMMENTS
Epidemiology/Pathogenesis
With a complex life cycle that requires one or two intermediate hosts, cestodes are relatively uncommon in cultured fish. Fish can be an intermediate host, definitive host, or both (Fig. II-57, *E*).

While a few cestodes that infect elasmobranchs and sturgeons are in the Cestodaria, the great majority of fish-infecting cestodes are in the Eucestoda, which are characterized by having an attachment organ (scolex), as well as internal and external segmentation (proglottids) (Fig. II-57, *F*). Proglottids increase in size and maturity toward the end of the parasite's body. The scolex may have hooks, suckers, grooves, and/or spines (Fig. II-57, *F*). The less common Pseudophyllidea usually infect elasmobranchs as adults, but the larvae of one species can damage salmonids (Kent, 1992).

Pathogenesis
A few freshwater cestodes cause serious disease in wild fish. Larval cestodes (plerocercoids), also known as *metacestodes* (Freeman, 1973), are some of the most damaging parasites to viscera of freshwater fish and decrease carcass value if present in muscle. Migrating plerocercoids may cause adhesions and damage viscera or muscle because of pressure necrosis. Impaired reproduction is a common sequela. *Ligula* (Fig. II-57, *A*) causes peritoneal adhesions and pressure atrophy of the liver, gonads, and body wall musculature of cyprinids worldwide. Many piscivorous birds or mammals can act as a final host for *Ligula*. *Gilquinia squali* metacestodes infect the eyes (vitreous humor) of net-pen cultured chinook salmon, causing blindness and idiopathic mortality (Kent et al., 1991).

Adult cestodes infect the intestine or pyloric ceca and almost all species are asymptomatic. However, adult *Eubothrium* species have caused poor growth and chronic mortality in marine-cultured Atlantic salmon (Bristow & Berland, 1991) and juvenile sockeye salmon (Boyce & Clark, 1983).

One of the most serious adult cestodes that affect fish is the Asian tapeworm, *Bothriocephalus acheilognathi* (formerly known as *B. gowkongensis*), having an unusually wide host range (minnows, golden shiner, various carp species, channel catfish, and possibly aquarium fish, such as discus and other cichlids). It was introduced into the United States with grass carp and has caused serious problems with bait minnow producers. It can cause up to 90% mortality in grass carp and juvenile common carp.

The Asian tapeworm is large, with two long, deep grooves (bothria) (Fig. II-57, *C*). Worms accumulate in the anterior intestine, which may become obstructed (Fig. II-57, *D*) or perforate, resulting in high mortalities (Hoffman, 1980). The entire life cycle requires about 1 year in warm water environments and 2 or more years in cold waters. Development ceases at < 12° C (54° F). Worms mature in about 21 days at 28° C (82° F) and in 2 months at 15° C (59° F) (Paperna, 1991). The plerocercoids are transmitted by copepods. Several copepod genera can be intermediate hosts and the distribution of infections depends largely on the abundance of the intermediate host (Paperna, 1991).
Diagnosis
Worms are easily identified as cestodes from wet mounts or histology. Large worms can be identified grossly. Larval cestodes may not have segmentation, but a recognizable (Fig. II-57, *B*), although often rudimentary, scolex is usually present. Diagnosis of intestinal cestode infections can presumably also be made from wet mounts of fecal contents having proglottids or eggs.

Identification of adult cestodes to species uses features of the scolex and organs of the mature proglottid; immature cestodes might only be classifiable to order. Schmidt (1986) provides identification of

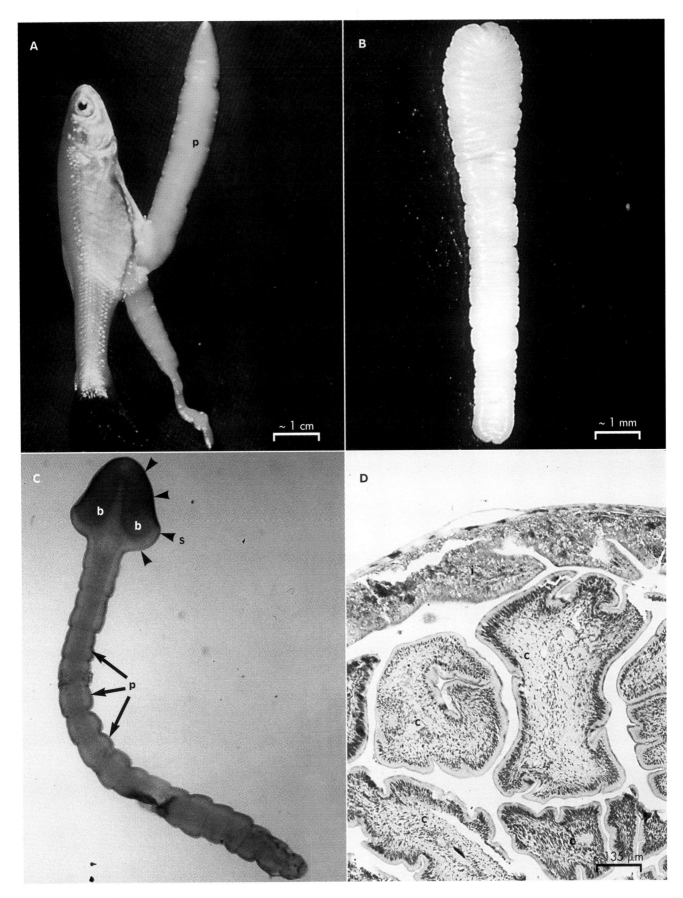

Fig II-57   *For legend see page 172.*

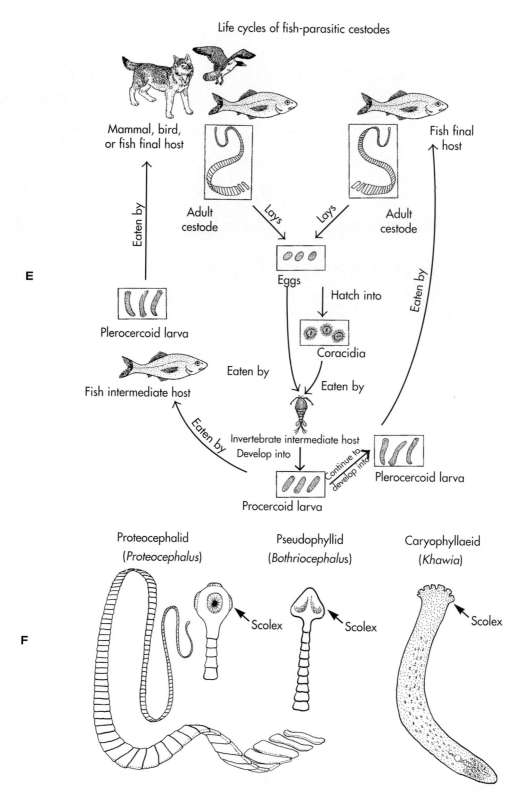

Life cycles of fish-parasitic cestodes

E

Mammal, bird, or fish final host

Eaten by

Adult cestode

Lays

Lays

Adult cestode

Fish final host

Eaten by

Plerocercoid larva

Eggs

Hatch into

Coracidia

Fish intermediate host

Eaten by

Eaten by

Eaten by

Invertebrate intermediate host

Develop into

Continue to develop into

Plerocercoid larva

Procercoid larva

F

Proteocephalid (*Proteocephalus*)

Pseudophyllid (*Bothriocephalus*)

Caryophyllaeid (*Khawia*)

Scolex

Scolex

Scolex

Fig. II-57 A, *Ligula intestinalis* in a cyprinid. The body wall has been cut, revealing the peritoneal cavity filled with a single plerocercoid (*P*). Part of the worm remains in the peritoneal cavity. **B,** Plerocercoid of *Diphyllobothrium latum.* **C,** *Bothriocephalus acheilognathi.* The pit viper–shaped scolex(s) with bothria (*B*) (grooves) is diagnostic. *P* = proglottids. **D,** Histological section through a cestode (*C*), *Bothriocephalus acheilognathi,* filling the lumen of the intestine (*I*) of a minnow. Giemsa. **E,** Life cycles of cestodes infecting fish. **F,** Diagram of typical cestodes (Eucestoda).

[*A* photograph courtesy of A. Mitchell; *B* photograph courtesy of H. Moller; *C* photograph courtesy of G. Hoffman.]

specific groups. Specimens are best sent to a reference laboratory if determining species is desired.

Treatment
Praziquantel is effective in treating adult cestode infections. There are no published studies of metacestode treatment. Aquarium fish should not be fed live foods that might transmit larval cestodes, especially if *Bothriocephalus acheilognathi* is prevalent. Ponds can be disinfected to eradicate the Asian tapeworm's intermediate host.

PROBLEM 58
Acanthocephalan Infections (Thorny-Headed Worm Infection)

Prevalence Index
WF - 4, WM - 4, CF - 4, CM - 4
Method of Diagnosis
Wet mount of affected tissue having acanthocephalans
History
Wild-caught fish
Physical Examination
Adult worms in intestine; larvae in mesentery or liver
Treatment
None reported

COMMENTS
Epidemiology/Pathogenesis
Acanthocephalan infections (~400 species affecting fish) are rare in cultured fish. With a complex life cycle that requires one or two intermediate hosts, fish may be intermediate or final hosts, depending on the acanthocephalan species. The egg that contains the larva (acanthor) is passed into the water, where it is ingested by an intermediate host (usually an amphipod or other crustacean). The acanthor enters the hemocoel of the intermediate host, forming a cystacanth. When the intermediate host is ingested by a fish, the cystacanth either matures into an adult or encysts in the fish's tissue. The fish may thus act as an intermediate or paratenic host, which is eventually ingested by the final host (fish, bird, or mammal).

Larval infections are usually located in the mesentery or liver, while adults always infect the intestine. Very little disease has been associated with acanthocephalan infections in fish, although heavy worm burdens would presumably have the potential to cause serious intestinal damage (Fig. II-58, *B*).
Diagnosis
Diagnosis of intestinal acanthocephalan infection can be made from wet mounts of intestinal tract. Species are identified mainly by the arrangement of hooks on the proboscis. Yamaguti (1963) and Petrochenko (1971) provide identification of specific groups. Specimens are best sent to a reference laboratory if determining species is desired.

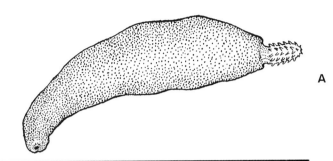

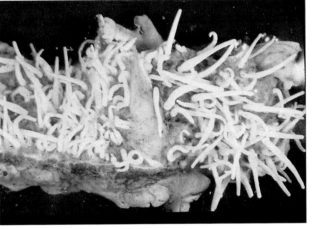

Fig. II-58 **A,** Diagram of typical adult acanthocephalan. **B,** Acanthocephalans embedded in the intestinal mucosa of a fish.

(*B* photograph courtesy of Armed Forces Institute of Pathology.)

PROBLEM 59
Myxozoan Infections: General Features

Prevalence Index
WF - 2, WM - 3, CF - 2, CM - 2
Method of Diagnosis
1. Wet mount of affected tissue having spores
2. Stained smear of affected tissue having spores
3. Histology of affected tissue having spores
History
Usually wild-caught or pond-raised fish; various-sized nodules that enlarge slowly, if at all
Physical Examination
Often white or yellowish, variously sized nodules (pseudocysts) that have firm-to-soft material; in species not forming pseudocysts, clinical signs depend on the organ system(s) affected
Treatment
Disinfect and quarantine

COMMENTS
General Life Cycle: Types of Myxozoans
The Phylum Myxozoa is restricted to invertebrates (mostly annelids) and poikilothermic vertebrates; the vast majority infect fish. The Myxozoa that infect fish are

all members of the Class Myxosporea. They are obligate parasites of tissues (histozoic forms that reside in intercellular spaces or blood vessels or reside intracellularly) and organ cavities (celozoic forms that live primarily in the gall bladder, swim bladder, or urinary bladder). Most are intercellular parasites that are typically site specific, infecting only certain target organs, and taxonomically specific, usually infecting only one species or a closely related group.

Myxozoan Characteristics

Key characteristics of the Myxozoa include development of a multicellular spore, presence of polar capsules in their spores, and endogenous cell cleavage in both the trophozoite and sporogony stages. One of the most important characteristics of myxosporeans is that, except during autogamy (sexual reproduction), all of the stages are multinucleated forms that have enveloping (primary) cells that contain enveloped (secondary) cells.

Developmental Stages

Spores have one binucleate or two uninucleate sporoplasms, one to six (usually two) polar capsules (refractile in live spores; each has a polar filament), and a shell with two to six valves. When a host ingests the spore, this triggers the rapid release of the coiled polar filaments, which probably facilitates the adherence of the spore to the intestinal mucosa. The spore valves separate, releasing the infective sporoplasm. When the parasite hatches, fusion of the two uninucleate sporoplasms occurs, producing the only uninucleate stage in the parasite's life cycle. This zygote or synkaryon was previously believed to then migrate to the target tissue of the fish host. However, there is now increasing evidence that these events may instead occur in an intermediate host (Fig. II-59, A). Once in the fish host, the trophozoite usually migrates immediately to the final target tissue. However, in some species (e.g., *Sphaerospora*), a separate proliferative phase may also be evident in organs other than the final target tissue that increase the number of parasites in the host without involving sporogenesis (extrasporogonic stages).

In the final target tissue, the trophozoite may reproduce in one of two ways. In some species the nucleus divides to produce a massive plasmodium containing generative cells, as well as many (vegetative) nuclei belonging to the plasmodium itself (Fig. II-59, A). In other species there are a large number of small plasmodia, each with only one vegetative nucleus that divides to produce many parasites before sporogony; each gives rise to one to two spores. In coelozoic species the plasmodia cover the walls of the lumen or attach to the epithelial surface, where they usually divide by cleaving into two or more parts or by producing multinucleate buds.

In coelozoic species (see *PROBLEM 61*) the plasmodia constantly divide and produce spores continu-

ously, resulting in infections that may last a long time. Conversely, spore production in histozoic plasmodia is synchronous, and thus eventually the plasmodium matures into a large packet of spores (Fig. II-59, A and G). Plasmodia situated near an external surface, such as the gills, skin, or intestine, may rupture, releasing the spores. Dissemination of spores from deeper tissue sites probably depends on the death of the host by predation or other means. Spores are typically resistant to environmental conditions.

Mode of Transmission

The method of transmission for almost all myxozoans is unknown, but evidence suggests that at least some fish-pathogenic myxozoans have an indirect life cycle (Fig. II-59, A). What is quite amazing is that this life cycle may require the completion of two different life cycles involving a vertebrate (fish) and an invertebrate (annelid) host, with each life cycle having its own sexual and asexual stages (Wolf et al., 1986). Such an alternation of life cycles has never been documented in any other parasite group (Wolf & Markiw, 1984; Wolf et al., 1986; Markiw & Wolf, 1983).

Pathogenesis

Most myxozoan infections of fish are relatively innocuous, inciting only moderate host reactions. But heavy infections can be quite serious, resulting in mechanical damage from the pseudocysts or tissue necrosis and inflammation from trophozoite feeding. Young fish are usually most seriously affected by myxozoan infections. Histozoic forms usually cause more serious diseases.

The early stages of the life cycle usually incite little host reaction, but plasmodia with mature spores often induce considerable inflammation. Interestingly, in many cases, tissue damage is greatest after death of the host, when enzymes released by the parasites are believed to cause massive muscle liquefaction (e.g., tapioca disease of mackerel and tuna; see *PROBLEM 65*). Muscle lysis can cause serious reduction in carcass value.

Taxonomic Identification

The taxonomy of the Myxosporea is based solely on spore structure, including spore size and shape, and the number and position of polar capsules. Spores usually range from about 8 to 25 μm (rarely as high as 100 μm), which is considerably larger than the typical microsporidian spore (see *PROBLEM 66*). The Order Bivalvulida (e.g., *Myxobolus*) has spore walls with two valves. The Order Multivalvulida has spore walls with three to six valves; most live intracellularly in myocytes (e.g., *Kudoa*). Spores may have projections of various sorts (Fig. II-59, B) that may facilitate their maintenance in the water column or passive attachment to food of potential hosts.

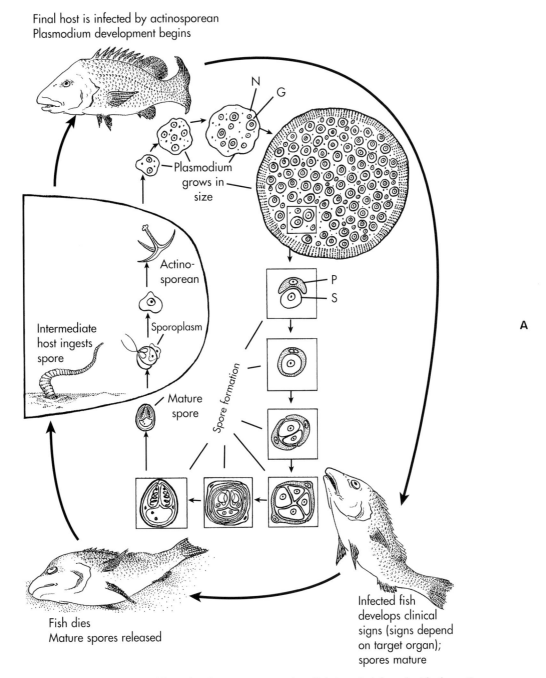

Final host is infected by actinosporean
Plasmodium development begins

Plasmodium grows in size

Intermediate host ingests spore

Actino-sporean

Sporoplasm

Mature spore

Spore formation

Fish dies
Mature spores released

Infected fish develops clinical signs (signs depend on target organ); spores mature

A

Fig. II-59   A, Generalized life cycle of myxozoan parasites. Fish host is infected with the acti-nosporean stage (infection is either by direct penetration of actinosporean into fish or by fish eating the intermediate host). Actinosporean transforms into a plasmodium, which grows in size in the fish. Plasmodium has generative cells (*G*), as well as many vegetative nuclei (*N*). Cells within the plasmodium then begin spore formation, first forming pansporoblasts, consisting of the union of two cells, a pericyte (*P*) and a sporogonic cell (*S*). These cells then divide, forming the various structures of the mature spore. As plasmodium grows and matures, fish develop clinical signs of infection. Signs depend on target organ infected. Eventually, the spores are released, usually when the fish dies. Spore is ingested by the intermediate host and the sporo-plasm is released from the spore; it transforms into an actinosporean. Note that an intermedi-ate host has not yet been identified for most myxozoan species.

Continued.

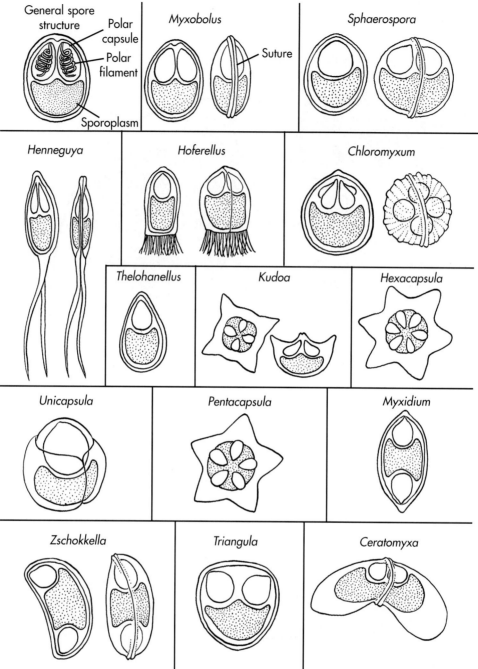

B

Fig. II-59—cont'd.   B, Spores of important myxozoan parasites. Key diagnostic features of myx-ozoan spores include: size (~10 to 100 μm), presence of polar capsules, and polar filaments. Polar filaments are not drawn for most spores. Polar filaments are not visible with routine light microscopy. C, Pseudocysts (*p*) of *Myxobolus argenteus* in golden shiner. D, Pseudocysts (*arrows*) of *Henneguya* in channel catfish fin. E, Wet mount of a typical myxozoan spore (*Myxobolus* sp.). Note that polar capsules (*c*) may be difficult to see on some fresh spores. Polar filaments (within the polar capsule) are not visible without special microscopic techniques. F, Modified Wright's stain of *Henneguya* spores. Note the well-stained polar capsules (*c*). Polar filaments (*f*) have discharged during sample preparation. *P* = caudal process. G, Histological sec-tion of intralamellar *Henneguya* infection in channel catfish gill. Note enlarged secondary lamella (*l*) filled with spores (*S*). Hematoxylin and eosin. H, Histological section of *Henneguya* lesion in Atlantic menhaden muscle, showing spores with polar capsules (*c*). Giemsa. I, *Sphaerospora molnari* spores (*s*) filling the primary lamella (*pr*) of a goldfish gill. Hematoxylin and eosin. J, Histological section through the gall bladder of a naso tang with a *Ceratomyxa* infection (coelozoic myxozoan). Developing spores are attached to the epithelium; maturing spores are in the lumen (*arrows*). E = gall bladder epithelium. Hematoxylin and eosin.

[*A* modified from Lom & Dykova, 1992; *C* and *E* photographs courtesy of G. Hoffman; *D, F,* and *I* pho-tographs by L. Khoo and E. Noga.]

Continued.

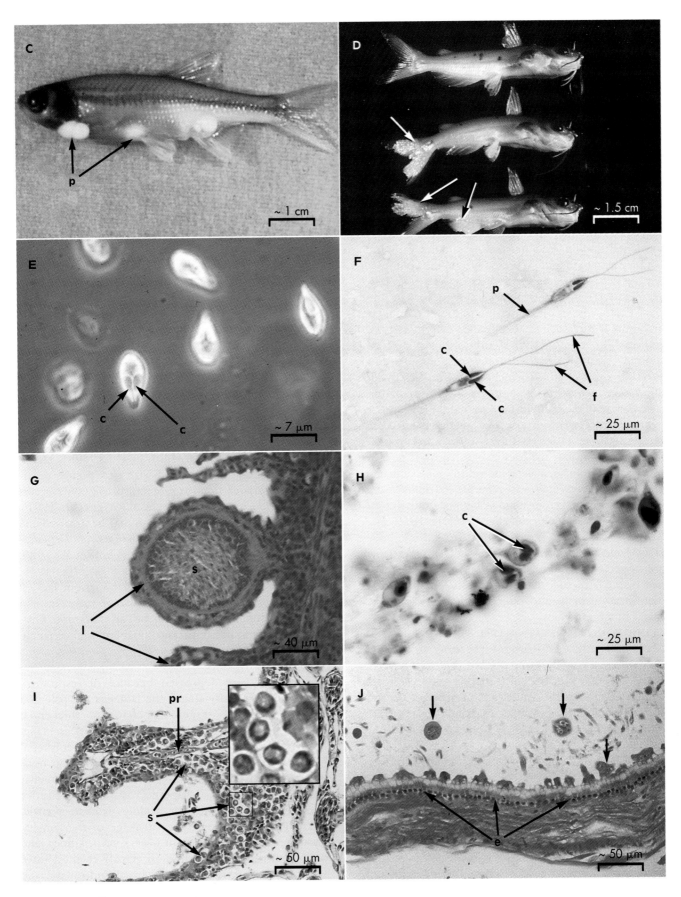

Fig. II-59—cont'd   *For legend see opposite page.*

Diagnosis
GROSS LESIONS
Myxozoan lesions (e.g., Fig. II-59, *C* and *D*) can look
grossly similar to other diseases that cause focal masses,
including microsporideans (see *PROBLEM 66*), ich (see
PROBLEM 19), lymphocystis (see *PROBLEM 39*), and
dermal metacercariae (see *PROBLEM 55*). Internal
lesions may resemble focal granulomas (see Fig. II-53, *C*)
and neoplasia (see *PROBLEM 72*); differentiation is easily
done by examining wet mounts or histological material.

DEFINITIVE DIAGNOSIS
Diagnosis of myxozoan disease is based on identifying
myxozoan spores in target tissues with appropriate clinical signs. Note that myxozoan pseudocysts are often an
incidental finding. Counterstaining samples with India
ink may help to identify spores in wet mounts but is usually not necessary. Spores with polar capsules (Fig. II-59,
E, *F*, and *H*) are pathognomonic for myxozoan infection. Polar capsules can be seen in fresh wet mounts but
are more easily seen in Giemsa or Wright's stained
smears (Fig. II-59, *F*). If identification to species is
desired, fresh (unfixed) spores are often needed.
Fixation causes artifacts, including shrinkage, which
affects size measurements. Note that spore size within a
species may vary slightly from reported dimensions.

Histopathology may be better for detecting certain
infections (Fig. II-59, *G* through *J*), especially when
inflammation against the parasite is extensive (e.g., when
pseudocysts rupture), making individual spores difficult to
find in wet mounts. Spores are refractile and difficult to see
in hematoxylin and eosin sections, but polar capsules stain
intensely with Giemsa or toluidine blue (Fig. II-59, *H*).

In a few diseases (i.e., proliferative kidney disease
[PKD] and proliferative gill disease [PGD]) myxozoans
are suspected to be responsible, but mature spores are
not formed. In such cases, diagnosis is based on the
identification of trophozoites or other developmental
stages in target tissues.

CLINICAL INTERPRETATION OF INFECTIONS
Many wild-caught fish harbor myxozoans. In aquarium
fish, *infection* is fairly common, but *epidemics* have not
been reported, possibly since the life cycle cannot be
completed in aquaria because of the absence of an essential intermediate host (Wolf & Markiw, 1984). In more
natural environments, such as ponds (see *PROBLEM
60*), or where fish are exposed to natural waters (see
PROBLEMS 61 and *64*), myxozoans can be serious.

Treatment
Aside from disinfection and quarantine, there are no well
established remedies for myxozoan infections (Molnar,
1993), although fumagillin (Hedrick et al., 1988) and
malachite green (Alderman & Clifton-Hadley, 1988)
have shown some promise. Myxozoan spores are long-
lived; some can survive for well over 1 year (Hoffman et
al., 1962), so disinfection is mandatory for eradication.

PROBLEM 60
Proliferative Gill Disease (PGD, Hamburger Gill Disease)
Prevalence Index
CF - 2
Method of Diagnosis
1. Wet mount of affected tissue having life stages of
   PGD organism
2. Histology of affected tissue having life stages of PGD
   organism
History
Pond-raised channel catfish
Physical Examination
Pale, grossly thickened ("clubbed") and broken gill
lamellae; dyspnea
Treatment
Supplemental oxygen for affected fish

COMMENTS
Epidemiology
Proliferative gill disease (PGD) causes acute branchitis
and low-to-high mortality (1% to 95%) in all ages of
channel catfish throughout the southeastern United
States and California (Hedrick et al., 1990). PGD occurs
most commonly at 16° to 20° C (61° to 68° F),
although epidemics have been seen between 14° and 26°
C (57° and 79° F) (MacMillan et al., 1989b). Development of PGD is associated with new ponds; recurrence in the same pond is rare and usually only occurs
after it has been drained and refilled (Styer et al., 1991).

Evidence exists that a myxozoan may be involved and
that a microscopic aquatic oligochaete worm (*Dero digitata*) may be an intermediate host (Groff et al., 1989;
Styer et al., 1991).

Because of the severe, acute inflammation, lack of
mature myxozoan spores, and lack of recurrence in
ponds, channel catfish may be an aberrant host.
However, the source of parasite inoculum is uncertain in
a monoculture pond.
Pathogenesis
Affected fish are depressed because of respiratory
impairment. In early stages the lamellae are pale and
swollen. In later stages, lamellae are thickened,
blunted, and bleed easily (*hamburger gill disease*) (Fig.
II-60, *A*). Histologically, there is severe epithelial
hyperplasia and granulocytic infiltrate, forming nodules around parasitic cysts (Fig. II-60, *C*). Lamellar
fusion is common. Cartilage necrosis and liquefactive
necrosis of cells within the nodules is characteristic.
Cartilage necrosis results in breakage of the lamella.
Cysts have also been seen in liver, spleen, kidney, and
brain, with little inflammation (Groff et al., 1989).
Later, healing is characterized by chondroplasia and
absence of cysts.

Diagnosis

While swollen, clubbed, and broken lamellae in channel catfish provide a presumptive diagnosis of PGD, it is advisable to perform histopathology to identify the characteristic inflammatory response and parasites in the gill parenchyma (Fig. II-60, *C*). Parasite cysts can be seen in wet mounts, but only if samples are examined within minutes of excision. In early stages, focal areas of cleared cartilage are strongly suggestive of PGD (Fig. II-60, *B*).

Treatment

Fish with PGD are intolerant of stresses, such as handling, low dissolved oxygen, or high ammonia, so increased aeration and possibly water changes can be helpful. Treatment with chemical irritants, such as formalin, are contraindicated, since they can increase mortality. Many fish can recover spontaneously if undisturbed. Pond disinfection should be considered but may be contraindicated, since it may precipitate a new disease cycle.

PROBLEM 61

Ceratomyxa Shasta Infection (Ceratomyxosis)

Prevalence Index

CF - 3

Method of Diagnosis

1. Wet mount of affected tissue having *Ceratomyxa shasta* spores
2. Histology of affected tissue having *Ceratomyxa shasta* spores

History

Salmonids exposed to parasite-endemic waters

Physical Examination

Swollen abdomen; necrotic muscle lesions

Treatment

1. Avoidance and quarantine
2. Disinfect incoming water

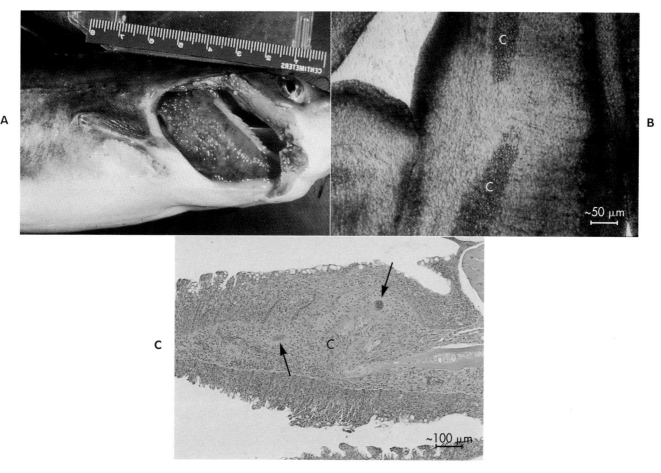

Fig. II-60 **A,** Gills of a channel catfish with PGD. Lamellae are pale and highly thickened. **B,** Wet mount of PGD-affected primary lamella that has clear areas where cartilage (*C*) has broken. **C,** Histological section of gill with PGD, with severe lamellar hyperplasia, chondrodysplasia of cartilage (*C*), and PGD organisms (*arrows*). Hematoxylin and eosin.

(*A* and *B* photographs courtesy of A. Mitchell; *C* photograph by L. Khoo and E. Noga.)

COMMENTS

Epidemiology

Ceratomyxa shasta affects salmonids, especially anadromous species, in the western United States and Canada (primarily the Columbia River basin, including Oregon, Idaho, California, Washington, and British Columbia). It can cause up to 100% mortality in young fish and is also an important cause of prespawning mortality in adult salmon. The most susceptible species are rainbow trout, cutthroat trout, chinook salmon, and chum salmon. Coho salmon, sockeye salmon, brown trout, and brook trout are less susceptible.

Endemic strains of salmonids from the Columbia River basin are relatively resistant, while *exotic* strains and the native-endemic crosses are more susceptible (Bartholomew et al., 1989; Hoffmaster et al., 1985). Thus, introducing susceptible strains into parasite-endemic areas could endanger the native stocks. Many naive, native stocks with no prior exposure are also vulnerable.

Fish can be infected at as low as 4° to 6° C (39° to 43° F) (Ching & Munday, 1984a); however, at such low temperatures, the disease progresses slowly. Higher temperatures cause a faster onset of clinical signs, which can occur as quickly as 7 days at 18° C (64° F). At 10° C (50° F), infections may take over 3 months to kill fish. The temperature dependence accounts for the seasonal nature of the disease, peak prevalence being in warmer months (May to November).

The inability to transmit ceratomyxosis via fish-to-fish contact, feeding spores, or feeding-infected tissues suggests that an intermediate host may be required. Fish are readily infected (within minutes) if exposed to parasite-endemic waters or mud (Johnson et al., 1979). Spores require *aging* before being infective and are not directly transmissible.

Pathogenesis

Clinical signs vary with fish species, but the main target tissue is usually the gastrointestinal tract, especially the intestine. Developing parasites incite a diffuse granulomatosis in many host tissues, including intestine, liver, kidney, spleen, gonads, and muscle. The abdomen is often distended because of granulomatous peritonitis (Fig. II-61, *A*), with many conical, widely arched spores in the exudate (Fig. II-61, *B*). The vent may be swollen, and necrotic abscesses ("boils") have been reported in muscle of some species (Wood et al., 1989).

Diagnosis

Diagnosis is based upon identification of typical spores in lesions or in scrapings of the intestinal lumen or gall bladder. With Ziehl-Neelsen stain, polar capsules stain red and sporoplasm, blue. Note that mature spores may not develop until the terminal stages of the infection. In such cases, trophozoites can be identified by electron microscopy (*C. shasta* trophozoites cannot be differentiated from those of other myxozoans by light microscopy). Monoclonal antibodies have also recently been developed that can identify mild infections in fixed tissues by using antibodies that recognize the prespore stage (Bartholomew et al., 1989).

Treatment

There are no proven chemotherapies. Disease progression can sometimes be reduced by transfer to saltwater (Hoffmaster et al., 1985). This also prevents further infection. However, salmonids infected in freshwater and transferred to seawater may still exhibit high mortalities (Ching & Munday, 1984b). Susceptible fish can

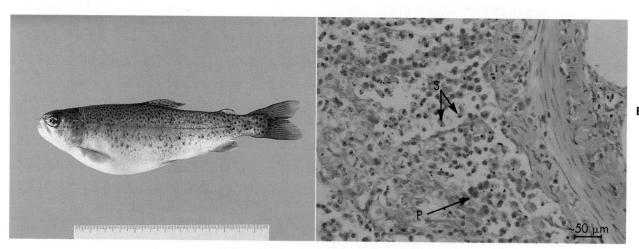

Fig. II-61 **A,** Rainbow trout with experimental *Ceratomyxa shasta* infection. Pronounced abdominal swelling caused by peritonitis. **B,** Histological section with severe, chronic peritonitis, with disporic, 13 × 19 μm plasmodia (*P*) and spores (*S*). Key diagnostic features of spores: size (14 to 23 μm long and 6 to 8 μm wide at the suture line), winged shape (ends of spores are rounded and reflect posteriorly), and polar capsules 2.2 μm. Hematoxylin and eosin.

[*A* photograph by J. Landsberg and E. Noga; *B* photograph by L. Khoo and E. Noga.]

be protected by filtration of infective water, followed by ultraviolet sterilization or chlorination (Sanders et al., 1972). Fish from *C. shasta*-endemic areas should not be moved to other areas unless certified free of the disease.

PROBLEM 62
Hoferellus Carassii Infection (Kidney Enlargement Disease, KED, Kidney Bloater)
Prevalence Index
WF - 2
Method of Diagnosis
1. Wet mount of affected tissue having spores
2. Histology of affected tissue having spores or developmental stages
History
Pond-raised goldfish
Physical Examination
Moderate to severe abdominal swelling, often asymmetrical; usually normal otherwise

Treatment
None known

COMMENTS
Epidemiology
Hoferellus carassii, formerly known as *Mitraspora cyprini*, causes *kidney bloater*, a chronic renal infection that results in massive renal hypertrophy and concommitant abdominal distension in goldfish. The disease occurs in North America and Asia (Hoffman, 1981), especially goldfish-producing areas (e.g., Japan, Israel). Fish typically become infected in ponds during summer but usually do not exhibit clinical signs until fall. Spores are produced in early spring, when fish most often tend to die. The life cycle is believed to be about 1 year. An oligochaete worm *Branchiura sowerbyi* has been implicated as an intermediate host (Yokoyama et al., 1993).
Pathogenesis
While infections are invariably fatal, infected fish can live for months, especially if they are over 1 year old when

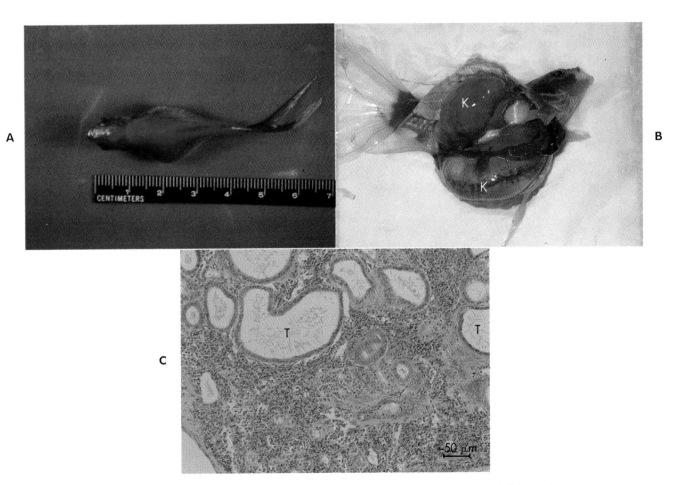

Fig. II-62 A, Goldfish with *Hoferellus carassii* infection. Pronounced asymmetrical abdominal swelling. **B,** Goldfish with *Hoferellus carassii* infection. Massively enlarged, cystic kidneys (*K*). **C,** Histology of goldfish kidney with *Hoferellus carassii* infection. Note massively dilated kidney tubules (*T*). *P* = plasmodia. Giemsa.

(*A* photograph courtesy of G. Hoffman; *B* and *C* photographs by L. Khoo and E. Noga.)

clinical signs develop. Fish usually act and eat normally. The abdomen often protrudes asymmetrically (Fig. II-62, A) because of the swelling of the kidneys and ureters (Egusa, 1978). The swim bladder may be displaced, causing balance problems, with the fish then floating on its side. There are no other internal lesions, despite the space-occupying, swollen kidney. The kidney appears cystic grossly (Fig. II-62, B) and is hypertrophic because of the extensive swelling of renal tubules. In the advanced stage a yellow fluid is found in the dilated tubules. Only some tubules are affected. After several developmental stages, trophozoites line the tubular epithelium and differentiate into spores in early spring, which are shed in the urine (Molnar et al., 1989).

Diagnosis

Diagnosis is based upon identification of typical spores in lesions. Spores are mitre-like, ~7.5 × 13 μm, with 4.5 to 6.0 μm long bristles (see Fig. II-59, B). If spores have not yet developed, identification of myxozoan trophozoites in typical lesions provides a strong presumptive diagnosis.

Treatment

There are no proven treatments. Disinfecting ponds and restocking with known, uninfected goldfish may break the transmission cycle.

PROBLEM 63
Proliferative Kidney Disease (PKD, PKX)

Prevalence Index

CF - 2

Method of Diagnosis

1. Histology of affected tissue having PKX life stages
2. Impression smear of affected tissue having PKX life stages

History

Chronic morbidity/mortality in salmonids

Physical Examination

Hypertrophic kidney; anemia; swollen abdomen; splenomegaly

Treatment

1. Disinfection, avoidance and quarantine
2. Malachite green bath
3. Salt bath

COMMENTS

Epidemiology

Proliferative kidney disease (PKD) is a serious disease of salmonids reported in the Pacific Northwest of the United States, including California, Idaho, and Washington, as well as British Columbia, Canada, and Europe (Hedrick et al., 1986, 1993). It affects rainbow trout, steelhead trout, Atlantic salmon, brown trout, grayling, coho salmon, and chinook salmon.

While there has been controversy concerning the taxonomic identification of this organism, most data suggests that it is a myxozoan. The pronounced inflammatory response and lack of typical mature myxozoan spores has also made some speculate that salmonids may be an aberrant host; however, no definitive host has been identified.

PKD primarily occurs during summer. The infection is typically contracted between April and June, when fingerlings are stocked into infected waters (Foott & Hedrick, 1987). Mortalities may range from 10% to 95%. Highest mortalities occur at 12° to 14° C (54° to 57° F). High parasite intensities are not always strongly correlated with high mortalities, suggesting that other factors (e.g., complicating infections) influence morbidity (Hedrick et al., 1985a).

Pathogenesis

Most pathology can be attributed to damage of the kidney, which is the primary target organ. Gross lesions include darkened body color, exophthalmos, pale gills (anemia), abdominal swelling, ascites, splenomegaly, and renal hypertrophy (Fig. II-63, A) (Ferguson & Needham, 1978). The kidney may be so enlarged that it forms a swelling just beneath the lateral line. Multifocal swellings give the kidney a nodular appearance.

There is a diffuse, chronic inflammatory response, consisting primarily of macrophages and lymphocytes, often surrounding the amoeboid parasites (Fig. II-63, B and C). This results in vasculitis and tubular atrophy. Other organs, especially spleen, but also intestine, gill, liver, and muscle, may be infected, presumably hematogenously.

Parasites penetrate the kidney tubule lumen and begin sporogenesis but do not produce mature spores. Parasites are often found singly or in aggregates in the renal portal vessels. Fish in North America that are recovering often have sporoblasts in the tubules that resemble *Sphaerospora* sp., providing evidence that PKD may be caused by the prespore stage of a myxosporean (Kent & Hedrick, 1985). Stickleback and common carp have been speculated to be the definitive host (Kent & Hedrick, 1986).

Diagnosis

Diagnosis of PKD is based on the identification of typical amoeboid parasites in stained tissue smears (Fig. II-63, B) (Clifton-Hadley & Richards, 1983) or histological sections (Fig. II-63, C). The primary cell is up to 15 μm, with one or more secondary (daughter) cells. They can be found within and between host cells. Recently, monoclonal antibodies and lectin probes that can specifically identify both the extrasporogonic (interstitial) and sporogonic (intraluminal) stages of the parasite have been developed (de Mateo et al., 1993).

Treatment

Malachite green bath shows some efficacy (Alderman & Clifton-Hadley, 1988). Fumagillin slows but does not stop disease progression (Hedrick et al., 1988). Increasing salinity to 8 to 12 ppt decreases morbidity and mortality. Fingerling salmonids should not be stocked into PKD-infected waters until at least July to

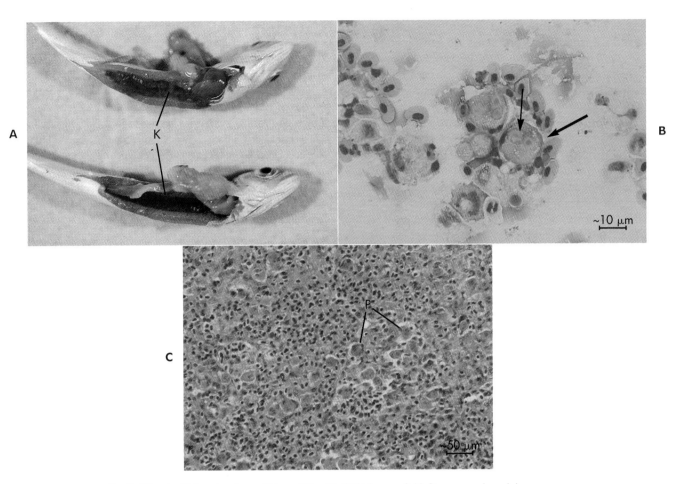

Fig. II-63   **A,** Chinook salmon kidney (*K*) with PKD (upper fish). Pronounced, nodular swellings. Compare with kidney in healthy fish. **B,** Kidney imprint with the PKD organism. Diagnostic feature is secondary cell (*small arrow*) within the *mother* or *primary* cell (*large arrow*). Leishman-Giemsa. **C,** Histological section of fish with PKD. A thin, basophilic ring of macrophage and lymphocyte host cells (*H*) surrounds some of the large, eosinophilic parasites (*P*). Hematoxylin and eosin.

(*A* and *B* photographs courtesy of R. Hedrick; *C* photograph by L. Khoo and E. Noga.)

avoid clinical disease. Recovered fish are resistant to reinfection (Foott & Hedrick, 1987).

PROBLEM 64
Whirling Disease (Black Tail)

Prevalence Index
CF - 2

Method of Diagnosis
1. Wet mount of cartilage digest having typical spores
2. Histology of cartilage having typical spores

History
Whirling or *tail-chasing* behavior in young salmonids; fish raised on mud bottom

Physical Examination
Scoliosis, kyphosis, other axial skeletal deformities; postural deficits; regional pigment abnormalities

Treatment
1. Disinfect and quarantine
2. Raise stock in parasite-free water for first 6 months of life
3. Disinfect water source

COMMENTS
Epidemiology
Whirling disease is a chronic, debilitating disease caused by *Myxobolus* (syn. *Myxosoma*) *cerebralis*. It has been reported worldwide, including in Europe, Asia, North and South America, and New Zealand. All salmonids (especially rainbow trout) are susceptible to varying degrees. Nonsalmonids have also been reported to be hosts, but this information awaits confirmation. The severity of the disease is inversely related to the age of the fish when exposed, varying from 100% mortality in newly hatched fry to little or no clinical signs in fish over 6 months old. After 1 year there is

little cartilage available in the skeleton for infection, but even fish that are several years old can be infected via the gill cartilage and thus become carriers. In endemic areas, *M. cerebralis* typically causes a mild disease that is restricted to hatcheries and is not usually evident in feral populations.

Depending on temperature the entire life cycle may require over 1 year (Hoffmann, 1976), making it an insidious problem that may go undetected for a long time. Clinical signs usually develop 2 to 8 weeks after infection (longer at low temperatures). Spore formation in infected fish requires 4 months to complete at 7° C (45° F), 3 months at 12° C (54° F), and about 50 days at 17° C (63° F) (Halliday, 1973).

Spores released from necrotic cartilage can pass in the feces, but most spores remain trapped in the skeletal tissues until the fish dies (Hoffman & Putz, 1969). Spores can be spread in the feces of piscivorous birds. Spores must be ingested by an annelid intermediate host, the sludge worm (*Tubifex tubifex*), which is common in organically polluted sediment. The spore releases the sporoplasm, which transforms into an actinosporean. After completion of both sexual and asexual stages in the annelid (this requires about 3 to 4 months) the actinosporean either directly penetrates a new host or is ingested with the infected worm (see Fig. II-59, *A*).

Pathogenesis
The parasite feeds on cartilage of the axial skeleton and clinical signs are related to this damage. The first clinical sign is usually a black tail (Fig. II-64, *A*) caused by vertebral instability and the resultant damage to sympathetic nerves near the spinal cord. These nerves control melanin pigmentation. Black tail occurs only in 3- to 6-month-old fish.

Predilection for cartilage of the auditory capsule causes impaired balance and a frenzied, tail-chasing behavior (*whirling*). Whirling is most obvious when the fish are fed or disturbed. Both black tail and whirling eventually disappear with time. However, survivors of these episodes often develop spinal curvature, pug-headedness, or an undershot jaw because of cartilage damage. Clinical signs seem to be more evident at ~17° C (63° F). Heavy infections may cause acute mortalities without clinical signs.

The parasites feed on chondrocytes and histologically, there is a reactive chondrosteal proliferation to infection. Damaged cartilage often has a chronic inflammatory response.

Diagnosis
Because spores are trapped in cartilage, it is difficult to make wet mounts of fresh tissues. Thus, diagnosis is usually made by histopathology of head, gill, or vertebral cartilage. To sample for *Myxobolus cerebralis*, a cross-section should be taken just behind the eye (approximately 5 mm posterior), so that the cartilage around the auditory capsule is included (this is a highly common site for *M. cerebralis* infection). Note that other *Myxobolus* species may be found in the connective tissues *outside* the cartilage, especially in brown trout and grayling (Bucke, 1989). For asymptomatic infections, a more sensitive method is to enzymatically digest head cartilage and concentrate spores by sedimentation (Markiw & Wolf, 1980) (Fig. II-64, *B*). Spores are highly variable, oval to circular in front view, 7.4 to 9.7 µm long × 7 to 10 µm wide × 6.2 to 7.4 µm thick, with a mucus envelope on the posterior half of the spore (Lom & Dykova, 1992). The sporoplasm has an iodinophilous (glycogen) vacuole, which is best seen in fresh spores. This vacuole is characteristic of the genus *Myxobolus*.

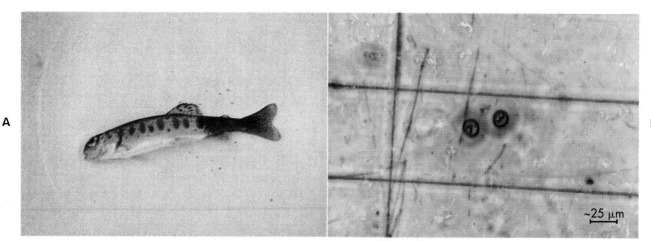

Fig. II-64 A, Rainbow trout with whirling disease. Black tail. **B,** Wet mount of cartilage digest from a fish with whirling disease, showing the characteristic spores that are almost round in front view, with two pyriform polar capsules.

[*A* and *B* photographs courtesy of G. Hoffman.]

Treatment

Whirling disease can be eliminated in culture facilities only by thorough disinfection and quarantine and repopulation with specific-pathogen-free stock. Raising fish in concrete raceways to avoid exposure to mud is also useful. When whirling disease is endemic in a watershed, eradication is impossible; thus, management of the disease requires stocking fish into affected waters only after 6 months of age or at least raising them in concrete vats during this time to reduce infective inoculum. Ultraviolet sterilization of incoming water has shown some success in eliminating the infective stage (Hoffman, 1974) but is almost never practical.

Whirling disease is a reportable disease in the United States and exotic salmonids must be certified free of the disease. The disease has been reported from 19 countries, including the United States, and it probably exists in all countries that have imported live or frozen salmonids or salmonid products. Spores can survive in fresh and frozen fillets (over 3 months at −20° C [−4° F]), posing a danger to nonendemic areas (El-Matbouli & Hoffman, 1991). Spores are killed after 10 minutes at 60° C (140° F), and thus are killed by hot smoking. They survive drying. Spores can survive in water for over 1 year. They also survive passage through the alimentary tract of northern pike and mallard ducks, which means that they could be spread via this route (El-Matbouli & Hoffman, 1991). All spores are killed in 2 days by treating with 25% unslaked lime in 3-cm-deep soil, by adding 380 g unslaked lime/m² (Hoffman & Hoffman, 1972).

PROBLEM 65
Miscellaneous Important Myxozoan Infections
Prevalence Index
WF - 2, WM - 3, CF - 2, CM - 2
Method of Diagnosis
1. Wet mount of affected tissue having typical spores
2. Histology of affected tissue having typical spores

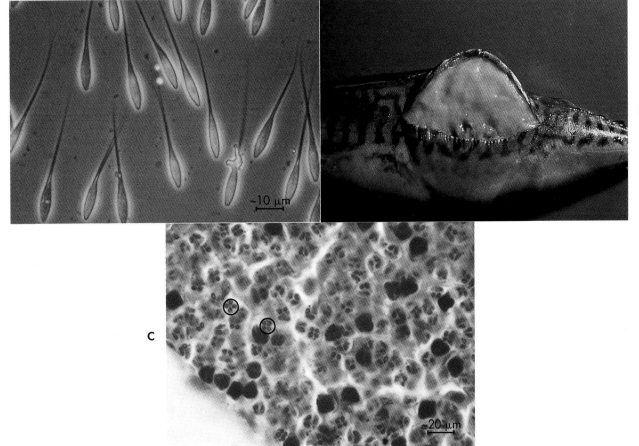

Fig. II-65   **A,** Wet mount of *Henneguya* spores. **B,** *Kudoa histolyticum* infection of Atlantic mackerel (head is to the left), causing tapioca disease or jellied flesh. The skin has been cut lengthwise, revealing soft, liquified muscle. **C,** Histological section of Atlantic menhaden muscle. *Kudoa* pseudocyst within myofibril. Note individual spores (*circles*), each with four polar capsules. Giemsa.

[*A* photograph courtesy of G. Hoffman; *B* photograph courtesy of H. Moller.]

Table II-65 Miscellaneous important myxozoan infections of fish.

Pathogen/disease	Host(s)	Sites	Geographic range	Diagnostic features	References
Henneguya (several species)	Channel catfish	Skin, gills	USA	Macroscopic and/or microscopic pseudocysts; inter- and intralamellar pseudocysts in gills; interlamellar lesions most pathogenic (can cause severe branchitis and respiratory impairment); skin pseudocysts or diffuse cutaneous masses (Fig. II-59, D) usually not important (no effect on carcass quality) (Fig. II-65, A)	Minchew, 1977 McCraren et al., 1975
Myxobolus koi	Goldfish, koi	Gills	Japan; Europe	Proliferative branchitis; can be fatal; infects connective tissue of gill filaments and subcutaneous tissue of head	Hoshina, 1952 Cranshaw & Sweeting, 1986
Chloromyxum truttae	Salmonids	Gall bladder, bile ducts	Europe	Hypertrophy of gall bladder; inflammation of gastrointestinal tract; emaciation; icterus	Bauer et al., 1981
Hoferellus cyprini	Common carp	Kidney	Europe; Asia	Infects renal tubular epithelium in summer, produces trophozoites in fall, spores in winter; abdominal distension; exophthalmos	Bauer et al., 1981 Alvarez-Pellitero et al., 1982
Henneguya zschokkei [= *H. salminicola*; milky flesh]	Salmonids	Muscle	Europe; North America	Ulcers from breakdown of large pseudocysts; cysts with milky fluid; fillets unmarketable	Petrushevski & Shulman, 1961 Boyce et al., 1985
Kudoa, Hexacapsula, Unicapsula, Pentacapsula (various species); [tapioca disease; jellied flesh]	Various pelagic and benthic fish	Muscle	Worldwide	Microscopic to small macroscopic white pseudocysts; cause rapid muscle autolysis on death of fish (within hours of capture); decreases carcass value; *soft, milky,* or *jellied* flesh (Fig. II-65, B and C); cysts turn dark (black) with age because of melanization; cooking may stop enzyme activity, but for some, cooking softens flesh; *Kudoa* has most muscle-invading myxozoans	Egusa, 1978 Lom & Dykova, 1992
Myxidium giardi (=*Myxidium matsui*)	American eel, Japanese eel	Skin, gill, viscera	USA; Japan	Pseudocysts usually not fatal but disfiguring; decrease carcass value	Ghittino et al., 1974 Paperna et al., 1987
Myxidium minteri	Salmonids	Kidney	Northwest USA	Renal tubular degeneration	Yasutake & Wood, 1957
Chloromyxum majori	Rainbow trout, chinook salmon	Kidney	Northwest USA	Glomerulonecrosis	Yasutake & Wood, 1957
Myxobolus pavlovskii	Bighead carp	Gills	Asia; Europe	Branchial necrosis	Molnar, 1979
Myxobolus exiguus	Cyprinids, mullets	Gills, skin, stomach, pyloric ceca	Asia; Europe; Africa	Has caused mass mortalities in mullet	Pulsford & Matthews, 1982
Myxobolus sandrae	Pike-perch, redfin perch	Subcutaneous tissue of head; branchial cavity and gills; spinal cord	Europe	Severe vertebral deformities; unmarketable	Lom et al., 1991b

Species	Host	Site	Signs/Pathology	Geographic location	Reference
Myxobolus notemigoni	Golden shiner	Skin	Pseudocysts lift scales, causing bristled appearance; decreased market value as bait fish	USA	Lewis & Summerfelt, 1964
Myxobolus buri	Yellowtail	Brain	Severe scoliosis	Japan	Egusa, 1985
Sphaerospora renicola (swim bladder inflammation)	Common carp, goldfish	Swim bladder, kidney, blood	Swim bladder inflammation, hemorrhage, thickening, hypertrophy in 0+ carp; locomotion dysfunction; peritonitis; renal hypertrophy; don't confuse with viral swim bladder inflammation (see PROBLEM 78)	Eurasia	Lom & Dykova, 1992
Sphaerospora molnari	Common carp, goldfish	Gills, skin	Infects skin and gill epithelium, causing hyperplasia/necrosis; can be fatal (Fig. II-59, J)	Europe; Israel; USA	Svoboda & Groch, 1986 Paperna, 1991
Myxobolus encephalicus	Common carp	Brain	Encephalitis; locomotion dysfunction; emaciation	Europe	Lom & Dykova, 1992
Thelohanellus nikolskii (= T. cyprini)	Common carp	Fins	Pseudocysts on fin rays; rays may break off, causing secondary infection and impaired ambulation	Europe; Asia	Molnar, 1982
Thelohanellus kitauei	Common carp	Intestine	Pseudocysts occlude intestine; emaciation; pressure atrophy of adjacent viscera	Japan	Lom & Dykova, 1992
Chloromyxum cristatum	Cyprinids	Liver	Liver necrosis	Eurasia	Lom & Dykova, 1984
Zschokkella nova	Goldfish, other cyprinids	Liver	Bile ducts distended with plasmodia; liver atrophy	Eurasia	Lom & Dykova, 1992
Triangula percae	Redfin perch	Brain	Spinal curvature; brain damage	Australia	Langdon, 1987b
Sphaerospora tincae	Tench	Kidney	Externally visible renal hypertrophy	Europe (France, Germany)	Lom & Dykova, 1992
Sphaerospora ictaluri	Channel catfish	Gill (mainly)	See PGD (see PROBLEM 60)	USA	Hedrick et al, 1990
Sphaerospora testicularis	European sea bass	Testes	Damages seminiferous tubules; impairs male reproduction	Mediterranean Sea	Sitja-Bobadilla & Alvarez-Pellitero, 1990
Parvicapsula sp.	Salmonids	Kidney	Renal tubular necrosis; nephritis	Northwest USA	Johnstone, 1985

History
Usually wild-caught or pond-raised fish; variously sized nodules that enlarge slowly, if at all
Physical Examination
Usually white or yellowish-colored, variously sized nodules having firm to soft material; other clinical signs depend on the organ system(s) affected
Treatment
None proven

PROBLEM 66
Microsporidian Infections
Prevalence Index
WF - 3, WM - 4, CF - 3, CM - 4
Method of Diagnosis
1. Wet mount of affected tissue having typical spores
2. Histology of affected tissue having typical spores
History
Usually wild-caught or pond-raised fish; variously sized nodules that enlarge slowly, if at all
Physical Examination
Usually white or yellowish, variously sized nodules having firm to soft material; other clinical signs depend on the organ system(s) affected
Treatment
Disinfect and quarantine

COMMENTS
Life Cycle
Microsporidians (Order Microsporidia) are not as common as myxozoans, but they are responsible for a number of serious diseases in cultured fish (Table II-66). They are often taxonomically specific, infecting only one fish species or a closely related group. However, some species (e.g., *Pleistophora hyphessobryconis*, *Glugea stephani*) can infect a broad range of fish.

All microsporidians are intracellular parasites, with a direct life cycle. They form a characteristic, thick-walled spore, which contains a sporoplasm. When a host ingests the spore, the sporoplasm is discharged through the channel of a tubular polar filament that is stored coiled within the spore. The sporoplasm then migrates to the target organ and starts a proliferative phase (merogony), producing a large number of cells (meronts) by binary or multiple fission. In the final stages of development, meronts give rise to sporonts, which undergo sporogony, producing mature spores (Fig. II-66, *I*). Mature spores may be released from lesions on body surfaces (e.g., skin, gills, intestine) or after death of the host.
Epidemiology
Depending on the parasite species and the particular tissue predilection, microsporidian infections may be widely disseminated throughout various organs. They appear to be cell-specific, infecting only certain cell types in a host but may infect many organs if that cell is widespread throughout the body. How infections spread within a host is unknown; possibilities include migration of meronts and autoinfection, where spores hatch in the individual where they were formed, beginning another propagation cycle.
Pathogenesis
Clinical signs depend on the organ(s) infected (Table II-66) and can range from asymptomatic lesions to mortality. While mild infections may be innocuous, mechanical displacement and tissue disruption caused by parasite growth can lead to serious organ dysfunction (e.g., intestinal blockage, parasitic castration, muscle loss) with severe morbidity and/or mortality.

All microsporidians infect a host cell, but some (e.g., *Glugea*) also induce the formation of a tremendously hypertrophied cell that, together with the parasite, forms a xenoma, or xenoparasitic complex. Xenomas appear as whitish, cyst-like structures up to several millimeters in diameter (Fig. II-66, *A* and *B*). Some species (e.g., *Ichthyosporidium giganteum*) may form large (up to 2 cm or more) pseudotumors, consisting of many individual xenomas.
Taxonomy
Classification of the Microsporidia is based on the life cycle, type of spore formation (sporogony), and spore morphology. There are two suborders in the Microsporidia. In the Suborder Pansporoblastina (e.g., *Glugea*, *Pleistophora*, *Thelohania*, *Loma*, *Heterosporis*), spores develop in membrane-bound packets known as sporophorous vesicles (SPV, pansporoblast membranes), which may be seen in wet mounts of lesions (Fig. II-66, *C*). The number of spores per vesicle is diagnostic. In the Suborder Apansporoblastina (e.g., *Nosemoides*, *Ichthyosporidium*, *Spraguea*, *Microfilum*, *Enterocytozoon*, *Tetramicra*, *Microgemma*), spores are free within the host cell cytoplasm.
Diagnosis
Microsporidian lesions may grossly resemble other pathogens that cause masses, including myxozoans (see *PROBLEM 59*), ich (see *PROBLEM 19*), lymphocystis (see *PROBLEM 39*), dermal metacercariae (see *PROBLEM 55*), granulomas (see Fig. II-53, *C*), and neoplasia (see *PROBLEM 72*); they are easily distinguished by examining wet mounts or histological material for spores.

Diagnosis of microsporidian disease is based on the identification of microsporidian spores in target tissues that have appropriate clinical signs (Fig. II-66, *D* through *G*). The presence of spores that are small (2 to 10 μm, usually 7 μm or less), egg-shaped to elliptical, and have a prominent posterior vacuole (Fig. II-66, *E*) is diagnostic for microsporidia.

Table II-66   Important microsporidian infections of fish.

Pathogen / disease	Host(s)	Site(s)	Geographic / ecological range	Diagnostic features	References
Glugea stephani	Flatfishes (*Pleuronectes flesus; Platessa platessa;* English sole; *Rhombus maximus;* seven other spp.)	Gastro-intestinal tract	North Atlantic (M)	Xenomas in connective tissue of gastro-intestinal tract; may be important cause of natural mortality	Cali et al., 1986
Tetramicra brevifilum	Turbot	Muscle	England; Spain (M)	0+ fish with muscle nodules that show through skin; degenerate muscle fibers impair swimming	Matthews & Matthews, 1980
Icthyosporidium giganteum	*C. melops* wrasse; *C. ocellatus* wrasse; spot		France; Black Sea; East USA (M)	Large masses in subcutaneous and adipose tissues; can produce large ventral body swelling with xenomas	Sprague & Hussey, 1980
Glugea hertwigi	Smelts	Viscera	Holarctic (F,E)	Xenomas mainly in intestine; intestinal obstruction; lower fecundity; fish kills in late spring after spawning	Nepszy et al., 1978
Glugea luciopercae	Pike perch	Intestine	Asia; Europe (F,E)	Intestinal damage in pike perch	Dogel & Bykhovski, 1939
Heterosporis anguillarum (= *Pleistophora anguillarum*; Beko disease)	Japanese eel	Muscle	Japan	Yellowish nodules on body surface, forming irregular indentations; chronic mortality; slow growth; decreased market value	T'sui & Wang, 1988
Glugea plecoglossi	Ayu; rainbow trout	Most tissues	Japan (F)	Xenomas may bulge from body surface	Takahashi & Egusa, 1977
Loma salmonae	Salmonids	Gill	North America; Japan; France (F)	Xenomas on gill; heavy infections cause high mortalities	Putz, 1964
Microsporidium takedai	Salmonids	Muscle	Japan	Very common; only infects heart in chronic form (low temperature); also in skeletal muscle in acute form	Awakura, 1974
Microsporidium seriolae	Yellowtail	Muscle	Japan	Beko disease	Egusa, 1982
Heterosporis finki	Freshwater angelfish	Esophagus muscle	(F)	Infects connective tissue of esophagus, forming nodules; infected muscles are milky white, with creamy consistency; emaciation; up to 5 mm necrotic foci on body surface	Michel et al., 1989
Heterosporis schuberti	*Pseudocrenilabrus multicolor, Ancistrus cirrhosis* (aquarium fish)	Muscle	France (F)	Emaciation; myocytes not very hypertrophied	Lom et al., 1989
Pleistophora hyphessobryconis (neon tetra disease)	Sixteen species; mostly tetras; also lineatus barb, zebra danio, goldfish	Muscle	Worldwide (F)	Focal color loss / fading with white patches under skin; body contorted from muscle damage; emaciation; in heavy infection, may spread to connective tissue of intestine, ovary, skin: sometimes can detect spores in skin scrapings; clinical signs for 2-4 weeks	Nigrelli, 1953 Dykova & Lom, 1980
Glugea anomala	Three-spined stickleback, ten-spined stickleback tropical killies	Most tissues	USA; Europe; Asia	Xenomas in virtually any tissue; may bulge from surface	Canning et al., 1982 Noga & Lom, unpublished data
Glugea pimephales (= *Nosema pimephales*)	Fathead minnow	Viscera	USA (F)	Xenomas in viscera of fry; high mortality	Morrison et al., 1985
Pleistophora ovariae	Golden shiner; fathead minnow	Ovary	USA (F)	Ovary mottled with white spots and streaks; parasitic castration; very common, especially spawning season (May-June)	Nagel & Summerfelt, 1977
Glugea cepedianae (= *Pleistophora cepedianae*)	Gizzard shad	Viscera	Ohio, USA (F)	Xenomas in peritoneal cavity; protrude from 0+ fish; only 1 xenoma / fish	Price, 1982

F = freshwater; *M* = marine; *E* = estuarine.
See Canning & Lom, 1986; Lom & Dykova, 1992, for more details on microsporidians

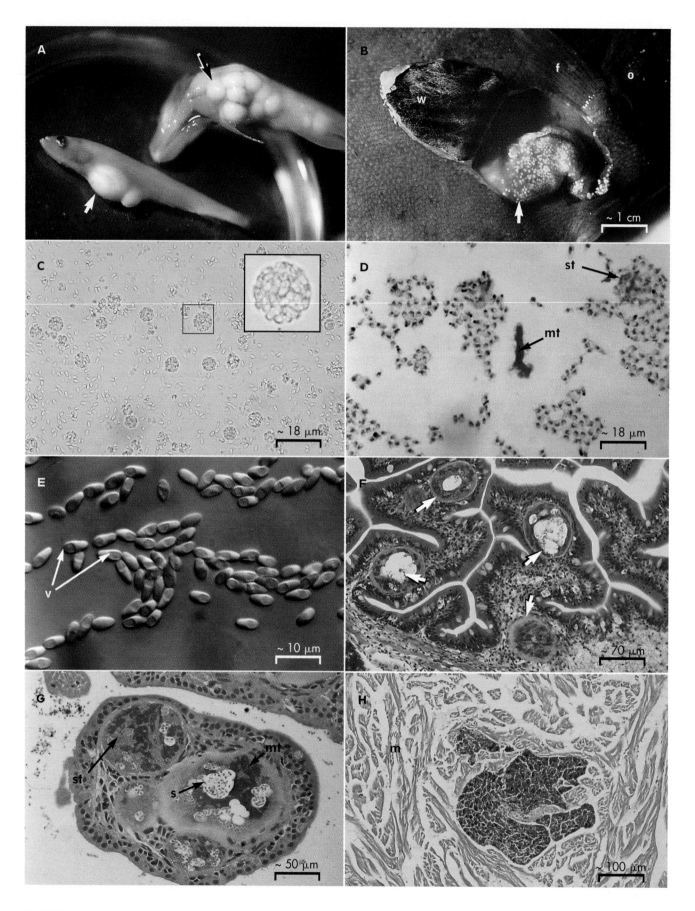

Fig. II-66   *For legend see opposite page.*

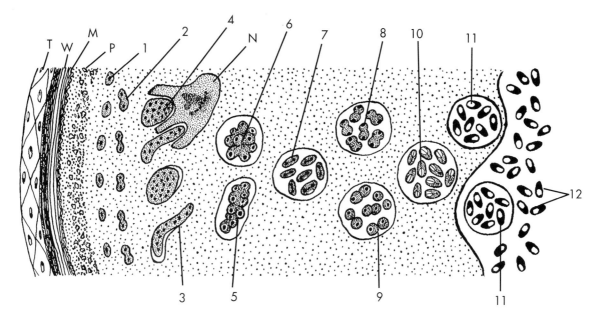

Fig. II-66—cont'd.   **A,** *Glugea hertwigi* infection that produces large pseudotumors (*arrows*) in the viscera of European smelt. **B,** *Glugea stephani* infection of dab. The abdominal wall (*w*) has been cut away, revealing the intestine with numerous xenomas (*arrow*). Head is to the right; *f* = pectoral fin; *o* = gill operculum. **C,** Wet mount of sporophorous vesicles (SPVs) (inset) of a *Glugea* sp. Some SPVs are breaking up, releasing individual spores. **D,** Stained smear of a *Glugea* xenoma with developmental stages; *mt* = meront; *st* = sporoblast. Modified Wright's. **E,** Individual microsporidian spores. Note egg shape and vacuole (*v*) at posterior end of spore. **F,** Histological section through xenomas (*arrows*) in the intestine of a killifish. Hematoxylin and eosin. **G,** Grazing histological section through wall of a xenoma; *mt* = meronts; *st* = sporonts; *s* = spores. Hematoxyin and eosin. **H,** Histological section through muscle (*m*) of Atlantic menhaden, with gram-positive spores of a *Pleistophora* sp. Gram's. **I,** Diagram of a xenoma (*Glugea anomala* type), showing sequential development to form mature spores. Various developmental stages are similar in all microsporidians; *1* = uninucleate meront; *2* = dividing meront, forming multinucleated meront (*3*); *4* = multinucleated meront rounding up; *5* = elongate sporogonial plasmodium beginning to segment into sporoblast mother cells within a sporophorous vesicle (SPV; indicated by clear space); *6* = sporogonial plasmodium segmenting into sporoblast mother cells: *7* = sporoblast mother cells, which divide (*8* and *9*), producing sporoblasts (*10*); *11* = SPV with spores (*12*); spores are also free within the center of the xenoma. Note the spore's typical egg shape and prominent posterior vacuole; *T* = host connective tissue; *W* = xenoma cell wall; *M* = cell membrane of xenoma; *P* = periphery of xenoma, with increased pinocytotic activity; *N* = host cell nucleus.

[*A* and *B* photographs courtesy of H. Moller; *C, D, F, G,* and *H* photographs by L. Khoo and E. Noga; *E* photograph courtesy of J. Lom; *I* from Lom & Dykova, 1992.]

Spores have a polar tube (typically not seen when using routine light microscopy) and, unlike the Myxozoa, have no polar capsule. Microsporidian spores are the only protozoan spores that are gram-positive (Fig. II-66, *H*). Not all spores within a lesion may be gram-positive. Birefringence also differentiates them from other protozoan spores (Tiner, 1988).

Treatment

Spores are typically resistant to environmental conditions and can often survive for over 1 year at low temperatures. Aside from disinfection and quarantine, there are no proven remedies for microsporidian infections. Toltrazuril has shown some efficacy experimentally (Schmahl et al., 1990).

PROBLEM 67
Ichthyophonosis (Swinging Disease)

Prevalence Index

WF - 4, WM - 4, CF - 4, CM - 4

Method of Diagnosis

1. Culture of *Ichthyophonus*
2. Wet mount of lesion (skin or viscera) with sporulating fungus
3. Histopathology of pathogen

History/Physical Examination

Emaciation; usually shallow skin ulcers; *sandpaper-like* texture to skin; vertebral curvature

Treatment

Avoid exposure to contaminated feed

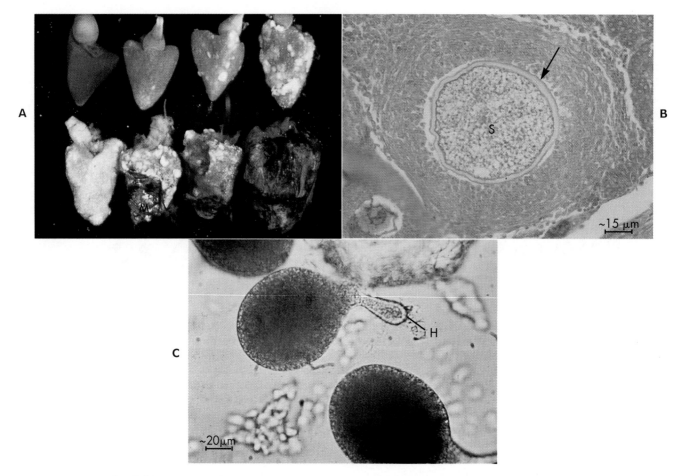

Fig. II-67 **A,** Hearts from menhaden with various degrees of ichthyophonosis. Normal heart is on the upper left. Note numerous, raised, white nodules of chronic inflammation. More advanced cases also have considerable melanization. **B,** Chronic inflammation surrounding an *I. hoferi* spore (*S*). Diagnostic features: size (10 to 250 μm); thick double wall (*arrow*); multinucleated cytoplasm. Hematoxylin and eosin. **C,** Wet mount of a germinating *I. hoferi* spore. The nonseptate hypha (*H*) usually develops after death of the fish.

(*A* photograph courtesy of C. Sindermann; *C* photograph courtesy of C.L. Davis Foundation for Veterinary Pathology.)

COMMENTS

Epidemiology

Ichthyophonus is a fungus-like agent that causes a chronic, systemic, granulomatous disease. It is endemic in many feral, cold water marine fish populations (McVicar, 1982). Epidemics have occurred in Atlantic herring and yellowtail flounder in the northwest Atlantic Ocean, haddock and plaice in the northeast Atlantic, and cod in the Baltic Sea (Noga, 1993c). It is probably a significant cause of chronic mortality in some feral marine fish populations (McVicar, 1982).

While it is rarely a problem in cultured fish, *Ichthyophonus* has infected freshwater fish that were fed contaminated marine offal (Wood, 1974). It is thought to be common in aquarium fish (Reichenbach-Klinke, 1973), but there are no recent published reports substantiating this claim. Its supposedly high prevalence

may be due to the misidentification of mycobacteriosis (see *PROBLEM 53*).

Life Cycle

The life cycle of *I. hoferi* is complicated, involving production of multinucleated spores (Fig. II-67, *B*), which produce endospores. Hyphae may or may not be produced before endospore formation. Endospores are disseminated to new hosts or to other parts of the same host. The endospores then produce multinucleated spores. McVicar (1982) discusses the life cycle in detail. *Ichthyophonus* is an obligate pathogen.

Pathogenesis

Lesions of ichthyophonosis are most common in highly vascularized organs, such as heart, spleen, kidney, and liver. The *acute* form, which takes several weeks to develop, involves fungal invasion of tissue with little inflammatory response. In the *chronic* form, there is a strong, chronic inflammatory response to invasion (Fig. II-67, *B*). White or dark (pigmented) nodules may be present on various organs (Fig. II-67, *A*). Lesions on the skin may be rough ("sandpaper-like") or ulcerated. Neurological signs (*swinging disease*) are common in freshwater salmonids because of central nervous system involvement (Wood et al., 1955). Fish may also have spinal curvature and darkening of the skin.

Diagnosis

Ichthyophonus can often be identified from fresh lesion material; spores in affected flounder tissue readily germinate within 30 minutes (McVicar, 1982). The germinating spore is flask-shaped, with a neck that consists of a hypha that breaks through the outer wall (Fig. II-67, *C*). The germinating spore is pathognomonic. Characteristic life stages can also be identified in histological sections, including the spore (usually the most common stage; Fig. II-67, *B*), germinating spore with hyphae, and hyphae. *Ichthyophonus* is PAS- and silver-positive. Lesions can also be cultured using Sabouraud dextrose agar with 1% serum (McVicar, 1982).

Treatment

There is no treatment. Avoidance or pasteurization of contaminated feed should be advocated. Ichthyophonosis can render fillets unmarketable, with a foul odor and poor flesh texture (e.g., muscle liquefaction, nodules in muscle). Infected fillets should be culled, since they can contaminate normal fillets by contact.

PROBLEM 68
Miscellaneous Systemic Fungal Infections

Prevalence Index
WF - 4, WM - 4, CF - 4, CM - 4
Method of Diagnosis
1. Wet mounts or histology with fungus
2. Culture of fungus
History
Varies with organ affected
Physical Examination
Varies with organ affected
Treatment
None proven

COMMENTS

All systemic fungal infections (Table II-68) are rare; most have been encountered as sporadic cases, although some have caused localized epidemics. Virtually all of these diseases are chronic infections, although some can eventually cause high mortalities. Most are probably taking advantage of a stressed host (Noga, 1990). Presumptive diagnosis of at least the major group responsible (e.g., yeast, dematiaceous fungus) can often be discerned from histology or wet mounts of lesions.

For example, *Ochroconis* and *Exophiala* are dematiaceous fungi, which have pigmented hyphae (chromomycoses). Thus, a wet mount with pigmented hyphae would suggest that one of these agents may be involved.

Definitive identification of the specific fungus responsible requires fungal isolation. Sabouraud's dextrose agar is a good general-purpose medium for isolation. See p. 35 for details on culture. Many of these fungi are common soil saprophytes. Thus multiple samples, preferably from aseptically cultured internal lesions, should be done to reduce the chance that contaminants are cultured instead of the pathogen. Histological confirmation of tissue damage by specific fungi is also advisable.

PROBLEM 69
Hexamitosis (Spironucleosis)

Prevalence Index
WF - 2, CF - 2, CM - 4
Method of Diagnosis
1. Wet mount of skin, feces, or viscera with parasites
2. Histopathology of lesion with parasites
History
Anorexia, chronic mortalities
Physical Examination
Abdominal swelling, exophthalmos, cachexia
Treatment
1. Metronidazole oral
2. Metronidazole prolonged immersion
3. Magnesium sulfate oral
4. Raise temperature to 35° C (95° F) for 7 days

COMMENTS
Epidemiology/Pathogenesis

Hexamita and the related flagellate *Spironucleus* have been associated with gastrointestinal disease in salmonids and aquarium fish. Predisposing stress appears to play an important role in initiating disease, since *Hexamita*, *Spironucleus*, and similar flagellates (*Chilomastix*, *Trimitus*, *Tritrichomonas*, *Protrichomonas*, *Monocercomonas*) often reside in the gastrointestinal tract of clinically normal fish (Brugerolle, 1980; Noble & Noble, 1966; Lom & Dykova, 1992).

SALMONID INFECTIONS

Hexamita salmonis (syn. *Octomitus salmonis*) infects debilitated or stressed freshwater salmonids and has recently been reported from seawater-cultured Atlantic salmon (Mo et al., 1990). It primarily infects the anterior intestine and pyloric ceca, but, in advanced cases, it can spread to the gall bladder and other organs, causing high mortality (Wood, 1976). Fish may have abdominal distension caused by fluid accumulation in the gut or

Table II-68 Miscellaneous systemic fungal infections of fish.

Pathogen	Hosts	Geographic range	Key diagnostic features	References
HYPHOMYCETES				
Fusarium solani	Vidua triggerfish, bonnethead shark	Canada; Maryland, USA (aquaria); marine	Deep mycosis with chronic inflammation	Ostland et al., 1987 Muhvich et al., 1989
Fusarium culmorum	Common carp	Europe; freshwater	Infection of eyes and skin	Horter, 1960
Fusarium oxysporum	Red sea bream	Japan; marine	Deep mycosis	Hatai et al., 1986b
Exophiala salmonis (cerebral mycetoma)	Atlantic salmon, lake trout, cutthroat trout	Alberta, Canada; Scotland; North Carolina, USA; freshwater, marine	Ataxia; erratic swimming; exophthalmos; cranial ulcers; chronic inflammation with many giant cells, especially in posterior kidney	Carmichael, 1966 Richards et al., 1978 Alderman, 1982
Exophiala piscifila	Saltwater catfish; smooth dogfish shark, other species; channel catfish	New York, USA, (aquarium); Alabama, USA; freshwater, marine	Skin ulcers and focal necrosis of viscera, often with chronic inflammation	Gaskins & Cheung, 1986 Fijan, 1969
Exophiala jeanselmei-like	Rainbow trout	England; freshwater	Kidney infection	Alderman & Feist, 1985
Exophiala sp.	Atlantic salmon	Norway		Langvad et al., 1985
Exophiala-like	Atlantic cod; seahorse; porgy; sargassum triggerfish; sebae anemonefish; cunner (E); winter flounder (E); mummichog (E)	Connecticut, USA (aquarium); marine	Nonulcerated dermal masses; raised white to yellow foci on viscera; acute necrosis or chronic inflammation in response to fungus	Blazer & Wolke, 1979
Cladosporium sp.	Atlantic cod	Marine		Reichenbach-Klinke, 1956
Ochroconis humicola	Silver salmon; coho salmon; rainbow trout	USA; freshwater	Low, chronic mortality with occasional skin ulcers; fluid in peritoneal cavity; adhesions; kidney often affected; necrosis with lymphocytic infiltrate	Ross & Yasutake, 1973 Ajello et al., 1977
Ochroconis tshawytshae	Chinook salmon	California, USA; freshwater	Infects posterior kidney	Doty & Slater, 1946
Ochroconis sp.	Yamame salmon; masu salmon	Japan; freshwater	Kidney infection that may spread to other organs (visceral mycosis); chronic inflammation	Kuroda et al., 1986 Hatai & Kubota, 1989
Phialophora sp.	Atlantic salmon	Scotland		Ellis et al., 1983
Aureobasidium sp.	Stingray	Germany (aquarium); marine	Hepatomegaly and fluid in peritoneal cavity; disease experimentally reproduced in common carp	Otte, 1964
Paecilomyces farinosus	Atlantic salmon	Scotland; marine	Reddened vent; swollen abdomen; may be infected from insect larvae; infects swim bladder	Bruno, 1989
Paecilomyces marquandii	Hybrid red tilapia	USA; freshwater	Infects kidney	Lightner et al., 1988
Aspergillus flavus	Tilapia	Freshwater	Contracted from contaminated feed	Olufemi, 1985
Aspergillus niger	Tilapia	Freshwater	Contracted from contaminated feed	Olufemi, 1985
Candida sake	Amago salmon	Japan; freshwater	Distended stomach with viscid, turbid fluid, having many yeast cells	Hatai & Egusa, 1975
Candida albicans	Grey mullet	Italy; marine	Isolated from skin lesions and muscle	Macri et al., 1984
Cryptococcus sp.	Tench	Italy; freshwater	Bilateral exophthalmos	Pierotti, 1971
COELOMYCETES				
Phoma herbarum	Silver salmon; chinook salmon; rainbow trout	Northwest USA; England; freshwater	Chronic infection of swim bladder that may extend to other tissues, causing necrosis and chronic inflammation	Ross et al., 1975
Phoma sp.	Ayu	Japan; freshwater	Infects swim bladder	Hatai et al., 1986a
UNCERTAIN TAXONOMY				
Sarcinomyces crustaceus	Cantharus black sea bream	Italy; marine	Exophthalmos	Todaro et al., 1983
Rosette agent	Chinook salmon	Washington, USA; marine	Chronic, high mortality; spherical, 3 to 7 μm, Gram +, PAS +, GMS +, clusters (rosettes) in macrophages	Harrell et al., 1986

All of these fungal infections are usually associated with chronic morbidity/mortality.
E = Experimental host.

may have exophthalmos. Fish may be emaciated and thus the head may appear relatively large (*pinheads*) (Wooten, 1989). Histologically, gastrointestinal lesions may range from no visible damage to severe enteritis.

AQUARIUM FISH INFECTIONS

In aquarium fish, related parasites of the genus *Spironucleus* infect primarily cichlids and anabantids, causing cachexia, gastroenteritis, and peritonitis (Lom & Dykova, 1992). Parasites may eventually spread to other organs. Many cases of spironucleosis in aquarium fish are mixed infections that involve other parasites or bacterial opportunists (e.g., *Capillaria* infections in angelfish) (Ferguson & Moccia, 1980). *Spironucleus* also commonly infects grass carp and other cyprinids (Molnar, 1974). There is evidence that some amphibians can act as vectors (Lom & Dykova, 1992).

Hexamitosis has also been associated (mainly in the aquarium literature) with an idiopathic syndrome known as hole-in-the-head disease (see *PROBLEM 89*). However, *Hexamita*'s importance in the syndrome is unclear.

Diagnosis

Fecal exam may reveal the presence of typical trophozoites, but necropsy will give a more accurate indication of the degree of infection, since trophozoites are often localized in the anterior intestine. Determining degree of infection is important, as *Hexamita* and

Spironucleus are often present subclinically. Post (1987) has the following recommendations for grading severity of infections in salmonids when observed in the low power field of a microscope:

1. Occasional field with one to five organisms: no treatment needed
2. Average of five to fifteen organisms in the field: no treatment needed unless no other cause of poor health is identified; watch closely for more serious infections
3. Average of 15 to 30 organisms in the field: treatment needed
4. Average of 30 to 100 organisms in the field: severe infection and therapy essential

Trophozoites are active, swimming rapidly forward; therefore, preparing fixed smears may facilitate definitive identification. However, clinical diagnosis is often presumptively based on the characteristic morphology (Fig. II-69, *A*) and hyperactive motility in live preparations. *Spironucleus* and *Hexamita* are similar (Fig. II-69, *B*) and are often confused (Lom & Dykova, 1992). Whether there are differences in response to treatment is unknown. A cyst is produced by some species but is more difficult to identify in clinical specimens than the trophozoite. *Hexamita* cysts are ~7 × 10 μm and filled with glycogen (turn brown when treated with iodine).

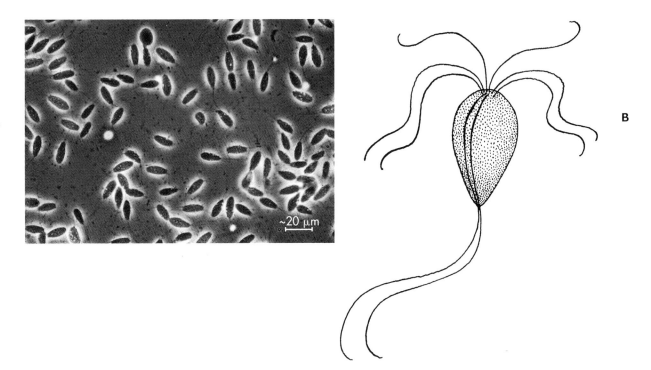

Fig. II-69 **A,** Wet mount of hexamitids. **B,** Diagram of a typical hexamitid with diagnostic features: size (from 5 to 11 μm long × 2 to 5 μm wide for *Spironucleus* to 8 to 14 μm long × 3 to 10 μm wide for *H. salmonis*); eight flagella (three pairs anteriorly, one pair posteriorly); pyriform to ellipsoidal to egg shape to tapering body.

(*A* from Reichenbache-Klinke, 1973.)

In discus, do not confuse *Spironucleus* with *Protoo-palina* (see *PROBLEM 71*), which is easily differentiated by its larger size and slower, ciliate-like movement.

Treatment
Metronidazole is usually effective. Magnesium sulfate has successfully treated freshwater salmonids, presumably acting as a cathartic. Raising the temperature has also been suggested for aquarium fish tolerant of this treatment. *Hexamita* is probably capable of a free-living existence. Treatment should always include improving environmental problems.

PROBLEM 70
Tissue Coccidiosis
Prevalence Index
WF - 4, WM - 4, CF - 4, CM - 4
Method of Diagnosis
1. Wet mount of affected tissue having oocysts
2. Histological section of affected tissue with parasite life stages
History
Varies with organs affected; may be acute or chronic
Physical Examination
Varies with organs affected (Table II-70)
Treatment
Monensin oral

COMMENTS
Epidemiology
Some coccidia are hemoparasites (see *PROBLEM 43*), but the most important fish pathogens affect solid tissues. Virtually all tissue coccidians that infect fish belong to the Family Eimeriidae (*Eimeria, Epieimeria, Goussia, Crystallospora, Calyptospora, Octosporella* and *Isospora*) (Lom & Dykova, 1992). They are completely intracellular (Fig. II-70, *A*). Nearly 200 species of eimeriids have been identified from fish, and their prevalence is probably underestimated. They are uncommon problems in most cultured fish but have caused serious disease in some (e.g., common carp).

The infective stage (sporozoite) is formed within an oocyst (Fig. II-70, *A*). After ingestion by the host the sporozoite penetrates the intestinal wall to reach the final site of infection. In the host cell the parasite forms a schizont, which produces many merozoites by asexual reproduction (merogony). Merozoites produce flagellated microgametes and oocyte-like macrogametes, which mate, producing a zygote (gametogony). The zygote then forms an oocyst (Fig. II-70, *B*), containing sporocysts with the sporozoites (sporogony). The life cycle is usually direct, but an intermediate host is required in at least one species, *Calyptospora funduli* (Solangi & Overstreet, 1980).

The rarely encountered Family Cryptosporidiidae (*Cryptosporidium* species; only reported from tilapia and naso tang) is similar to the Eimeriidae, but infection occurs in a parasitophorous vacuole of the epithelial microvillus (Hoover et al., 1981; Landsberg & Paperna, 1986). Also, microgametes are not flagellated.

Pathogenesis
The pathogenesis of tissue coccidia infections is poorly studied, but there is increasing evidence that they can be serious pathogens. Intestinal infections are often asymptomatic but can cause epithelial necrosis and enteritis (Fig. II-70, *C* through *F*). Inflammation may encapsulate oocysts. Extraintestinal parasites can also cause lesions (Dykova & Lom, 1981; Lom 1984), with characteristically destruction of target cells, followed by inflammation. Common infection sites include reproductive organs, liver, spleen (Fig. II-70, *G*), and swim bladder (Table II-70).

Diagnosis
A definitive diagnosis of tissue coccidia is based on identification of oocysts (Fig. II-70, *B* and *H*). Oocysts are thin walled compared with those of coccidia infecting mammals; they are usually sporulated (i.e., sporozoites are present) when shed, and in such cases they sporulate while still in the host cell. Coccidia that infect fish typically have oocysts with four sporocysts, each with two sporozoites. Exceptions include *Isospora* (two sporocysts), *Octosporella* (eight sporocysts) and *Cryptosporidium* (sporozoites free). Genera are also differentiated by using sporocyst structure.

Presumptive diagnosis of coccidiosis is based on histopathological identification of developmental stages (meronts, macro- and microgamonts; Fig. II-70, *C* through *F*) in target tissues.

Treatment
There are few published studies of chemical control of fish coccidiosis. The coccidiostat monensin significantly reduces infection burdens of *Calyptospora*. Toltrazuril has also shown efficacy experimentally (Melhorn et al., 1988). The coccidiostat sulfadimidine (33%, 1 ml/32l water; repeat weekly) (Langdon, 1990; Gratzek et al., 1992) has also been advocated, but there are no published clinical trials on the latter. *Calyptospora funduli* has been successfully treated with either amprolium (.63 ml/l of a 9.6% solution given over 2 days) in water or the antibiotic narasin (< 0.005 g/moderate-sized *Fundulus*) in the food. Treatment has been successful when initiated soon after the fish are infected (Overstreet, 1988). Maintaining a proper environment and reducing stress appear to be important in preventing outbreaks in cultured fish (Lom & Dykova, 1992).

Table II-70 Common and/or pathogenic coccidian infections of fish.

Pathogen / disease	Host(s)	Site(s)	Geographic / ecological range	Diagnostic features	References
INTESTINAL FORMS					
Eimeria truttae	Brown trout; brook trout; masu salmon	Intestine	Europe; Canada; Japan, (F)	No reported pathogenicity, but common	Molnar & Hanek, 1974
Epieimeria anguillae	Anguillid eels		Europe	Epithelial infection causes erosion, ulceration; can lead to emaciation and death	Hine, 1975
Goussia subepithelialis	Common carp	Intestine	Europe, (F)	Common cause of nodular coccidiosis; usually 1+ carp; sporulation at > 14° C	Marincek, 1973; Studnicka & Siwicki, 1990
Goussia carpelli	Cyprinids	Intestine	Europe; USA, (F)	Common in carp and crucian carp; most severe with overwintering stress; can cause high mortalities in goldfish fry after transport stress; can transmit directly and via tubificids or small crustaceans; infects epithelial cells, causing necrosis, ulceration, diffuse enteritis; *Goussia cheni* and *G. mylophanyngodoni* are similar, from east Asian herbivorous cyprinids	Steinhagen et al., 1989
Goussia iroquoina	*Notropis* sp.; *Pimephales* sp.; other minnows	Intestine	Canada, (F)	Primarily affects fry	Paterson & Desser, 1982
Goussia vanasi	Tilapia spp.; *Pseudocrenilabrus*	Intestine	Israel; S. Africa, (F)	Emaciation; slow growth; occasional mass mortalities in fry	Landsberg & Paperna, 1987
BOTH INTESTINAL AND EXTRAINTESTINAL FORMS					
Calyptospora funduli	Topminnow (*Fundulus*); silverside	Viscera, skin	USA Atlantic and Gulf of Mexico coasts	In heavy infections, white or black foci of oocysts in liver; also infects pancreatic acini, adipose tissue, mesentery, ovary, gall bladder and dermis; can be fatal; recovered fish may be immune; requires shrimp (*Palaemonetes*) intermediate host	Fournie & Overstreet, 1983; Solangi & Overstreet, 1980
EXTRAINTESTINAL FORMS					
Eimeria rutili	Roach	Kidney	Eurasia, (F)	Infects tubules and interstitium, causing tubular necrosis	Dogel & Bykhovski, 1939
Eimeria sardinae	Herring; sardines (*Engraulis*)	Testes	North Sea; N. Atlantic; N. Pacific, (M)	High prevalence; damage (hemmorhage and fibrosis) to seminiferous tubules; can cause parasitic castration	Kabata, 1963
Goussia clupearum	Clupeids	Liver	N. Atlantic; N. Pacific; Mediterranean Sea; North Sea, (M)	Oocysts associated with necrosis, inflammation, and fibrosis	Kabata, 1963
Goussia gadi	Codfish	Swim bladder	N. Atlantic; North Sea; Baltic Sea, (M)	Yellow creamy or waxy material (mass of parasites, fibrous debris and lipid); may eventually fill entire swim bladder, making nonfunctional; might cause death; most prevalent in fall	Odense & Logan, 1976
Goussia spraguei	Codfish; haddock	Kidney	Canada, (M)	Tubular epithelial necrosis; granulomas around infected tubules	Morrsion & Poynton, 1989
Goussia metchnikovi	Goby (*Gobio* sp.)	Spleen, liver, kidney	Europe, (F)	Heavy infections have white foci on spleen surface; inflammation and fibrosis around oocysts	Pellerdy & Molnar, 1968
Goussia cichlidarum	Tilapia spp.	Swim bladder	Israel; Uganda, (F)	Epithelium covered by mass of gamonts	Paperna et al., 1986

F = freshwater; M = marine.
See Lom & Dykova, 1992 for details on other coccidia.

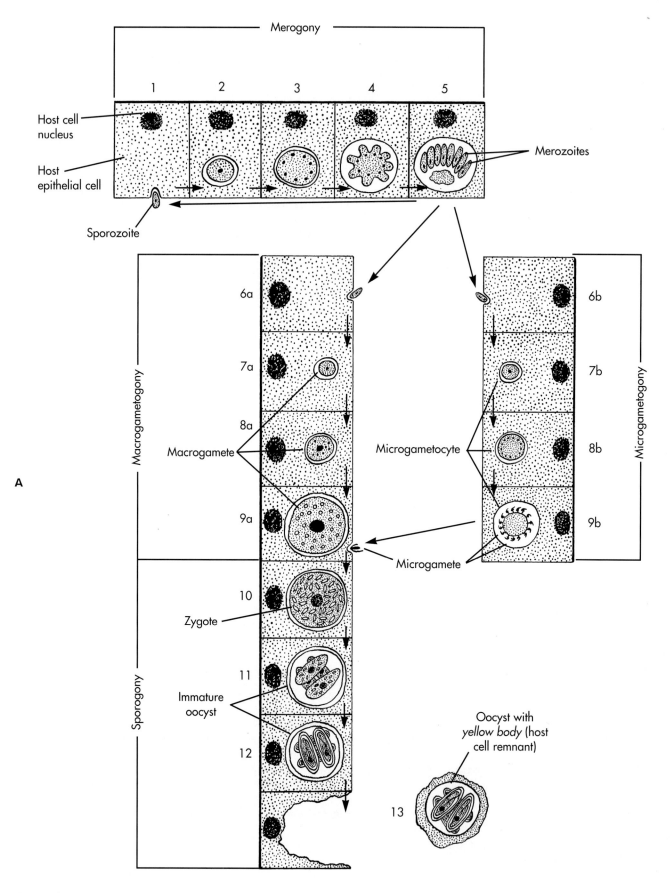

Host cell nucleus

Host epithelial cell

Sporozoite

Merogony

Merozoites

Macrogametogony

Microgametogony

Macrogamete

Microgametocyte

Microgamete

Sporogony

Zygote

Immature oocyst

Oocyst with *yellow body* (host cell remnant)

A

Fig. II-70   *For legend see opposite page.*

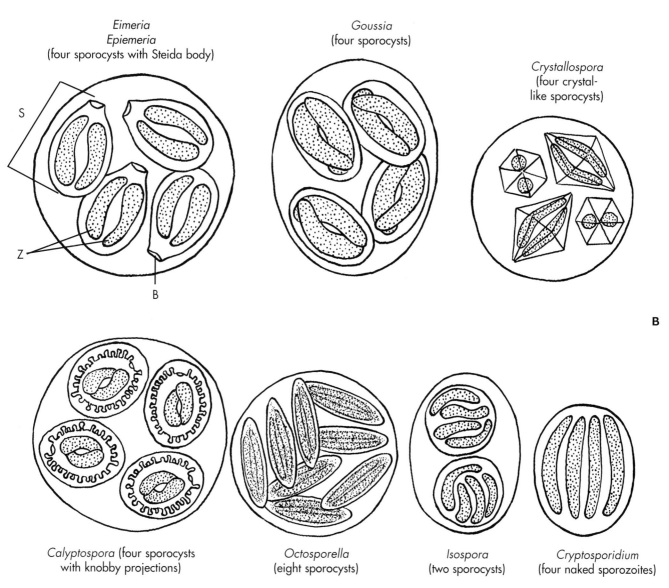

Eimeria
Epiemeria
(four sporocysts with Steida body)

Goussia
(four sporocysts)

Crystallospora
(four crystal-
like sporocysts)

B

Calyptospora (four sporocysts
with knobby projections)

Octosporella
(eight sporocysts)

Isospora
(two sporocysts)

Cryptosporidium
(four naked sporozoites)

Fig. II-70   **A,** Life cycle of a typical fish-pathogenic coccidia of the Family Eimeriidae (endocy-toplasmic, intestinal species; adapted from Lom & Dykova, 1992). The sporozoite invades an epithelial cell (*1*) and grows within a parasitophorous vacuole (*2*), forming a multinucleated stage (*3* and *4*), which produces merozoites (*5*) by asexual reproduction. The merozoite then infects another host cell and either produces more merozoites or undergoes sexual reproduction, pro-ducing a single macrogamete (*6a* through *9a*) or many microgametes (*6b* through *9b*). A microgamete fertilizes a macrogamete, producing a zygote (*10*), which forms an oocyst (*11* and *12*). The oocyst may leave the host cell unsporulated, or it may undergo intracellular sporulation (as shown in *11* and *12*). A degraded remnant of host cell (*yellow body*) is often present (*13*). **B,** Oocysts of various coccidian genera infecting fishes. S = sporocysts; Z = sporozoites; B = Steida body. **C,** Histological cross-section of yellow perch intestine infected with *Goussia* sp. The entire intestine is occupied by macrogametes and microgametocytes. *V* =intestinal villus; *W* = intestinal wall. **D,** Close-up view of a single villus in Fig. II-70, *C,* showing macrogametes (*ma*) and microgametocytes (*mi*); the latter is filled with microgametes. **E,** Histological section of blue tilapia intestine infected with *Goussia vanasi.* Various parasite stages are present (*dark arrows*). Note the detachment (*light arrows*) of infected epithelium, before it sloughs into the lumen. Hematoxylin and eosin. **F,** Close-up of infection in Fig. II-70, *E,* showing meronts (*me*) and macrogametes (*ma*). Hematoxylin and eosin. **G,** Histological section of goby spleen infected with *Goussia metchnikovi.* Light-colored area is an aggregation of oocysts (*o*). **H,** Wet mount of *Eimeria* oocysts. Each oocyst (*o*) has four sporocysts (*S*). Each sporocyst has two sporozoites.

(*C, D, G,* and *H* photographs courtesy of J. Lom; *E* and *F* photographs by L. Khoo and E. Noga.)

Continued.

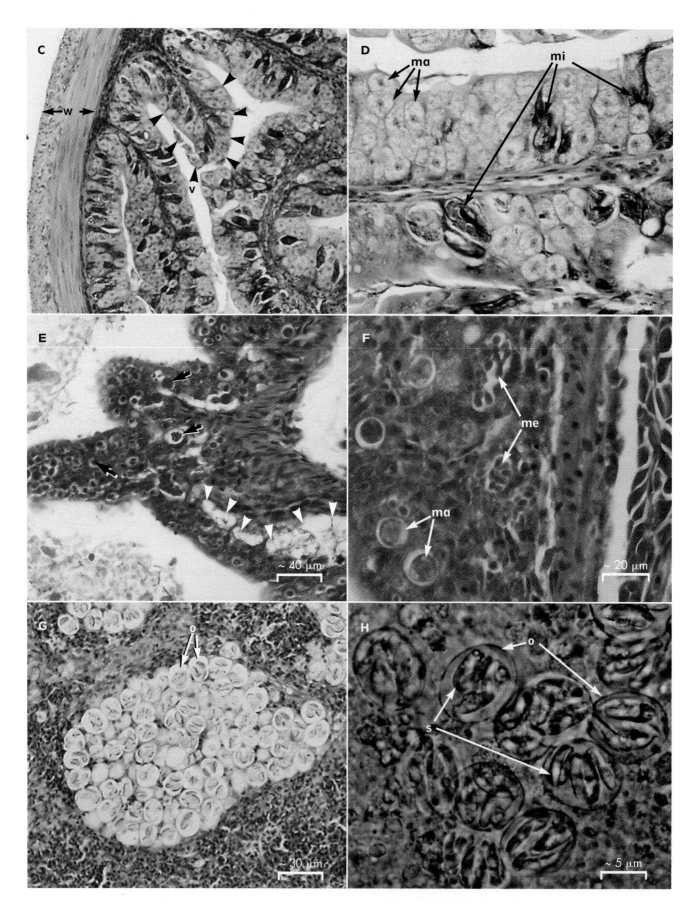

Fig. II-70—cont'd.   *For legend see page 199.*

PROBLEM 71
Miscellaneous Endoparasitic Infections

Prevalence Index

WF-4

Method of Diagnosis

1. Wet mount of viscera with parasite
2. Histology of viscera with parasite

Systemic Cryptobiosis

Cryptobia iubilans causes submucosal granulomas in cichlids. It is the only endozoic *Cryptobia* species (see *PROBLEM 29* for morphology of the genus). Chichlids (*Heterichthys* and *Cichlasoma* species) are infected, with parasites both inter- and intra-(macrophages)cellular. They incite granulomas (spleen, liver) and peritonitis (Dykova & Lom, 1979a). This organism is probably responsible for some cases of Malawi bloat reported in African rift lake cichlids (see *PROBLEM 92*; Ferguson et al., 1985).

Granulomatous Amoebic Disease

This disease affects various internal organs, causing chronic granulomatous lesions in goldfish, especially in the kidney and spleen. The organism responsible has not been isolated (Voelker et al., 1977).

Miscellaneous Amoebae

Valkamphia, *Naegleria*, *Acanthamoeba*, *Hartmanella*, *Schizamoeba*, and *Entamoeba* occasionally have been isolated from the internal organs of fish. In most cases these have been asymptomatic infections (Lom & Dykova, 1992). However, Nash et al. (1988) described a severe systemic amoebiasis in cultured European catfish.

Intestinal Protozoa

Protoopalina is a large (60 to 100 μm), ciliate-like protozoan that is a common, nonpathogenic commensal in discus (Lom & Dykova, 1992). Some claim that it may cause debilitation in young fish (Untergasser, 1991).

PROBLEM 72
Idiopathic Epidermal Proliferation / Neoplasia

Prevalence Index

WF - 4, WM - 4, CF - 4, CM - 4

Method of Diagnosis

Rule-out of other problems combined with histology of lesion

History

Various-sized mass that has often increased slowly in size

Physical Examination

Varies, depending on organ affected

Treatment

Surgery if superficial mass (i.e., on skin)

COMMENTS
Epidemiology/Pathogenesis
IDIOPATHIC EPIDERMAL PROLIFERATION (IEP)

Idiopathic epidermal proliferation has been reported in several fish, mainly feral individuals (Table II-72). IEP is usually a benign disease that typically presents as various-sized, flattened-to-papillary, epidermal thickenings (Fig. II-72, *A* and *B*). Lesions may be simply hyperplastic or show evidence of early neoplastic change. Some IEP lesions are viral-associated, but all are idiopathic. Some are pollution-associated, but others occur in fish from relatively pristine environments. Most idiopathic proliferative skin lesions reported from fish are benign. However, stomatopapilloma (Fig. II-72, *C*) has caused serious problems in European eels. Growths may be so large that they prevent eating, causing starvation.

NEOPLASIA

Many types of neoplasms have been documented in fish (see Table II-72, *B*) (Mawdesley-Thomas, 1972, 1975; Harshbarger & Clark, 1990; Harshbarger et al., 1993), mainly from feral fish. Some neoplasms have been highly prevalent (> 25%) in feral populations. Environmental contaminants have been strongly suspected as the cause in many cases, although a cause-and-effect relationship has not been proven (Mix, 1985).

Virtually any tissue can be affected by neoplasia. Skin tumors are the most common neoplasms that affect fish (Wellings, 1969), especially papillomas (see Idiopathic Epidermal Proliferation). Liver tumors are also prevalent in polluted environments and were common in salmonids in the 1960s because of feed contamination by carcinogenic aflatoxins (see *PROBLEM 79*). Several types of tumors can be experimentally induced in fish by exposure to carcinogens.

Neoplasia is rare in cultured fish, especially food fish. Tumors are occasionally seen in aquarium species. Thyroid growths are probably the most common tumors affecting tropical marine aquarium fish. Thyroid growths (ranging from benign hyperplasia to adenomas to carcinomas) (Hoover, 1984; Moccia et al., 1977) often result in grossly enlarged thyroid glands (Fig. II-72, *G*) that may interfere with breathing. Goldfish are one of the most common aquarium species affected by neoplasia (Fig. II-72, *E* and *F*), possibly because they are long-lived. Pigment cell tumors have also been seen in several aquarium species. Some proliferative lesions are apparently of no serious consequence (Fig. II-72, *H*).

Diagnosis

Histology is used for definitive diagnosis of idiopathic epidermal hyperplasia. Note that reactive hyperplasia is an extremely common reponse of fish epidermis to insults, such as parasite infestation or chronic trauma. Thus, chronic irritation caused by some exogenous agent must be ruled out.

Table II-72, A   Idiopathic, proliferative, epidermal responses in fish.

Disease	Species affected	Geographic range	Diagnostic features	References
HYPERPLASIA				
Diffuse epidermal hyperplasia	Walleye	North America	Thin epidermal plaque up to several cm in diameter; somewhat disorganized epithelium; herpesvirus-associated	Yamamoto et al., 1985
Blue spot disease	Northern pike	Manitoba and Saskatchewan, Canada	3 to 10 mm × 0.25 mm raised foci; herpesvirus-associated	Yamamoto et al., 1984
Esox epidermal hyperplasia	Northen pike; muskellunge	Canada; Sweden	5 to 10 × 1 to 3 mm plaques; undifferentiated cuboidal epithelial cells; retrovirus-associated	Yamamoto et al., 1984 Yamamoto et al., 1985
Discrete epidermal hyperplasia	Walleye	Lake Oneida, NY; Saskatchewan and Manitoba, Canada	Up to several cm plaque; retrovirus-associated	Yamamoto et al., 1985
Lake trout epidermal hyperplasia	Lake trout	Lake Superior; Lake Michigan		McAllister & Herman, 1989
Hybrid striped bass epidermal hyperplasia	Hybrid striped bass	North Carolina, USA	2 to 10 mm plaques (Fig. II-72, *B*)	E. Noga (unpublished data)
Atlantic cod epidermal hyperplasia	Atlantic cod	Baltic Sea	3 to 20 mm plaques; only seen once; herpesvirus-associated	Jensen & Bloch, 1980
Carp pox (*Herpesvirus cyprini* disease)*	Common carp; crucian carp; barbel; bream; golden ide; rudd; smelt; carp × goldfish; aquarium fish	Europe; Asia; Russia; Israel; Great Lakes, USA	Smooth to rough, milky white-to-grey plaques; up to 2 mm thick; this is not an idiopathic lesion (see *PROBLEM 78*)	
Dab epidermal hyperplasia	Dab	North Sea	2 to 10 mm plaques progressing to 5 to 15 mm papules (Fig. II-72, *A*); adenovirus-associated	Bloch et al., 1986
PAPILLOMA				
Stomatopapilloma* (cauliflower disease)	European eel	Baltic, North, and Black Seas; England and Scotland rivers	Mostly mouth and head growths (Fig. II-72, *C*) can interfere with eating, breathing; virus suspected, but not proven	Wolf, 1988
Smelt papillomatosis	Smelt	Europe	Cowdry-type intranuclear inclusions; herpesvirus-associated	Anders & Moller, 1985
Black bullhead papilloma	Black bullhead	USA	Papillary tumors	Grizzle et al., 1981
Gilthead sea bream papilloma	Gilthead sea bream	Spain	Maxillary tumors; may interfere with feeding	Guttierez et al., 1977
Pleuronectid epidermal papilloma (X-cell disease)*	Flatfish	Europe; North America	1 mm nodules to 5 cm polyps; virus suspected; X-cells also suspected to be protozoans; also found in pseudobranch and gills of Atlantic cod and blue whiting (Fig. II-72, *D*)	Wellings et al., 1976 Diamant, 1990
Winter flounder papilloma	Winter flounder	Newfoundland, Canada	Blister-like swellings, with spongiosis and hydropic degeneration; virus suspected	Emerson et al., 1985

*Clinically important diseases.

Table II-72, *B* Common neoplasms in fish.

Organ or tissue	Species commonly affected
EPIDERMIS	
Hyperplasia	See Table II-72, *A*
Papilloma	Yellow bullhead, American eel, Atlantic salmon, white sucker; also see Table II-72, *A*
Carcinoma	Yellow perch, brown bullhead
Pigment cell tumors	Goldfish, common carp, *Corydoras* catfish, platy × swordtail hybrids, melanomas most common
CONNECTIVE TISSUE	
Lipoma	Largemouth bass
Fibroma	Mullet, many salmonids (common)
Fibrosarcoma	Coho salmon, walleye, goldfish (Fig. II-72, *E* and *F*) (common)
MUSCULOSKELETAL	
Chondroma ("osteoma")	Many species; "osteoma" (Fig. II-72, *H*) is often an idiopathic, nonneoplastic, foreign body reaction
NERVOUS TISSUE	
Schwannoma	Goldfish, bicolor damselfish
Neurofibroma	Gray snapper
Neurilemmoma / neurofibroma	Goldfish
HEMATOPOIETIC TISSUE	
Lymphoma / lymphosarcoma	Northern pike, muskellunge, rainbow trout
CARDIOVASCULAR	
Hemangioma	Salmonids, Atlantic cod, mackerel, pollock, plaice
RESPIRATORY	Gill neoplasia is rare
THYROID	
Hyperplasia / adenoma / adenosarcoma	Salmonids, carp, koi, goldfish, aquarium fish (Fig. II-72, *G*), yellow perch, coho salmon; normal thyroid tissue may be found in kidney, spleen, or epicardial surface
GASTROINTESTINAL TRACT	
Ameloblastoma	Salmonids, cunner
LIVER	
Hepatoma / hepatocarcinoma	Many salmonids, brown bullhead, English sole, Atlantic tomcod, winter flounder (one of the few fish tumors that metastasize)
Cholangioma / cholangicarcinoma	Salmonids, English sole, winter flounder
KIDNEY	
Nephroblastoma	Rainbow trout (rare)
REPRODUCTIVE TISSUE	
Testicular adenoma	Goldfish × carp

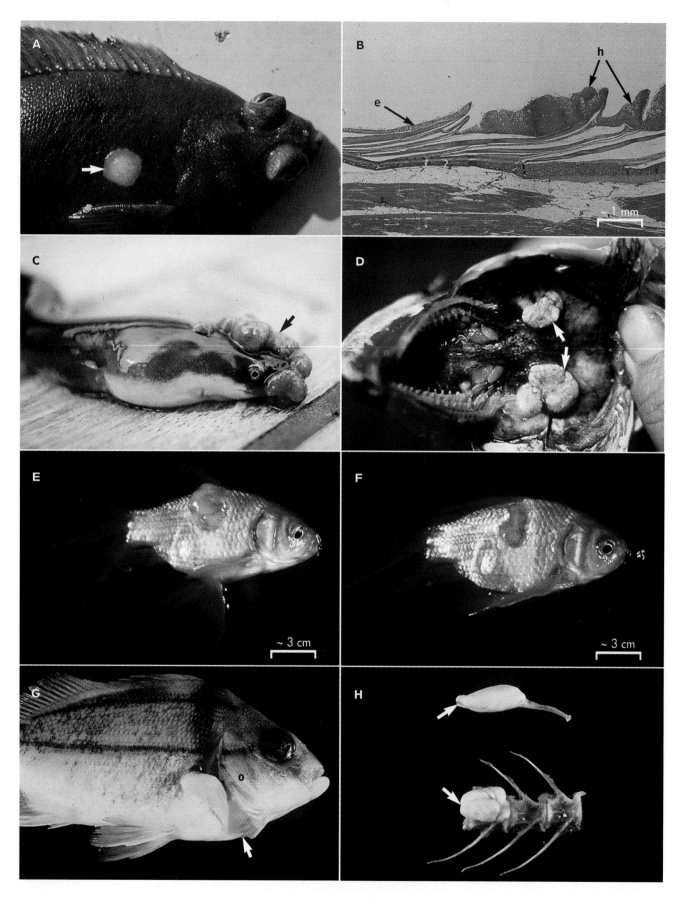

Fig II-72 *For legend see opposite page.*

Fig. II-72 A, Idiopathic epidermal hyperplasia (*arrow*) in dab. **B,** Hybrid striped bass with idiopathic epidermal hyperplasia (*h*). Compare with normal epithelium (*e*). **C,** Stomatopapilloma (*arrow*) in a European eel. **D,** X-cell lesions (*arrows*) in the gill cavity of a blue whiting. **E,** Fibrosarcoma on a goldfish. **F,** Fish in Fig. II-72, *E,* 2 months after tumor resection. **G,** Mass (*arrow*) in the throat region of a porkfish caused by a thyroid tumor. The operculum (*o*) cannot entirely close because of swelling. Preserved specimen. **H,** Osteomas (*arrows*) on the rib and vertebral column of an Atlantic croaker.

(*A, C,* and *D* photographs courtesy of H. Moller; *B* photograph by L. Khoo and E. Noga; *E* and *F* photographs by D. Probasco and E. Noga.)

Histology is also used for definitive diagnosis of neoplasia. Note that fish neoplasms do not always conform to mammalian criteria used to classify lesions. Hayes and Ferguson (1989) provide details on tumor biology and classification. Metastasis is rare, even for tumors that appear malignant histologically, although neoplasms may be locally invasive. Some proliferative, parasitic infections have been mistaken for neoplasia (Harshbarger, 1984).

Treatment

Neoplastic growths on the fins or body surface are often amenable to surgical excision (Probasco et al., 1994; Fig. II-72, *F*). Some may recur. Fish can often live a long time with many cancers.

CHAPTER 18

Problems 73 through 78

Rule-out diagnoses: *presumptive* diagnosis is based on the absence of other etiologies combined with a diagnostically appropriate history, clinical signs, and/or pathology; *definitive* diagnosis is based upon presumptive diagnosis combined with confirmation of viral presence (e.g., culture, immmunodiagnosis)

73. Systemic viral diseases: general features
74. Channel catfish virus disease
75. Infectious pancreatic necrosis
76. Infectious hematopoietic necrosis
77. Viral hemorrhagic septicemia
78. Miscellaneous viral infections

PROBLEM 73
Systemic Viral Diseases: General Features

Prevalence Index
See Group headings
Method of Diagnosis
1. Culture of specific virus from lesions
2. Immunological probe
3. Histopathology of diagnostic lesions
History
Varies with etiological agent and environmental conditions (especially temperature)
Physical Examination
Varies with etiological agent and environment
Treatment
1. Disinfect and quarantine
2. Eliminate source of contamination (i.e., water or fish)

COMMENTS
Systemic viral infections are common and important diseases. Many different types of viruses have been identified. General characteristics of viral infections of fish include: often temperature-dependent pathogenicity; host-specific (usually affecting only one species or a closely related group of species); usually young fish get sick, while older fish become carriers; no medications are available, only disinfection and quarantine can be used. Avoidance is the best method of control. This includes obtaining fish only from certified virus-free stocks and raising fish in virus-free water (spring, well, or disinfected). When exposure to virus-infected water is unavoidable (e.g., using contaminated surface waters), stocking fish that are past the age of greatest susceptibility is an option, since most important viral diseases are most damaging to young fish. Various antiviral compounds have been tried with varying success, but none are commercially available for use in fish. Considerable experimental work has been done with vaccines and several live attenuated vaccines hold promise (Walczak et al., 1981; Fryer et al., 1976), but none are presently licensed for use.

Definitive diagnosis of systemic viral disease is based on observation of relevant clinical signs and history in combination with virus isolation. Some viruses may be present in low numbers without causing disease (e.g., IPN), requiring quantification to determine its importance in causing disease. Some viruses may be shed from asymptomatic carriers during spawning time (e.g., IPN, IHN, VHS, HVS). See viral isolation techniques (p. 36) for details on sampling for systemic viruses.

PROBLEM 74
Channel Catfish Virus Disease (CCVD)

Prevalence Index
WF - 2
Method of Diagnosis
Culture of channel catfish virus from fish displaying typical clinical signs
History
Acute to chronic morbidity/mortality; corkscrew spiral swimming
Physical Examination
Reddening on body and base of fins; depression; exophthalmos; swollen abdomen; equilibrium deficit
Treatment
1. Disinfect and quarantine
2. Reduce temperature to less than 15° C (59° F)
3. Treat secondary infections

COMMENTS

Epidemiology

Channel catfish virus is the most important viral disease affecting channel catfish. Except for its accidental introduction into Honduras, it is restricted to the channel catfish-producing areas of the United States (Wolf, 1988). It is a highly species-specific herpesvirus and only naturally affects channel catfish, although it can experimentally infect some other ictalurids (blue catfish, channel × blue catfish hybrid) and possibly some clariid catfishes (Galla & Hartmann, 1974). Different strains of channel catfish vary in their susceptibility (Plumb & Chappell, 1978).

During CCVD epidemics, the younger, more robust fish typically die first. Only young (< 1 year) and small (< 15 cm) fish become clinically sick. Mortalities are most rapid and severe with higher temperatures, being highest at 25° to 30° C (77° to 86° F). Clinical signs may be evident in as little as 1 day at 30° C (86° F), taking 10 days at 20° C (68° F). No mortalities occur at < 15° C (59° F). There is also some evidence that young fish (Amend & McDowell, 1983) or broodfish (Bowser et al., 1985) may develop a chronic infection.

During epidemics, virus is readily transmitted horizontally in the feces and urine of clinically affected fish. There is also evidence for vertical transmission (Wise et al., 1985). Virus can usually only be isolated during an active epidemic. However, virus can be isolated from clinically normal adult broodstock after dexamethasone injection (Bowser et al., 1985). There is evidence for recrudescence of latent infections.

Clinical Signs/Pathogenesis

GROSS LESIONS

Clinical signs include hanging head up in the water, disorientation (corkscrew spiral swimming), abdominal distension, exophthalmos, and hemorrhages on the body, gills, and at the bases of the fins (Fig. II-74, *A*). Internally, there is a yellowish fluid in the peritoneal cavity and punctate hemorrhage in the viscera.

HISTOPATHOLOGY

Channel catfish virus attacks all major organ systems. Focal necrosis begins in the posterior kidney and quickly develops into diffuse necrosis of both hematopoietic and excretory tissues, accompanied by hemorrhage and edema (Fig. II-74, *B*). Necrosis also affects the liver, spleen, gastrointestinal tract, pancreas, and skeletal muscle (Yasutake, 1975). Neurological damage includes vacuolated neurons and edematous neurofibers (Major et al., 1975).

Diagnosis

The typical presentation of a CCVD epidemic is a rapid, abrupt increase in mortality in young-of-year channel catfish when the temperature is at least 25° C (77° F). Definitive diagnosis of clinical CCVD requires identification of virus from target tissues, with appropriate clinical signs. Peak viral titers correspond with the peak in tissue damage (Wolf, 1988). Kidney is the best organ for isolation. Ictalurid cell lines (BB or CCO) are most commonly used for isolation; syncytia formation and presence of intranuclear Cowdry type A inclusion bodies are strong presumptive evidence for CCV. Serum neutralization of cell culture-isolated virus is the most widely used method for definitive diagnosis. Fluorescent antibody of frozen tissues (Plumb et al., 1981) or DNA probes (Wise et al., 1985) have also been developed. None of these reagents are commercially available. Identification of anti-CCV antibody titers in convalescent sera of recovering fish can also be used for presumptive diagnosis. Serum should probably be collected 1 or 2 months after exposure. False negatives are common.

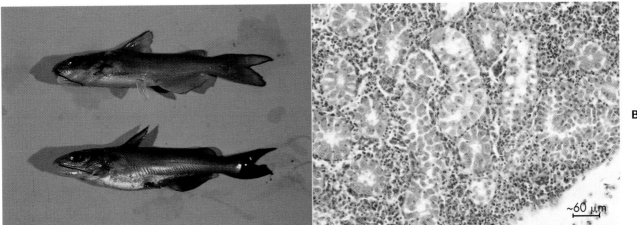

A
B

Fig. II-74 A, Channel catfish with CCV infection. Note hemorrhage in the fins (*bottom fish*) and abdominal swelling caused by fluid accumulation in the peritoneal cavity. Clinically normal fish above. **B,** Histological section showing acute necrosis of kidney caused by CCV infection. Hematoxylin and eosin.

Many CCVD epidemics are accompanied by secondary bacterial infections (*Aeromonas, Flexibacter, Edwardsiella*), which can mask the primary diagnosis. Virus cannot be isolated from a fish population within days after an epidemic ends (Wolf, 1988). The CCVD virus is also relatively unstable in the environment. There is a 50% loss of infectivity in fish stored for 100 days at approximately 20° C and 90% loss after 3 days on ice. It survives for less than 3 days in dead fish at room temperature (Plumb, 1973). Freezing and thawing rapidly destroys activity.

Treatment

Disinfection and quarantine is the most effective means of controlling CCVD epidemics. The virus can persist in water up to 1 or 2 months at 4° C (39° F) but less than 2 weeks at 25° C (77° F) (Plumb, 1978). Treating ponds with 20 to 50 mg/l chlorine will ensure that the virus is eliminated. Thorough drying also inactivates it.

All fish surviving an outbreak should be destroyed. Surviving fish are often stunted (McGlamery & Gratzek, 1974). By reducing the temperature to less than 15° C (59° F) epidemics can be stopped, but this method is impractical and probably does not eliminate the carrier state. There is evidence that many commercial catfish broodstock carry CCV DNA in a latent carrier state (Wise et al., 1985), making it difficult to obtain virus-free broodstock. Only broodstock without anti-CCV serum neutralization titers and no history of prior exposure to CCV should be used for spawning. Note that some fish do not produce neutralizing antibody titers after exposure to CCV.

Stress reduction is considered to be important in managing the disease, including preventing overcrowding, adequate oxygen and nutrition, and not handling fish when temperatures exceed 20° C (68° F). However, the highly infectious nature of the virus suggests that stress is not essential for virus dissemination (Wolf, 1988). Controlling concurrent secondary infections is mandatory. Both live, attenuated (Walczak et al., 1981) and subunit (Awad et al., 1989) vaccines experimentally provide protection, but neither is yet available commercially. Using resistant channel catfish strains may reduce severity of outbreaks (Plumb & Chappell, 1978).

PROBLEM 75
Infectious Pancreatic Necrosis (IPN)

Prevalence Index
CF - 1, CM - 3
Method of Diagnosis
Culture of IPN virus (IPNV) from fish displaying typical clinical signs
History
Usually acute, sometimes chronic, morbidity/mortality

Physical Examination
Neurological signs; trailing white feces; dorsal darkening; abdominal distension; exophthalmos; hemorrhage; pale gills; catarrhal exudate in stomach
Treatment
1. Disinfect and quarantine
2. Raise fish in virus-free water for first 6 months of life

COMMENTS: SALMONIDS
Epidemiology
Infectious pancreatic necrosis virus, a birnavirus, is a major cause of mortality in salmonids in freshwater. Its geographic range is the United States, Canada, Chile, Japan, Taiwan, Korea, and Europe. It infects rainbow, brook, and cutthroat trout; Atlantic, coho, and Kokanee salmon; Arctic char; and other salmonids. Brook and rainbow trout are most susceptible. Only young fish become clinically ill (mortality in fish < 6 months old is rare), but any age fish can become infected, forming chronic carriers.

The time course of clinical disease varies with fish age, species, temperature, and other conditions, but clinical signs typically appear on day 3 to 5 (fry) or on day 8 to 10 (fingerlings) after exposure to the virus. Peak mortality usually occurs on day 12 to 18.

Mortality is most rapid and severe at high temperatures (e.g., 10° to 14° C [50° to 57° F]); at lower temperatures, mortality is prolonged and often reduced (Frantsi & Savan, 1971). There is also usually less mortality above 14° C (57° F), possibly because of interferon production.

Even the most virulent outbreaks have at least a few survivors. Surviving fish often become stunted because of pancreatic fibrosis and up to 90% may become carriers. Survivors may shed virus in the feces and urine for over 2 years. Not all fish shed; some only shed intermittently (Billi & Wolf, 1969). Chronic shedding does not occur with other salmonid viral diseases.

The virus is highly contagious. During epidemics, virus is readily transmitted horizontally by contact and by ingestion of infected tissue; the fecal pseudocast (see *CLINICAL SIGNS*) is a major source of virus. Vertical transmission readily occurs via transport in reproductive fluids and on (or possibly in) the egg. IPNV is also suspected of contributing to embryo mortality (Wolf, 1988).

Clinical Signs/Pathology
GROSS LESIONS
A typical presentation of IPN is a sudden increase in mortality of fry or fingerling trout, with larger, more robust fish dying first. Clinical signs include dorsal darkening, trailing white feces, abdominal distension (Fig. II-75, *A*), exophthalmos, hemorrhage on the ventrum, and pale gills. Neurological signs (corkscrew spiral swimming, whirling) can often be initiated by startling the

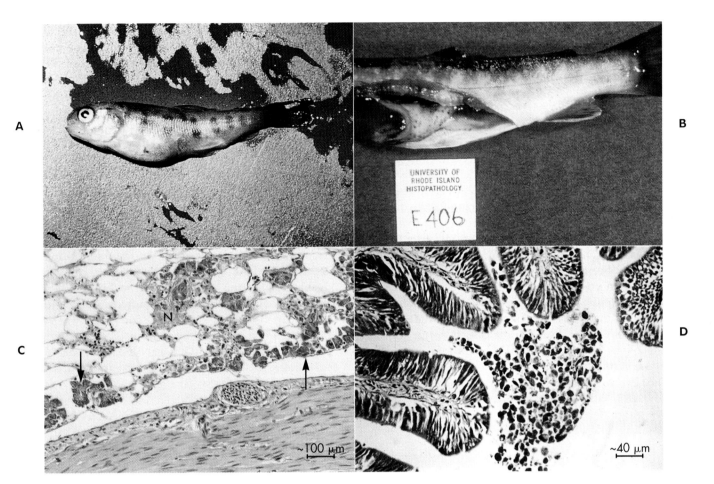

Fig. II-75 A, Rainbow trout with IPN. Note the swollen abdomen caused by accumulation of fluid in the peritoneal cavity. **B,** Rainbow trout with IPN. Note the punctate hemorrhages in the viscera. **C,** Histological section showing acute necrosis (*N*) of pancreatic acinar tissue caused by IPN infection. A few areas of more normal tissue remain (*arrows*). Hematoxylin and eosin. **D,** Histological section of pyloric ceca with McKnight cells sloughing into the lumen. Hematoxylin and eosin.

(*A* and *D* photographs courtesy of R. Roberts; *B* photograph courtesy of R. Wolke; *C* photograph by L. Khoo and E. Noga.)

fish. In older fingerling trout, there may be many petechial hemorrhages in the viscera (Fig. II-75, *B*). In contrast, fry have pale viscera with few petechiae. A catarrhal exudate in the stomach and intestine produces the mucoid, cohesive fecal pseudocast.

HISTOPATHOLOGY

The prime target of viral infection is the pancreatic acinar cells, which undergo acute necrosis (Fig. II-75, *C*) and have basophilic, intracytoplasmic "inclusions" ("inclusions" are actually products of cell degeneration). Adjacent adipose tissue may be damaged. Another diagnostic feature is the presence of McKnight cells, epithelial cells of the pyloric ceca, which swell and develop a fragmented nucleus; the eosinophilic cytoplasm is then shed into the lumen (McKnight & Roberts, 1976). Renal tubular and hematopoietic tissue, as well as liver, may also be necrotic in terminal cases.

Diagnosis

CLINICAL IPN

Definitive diagnosis of clinical IPN requires isolation of high titers (~10^6 to 10^9 infective units/gram-of-tissue) of virus from target tissues, with appropriate clinical signs in susceptible species. High titers are needed for a definitive diagnosis because IPNV is often present in a subclinical carrier state. The best tissue for isolation is posterior kidney; pyloric ceca are also useful. If sampled within 24 hours, whole tissues are best stored on ice, while homogenates are best frozen. If samples must be stored longer, it is best to freeze at the lowest possible temperature.

Presumptive diagnosis of clinical IPN is based on the presence of typical clinical signs and pathology in susceptible species. Major differentials include other salmonid viral infections, including IHN (see *PROB-*

LEM 76), VHS (see *PROBLEM 77*), and HVS (see *PROBLEM 78*). Especially diagnostic features include presence of white feces (which are more fragile than those seen with IHN or HVS) accompanied by the presence of clear to milky mucus in the stomach and anterior intestine (may be pathognomonic). Since the mucoid material does not coagulate in 10% neutral buffered formalin, it can also be detected in preserved specimens (Wolf, 1988). Key microscopic features include acute pancreatic necrosis and presence of McKnight cells (Fig. II-75, *C* and *D*). When the above lesions are present in salmonids, there is over a 90% probability of the disease being IPN. However, caution is warranted if there are lesions in other tissues, such as kidney and liver, since other viruses can cause similar lesions. There is also the possibility of more than one virus being present.

IPNV may co-occur with other pathogens, so a clinical decison must be made as to whether the pathogens detected in the clinical work-up can explain the severity and clinical signs of disease in the case. If not, it may be justifiable to examine fish for IPN, especially if the history suggests it.

SUBCLINICAL CARRIERS OF IPN
The most reliable method for detecting carriers is to sacrifice a significantly relevant number of fish (Tholsen, 1994) and take a culture of the posterior kidney, which has the highest virus titers. Other viscera yield lower, but still significant, amounts of virus. While techniques for kidney biopsy have been developed for bacterial pathogens (Noga et al., 1988b), this procedure has not yet been examined for diagnosing IPN carriers. Thus, nonlethal sampling is most reliable when sex products are examined, especially ovarian fluid sediment (McAllister et al., 1987). Blood, feces, and peritoneal washes are less sensitive (Yu et al., 1982). Adding 2% bovine serum albumin to body fluids helps to stabilize the virus, which can then be stored frozen. There is higher probability of virus recovery from stressed fish.

Treatment
Disinfection and quarantine is the only practical method of controlling an IPN epidemic. Extreme caution should be taken to avoid spreading virus to uncontaminated areas, both on and outside the farm. The IPN virus is one of the most stable fish viruses. It can survive for months in frozen viscera. In freshwater, it can survive for 5 days at 15° C (59° F), for 10 days in a 4° C (39° F) stream, and for 3 months in sterile water (Toranzo et al., 1983). It is even more stable in brackish water (Toranzo et al., 1983). It survives air drying at 10° C (50° F) for over 1 month.

The virus is readily inactivated by 40 mg/l chlorine for 30 minutes, 20,000 ppm formalin for 5 minutes, 35 ppm iodine for 5 minutes, pH 12.5 for 10 minutes, or 90 ppm ozone for 0.5 to 10 minutes. However, it is resistant to ultraviolet irradiation (only partially inactivated by $330,000$ mWs/cm^2), making this impractical for control (Wolf, 1988).

Avoidance is the most useful prophylactic measure, but this may not be possible in many cases. Many watersheds have feral IPNV-infected salmonids. Other fishes (e.g., striped bass) that are known to harbor IPNV may also transmit the virus to salmonids (McAllister & McAllister, 1988). To avoid clinical IPNV in such cases, young fish can be raised in a virus-free water source (e.g., spring or well water) for the first 6 months of life, after which they may be stocked in IPNV-infected, grow-out waters. While the young fish may still become infected, they will not usually become sick. Lowering the temperature will also reduce the severity of outbreaks (Frantsi & Savan, 1971), but this is usually impractical.

Aside from epidemics, the principal risk of IPNV infection is infected broodstock. Vertical transmission of IPNV cannot be controlled with antiseptic egg baths, possibly because the virus is carried within the egg or somehow sheltered on the egg's surface. Carriers that survive an outbreak are less commonly a risk. Populations that have recovered from IPN are susceptible to recrudescence of clinical disease if stressed. Maintaining a healthy environment can reduce the impact of IPN outbreaks.

IPNV is a potent immunogen and fish develop high titers of neutralizing antibody after exposure. However, the large amount of serological variation among various strains and apparent lack of cross-protection has hindered development of a practical vaccine. There are three major serotypes of IPNV (VR-299, Sp, and Ab) and many subtypes (Wolf, 1988).

COMMENTS: NONSALMONID FISHES
While freshwater salmonids are the group most commonly afflicted with clinical IPN, IPNV has been isolated from many species of fishes and aquatic invertebrates, including some marine species. Infectious pancreatic necrosis virus can infect at least one member of 20 families of fish, including those of the lamprey, herring, salmon, whitefish, grayling, true eel, sucker, carp, loach, pike, poeciliid, lefteye flounder, bastard halibut, sole, silverside, cavalla, perch, percichthyid bass, drum, and cichlid families (Wolf, 1988). Virus has also been isolated from oysters, crabs, and digenean trematodes. In almost all cases, these isolates have not been proven to be pathogenic for the host species, although they have occasionally been pathogenic to trout. Thus, at present, these aquatic species are most clinically important in acting as nonsusceptible viral reservoirs.

Clinical Disease in Nonsalmonid Fish
EELS
In young Japanese eels, IPNV causes muscle spasms, a retracted abdomen, congestion of the anal fin, and, in some fish, congestion of the abdomen and gills. Food is absent from the gut, and there can be ascites. The kidneys are hypertrophied, with exudative glomerulonephritis, congestion of renal interstitium, nephrosis

with hyaline droplet degeneration, and sloughing of tubule cells into the lumens. There is focal necrosis of the liver and spleen. The disease can be reproduced experimentally (Sano et al., 1981).

YELLOWTAIL
In Japan, both spontaneous and experimentally infected fry and fingerlings develop an important, acute disease (*pancreatic-hepatic necrosis*) with ascites (Sorimachi & Hara, 1985). Epidemics usually occur in May through June at 18° to 22° C (64° to 72° F) (Kimura & Yoshimizu, 1991).

OTHER SPECIES
IPNV infection has also been suspected of causing disease in European sea bass (Bonami et al., 1983), Atlantic menhaden, and striped bass (Schultz et al., 1984), but the data is less convincing for these species.

PROBLEM 76
Infectious Hematopoietic Necrosis (IHN, Chinook Salmon Disease Virus, Sacramento River Chinook Disease, Columbia River Sockeye Disease, Oregon Sockeye Disease)

Prevalence Index
CF - 2

Method of Diagnosis
Culture of IHN virus from fish displaying typical clinical signs

History
Variable; acute to chronic morbidity/mortality

Physical Examination
Lethargy; sporadic hyperactivity; long, thick, trailing white feces; dorsal darkening; abdominal distension; exophthalmos; hemorrhage; pale gills; mucoid fluid in stomach

Treatment
1. Disinfect and quarantine
2. Raise temperature above 15° C (59° F)
3. Treat eggs with iodophore

COMMENTS
Epidemiology
Infectious hematopoietic necrosis virus, a rhabdovirus, is a major cause of mortality in salmonids in freshwater. It is probably endemic to the Pacific northwest coast of North America but has been inadvertently introduced into and become established in Japan, Taiwan, Italy, France, and Germany, as well as other areas of the United States (Snake River Valley, Idaho).

In North America, natural IHN outbreaks have occurred in rainbow (steelhead) trout, Kamloops rainbow trout, and brown trout and in Atlantic, chinook, pink, and sockeye salmon. In Japan, epidemics have occurred in chum, amago, and yamame salmon (Wolf, 1988). Viral strains vary in pathogenicity for different salmonids. Coho salmon and brook, brown, and cut-

throat trout are considered refractory, although the virus has been isolated from asymptomatic coho salmon and from brook and cutthroat trout.

During IHN epidemics, only young (< 2 years old) fish become clinically ill. High mortality can occur in fish less than 6 months old, while older fish have lower mortality and may not show clinical signs (Yasutake, 1978). Prodromal period is about 5 to 14 days. Temperature has an important influence on epidemics. Peak mortalities (to 100%) occur at 10° C (50° F); fewer and more chronic mortalities occur at less than 10° C, while fewer and more acute mortalities occur above 10° C. No disease occurs above 15° C (59° F) (Amend, 1970).

During epidemics, virus is readily transmitted horizontally by ingestion of infected tissue, as well as by the feces and urine of infected fish. Survivors can become carriers, but the virus is not detectable until sexual maturity. Vertical transmission probably occurs via transport in reproductive fluids and on the outside of the egg. Virus is abundant in the water during spawning and horizontal transmission between carriers and uninfected adults is also considered a distinct possibility. The gills are implicated as a major portal of entry and gill tissue has large amounts of virus just before spawning. Virus has also been isolated from leeches, copepods, and mayflies (Winton, 1991).

Clinical Signs/Pathology
GROSS LESIONS
The typical presentation of IHN is increased mortality among fry or fingerlings of susceptible species at the appropriate temperature. Larger, more robust individuals die first. Fry are lethargic (swim feebly and avoid current by moving to the edge of the raceway) with sporadic hyperactivity. A long, thick, off-white fecal pseudocast trailing from the rectum (Fig. II-76, *A*) is diagnostic. Other clinical signs include darkening, abdominal distension, exophthalmos, and hemorrhage at the base of the fins. Gills are pale, and internally, there is visceral pallor, caused by anemia. There is no food in the gastrointestinal tract, which is distended with an off-white, translucent, mucoid, fluid. There may be petechiation of the visceral fat, mesenteries, peritoneum, swim bladder, meninges, and pericardium (Wolf, 1988). In sockeye salmon, 5% or more of surviving fish may have spinal deformities (Amend et al., 1969). Clinical signs are less severe in older fish and may be absent or simply appear as lateral compression because of anorexia (Yasutake, 1978).

CLINICAL PATHOLOGY
IHN causes profound changes in cellular and chemical blood constituents, primarily because of renal damage. The most clinically useful change is the presence of remnants of necrotic cells ("necrobiotic bodies"), probably erythrocytes, in kidney smears (Fig. II-76, *B*) (Yasutake, 1978). These cells are less frequent in peripheral blood (Yasutake, 1978). Fish are anemic and leukopenic, and there is evidence of osmotic imbalance (hypoosmolality) (Amend & Smith, 1974).

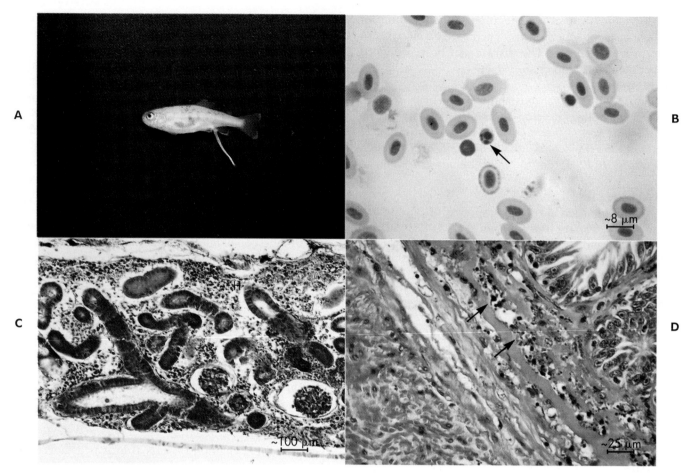

Fig. II-76 **A,** Salmonid with IHN. Note the characteristic, thick trailing fecal cast. **B,** Blood smear with *necrobiotic bodies* (*arrow*) caused by IHN. Giemsa. **C,** Histological section showing acute necrosis of kidney hematopoietic tissue (*H*) caused by IHN. Note the lack of damage to renal excretory tissue. Hematoxylin and eosin. **D,** Histological section showing acute necrosis of eosinophilic granular cells (*arrows*) of the intestinal submucosa. Hematoxylin and eosin.

[*A* photograph courtesy of K. Wolf; *B* and *D* photographs courtesy of C. Smith; *C* photograph by L. Khoo and E. Noga.]

HISTOPATHOLOGY

In affected fry, major changes are necrosis of the kidney, hematopoetic tissue, pancreas, gastrointestinal tract, and interrenal tissue (adrenal cortex). Splenic and renal hematopoetic tissues are usually affected first and most severely (Fig. II-76, *C*); inter-renal tissue may eventually be involved, as well as glomeruli and tubules. Pancreatic necrosis is common. Pleiomorphic intracytoplasmic and intranuclear inclusions are present in the pancreatic acinar and islet cells. Hepatic necrosis has been reported in some cases. Necrosis of the eosinophilic granule cells of the intestinal submucosa (Fig. II-76, *D*) is highly diagnostic but is only evident in fish at least 3 to 4 months old (Yasutake, 1978).

In older fingerlings, lesions are similar (splenic and renal hematopoetic necrosis, moderate sloughing of intestinal mucosa, degeneration of pancreas) but more subtle. One distinguishing feature may be the presence of gill lesions (branchial hyperplasia and fusion) (Burke & Grischkowsky, 1984).

Diagnosis

CLINICAL IHN

Definitive diagnosis of clinical IHN requires isolation of virus from target tissues with appropriate clinical signs and history in susceptible species. Note that there may be few clinical signs or histopathological changes in fish over 6 months old. Virus is usually abundant in organ homogenates from clinical cases. Virus can also be isolated from dead eggs and dead, partly developed, embryos. The IHN virus is stable in frozen viscera (months) and tissue samples can be stored at 4° C (39° F) before processing.

Presumptive diagnosis of clinical IHN is based on the presence of typical clinical signs and pathology in susceptible species kept at low temperature. Major differentials include other salmonid viral infections, including IPN (see *PROBLEM 75*), VHS (see *PROBLEM 77*), and HVS (see

PROBLEM 78). Especially diagnostic features include the presence of white feces (which are thicker and longer than those seen with IPN). Key microscopic features include renal and hematopoietic necrosis. Degeneration and necrosis of the granular cells of the stratum compactum and stratum granulosum are pathognomonic. The presence of *necrobiotic bodies* is also supportive, although such cells also are present to a lesser extent in IPN and VHS.

When the above lesions are present in salmonids, there is a high probability of the disease being IHN. However, caution is warranted if there are lesions in other tissues, such as pancreas, since other viruses can cause similar lesions; although rare, dual virus infection does occur (Mulcahy & Fryer, 1976).

Histopathology should be supported by at least immunological confirmation, when possible. Virus-infected cells can be immunologically identified in histological sections or tissue smears from target organs or blood (Yamamoto et al., 1989). IHNV is a relatively weak immunogen. However, there is little antigenic variation among various isolates, making serological identification of the virus relatively simple.

SUBCLINICAL CARRIERS OF IHN

Adult carriers are asymptomatic. In female carriers the most sensitive tissues for virus isolation are ovarian fluid, gills, pyloric ceca, and kidney. Postspawning examination of a carrier's ovarian fluid is best, since no virus may be detectable for as little as 2 weeks before spawning. In spawning males, kidney and spleen are best. Sperm strongly adsorbs IHNV (Mulcahy & Pascho, 1984) but appears to be inactivated by yolk components, reducing the chance of vertical transmission (Yoshimizu et al., 1989).

Treatment

Disinfection and quarantine is the only proven means of controlling IHN epidemics. Extreme caution should be taken to avoid spreading virus to uncontaminated areas, both within and outside the hatchery. Aside from epidemics, the principal risk of IHNV infection is infected broodstock. Carriers that survive an outbreak do not shed virus until immediately before and after spawning.

Avoidance is the most useful prophylactic measure. Use of specific pathogen-free water (i.e., spring, well, or disinfected surface water) can be used for rearing susceptibles (Wedemeyer et al., 1979). However, a high percentage of many salmonid stocks carry latent IHNV infections, making avoidance of the virus virtually impossible in many cases, especially when propagating feral salmonids. Infection incidence among various feral American Pacific salmon stocks ranges from 5% to 94% (Grischkowsky & Amend, 1976). Infection incidence is higher in females than males.

Infection incidence can be reduced with broodstock culling (Mulcahy, 1983), where eggs and ovarian fluid of individuals or small groups (three to five fish) of females

are sampled for virus. Each group's eggs are maintained under quarantine until virus status is determined. While males have a much lower incidence of infection, it is also advisable to screen them, as well. Infected lots are destroyed and only virus-negative progeny are combined for rearing. While it is labor intensive and does not totally eliminate the virus, this procedure can dramatically reduce the incidence of viral infection and subsequently greatly increase fish yield (Mulcahy, 1983).

Elevating the temperature over 15° C (59° F) can stop epidemics but is only effective for some strains (Mulcahy et al., 1984). For example, the Buhl, Idaho, strain of IHNV is resistant to high temperature. Elevated temperature is also much less effective in fish that show clinical signs and does not eliminate the carrier state. Elevating temperature is only practical for small volumes of water (eggs or fry). A recombinant subunit vaccine is nearing commercialization (Leong et al., 1993).

The IHN virus can survive well in frozen viscera. Virus can remain infectious in water for months (Toranzo & Hetrick, 1982). It is less stable in brackish or seawater compared to freshwater. The virus is readily inactivated by 25 ppm iodine for 5 minutes (Amend & Pietsch, 1972). Treating eggs with iodophore will greatly reduce the chance of vertical transmission, but there have been cases where this treatment did not eliminate IHNV (Wolf, 1988).

Ectoparasites (e.g., leeches) and insects are considered potential reservoirs for the virus (Mulcahy et al., 1990). Exposure to copper (Hetrick et al., 1979) or other stressors increases susceptibility.

PROBLEM 77
Viral Hemorrhagic Septicemia (VHS, EGTVED Disease)

Prevalence Index
CF - 2
Method of Diagnosis
Culture of VHS virus from fish displaying typical clinical signs
History
Acute to chronic morbidity/mortality
Physical Examination
Neurological signs: lethargy; darkening; exophthalmos; swollen abdomen; hemorrhage
Treatment
Disinfect and quarantine

COMMENTS
Epidemiology
Viral hemorrhagic septicemia is a major cause of mortality in salmonids in freshwater. It is primarily a disease of rainbow trout and brown trout. Other naturally susceptible species include grayling, whitefishes, and northern

pike. Atlantic salmon, brook trout, golden trout, giebel, European sea bass, and turbot are experimentally susceptible (Wolf, 1988). Previously confined to Europe, it has recently been isolated from asymptomatic steelhead trout, coho and chinook salmon, and Pacific cod in Puget Sound and the Gulf of Alaska.

During VHS epidemics, any age fish can become clinically ill, but young fish are most severely affected. Prodromal period is usually 1 to 2 weeks but may be 3 to 4 weeks at low (e.g., 2° C [36° F]) temperatures (Yasutake & Rasmussen, 1968). Epidemics occur at 3° to 12° C (37° to 54° F), with highest mortalities at about 8° to 10° C (46° F to 50° F). Outbreaks rarely occur above 15° C (59° F).

During epidemics, virus is readily transmitted horizontally by water-borne transmission; virus is shed in the urine and possibly from the gills but not from the feces. Ingestion of virus does not appear to be a route of transmission in salmonids, but pike can contract the infection from feeding (Wolf, 1988). Survivors can become carriers, shedding virus in urine or sex products, but virus is not consistently detectable in carriers until they are sexually mature. The surface of eggs released by latent carriers can carry virus, but it is lost within hours; thus, vertical transmission has not been demonstrated. Shedding only occurs in winter, when temperatures are low (Vestergard Jorgensen, 1982). Low temperature appears necessary to transfer the virus from one generation to the next (Wolf, 1988).

Wild strains vary in virulence. VHSV is serologically distinct from other rhabdoviruses, but there are three major serotypes, which only weakly cross-react. Polyvalent antiserum is needed for serological confirmation.

Clinical Signs/Pathology
GROSS LESIONS

The range of gross lesions seen with VHS is great. There are three phases to VHS outbreaks, which reflect the severity of infection, not the chronological stages. The **acute** phase involves high mortality. Fish are dark and lethargic (congregate away from the current on the edges of the pond or raceway, eventually massing near the outlet screen), with reddening at the base of the fins and gills caused by injection of vessels and punctate hemorrhage. There is also hemorrhage in the abdominal cavity and a leucopenia.

In the **chronic** phase there is moderate, protracted mortality. Fish are black, with anemia, exophthalmos, and a swollen abdomen. The organs are pale, with organizing hemorrhages. In the **nervous** phase, there are low mortalities. Fish exhibit a looping swimming behavior, darting through the water and spiraling at the bottom of the pond.

HISTOPATHOLOGY

While hemorrhage is a feature of VHS, degeneration and necrosis are the most common findings. Kidney is the prime target, with mostly damage to hematopoietic tissue.

Liver necrosis and degeneration (vacuolation) is common. There is anemia, leukopenia, and thrombocytopenia.

In the acute phase there is focal hemorrhage, necrosis, and lymphocytic inflammation in all tissues, especially well-vascularized organs, such as spleen and kidney. Hemorrhage may be occasionally seen in skeletal muscle. In the chronic phase there is heavy hemosiderin deposition in melanomacrophages because of the anemia. There is also focal hyperplasia and degeneration of hematopoietic tissue; lesions that resemble membranous glomerulonephritis of mammals are also present. Exophthalmos is due to choroidal retrobulbar hemorrhage.

Diagnosis
CLINICAL VHS

Definitive diagnosis of clinical VHS requires isolation of virus from target tissues with appropriate clinical signs and history in susceptible species. Note that there may be few clinical signs or histopathological changes in fish over 6 months old. Kidney and spleen have the highest titers in the acute or chronic phase. Brain should also be sampled in fish in the convalescent stage. The VHS virus is stable for months in frozen viscera and tissue samples can be stored before processing.

Presumptive diagnosis of clinical VHS is based on the presence of typical clinical signs and pathology in susceptible species kept at low temperature. Major differentials include other salmonid viral infections, including IHN (see PROBLEM 76), IPN (see PROBLEM 75), and HVS (see PROBLEM 78). Until recently, the restriction of VHS to Europe and absence of IHN and HVS from Europe made IPN the primary differential in Pacific coast salmonids. However, VHS must now be seriously considered as a possible differential in fish from the Pacific Northwest of the United States, although clinical disease from VHS has not yet been reported in this area.

Especially diagnostic features include relative lack of pancreatic damage (compared with IHN or IPN), relatively normal intestine and gills, and lack of damage to eosinophilic granular cells of stratum compactum (compared with IHN). Clinical signs and pathology are similar in salmonid and nonsalmonid hosts.

When possible, histopathology should be supported by at least immunological confirmation, with submission of samples to a qualified reference laboratory. Note that VHS may be complicated by concurrent infections of IPN or bacterial infections, which can confound the clinical presentation.

SUBCLINICAL CARRIERS OF VHS

In carriers the most senitive tissue for isolation is ovarian fluid, then pyloric ceca, then kidney. The brain should also be sampled. Postspawning examination of a carrier's ovarian fluid is best.

Treatment

Disinfection and quarantine is the most effective means of controlling VHS epidemics. VHSV is stable in water (over 1 week at 14° C [57° F]) and survives drying for up to 1 week at 4° C (39° F). There is no evidence for transmission by parasite vectors, but fish-eating birds can carry infected fish to other farms. The virus does not survive in the gut of homeotherms because of the low pH and high temperature.

Obtaining fish from certified VHS-free stock is the surest method of avoiding the disease. Iodophore treatment will readily eliminate the virus from eggs of carriers, making it reasonably certain that the progeny will be free of VHS. Fish at risk because of environmental contamination should be raised in virus-free water (e.g., spring, well, or disinfected [Maisse et al., 1980]). The ability of VHS to cause disease in any age fish makes it a serious threat to salmonid culture and possibly other susceptible species. Because of the potentially devastating nature of this disease to North American salmonid stocks and its recent discovery off the coast of the United States, all suspect cases of VHS in the United States or Canada should be reported immediately to regional fish health authorities. The virus has been successfully eradicated from some parts of Europe (Vestergard Jorgensen, 1974).

PROBLEM 78
Miscellaneous Systemic Viral Infections
Prevalence Index: See specific agents

Method of Diagnosis
Rule-out of other problems combined with the following:
1. Culture of specific virus from typical lesions
2. Morphological identification of virus with typical histopathology

History
Variable; acute to chronic morbidity/mortality

Physical Examination
Varies with target organ(s)

Treatment
1. Disinfect and quarantine
2. Prophylactic therapies for secondary invaders

COMMENTS
Clinically important diseases (e.g., Fig. II-78, *A* through *C*) are defined as those that have consistently been responsible for morbidity or mortality in wild or cultured fish. Not included in the group of clinically important diseases are viruses that have caused disease but have only been observed or isolated once or twice or are agents that have not been shown to cause any clinically obvious sickness in naturally infected fish (even if histopathological lesions can be seen in infected fish).

Note that for some important *diseases*, there is little evidence that the virus(es) isolated from affected fish is(are) responsible for that disease (e.g., EUS).

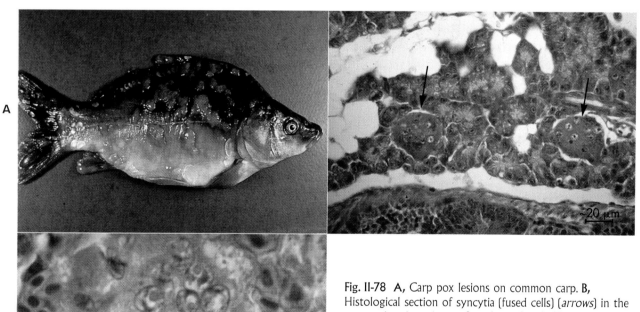

Fig. II-78 **A,** Carp pox lesions on common carp. **B,** Histological section of syncytia (fused cells) (*arrows*) in the pancreatic acinar tissue of a salmonid with *Herpesvirus salmonis.* Hematoxylin and eosin. **C,** Intranuclear, Cowdry type A inclusions (*arrows*) in pancreatic cells infected with *Herpesvirus salmonis.* Hematoxylin and eosin.

(*A, B,* and *C* photographs courtesy of National Fish Health Research Laboratory, USA.)

Table II-78 Miscellaneous systemic viral infections of fish.

Disease/pathogen	Hosts	Geographic range	Morbidity/mortality; significance	Diagnostic features	References
Sturgeon wasting disease* (adenovirus-like)	White sturgeon	Sacramento River, California, USA	Chronic 1	Enlarged nuclei in intestinal and spiral valve epithelium; epithelial cells eventually rupture	Hedrick et al, 1985b
Eel rhabdoviruses (eel virus European X, eel virus American)	American eel (H); European eel (H); rainbow trout (E)	Japan; France; Cuba	None 2	Hemorrhage and necrosis of viscera; isolated from all ages of eels; clinical disease not yet proven experimentally for eels	Sano, 1976 Wolf, 1988
EV-102 (iridovirus, ICDV, icosahedral, cytoplasmic, deoxyribovirus)	Japanese eel (E)	Japan	Acute 1	Only isolated once; pathogenic to young eels: congested fins, increased mucus production; highest mortality at lower temperature (<24° C)	Sorimachi, 1984 Sorimachi & Egusa, 1987
Eel birnaviruses* (eel virus European, branchionephritis, eel virus kidney disease)	Japanese eel	Japan; Taiwan	Acute 1	IPN-like (see *PROBLEM 75*)	Sano & Fukuda, 1987
Rainbow smelt picornavirus	Rainbow smelt	New Brunswick, Canada	Acute 2	Isolated from sick fish but not yet proven pathogenic	Moore et al, 1988
Pike fry rhabdovirus disease* (hydrocephalus, red disease of pike, grass carp rhabdovirus)	Northern pike; brown trout; grass carp; white bream; gudgeon; tench	Europe	Subacute-to-acute 1	Spontaneous disease only in young pike; two syndromes: (1) swelling on skull (hydrocephalus) or (2) hemorrhagic mass between pelvic fins and hemorrhage on flanks; hemorrhagic necrosis of viscera	Ahne, 1985
Herpesvirus salmonis* disease	Atlantic salmon (E); brook (E), brown (E), and rainbow trout; chum salmon (E); chinook salmon (E)	Washington, USA; California, USA	Subacute /chronic 1	Natural disease only in young rainbow trout at <10° C; exophthalmos, swollen abdomen; thick, white fecal casts; pale viscera; kidney is primary target (hematopoietic hyperplasia); **pathognomonic:** syncytia in pancreas (Fig. II-78, *B* and *C*) (not always present); little or no pancreatic necrosis (ddx from IPN, IHN, VHS)	Eaton et al, 1989 Wolf & Smith, 1981
Landlocked salmon virus disease	Masu salmon	Taiwan	Acute 1	None described	Hsu et al, 1989
Focal necrotizing hepatitis (reovirus)	Masu, chum (I, H), kokanee (I), and chinook (I) salmon; rainbow trout (E)	Japan	None 3	No clinical disease; some focal hepatic necrosis	Winton et al, 1981
Rhabdoviral salmonid hepatitis	Rainbow trout	Ukraine	2	Hyperactivity; splenomegaly; hepatitis	Osadchaya, 1981
Chinook salmon paramyxovirus	Chinook salmon (H)	Oregon, USA	None 3	No clinical disease	Winton et al, 1985
Epizootic epitheliotropic disease (EED)* (herpesvirus-like)	Lake trout; lake trout × brook trout	Great Lakes; USA	Acute 1	Sporadic flashing; corkscrew swimming; grey to white, mucoid foci on skin and fins; hyphema; splenomegaly; elevated hematocrit	Bradley et al, 1989

Virus	Host	Location	Clinical form / level	Signs and comments	Reference
Atlantic salmon picorna-like virus	Atlantic salmon	Washington	Chronic 3	Mild hematopoietic necrosis; focal hepatitis; only isolated once	McDowell et al., 1989
Picorna-like virus of salmonids	Brook, brown, rainbow and cutthroat trout; kokanee salmon (E)	California	None 2	No clinical disease except in experimentally infected kokanee salmon	Hedrick et al., 1991
Oncorhynchus masu virus* (OMV herpesvirus)	Masu, coho, chum, kokanee salmon; rainbow trout	Japan	Acute/chronic 1	Serious problem; to 100% mortality in fry (exophthalmos, petechiation); up to 60% of survivors develop epithelial tumors on mouth; Yamame tumor virus (YTV) causes similar disease	Kimura et al., 1981; Sano et al., 1983
Nerka virus in Towada Lake, Akita (NeVTA herpesvirus)	Kokanee, chum (E), pink (E), yamame (E) salmon; rainbow trout (E)	Japan	Acute 1	Mortality in fry; dark; anorexia; depression; secondary water mold infection	Sano, 1976
Salmon leukemia virus* (SLV retrovirus)	Chinook salmon; sockeye salmon (E); Atlantic salmon(E)	British Columbia, Canada; California, USA	Chronic 1	Sea-cultured fish, usually after 1 year at sea; infiltration/proliferation of immature plasma cells into viscera and retrobulbar tissue; anemia; exophthalmos; grossly resembles BKD (see *PROBLEM 52*); often follows BKD epidemics; avoid using progeny of fish with history of SLV (may be vertically transmitted)	Eaton & Kent, 1992; Kent, 1992
Golden shiner virus* (reovirus)	Golden shiner	USA	Chronic 1	Hemorrhage, especially in dorsal muscles, ventrum, eyes, visceral fat; most mortality in older fish	Plumb et al., 1979
Goldfish viruses 1 and 2 (GFV-1, GFV-2, iridovirus)	Goldfish	Massachusetts	None 3	Not associated with disease	Berry et al., 1983
Spring viremia of carp* (*Rhabdovirus carpio* infection, SVC; swim bladder inflammation, SBI)	Common, bighead, crucian and grass carp; sheatfish; guppy (E); northern pike (E)	Great Britain; Europe; Russia; Middle East	Acute 1	Acute mortalities in spring and early summer; decreased swimming ability; dark skin; hemorrhages on skin, vent, gills; peritonitis; enteritis; inflammatory exudate and hemorrhage in muscle and viscera, especially swim bladder; transmitted by *Argulus* (see *PROBLEM 14*) and leeches (see *PROBLEM 12*); secondary bacterial infections, especially with *Aeromonas hydrophila*, are common; SVC comprises the acute form of the syndrome *Infectious Dropsy of Carp*; see *PROBLEM 46* for a discussion of this syndrome; do not confuse this disease with myxozoan-induced swim bladder inflammation caused by *Sphaerospora renicola* (see *PROBLEM 65*)	Fijan, 1972

Continued.

Table II-78 Miscellaneous systemic viral infections of fish, cont'd.

Disease/pathogen	Hosts	Geographic range	Morbidity/mortality; significance	Diagnostic features	References
Rosy barb virus (birna-like virus)	Rosy barb	Singapore; Australia	Acute 3	Visceral necrosis; only seen once	Langdon, 1992b
Grass carp reovirus* disease (hemorrhagic virus of grass carp)	Grass carp; black carp; chebachek	China	Acute 1	Exophthalmos; hemorrhage in gills, mouth, fins, viscera; disease at 25° to 30° C; most severe in young fish; may be related to golden shiner virus	Nie & Pan, 1985 Chen et al., 1985
Grass carp virus CIVH 33/86	Grass carp	Hungary	None 3	No clinical disease	Ahne et al., 1987
Carp pox* (Herpesvirus cyprini disease, carp epithelioma)	Common carp; Crucian carp; barbel; bream; golden ide; rudd; smelt; carp × goldfish; aquarium fish	Europe; Asia; Russia; Great Lakes, USA; Israel	Acute/chronic 1	Smooth to rough, milky white-to-grey plaques up to 2 mm thick; may cause scarring, retard growth, lead to skeletal deformities; hyperplastic epithelium (may be papillomatous) intracytoplasmic and intranuclear (Cowdry type A) inclusions; plaques up to several cm along longest dimension; lesions eventually slough but can last for months; lesions may become dark pigmented, reducing value; lesions develop in low temperatures (winter/spring) and regress with high temperature (summer); transmission probably from wounds; acute disease in young fish; experimentally virulent in carp fry (Fig. II-78, A)	Sonstegard & Sonstegard, 1978 Wolf, 1988 Sano et al., 1990
Catfish reovirus	Channel catfish	California, USA	Chronic 3	Associated with gill lamellar hyperplasia and fusion; low mortality in naturally infected fish	Amend et al., 1984
Epizootic hematopoietic necrosis* (perch iridovirus, Nillahcootie redfin virus)	Redfin perch; rainbow trout (E); Atlantic salmon (E); native Australian fishes	Australia	Acute 1	Neurological signs; skin ulcers; hemorrhage; multifocal to diffuse necrosis in viscera, especially kidney, spleen, liver; high mortality in both juvenile and adult perch; basophilic to amphophilic intracytoplasmic inclusions in hepatocytes; virus persistent in environment; redfin can be carriers; virus possibly cycles through insects or amphibians; trout have low mortality but high morbidity in summer/fall; perch kills in late spring/summer	Langdon et al., 1988 Langdon, 1992b
Perch rhabdovirus infection	Eurasian perch; northern pike (E)	France	Chronic 1	Neurological signs, exophthalmos; only isolated once	Dorson et al., 1987
Bluegill virus infection	Bluegill	West Virginia and Kentucky, USA	None 3	No clinical disease	Wolf, 1988

Disease (agent)	Fish	Location	Course	Signs	Reference
13p2 Reovirus infection (bluegill hepatic necrosis reovirus)	Bluegill (E); golden shiner (E); rainbow trout (E)	Long Island Sound, New York, USA	Subacute 2	Only naturally isolated from oysters; clinical disease only in bluegill fry; focal necrotic hepatitis that can be lethal	Meyers, 1983
Ramirez's dwarf cichlid virus disease	Ramirez's dwarf cichlid	Uncertain (South America?)	Chronic 4	Dyspnea; neurological signs, hemorrhage in eyes, skin; focal necrosis of viscera; splenomegaly; eosinophilic inclusions in splenocytes; to 80% mortality after 4 weeks	Leibovitz & Riis, 1980
Rio Grande cichlid rhabdovirus disease	Rio Grande cichlid; convict cichlid; zilli cichlid	Uncertain (Florida, Mexico?)	Acute 1	Lethargy	Malsberger & Lautenslager, 1980
Deep angelfish disease (herpesvirus-like)	Deep angelfish	Uncertain (Amazon basin?)	Acute 4	Loss of equilibrium; headstanding; hemorrhage on surface; only seen once	Mellergaard & Block, 1988
Chromide cichlid anemia (iridovirus-like)	Chromide cichlid	Uncertain (Malaysia?)	Acute 4	Pale; weak; cachexic; ballooned cells with virus particles in renal hematopoietic tissue and other organs	Armstrong & Ferguson, 1989
Striped bass reo-like virus	Striped bass	Potomac River, Maryland, USA	3	Large hemorrhages along flanks and on swim bladder; "membranous" material connects liver to body wall; only isolated once	Baya et al, 1990b
Vacuolating encephalopathy* of sea bass (picorna-like virus)	Australian sea bass	Malaysia; Singapore; Indonesia; Thailand; Tahiti; Australia; Philippines	Acute 4	High mortality in 9- to 30-day-old fry; nervous signs; extensive vacuolation of brain grey matter, especially optic tectum and cerebellum; also other parts of brain and spinal cord; older fry may infect younger fish	Glazebrook et al, 1990
Tiger puffer virus* (kuchijiro-sho = white mouth disease)	Tiger puffer	Japan	1	Ulcers on mouth and snout; viral particles in brain; epidemics May through June (18° to 22° C)	Wada et al, 1986
MHLLE-associated virus*	Semicirculatus angelfish	Uncertain	Chronic 3	Isolated from fish with MHLLE (see PROBLEM 90); little evidence for viral involvement	
Turbot reovirus	Turbot	Spain	Chronic 3	Co-isolated with Vibrio	Lupiani et al, 1989
Turbot epithelial cell* gigantism (herpesvirus scophthalmi infection)	Turbot	Scotland	Acute or chronic 4	Hypertrophic (fused) epithelial cells in gills and skin	Richards & Buchanan, 1978

Continued.

Table II-78 Miscellaneous systemic viral infections of fish, cont'd

Disease/pathogen	Hosts	Geographic range	Morbidity/mortality; significance	Diagnostic features	References
Japanese flounder, rhabdovirus disease* (*Rhabdovirus olivaceus*; hirame rhabdovirus)	Japanese flounder; ayu; rainbow trout and other salmonids (E); black sea bream; red sea bream; black rockfish; red spotted grouper; spotbelly greenling; yellowfin goby; sunrise sculpin	Japan	Acute 1	Ascites; focal hemorrhage of muscles, fins, and viscera; exophthalmos; hematopoetic necrosis; highest mortality at low (< 5° C) temperature (keep temperature > 15° C)	Oseko et al, 1988 Kimura & Yoshimizu, 1991
Epidermal hyperplasia/necrosis*	Japanese flounder	Japan	4	Larvae and juveniles affected with opaque fins caused by epidermal hyperplasia; may be epidermal necrosis or ascites; disease at 18° to 20° C	Iida et al, 1989
Epidermal necrosis*	Fox jacopever	Japan	4	Larvae with necrotic epidermis having herpes-like particles	Kimura & Yoshimizu, 1991
Epithelial necrosis*	Schlegeli black sea bream	Japan	4	Larvae with rounded, necrotic epithelial cells of skin, mouth, gill and intestine; intracytoplasmic, enveloped virions	Miyazaki et al, 1989
Viral nervous necrosis* (picorna-like virus)	Japanese parrotfish; red-spotted grouper; striped jack	Japan	Acute 4	Larvae and juveniles with necrosis of CNS and ganglia; to 100% mortality in fish up to 40 mm; may be different viruses in different fish species	Yoshikoshi & Inoue, 1990 Langdon, 1992b
EUS viruses* (rhabdoviruses)	Striped snakehead; swamp eel	Southeast Asia	Acute/chronic 3	Virus isolated from viscera of fish with EUS (see *PROBLEM 34*); little evidence for viral cause	Frierichs et al, 1986

<u>Note</u>: Many viruses have been associated with various proliferative lesions, especially on the skin, but have not been proven to be the cause of these lesions. See *PROBLEM 72* for a discussion of the virus-associated lesions; see *PROBLEM 43* for virus-associated hemopathies.

* Clinically important diseases.

<u>Note</u>: A disease may be clinically important even if the virus isolated from the lesions has not proven to be clinically important in causing the disease.

1. Virus is a proven cause of disease in spontaneously affected fish (River's Postulates fulfilled).
2. Virus is proven to cause disease only in experimentally affected fish.
3. Virus has been isolated from fish but not yet proven to cause any disease.
4. Virus particles were seen in lesions of affected fish; virus has not yet been isolated.
H= In spontaneous cases, virus has been isolated only from clinically healthy individuals of this species.
E = Only shown to cause disease in experimentally challenged individuals of this species.
I = Fish can be experimentally infected with virus, but fish do not show clinical signs of disease (histopathological lesions may be present in some cases, but virus does not cause gross morbidity/mortality)

CHAPTER 19

Problems 79 through 88

Rule-out diagnoses: *Presumptive* diagnosis is based upon the absence of other etiologies combined with a diagnostically appropriate history, clinical signs, and/or pathology. *Definitive* diagnosis is based on presumptive evidence combined with further, more extensive work-up with a specific identification of the problem

79. Nutritional deficiency
80. Hypercarbia
81. Hydrogen sulfide poisoning
82. Chlorine/chloramine poisoning
83. Metal poisoning
84. Miscellaneous water-borne poisonings
85. Noxious algae
86. Environmental shock/delayed mortality syndrome
87. Traumatic lesions
88. Genetic anomalies

PROBLEM 79
Nutritional Deficiency

Prevalence Index

WF - 2, WM - 1, CF - 4, CM - 4

Method of Diagnosis

Rule-out of other problems combined with the following:

1. Measurement of specific low nutrient levels in feed and/or fish
2. History

History

Outdated or improperly stored feed; feeding a monotonous diet (i.e., single food item); not feeding often enough or enough food at one time; poor growth; chronic mortalities; depressed or otherwise abnormal behavior; cannot find food (blind)

Physical Examination

Varies with specific deficiency, but most common clinical signs include the following:

Skeletal abnormalities; cataracts or other ophthalmic lesions; hematopathologies (e.g., anemia)

Treatment

1. Adjust diet to requirements of that fish species (evaluate current dietary formulation)
2. Provide varied diet if appropriate

COMMENTS
General Nutritional Requirements of Fish

Fish are efficient feed converters, with many food fish species producing 1 kilogram of fish for every 1.6 kilograms of feed. Nutritional requirements of fish are similar to those of mammals, but there are some important differences.

PROTEIN

Protein provides a major source of energy for fish and subsequently fish require a higher percentage than warm-blooded animals (e.g., 30% to 36% for warm water fish vs 16% to 22% for poultry). Protein requirements vary with fish species and fish size (greater in small fish). While most fish use some plant protein (e.g., soybean meal), most fish also require a certain amount of animal protein. Carnivorous fish, such as salmonids, need more high-quality protein than omnivorous/herbivorous fish, such as tilapia.

ENERGY

The primary energy sources for fish are fats and proteins. Fish can digest simple sugars efficiently, but as the sugar molecule becomes large and more complex, digestibility decreases rapidly. For example, glucose is much more digestible than starch. This is especially true for cold water species (e.g., trout).

Adverse effects of high-energy diets include the following:

1. **Inadequate protein intake**: since fish eat to satisfy an energy requirement, a diet high in energy (in relation to the amount of protein present) will prevent fish from consuming enough protein for a maximal growth rate, even if fish are fed ad lib.
2. **Excess fat deposition**: reduces the dressing percentage (percent of live weight available after gutting), reduces the shelf life of frozen fish, and may cause pathological changes (fatty infiltration of liver), especially in salmonids.

Animal fats and highly saturated fats are poorly assimilated by fish. However, highly unsaturated fats, which

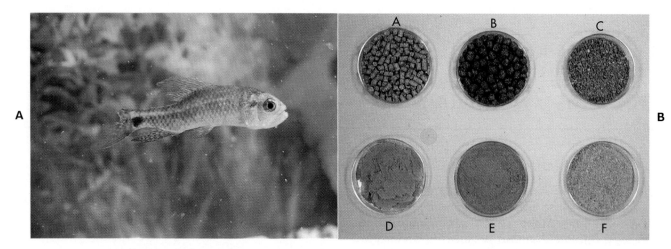

Fig. II-79 A, Chronic wasting in a killifish, as evidenced by the strongly concave abdomen. **B,** Major types of dry fish feeds: *A* = sinking pellet; *B* = floating (extruded) pellet; *C* = crumble; *D* = flake; *E* and *F* = mash.

[*A* photograph courtesy of T. Wenzel.]

are easily digested, are susceptible to auto-oxidation, resulting in feed spoilage. Thus, antioxidants are routinely added to fish diets. Vitamin E is the antioxidant of choice because of the often illegally high levels of synthetic antioxidants (e.g., butylated hydroxyanisol [BHA], ethoxyquin) that would be required and because it also prevents cellular auto-oxidation. Fish also have requirements for essential fatty acids (e.g., linolenic acid).

VITAMINS

Fifteen vitamins are essential for most fish, including vitamins A, D, E, K, thiamin, riboflavin, pyridoxine, pantothenic acid, niacin, folic acid, B_{12}, biotin, choline, ascorbic acid, and inositol. However, not all species require all 15 vitamins in the diet. Most commercial diets are overly fortified with vitamins because of the high levels of oxidizable fats in the diets that can result in their inactivation.

MINERALS

Fish probably require the same minerals as warm-blooded animals for various physiological functions. In addition, fish use inorganic ions to maintain osmotic balance between themselves and the external environment. It is important to note that minerals in the water can make significant contributions to a fish's dietary requirements. The availability and biological activity of aqueous minerals are highly dependent on the composition and properties of the chemical soup in which the fish swim. The presence of certain minerals influences the activity of others, all of which are influenced by temperature, pH, etc. Fish can meet much of their calcium requirements by absorbing it through the gills, provided that adequate calcium levels are present in the water. Conversely, most natural waters are low in dissolved phosphorus and thus dietary phosphorus is essential.

Growth can also be influenced by changing dietary levels of magnesium (Mg), potassium (K), copper (Cu),

iodine (I), selenium (Se), zinc (Zn), and iron (Fe). Goiter resulting from iodine deficiency has occurred in salmonids fed on all-meat diets. Fish feeds that are low in animal products may be deficient in trace minerals and thus may require supplementation.

Types of Feeds

While meal-type feeds can be used to feed some types of fish, feeds for most fish species must be in the form of large particles for them to be readily accepted by the fish. Thus feeds are processed to form pellets, extruded feeds, or flakes (Fig. II-79, *B*). Ninety days is the maximum storage time recommended for complete fish feed stored at ambient temperature; ascorbate is the most sensitive vitamin, although more heat-stable forms are now available.

Feeding Aquarium Fish

This group varies widely in their natural food habits and thus their nutritional requirements (i.e., herbivores, carnivores, insectivores, omnivores). Diet formulations for aquarium species have been based mainly on the nutritional requirements of warm water food fish. Aquarium feeds also contain carotenoids and similar compounds to enhance pigmentation.

Fortunately, most freshwater aquarium fish do well on a good brand of flake or pelleted feed as the staple. Flaked feeds are most commonly used, since diets with a hard texture or which sink rapidly may be poorly consumed (Lovell, 1980), especially by small fish. Dry diets should be used within 3 months of manufacture if they are stored at ambient temperature because vitamins may decay considerably by this time. Unfortunately, many companies that manufacture aquarium feeds do not place an expiration date or date of manufacture on their products. Flake or pellet feed should always be supplemented with other food items, such as various live or frozen products.

Live or frozen foods that are good supplements include larval ("baby") and adult brine shrimp (*Artemia salina*), microworms (a nematode), water fleas (*Daphnia* spp.), krill, and earthworms. Tubificid worms are also a good nutritional source but are collected from organically polluted water and thus may harbor pathogens or toxins. Live fish are an excellent source of nutrients for carnivorous fish but may also transmit many diseases; parasites, mycobacteriosis, and other bacterial diseases are usually the most serious problems. Frozen whole fish are safer to feed but may not be as well accepted by the fish. Note that many bacterial pathogens (e.g., *Mycobacterium*) are not killed by freezing.

The natural diets of marine reef fish are highly specialized and may not be satisfied by foods that are available in captivity. Owners should be aware of the natural food habits of potential pets, since this is a useful predictor of success in captivity. See Bower (1983) for marine species that do well in captivity. It is essential to provide a highly varied diet with emphasis on live or frozen preparations.

Feeding Larval Fish

In addition to the other important properties of practical diets already mentioned, diets for larval fish must also have the proper density to remain suspended by water currents to facilitate consumption by the fish. While fish with large yolk supplies, such as trout and channel catfish, can assimilate a wide range of nutrient sources, including artificial diets, immediately after absorption of the yolk sac, many other fish must begin feeding before their digestive system is well developed.

Many marine species begin feeding when they are a small size. There is at present no artificial feed that will completely replace live food for these individuals; this presents a number of problems:

1. There are trouble and expense involved in obtaining live food.
2. Some species require completely different types of food as they become older, requiring that a number of different live foods be available.
3. If the live food required cannot be cultured or for some other reason must be collected in the wild, there is the added danger of introducing pathogens along with the food, as well as introducing potential predators, such as aquatic insects (see *PROBLEM 87*); the live food most commonly used in raising larval fish is larvae of the brine shrimp (*Artemia salina*), but this is too large for some species that must be fed smaller food items such as rotifers.

There is evidence that inadequate hormone levels may lead to some developmental anomalies. For example, striped bass larvae often have a high incidence of failure to inflate the swim bladder. Treating prespawning female striped bass with thyroid hormone increased the incidence of normal swim bladder inflation and larval survival (Brown et al., 1988).

Young fish should be fed often. Some species need to have food constantly present to survive the early stages of life. The amount of food provided must also be constantly increased as the fish grow, requiring more total feed. But avoid overfeeding, which causes environmental problems.

Effect of Culture System on Nutritional Requirements

Fish in ponds are less at risk for nutritional problems if there is a sufficient amount of natural food in the pond. Thus, fish in *farm ponds*, which are relatively low density, rarely exhibit nutritional problems. However, commercial food fish ponds typically raise fish at high density, placing them at risk for nutritional disease. Many goldfish and koi ponds, especially those having filtration or aeration to allow greater fish densities, have little natural food available. Fish in raceways or cages have little access to natural food items and thus are totally reliant on the prepared diet for their nutritional needs (Hepher, 1988). Typical hobbyist aquaria also have little natural food items, although some hobbyists often encourage the growth of algae and invertebrate feed items.

Feeding Food Fish

Feeding fish, as in other animal agriculture industries, constitutes a major expense to the farmer. Up to 70% of the fish farmer's total costs are for feed. Fish culturists also face two problems unique among farmers: first, uneaten food quickly deteriorates in the water and makes relatively little contribution to fish production; second, uneaten food also contaminates the environment and may be detrimental to the fish's health (see *PROBLEM 4*). Feeding techniques are affected by a number of factors, including the following:

Physical factors: Rate of water exchange, type of rearing facility (e.g., pond, raceway), and size of fish will all influence feeding practices.

Temperature: All fish species have a temperature range at which optimum feed conversion is obtained. This occurs around 30° C (86° F) for warm water fish; below about 12° C (54° F) feeding is erratic. Thus warm water fish, such as catfish, are fed daily only when the temperature is above 12° C.

Water quality: Because of the intimate interrelationship between the aquatic environment and fish's metabolism, feeding practices must be used within the constraints that this relationship imposes. In warm water culture, dissolved oxygen (DO) levels in ponds that have heavy plant growth are related to photosynthetic activity, with the lowest DO levels in the early morning just before photosynthesis resumes. Thus feeding should be done after DO levels have risen. Feeding should not be done in late evening because DO begins to drop again and the nutrients in the feed simulate oxygen consumption (see *PROBLEM 1*).

DIETS FOR VARIOUS FOOD FISH SPECIES

Nutritional requirements for well-established food fish species, such as channel catfish, salmonids, carp, and

Japanese eel (among others) are well defined, and thus, nutritional problems in these species usually result from improper feed handling and/or storage or occasionally from improper formulation at the feed mill.

For many other food fish species, nutritional requirements are less defined, which may be responsible for many problems encountered in propagating these species. Lovell (1989), National Research Council (1981, 1983), Steffens (1989), Tacon (1992), and Wilson (1992) should be consulted for specific nutritional requirements for various fish species.

Food-Borne Toxins

Many food-borne toxins have been experimentally induced in fish. These are summarized by Tacon (1992). A few have caused disease in clinical situations. Trout are extremely sensitive to aflatoxins, associated with moldy feeds, and develop hepatomas when levels as low as one part per billion are fed for several months (Lovell, 1989). Unsaturated fatty acids, such as those found in fish oils, are readily oxidized, becoming rancid. Salmonids fed such rancid fats can develop lipoid liver disease, characterized by fatty infiltration of the liver and severe anemia (Tacon, 1992).

Antinutrients, such as thiaminase, are present in many aquatic animal tissues and can cause vitamin deficiencies if fed raw to fish. Many other food products, especially plant products, have other types of antinutrients (Tacon, 1992).

Some manufacturers reportedly add testosterone to their commercial aquarium feeds, since this enhances the color of many fish by stimulating breeding coloration. However, testosterone can have a major influence on sexual development. Exposure to high testosterone levels may cause sex reversal (from female to male) or sterility of some fish.

Taints

Muddy or earthy tastes in fillets are a serious problem in pond-cultured fish, especially channel catfish in the United States (Tacon, 1992). These taints are caused by soil bacteria (actinomycetes) or some cyanobacteria. Industrial wastes associated with taints include domestic sewage, phenols, or petroleum products (see PROBLEM 84).

Diagnosis of Nutritional Deficiency

Presumptive diagnosis of nutritional deficiency is based on compatible clinical signs, combined with evidence of an inadequate diet. Obviously, the diagnosis is much easier to make for species where the nutritional requirements are known. Unfortunately, deficiencies are most common in species with undetermined requirements. Definitive diagnosis requires identification of a specific nutritional deficiency in the diet.

Clinical signs of inadequate nutrition are most likely to be seen in young, rapidly growing fish that typically have the highest requirements for many nutrients. The most obvious sign of poor nutrition is starvation (Fig.

Table II-79   Characteristics of various types of fish feeds.

	Stability in water	Cost	Nutritional adequacy*
Flake	Excellent	Moderate	Moderate
Pellet	Poor to excellent*	Low	High
Freeze-dried	Good to excellent	Moderate to high	Moderate
Frozen	Poor	High	High
Live	Excellent	High	Highest

*Varies greatly with manufacturing process and commercial brand.

II-79, A). A number of pathological changes have been induced in fish by specific nutrient deficiencies; the most common clinical signs are vertebral anomalies (scoliosis or lordosis), cataract, exophthalmos, fin erosion, fatty liver, and skin hemorrhage (Tacon, 1992; Roberts & Bullock, 1989; Ghittino, 1989). Other common lesions are anemia and gill hyperplasia. All of these lesions are nonspecific.

Many of these lesions also occur with genetic defects (see PROBLEM 88) and have also been associated with a generally *poor environment* or husbandry.

Besides direct pathological changes, there is evidence that inadequate nutrition can increase susceptibility to disease, especially when fish are stressed (Blazer et al., 1989; Landolt, 1989). Furthermore, stress may increase vitamin requirements (Tacon, 1992). Vitamin E and C appear to play important roles.

Treatment of Nutritional Deficiency

Unless the case involves possible litigation (such as because of negligent feed preparation), a definitive diagnosis is almost never sought. Instead, the client is advised to obtain fresh feed or change the diet. Where nutritional requirements are uncertain (e.g., aquarium fish), it is important to provide a varied diet.

PROBLEM 80
Hypercarbia

Prevalence Index
CF - 3

Method of Diagnosis
Rule-out of other problems combined with the measurement of aqueous CO_2 concentration > 12 mg/l

History
Overcrowded system; use of liquid oxygen; poorly buffered ground water

Physical Examination
Dyspnea; chronic inflammation in kidneys and epaxial muscles

Treatment
1. Increase aeration
2. Decrease density
3. Run water through a packed column degasser
4. Add slaked lime (ponds only)

COMMENTS

Causes

Carbon dioxide (CO_2) is very soluble in water and levels can far exceed the atmospheric concentration. Hypercarbia can occur when using ground water, which may be low in pH and high in CO_2 (up to 100 mg/l may occur). Elevated CO_2 may also develop when using liquid oxygen, which allows a higher stocking density in raceways. The CO_2 concentration in ponds varies diurnally in parallel with pH, usually ranging from 0 mg/l in the late afternoon to 5 to 10 mg/l at daybreak (see Fig. II-1, *D*). Although CO_2 may exceed 10 mg/l in highly eutrophic ponds, diurnal hypercarbia peaks do not appear to be a problem. However, hypercarbia may exacerbate environmental hypoxia (see *PROBLEM 1*), and carbon dioxide is often much higher after a phytoplankton die-off.

Pathogenesis

Increased aqueous CO_2 inhibits diffusion of CO_2 out of the blood. High blood CO_2 reduces blood pH, which reduces hemoglobin's affinity for oxygen (Bohr effect). CO_2 also directly decreases the amount of oxygen that can be loaded by hemoglobin (Root effect). The net effect is reducing the amount of oxygen that can be transported to tissues. In salmonids, chronically elevated CO_2 has been associated with nephrocalcinosis and systemic granuloma, a multifocal deposition of chalky, white mineral in the stomach, kidney, and epaxial muscles (see *PROBLEM 92*).

Diagnosis

In a flow-through system, carbon dioxide is lowest at the inflow and highest at the outflow. In a pond, CO_2 is highest near the bottom of the pond. If samples are submitted to a reference laboratory for analysis, sample bottles must be filled completely to exclude air, kept below the temperature at which the water was collected (to prevent escape of CO_2), and analyzed within 2 hours of collection.

Treatment

Some fish can adapt to elevated CO_2 levels, but this adaptation must be gradual. There is also the risk of the fish developing nephrocalcinosis, at least in salmonids. Treating water with a buffer to increase the pH can also reduce dissolved CO_2. Above pH 8.34, free CO_2 is not present (see Fig. II-6).

Up to 10 to 12 mg/l of free CO_2 is usually tolerated if O_2 is high. Some fish can survive exposure to up to 60 mg/l (Hart, 1944), which approaches narcotic levels (see *PHARMACOPOEIA*). If the CO_2 concentration in a pond exceeds 10 to 15 mg/l (e.g., after an algae die-off) it may be advisable to remove the excess CO_2 with slaked lime. Vigorous aeration also removes CO_2 from ponds (Ver & Chiu, 1986). Aeration will reduce CO_2 levels in flow-through systems and is optimized by providing maximum surface area, such as through a packed column degasser (Aquatic Ecosystems, Inc.) that is used to eliminate gas supersaturation.

PROBLEM 81
Hydrogen Sulfide Poisoning

Prevalence Index

WF - 4, WM - 2, CF - 4, CM - 2

Method of Diagnosis

Rule-out of other problems combined with the following:

1. Chemical measurement of hydrogen sulfide in water
2. History

History/Physical Examination

Acute to chronic stress response

Treatment

1. Aerate water
2. Raise pH
3. Lower temperature
4. Add potassium permanganate (freshwater only)

COMMENTS

Epidemiology/Pathogenesis

Hydrogen sulfide (H_2S) forms from the reduction of sulfate ion under anaerobic conditions. It is more of a problem in brackish water or marine systems, where there is a large amount of sulfate that can be reduced to sulfide. It can form on pond bottoms that become anaerobic because of high concentrations of organic matter combined with high metabolism (i.e., especially summer). Disturbing the bottom (e.g., seining) can release the toxin from the mud. It is also a problem in marine aquaria if anaerobic areas develop under rocks or if filter beds are not totally aerated. Some coastal aquifers also have high concentrations of H_2S. Paper mills and tanneries are also sources of H_2S. Hydrogen sulfide's main toxic action seems to be interference with respiration, causing hypoxia (Schwedler et al., 1985).

Diagnosis

Concentrations between 0.5 to 10 mg/l can cause acute mortality (Langdon, 1988). Greater than 0.006 mg/l is toxic to some species; thus, any levels detectable with commercial test kits should be considered detrimental (Boyd, 1990). Recommended maximum standards are < 0.002 mg/l for fish and < 0.012 mg/l for eggs (Piper et al., 1982). Presence of H_2S can often be detected from the characteristic smell of rotten eggs. Levels detectable by smell are not necessarily toxic. The threshold for odor concentration of H_2S in clean water is 0.025 to 0.25 µg/l (A.P.H.A., 1992). It can also be tasted at relatively low concentrations. Acute poisoning is reportedly associated with the presence of purple-violet gills (Langdon, 1988), but water testing is the recommended method of diagnosis.

Treatment

Vigorously aerating water or passing it over a packed column degasser (e.g., Aquatic Ecosystems, Inc.; Engineered Products, Inc.) before use in flow-through systems will remove H₂S. In ponds, hydrogen sulfide formation can be prevented by maintaining aerobic conditions. It can be removed by oxidation with potassium permanganate, but permanganate cannot be used in seawater (see *PHARMACOPOEIA*). Raising the pH (e.g., liming) and lowering the temperature also reduce H₂S toxicity. In brackish or marine aquaria, filter beds should be closely monitored to prevent the development of anaerobic zones. If a filter has stopped working, even for a few hours, extreme care must be taken when turning it on again, because, if the water has become anaerobic, H₂S may have formed. Thus, animals may need to be moved temporarily to avoid acute mortality when the filters are turned back on again.

PROBLEM 82
Chlorine/Chloramine Poisoning
Prevalence Index
WF - 4, WM - 4, CF - 4, CM - 4
Method of Diagnosis
Rule-out of other problems combined with the following:
1. Chemical measurement of chlorine or chloramine in water
2. History
History
Acute to chronic stress response; fish added to tank within days of setting up tank; tap water used; recent water change in established tank; unrinsed chlorinated utensils; dyspnea
Physical Examination
See *HISTORY*
Treatment
1. Place immediately in chlorine-free, chloramine-free, highly oxygenated water
2. Aerate chlorinated make-up water for 24 hours
3. Treat make-up water with chlorine or chloramine neutralizer

COMMENTS
Chlorine Poisoning
Chlorine is added to municipal (tap) water supplies to kill microorganisms (Boyd, 1990). Like many toxins in water, chlorine is much more toxic to fish than to humans (Brooks & Bartos, 1984). The amount of chlorine added varies considerably among different municipalities and can also vary considerably from time to time. Combined chlorine residual is the total amount of *chlorine* present in various forms (e.g., chloramine, hypochlorous acid). Municipal water systems generally require a minimum of 0.20 mg/l of combined chlorine residual at the tap; in actuality, there is usually 0.50 to 1.0 mg/l present. Water mains are routinely treated with high chlorine concentrations after being repaired, but

this bolus of chlorine is rarely a problem because the chlorine is normally held out of the system and not allowed to reach a user's pipes. Inadequately rinsed, chlorine-disinfected utensils may contaminate water.

Chlorine toxicity can present as acute to subacute mortality associated with fish being added to a newly set-up tank or when fresh tap water is used for a water change. However, doing a partial water change with chlorinated tap water does not always cause toxicity because the chlorine may be quickly inactivated if a large amount of organic matter is present (e.g., in a long-established aquarium). Most aquarists are well aware of chlorine toxicity, making it uncommon. Chlorine is also used to treat industrial effluents (e.g., sewage, textiles, paper waste) before their discharge into waterways. Fish culture facilities should not be sited near chlorinated effluents.

Fish with acute chlorine poisoning will usually be dyspneic. Free chlorine reacts readily with organic matter, including gill tissue, causing acute necrosis and asphyxiation.

Chloramine Poisoning
Many municipal water sources have high levels of natural organic matter, such as humic acids and fulvic acids. Chlorine reacts with these organics, producing haloacetic acids (e.g., trichloroacetic acid) and trihalomethanes (e.g., chloroform). Trihalomethanes and possibly haloacetic acids are carcinogenic (U.S.E.P.A., 1989) and thus, potentially dangerous to humans (Christman et al., 1991). To eliminate trihalomethanes from drinking water, many municipalities now add ammonia to the chlorine during disinfection. Reaction of ammonia with chlorine produces a more chemically stable disinfectant: chloramine. Chloramines are created by adding an excess of chlorine, resulting in monochloramine (other chloramines impart a taste to the water, and so the chemicals' ratio is designed to avoid their production). Chloramine, like chlorine, is highly toxic to fish (Tompkins & Tsai, 1976).
Diagnosis
Commercial test kits for chlorine and chloramine are available (Chemetrics, Inc., Hach Company), but presumptive diagnosis can often be made from the history. It is important to determine if fish may have been exposed to chlorine or chloramine-treated water. The disinfectant used in a particular municipality can be determined by contacting the public works department (Kowalski, 1984). The threshold for smelling chlorine is 0.20 to 0.40 mg/l (Anonymous, 1989).

Chlorine levels of 0.10 mg/l are common in tap water and can be acutely fatal in aquaria with low organic matter (e.g., newly established aquaria). Any detectable amount of chlorine is undesirable, with 0.003 mg/l considered to be a maximum tolerable limit for continuous exposure (U.S.E.P.A., 1973; 1979 to 1980). Chloramines should be undetectable by commercial kits before water is used for fish.

Chlorine or chloramine poisoning must be differentiated from other poisons (see *PROBLEMS 81, 83,* and *84*) and from environmental shock (see *PROBLEM 86*).

Prophylaxis

Chlorine is easily removed from water by vigorous aeration for 24 hours or by adding commercial dechlorinating agents. Chloramines are not easily removed by aeration. The water must be filtered through activated carbon or treated with a chemical neutralizer, such as sodium thiosulfate, to break the chlorine-ammonia bond. Because the chemical neutralization releases ammonia, this must also be removed (see *PROBLEM 4*). Heating the water to near boiling will also drive off chloramines. Many commercial chloramine neutralizers do not remove ammonia but simply cause the ammonia test to read negative.

Treatment

Fish exposed to acute chlorine poisoning appear to have improved survival if the water is supersaturated with oxygen for several days. Lowering the temperature may also help (G. Lewbart, Personal Communication).

PROBLEM 83
Metal Poisoning

Prevalence Index

WF - 3, WM - 3, CF - 3, CM - 3

Method of Diagnosis

Rule-out of other problems combined with the following:

1. Chemical measurement of metal in water
2. History

History

Metal plumbing used to carry water source; metal in contact with water (e.g., rocks, ornaments); metal in the water supply; copper-containing medications

Physical Examination

Varies with toxicosis

Treatment

1. Remove fish to another system
2. Water change
3. Add EDTA
4. Add ion exchange filter

COMMENTS

Epidemiology/Pathogenesis

Fish are much more sensitive than humans to aqueous metals, which is one reason why water that is safe for human consumption may be highly toxic to fish. Metals are most toxic in low-alkalinity water, which allows a high concentration of metal to remain dissolved (and thus toxic).

Lead, copper, or galvanized (zinc-coated) iron plumbing may leach metals. Since more and more metal will dissolve into the water over time, the longer that water sits in a pipe, the higher the metal concentration. Thus, water that first comes out of a pipe has the highest metal concentration. Ground water, especially soft, acid water, may have toxic concentrations of metals. Rainwater runoff may also be a source of metal poisoning in poorly buffered soils that may leach aluminum or other metals from soils or mine waste.

Metals may be introduced into aquaria from metal aquarium hoods or from objects placed into the tank; this may include not only metal objects, but also ceramic ware that has lead glaze and certain rocks. Only items known to be safe for aquarium use should ever be placed into a tank. Overdosing with copper that is used as an algaecide or to treat ectoparasites may lead to poisoning. Over-the-counter aquarium remedies for freshwater fish that include copper may be toxic, even when the recommended dosage is used, because copper toxicity varies greatly depending upon water conditions (see *PHARMACOPOEIA*).

Water from the hypolimnion (see *PROBLEM 3*) of lakes or reservoirs used in fish hatcheries may be high in copper, zinc, iron, and manganese because of mobilization of the metals from anaerobic conditions (Grizzle, 1981). Oxidized manganese may be toxic (see *POTASSIUM PERMANGANATE* in *PHARMACOPOEIA*).

CLINICAL SIGNS

Clinical signs of metal poisoning vary with the element and somewhat with the fish species. As with most toxins, signs are mostly nonspecific. The most common cause of metal poisoning is copper. Like most heavy metals, copper toxicosis primarily affects the gills, resulting in osmoregulatory dysfunction. Kidney and liver may also be affected (Cardeilhac & Whitaker, 1988). Copper is also immunosuppressive and thus may potentiate infectious disease epidemics (Knittel et al., 1981). See the *PHARMACOPOEIA* for more information on copper. Sorensen (1991) discusses metal poisoning in detail.

Diagnosis

Definitive diagnosis of metal poisoning requires the measurement of toxic metal levels in water. However, determining whether a metal concentration is toxic is often more complicated than simply measuring the total amount of metal in the water, because the toxicity of a metal is primarily due to its dissolved ionic form rather than the total concentration. Some metals form oxides, hydroxides, and carbonates in water. Clay and organic material adsorb and/or chelate metals, inactivating (i.e., detoxifying) them. Calcium and magnesium also reduce heavy metal toxicity by competing with heavy metal binding sites on the gill (Pagenkopf, 1983). Thus, it is hard to assess the probable effect of a metal when the above complications are present (e.g., water from a high hardness, high

Table II-83 Metal concentrations associated with toxicity in freshwater fish (mg/l unless stated otherwise).

Metal/metal salt	Levels in water associated with fish kills	Acceptable continuous exposure levels in water for fish culture*	Sources	Diagnostic clinical features†	References
Aluminium	> 0.1 to 5 (low pH); also toxic at pH 8 (alumate form)		Tank fittings in low pH or saltwater; acid rain		Brown et al., 1983
Antimony (potassium tartrate salt)	> 12 to 20				
Arsenic	> 1 to 2	< 0.7			
Arsenite	> 14				
Cadmium	> 1.0–3.7 \ > 5.2	< 0.0005 (soft water) \ < 0.003 (hard water)	Electroplating; superphosphate; galvanized pipe[4]		
Cadmium salts	> 0.1				
Chromates	> 3.3 to 133		Corrosion inhibitor in cooling towers; metal plating/anodizing; leather tanning; hexavalent chromium most commonly used		
Cobalt	> 30				
Copper	> 0.03–0.7 (soft water) \ > 0.6–6.4 (hard water)	< 0.006	Mining waste; low-alkalinity ground water; plumbing pipes; bronze, brass fittings; also see PHARMACOPOEIA		Jeffree & Williams, 1975
Copper nitrate	> 0.02	< 0.002 maximum			
Copper sulfate	> 0.14	< 0.00005 average			
Iron	> 0.5	< 0.1	Well or spring water; anoxic reservoir water; rising pH, O_2; acid drainage; industrial effluents; corroding iron pipes	Precipitating iron (ferric hydroxide) on gills impairs respiration); stains laundry, porcelain, and concrete; some persons can detect a bittersweet, astringent taste at > 1 mg/l	Wedemeyer, 1976; Langdon, 1987a
Lead	> 1.0 to 31.5	< 0.02	Lead or galvanized plumbing pipes‡; red paint; lead solder joints; industrial, mine, or smelter discharge; weights used to hold aquarium plants	Sigmoid spinal curvature; caudal cutaneous melanosis; erythrocytic stippling (chronic); elevated ALAD enzyme levels	Hine, 1982; Bengtsson, 1975; Untergasser, 199l; Hodson et al., 1984
Lead salts	> 0.5				
Manganese	> 75	< 0.01	Well or spring water; anoxic reservoir water; batteries; steel or aluminum alloys	Manganese oxide precipitates on gills, impairs respiration; stains laundry and porcelain at > 1 mg Mn/l; permanganates are most toxic species	
Manganese chloride	> 0.5				

Mercury Mercuric chloride Methyl mercury	> 0.17 > 0.0008 > 0.07	< 0.0002	Mining waste		
Nickel Nickel salts	> 4.5-9.8 > 0.1	< 0.01	Metal plating baths; corrosion product of stainless steel and nickel alloys		
Selenium	> 8-72	< 0.05	Coal power stations [coal ash, fly ash]; drainage from seleniferous soils in semiarid areas		Gillespie & Bauman, 1986; A.P.H.A., 1992
Silver Silver sulfide/ thiosulfate complex	> 0.006-0.07 > 280-360	< 0.17 µg/l	Surface-finishing; photographic film manufacturers and processors		
Tin	> 55			Poorly soluble in natural waters (< 100 µg/l)	A.P.H.A., 1992
Tri-n-butyl tin (TBT)	> 0.0015-0.02 mg/l	< 0.02 µg/l	Antifouling paints for boats, nets		Short & Thrower, 1987
Uranium	> 3-135				
Zinc	> 0.4-1.76	< 0.005	Galvanized tanks; de-zincification of brass; white paint; mining waste; low-alkalinity ground water	Over 5 mg/l causes bitter, astringent taste and opalescence in alkaline water; mean concentration in United States drinking waters = 1.33 mg/l	A.P.H.A., 1992

Modified from Langdon (1988), with data provided in the listed references, as well as from U.S.E.P.A. (1973, 1979 to 1980), Wedemeyer et al. (1976), Bengtsson (1975), Chen et al. (1985), Sorenson (1991), A.P.H.A. (1992)

*Safe levels are generally concentrations that are 10-100 times lower than the lowest concentrations reported to kill fish. Thus, these are usually conservative estimates.

†Most signs of metal poisoning are nonspecific.

‡Lead and cadmium can enter water with deteriorating galvanized pipe because the zinc that is used for galvanizing is contaminated with these metals.

alkalinity, pond with considerable suspended clay and organic matter).

If metal toxicity is suspected and if it is economically justifiable to confirm the cause, it is best to send samples to a specialized laboratory. However, the clinician should be aware of the limitations of analysis. Atomic absorption spectroscopy is most commonly used for highly accurate metal analysis. This method determines the total amount of metal in a sample. However, more gentle extraction methods are gaining wider use (Riggs et al., 1989) because of the aforementioned considerations.

It can also be advisable to submit affected fish for determination of metal concentration in target tissues (usually gill, liver, and kidney). Extreme care must be taken to avoid contamination of tissue samples during preparation, so it is usually advisable to submit live fish or freshly iced, live fish and have the analytical laboratory prepare specific tissues.

Commercial test kits are available from aquarium suppliers and other sources (Aquarium Systems, Inc., Chemetrics, Inc., Hach Company, LaMotte Company) for measuring total copper, iron, and other metals. Such kits are relatively reliable for determining metal levels in waters low in organics and suspended sediment (e.g., typical aquarium water, tap water, or ground water).

IRON TOXICITY

Iron toxicity is not due to direct toxicity of the metal, but rather to the precipitation of iron oxides on the gills when anaerobic water (e.g., from a well) that has soluble, reduced iron is exposed to air (Langdon, 1992; Wedemeyer et al., 1976). Diagnosis can be presumptively based on typical clinical signs; however, measuring iron levels in the water is also advisable. Waters with high iron content often stain concrete and other structures brown. Manganese toxicity acts similarly.

Treatment

Avoiding exposure to contaminated water is the best approach. When necessary, water can be treated to remove toxic metals. Ion exchange filters (e.g. Cole-Parmer) adsorb copper, zinc, lead, and other heavy metals. Pumps delivering a measured amount of EDTA will chelate heavy metals (J. Hinshaw, Personal Communication). Ion exchange filters and metal chelators are less effective in high-hardness water. They also remove essential heavy metals (Ca^{++}, Mg^{++}) which may need to be readded to the water for some fish. They are also expensive, being feasible only for hatcheries, research facilities, or recirculating systems.

Iron toxicity can be avoided by allowing the iron to settle out in a pond (the water in the pond should have a 1- to 2-day transit time). A quicker method is to vigorously aerate the water in a tower and then run it through a sand filter to remove the iron precipitate. It can then be used immediately (Boyd, 1990).

PROBLEM 84
Miscellaneous Water-Borne Poisonings

Prevalence Index

WF - 3, WM - 3, CF - 3, CM - 3

Method of Diagnosis

Rule-out of other problems combined with the following:

1. Toxicological exam
2. History

History

Acute to chronic mortality with evidence of exposure of fish to toxin(s)

Physical Examination

Varies with poison

Treatment

1. Place fish in unpoisoned system, or add activated carbon, or change water
2. Eliminate exposure to toxin

COMMENTS
Epidemiology/Pathogenesis

A wide range of toxins can affect fish. Many are more toxic to aquatic organisms than they are to terrestrial animals. Thus, insecticides, herbicides, nicotine (cigarette smoke), and household cleaners can be lethal, even if they only reach the water as an aerosol. Objects that are not tested safe for aquarium use can be toxic. For example, various soft plastics can leach plasticizers (softening agents) or may be treated with insecticides or fungicides (e.g., foam padding used for furniture manufacture) (Untergasser, 1991). Clinical signs will obviously depend on the type of poisonous exposure.

In ponds or systems that use surface water (e.g., trout raceways), poisoning may occur after rainfall, which may wash acids or agricultural chemicals into the water. However, most fish kills caused by agricultural chemicals result from aerial spraying of crops. Because crop spraying pilots are well aware of the toxicity of agricultural chemicals to fish, poisoning caused by agricultural spraying is now rare. When it occurs, it is usually caused by either the use of new chemicals not before applied in an area, the use of emergency-use pesticides for unusually heavy outbreaks of some pests, or the use of pesticides contrary to label recommendations (Mitchell, 1995).

Susceptibility varies greatly among species, and not all react similarly. Invertebrates often exhibit quite different susceptibility to toxins than fish (may be more or less susceptible). Of the pesticides, chlorinated hydrocarbon insecticides have the greatest potential for harming fish. In general, poisons are more toxic at higher temperatures and may be affected by pH, hardness, alkalinity, and DO. Young fish are usually more susceptible than older fish (Cope, 1971).

Table II-84 Water quality standards and levels associated with fish kills in freshwater [mg/l unless specified].

Parameter	Levels in water associated with fish kills	Acceptable continuous exposure levels in water for fish culture	Sources	Diagnostic clinical features[a]	References
TOTAL HARDNESS AS $CaCO_3$	> 200 (chronic CO_2 excess) > 800 (all causes)	20 to 200			
TOTAL SUSPENDED SOLIDS	< 5000 to 100,000	< 80 (most fishes); Secchi disk reading < 25 cm (see PROBLEM 1); for salmonids, < 5 best, not > 50; Sharp particles such as mica, silicon, or iron may cause gill abrasion at even low concentrations; 2 to 5 μm particles may be most abrasive	Clay; silt; algae; floods; earthmoving; sawdust and other suspended matter; inadequate solids removal in intensive closed systems	If caused by algae: low DO (see PROBLEM 1); if caused by inanimate material: 1. Low fish production in ponds (inhibits algae growth) 2. Coughing to clear gills; gill epithelial hyperplasia 3. Settles on eggs, causing suffocation and secondary infection 4. Add calcium or alum to reduce turbidity in ponds	Frakes & Hoff, 1982 Moe, 1992a See PROBLEM 5
TOTAL DISSOLVED SOLIDS	> 5000 to 20,000	< 400			
NITRATE	> 1000	< 50 < 2 (marine reef aquaria)	Oxidation of nitrite to nitrate; fertilizers	Indicator of water quality [high levels indicate need for water change in aquaria]; very nontoxic compared with ammonia and nitrite, but can impair growth of some fish at high levels (> 100 mg/l); reef corals sensitive to low levels	
MISCELLANEOUS AGRICULTURAL CHEMICALS					
Potassium salts	> 1500		Fertilizer		Langdon, 1992b
Ammonium salts	> 50		Fertilizer		
Phosphorus (elemental)	> 0.02 to 4.0 (acute) > 0.0001 to 0.002 (chronic)		Industry		Fletcher et al. 1970
Lime (calcium oxide, hydroxide)	Causing pH > 9 to 10				See PHARMACOPOEIA
MISCELLANEOUS POISONS					
Chlorine	> 0.10 to 4.0	< 0.003			See PROBLEM 82
Fluoride salts	> 5.0				
Sodium arsenite, arsenic trioxide	> 2.0 to 20				

Continued.

Table II-84, cont'd   Water quality standards and levels associated with fish kills in freshwater (mg/l unless specified).

Parameter	Levels in water associated with fish kills	Acceptable continuous exposure levels in water for fish culture	Sources	Diagnostic clinical features[a]	References
Cyanides	> 0.03 to 0.23	< 0.005	Mining waste; gas works; steel mills; ferrocyanide (see SALT in PHARMACOPOEIA)		See PROBLEM 81
Hydrogen sulfide	> 0.5 to 10	< 0.002	Anaerobic organic decay: paper mills; tanneries	Purple-violet gills (acute)	McKee & Wolf, 1963; Boyd, 1990
Methane (marsh gas)		> 65 mg/l apparently not harmful	Anaerobic organic decay	Bubbles trapped in a glass jar are easily ignited with a match	
Nicotine	> 1				
Algal toxins					See PROBLEM 85
ORGANOCHLORINE (CHLORINATED HYDROCARBON) PESTICIDES					
Endrin	> 0.0003 to 0.002 mg/l	> 0.003 μg/l (ppb)	Agricultural discharges	Paralysis (acute); spinal deformities and vertebral fractures (chronic); decreased egg viability; lipophilic toxins that may be mobilized during fasting (e.g., winter); persistent pesticides in environment	Gilbertson, 1985; Westin et al, 1985
Chlordecone (kepone)	> 0.004 to 0.07 mg/l	< 0.001 μg/l			
Endosulfan	> 0.01 mg/L	< 0.01 μg/l			
Pentachloraphenate	> 0.1 mg/L	> 0.1 μg/l			
Aldrin	> 0.013 to 0.05 mg/l	< 0.01 μg/l			
Heptachlor	> 0.019 to 0.25 mg/l				
Dieldrin	> 0.008 to 0.05 mg/l	< .005 μg/l			
Chlordane	> 0.02 to 0.08 mg/l	< 0.004 μg/l			
Lindane (BHC)	> 0.23 to 0.8 mg/l	> 0.02 μg/l			
Toxaphene (camphenes)	> 0.003 to 0.018 mg/l	< 0.01 μg/l			
DDT	> 0.008 to 0.027 mg/l	> 0.003 μg/l			
CARBAMATE PESTICIDES					
Carbaryl (Sevin®)	> 0.5 to 10 mg/l	< 0.02 μg/l		Depressed brain acetylcholinerase; vertebral deformities; muscular/neural lesions; moderately persistent pesticides in environment	Post, 1987
Zectran	> 2.5 to 17				
ORGANOPHOSPHATE PESTICIDES					
Diazinon	> 0.2 to 5.2	< 0.002 μg/l	Agricultural discharges; livestock discharges	Depressed brain acetylcholinerase; weak ness; vertebral fractures; perivertebral hemorrhage (acute and chronic); relatively nonpersistent pesticides in environment; often most toxic to scaled fish	Schneider, 1979 See PHARMACOPOEIA Mitchell, 1995
Malathion	> 0.1 to 30	< 0.008 μg/l			
Parathion	> 0.3 to 1.6	< 0.001 μg/l			
Trichlorphon	> 0.8 to 100.0	< 0.001 μg/l			
Fenthion®	> 0.9 to 2.5				
Dursban®	> 0.01				
Guthion®	> 0.005 to 0.09				

Agent			Source/Use	Signs / Notes	Reference
PYRETHRIN INSECTICIDES	> 0.0005 to 0.001 mg/l	< 0.001 µg/l			
IVERMECTIN ANTHELMINTICS	< 0.1 mg/l		Livestock discharges		Palmer et al, 1987
PISCICIDES					
Rotenone (derris root, cube root)	> 0.006-4 mg/l			Rotenone: Gills bright red even though clinically hypoxic; natural decay takes days (high temperature) to weeks (low temperature)	Post, 1987
Antimycin	> 0.05-20 µg/l			Antimycin: Most persistent and toxic at low pH (persists for 1 day to over 1 week, depending on pH); temperature less important	
ALGICIDES, HERBICIDES, & FUNGICIDES					
Herbicides/algicides					
Copper sulfate	> 0.14 to 0.5		Agricultural discharges; treatment of plants in waterways	Some persist for months in sediment (e.g., diquat, paraquat), especially granular forms	Reid & Anderson, 1982
Simazine	> 10.0	< .01			
Acrolein	> 0.14				
Glyphosphate	> 12 to 130				
Chlorthalonil	> 10 to 20				Davies & White, 1985
2,4-D	> 2.0 to 96.5	< 0.004 µg/l			
Paraquat	> 840				
Diuron	> 4 to 152				
Diquat	> 8 to 350				
Silvex	> 1				
Fungicides					
Antimildew agent			Silicone sealant not approved for aquaculture use (bathroom caulk)		
Trifluralin				Muscular/neural lesions; vertebral deformities	
MOTHPROOFING AGENTS					
Eulan WA New (chlorophenylid)	> 0.5 to 5.4				
Mitin N/Mitin FF (fenurons)	> 0.07 to 11.2				
DETERGENTS					
Sodium dodecyl sulphate	> 28 to 32	< 0.1	Household and industrial laundering; other cleaning operations	Hemorrhage; excess mucus; gill subepithelial edema; epithelial disruption	Wedemeyer et al, 1976
Dodecyl benzosulphonate	> 5	< 0.1			
Sulphonates	> 4	< 0.1			

Continued.

Table II-84, cont'd Water quality standards and levels associated with fish kills in freshwater (mg/l unless specified).

Parameter	Levels in water associated with fish kills	Acceptable continuous exposure levels in water for fish culture	Sources	Diagnostic clinical features*	References
PHENOLS					
Phenol	> 7.5 to 56	< 0.10	Industrial effluents; landfills; coal, petroleum processing; wood distillation; municipal, animal wastes	Low taste threshold by humans	U.S.E.P.A., 1973
o-Cresol	> 2.3 to 29.5	< 0.10			
m-Cresol	> 6.4 to 24.5	< 0.10			
Resorcinol	> 14	< 0.10			
Hydroquinone	> 0.30	< 0.10			
POLYNUCLEAR AROMATIC HYDROCARBONS (PAH'S)					
Napthalene	> 165	< 1.5?	By-products of petroleum processing or combustion	Very insoluble in water, but many are very carcinogenic	
Anthracene					
Benzo(a)pyrene					
Phenanthrene	> 1 to 2				
MISCELLLANEOUS PETROCHEMICALS					
Diesel oils, car oils	> 50 to 1,000		Surface waters: Usually oil spills Ground waters: leaking underground fuel storage tanks; industrial wastes; landfills; underground waste dumps	Fish exposed to petroleum develop hemosiderosis (excess deposition of hemosiderin, a yellow-brown, Perl's Prussian blue–positive pigment)	Malins et al. 1984; Poirer et al., 1986; Khan & Nag, 1993; Smith, 1968
Diesel fuel	> 167				
Crude oil					
Toluene	> 10 to 260				
Benzene	> Toxicity than benzene				
Hexachlorobenzene	> 100				
Aniline, toluidine					
PHTHALATE ESTERS	731 to 1300	< 0.3 µg/l	Plasticizers (softening agents), especially for PVC (polyvinyl chloride) plastics		
PHOSPHATE ESTERS					
Pydraul 115E	> 45 to 100		Lubricants; oil additives; plasticizers	Depressed brain acetylcholinesterase activity	Nevins & Johnson, 1978
Pydraul 50E	> 0.72 to 3				
Houghotosafe 1120	> 1.7 to 43				
POLYCHLORINATED BIPHENYLS (PCBs, Arochlor®)	> 0.015 to 61 mg/l (acute) > 0.003 mg/l (chronic)	<0.002 µg/l	Transformer lubricants; heat exchangers; hydraulic fluids; plasticizers; many sources	Stable in environment; chronic problems most serious, especially reproductive impairment, egg mortality; transformer oils with PCB less toxic than PCB alone	Mayer & Mayer, 1985; Murty, 1986

Modified from Langdon (1988), with additional data provided in the listed references, as well as from U.S.E.P.A. (1973, 1979-80); Wedemeyer et al. (1976); Alabaster & Lloyd (1982); Hine (1982); Piper et al. (1982); Hellawell (1986); Murty (1986a, b); Meyers & Hendricks (1982); Bengtsson (1975); Wellborn et al. (1984); Johnson & Finley (1980); A.P.H.A. (1989, 1992).
*Toxin-induced lesions are typically nonspecific and are induced by many types of agents (Mallatt, 1985; Meyers & Hendricks, 1982).
Also see the PHARMACOPOEIA for details on various therapeutants.

Diagnosis

When a fish kill occurs, some type of poisoning, especially pesticide-related, is one of the first thoughts that come to the mind of a fish culturist. However, poisonings are rarely a cause of kills in fish culture, and the clinician should rule out other more common causes of kills, such as hypoxia (see *PROBLEM 1*), or an infectious disease epidemic. The history is critical in determining the cause of miscellaneous water-borne poisonings. Specifically, it is necessary to have some idea about the type of toxin that the fish are or were exposed to, since it is impossible to analyze for all possible toxins. The death of other animals, such as frogs, turtles, snakes, and birds, is strongly suggestive of poisoning. Lack of algae (killed by herbicides) or zooplankton (killed by insecticides) in the water may indicate a pesticide kill.

ACUTE VS CHRONIC POISONINGS

Both acute and chronic poisonings are often difficult to diagnose. Chronic, sublethal toxicity is often insidious, taking a long time to develop. Furthermore, whether certain low levels of poison are toxic can be hard to decide. Most poisons can cause chonic toxicity at 10- to 1000-fold less concentrations than the acute concentrations shown in Table II-84.

Acute toxicity (i.e., fish kill caused by poisoning) can also be difficult to definitively diagnose because many poisonings are onetime events where the poison quickly dissipates after the kill. For example, although short-acting pesticides are fortunately replacing long-acting toxins, they present a greater diagnostic challenge. Prompt response is often crucial to diagnosis.

SAMPLE COLLECTION/SUBMISSION

Collect samples quickly and preserve them in a fashion that will allow accurate analysis, if a definitive diagnosis is required. The methods for collection depend on the type of toxin that is suspected. Most miscellaneous poisonings probably go undiagnosed because it is difficult to obtain this information. It can also be advisable to submit affected fish to determine toxin concentration in target tissues (gill, liver, and kidney are common targets). Extreme care must be taken to avoid contamination of tissue samples during preparation, so it is best to submit live fish or freshly iced, live fish and have the analytical laboratory prepare tissues. Specific recommendations should also be sought regarding sample preparation, depending on which toxin will be sought. Such analyses can be expensive and may not be a viable option for the owner. Analysis costs may range from $100 if a specific toxin is suspected, to several thousand dollars if it is not known what the toxin might be.

Samples can also be preserved for histopathology. Most lesions induced by toxicants are suggestive of a toxic insult but are nonspecific (e.g., degeneration, necrosis, hyperplasia) (Meyers & Hendricks, 1982). Only a few toxicants cause lesions in aquatic animals that may be useful for diagnosis, although virtually none are pathognomonic (Table II-84).

Treatment

Separation of the fish from the toxin is essential and may be accomplished either by placing fish in a clean system or by diluting and/or removing the toxin by adding clean water or activated carbon, where this is feasible.

Avoidance is the best method of control. The use of pesticides in aquatic areas should be discouraged. Aquarium owners should be made aware of the exquisite sensitivity of fish to even airborne toxicants. For example, fish are highly susceptible to even small amounts of airborne nicotine in smoke. Pesticides sprayed over fields can also drift a considerable distance, reaching ponds. Advise owners to plant high vegetation to intercept airborne drift of pesticides and construct barriers (e.g., ditches) to divert runoff from treated fields. Advocate proper methods of pesticide application and dispense them in a proper manner (i.e., don't contaminate waterways).

PROBLEM 85
Noxious Algae

Prevalence Index
WF - 4, WM - 4, CF - 4, CM - 2
Method of Diagnosis
Rule-out of other problems combined with identification of specific noxious alga in concentration sufficient to be pathogenic
History
Acute to chronic mortality with evidence of exposure of fish to toxic alga; most commonly, behavioral abnormalities and/or dyspnea; floating algae ("scum") on water; red, brown, or green discoloration of water
Physical Examination
Varies with poison, but often neurological signs; dyspnea; algae lodged in gills
Treatment
1. Eliminate exposure to algae
2. Place fish in unpoisoned system or add activated carbon or change water

COMMENTS
Epidemiology/Pathogenesis
Noxious phytoplankton are becoming an increasingly serious threat to fish culture (Fig. II-85, *A*), with the great majority of problems occurring in near-coastal marine systems (e.g, cage culture or aquaculture operations that use coastal or estuarine water). There is evidence that eutrophication is responsible for many of the outbreaks (Smayda, 1990). Many algae have been implicated in fish kills (Table II-85), with toxins suspected in many cases.

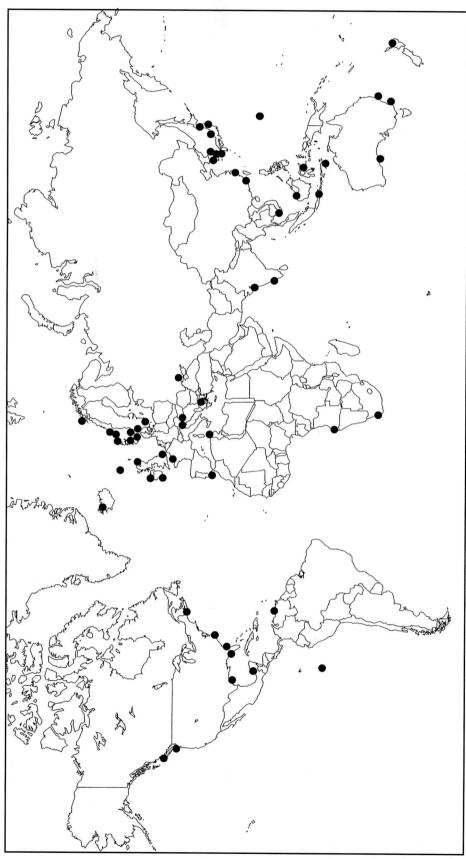

Fig. II-85 A, Global distribution of kills in wild and cultured fish associated with noxious phytoplankton.

(A from Sundstrom et al., 1990.)

Continued.

A

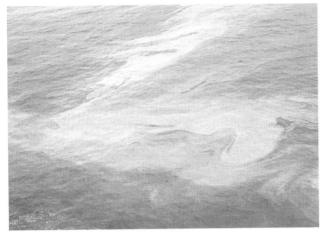

Fig. II-85—cont'd. B, Red tide caused by *Noctiluca miliaris* bloom.

(B photograph courtesy of H. Moller.)

Some algae produce potent toxins; neurotoxins are especially common. Clinical signs of algal neurotoxicity include disorientation, loss of equilibrium, and sporadic hyperactivity. Other algae mechanically obstruct or damage the gills, causing hypoxia (Kent, 1992).

DINOFLAGELLATES

Many dinoflagellates have been implicated or suspected in fish kills. The red tide dinoflagellate (*Gymnodinium breve* = *Ptychodiscus brevis*) causes mass mortalities of fish and invertebrates in states bordering the Gulf of Mexico (Steidinger & Baden, 1984).

Recently, a new dinoflagellate, *Pfiesteria piscicida*, has been discovered that causes acute mortality in both cultured and wild estuarine fish (Smith et al., 1988; Burkholder et al., 1992). Sublethal exposure also causes massive skin ulcers in surviving fish (Noga et al., In Press). This organism, a new genus and family of dinoflagellate, can kill fish from very dilute to full strength seawater. It has been identified in the Chesapeake Bay and Albemarle-Pamlico Estuary, the two largest estuaries in the United States. It may be a serious threat to coastal aquaculture, since it appears to be common in estuarine waters and can thus be easily introduced into a culture system with contaminated water or fish (Smith et al., 1988; Noga et al., 1993b; Noga et al., In Press).

Some dinoflagellate toxins are transferred up the food chain (e.g., *Alexandrium*) and have caused mortalities in wild fish that consume tainted zooplankton along the Northwest Atlantic coast (White, 1977 and 1981).

PRYMNESIOPHYTES

Prymnesium parvum causes mortality in brackish and marine pond fish in Europe and in the Middle East (Shilo, 1981).

DIATOMS

Chaetoceros spp. have been associated with mortality in seawater-cultured salmonids. The spines of the alga

Table II-85 Noxious algae associated with toxicoses to fish.*

TAXONOMIC GROUP

Dinoflagellates (Class Dinophyceae)

Alexandrium angustitabulatum†
Alexandrium catenella
Alexandrium excavatum
Alexandrium fundyense
Alexandrium monilatum
Alexandrium tamarensis
Amphidinium carterae
Amphidinium klebsii
Amphidinium rhynocephalum
Cochliodinium polykrikoides
Gambierdiscus toxicus
Gonyaulax spinifera
Gymnodinium breve
Gymnodinium galatheanum
Gymnodinium mikimotoi
Gymnodinium pulchellum
Gymnodinium sanguineum
Gymnodinium venificum
Gyrodinium cf. *aureolum*
Lingulodinium polyedra
Noctiluca miliaris
Peridinium polonicum (F)
Pfeisteria piscicida
Prorocentrum balticum
Prorocentrum concavum
Prorocentrum minimum
Pyrodinium bahamense var. *compressa*

Green Algae (Class Chlorophyceae)

Chaetomorpha minima

Cyanobacteria (*Blue–green algae*)

Anabaena flos-aquae (F)
Aphanizomenon flos-aquae (F)
Microcystis aeruginosa (F)
Nodularia spumigena
Oscillatoria agardhii (F)
Oscillatoria rubescens (F)
Schizothrix calcicola

Yellow-green Algae (Class Chrysophyceae)

Ochromonas danicum (F)
Ochromonas malhamensis (F)
Ochromonas minuta (F)

Prymnesiophytes (Class Prymnesiophyceae)

Chrysochromulina polylepis
Chrysochromulina leadbeateri
Prymnesium parvun
Prymnesium calathiferum
Prymnesium patelliferum

Rhaphidophyceans (Class Rhaphidophyceae)

Chatonella antiqua
Chatonella marina
Heterosigma akashiwo

Diatoms (Class Bacillariophyceae)

Chaetoceros convolutus
Chaetoceros concavicorinus
Corethron sp.

Data from Steidinger and Baden (1984), Davin et al. (1988), Kent (1992), Chang et al. (1990), and K. Steidinger (Personal Communication).
*Many of the listed algae have only been associated with fish kills and have not proven to be the cause of mortalities. The pathogenesis of most noxious algae in causing fish morbidity/mortality is uncertain.
†*Alexandrium* species were previously classified as *Gonyaulax*, *Protogonyaulax*, or *Gessnerium*.
F = freshwater alga.

apparently cause it to become lodged on or in the gills. Diatoms may become embedded in gill tissue, inciting a foreign body reaction. Epithelial hyperplasia causes hypoxia. In some cases, hyperactive mucus production appears to be primarily responsible for the hypoxia (Rensel, 1993).

CYANOBACTERIA

Cyanobacteria can be toxic to mammals but have not yet been proven to cause toxicosis in fish. However, die-offs of cyanobacteria can cause environmental hypoxia (see *PROBLEM 1*). A die-off appears as a change in the water's color from green or green-brown to light brown. The water often smells because of cyanobacteria decomposition.

Diagnosis

Any of the previously described clinical signs without evidence of another etiology suggests a possible algal toxicosis. The presence of an obvious *bloom* (Fig. II-85, *B*) is also supportive. Important differentials are other toxins (see *PROBLEMS 83* and *84*). Almost all documented toxic algae blooms have occurred in brackish or marine waters.

Many algae are *suspected* of causing fish morbidity/mortality but have not yet been proven as a cause. The *number*, as well as the *type* of algae present, is important in making a diagnosis. A certain minimum concentration (*bloom* concentration that varies with algal species) is required to implicate an algal organism as a cause of morbidity. Definitive identification of noxious algae requires examination of the sample by a trained expert, since to the untrained observer, noxious algae can look similar to closely related, nontoxic algae. Fresh samples are best for identification. Fresh samples should be kept at ambient water temperature or slightly lower but should not be iced. One of the best ways to do this is to wrap the container in wet newspaper and let evaporation cool the sample for transport (K. Steidinger, Personal Communication). If fresh samples cannot be examined within 24 hours of collection, they should be preserved in Lugol's iodine solution and kept refrigerated and in the dark until examination. Alternatively, samples can be preserved in 1% to 2% neutral buffered formalin. For delicate species (i.e., thinly armored or unarmored dinoflagellates), 2% gluteraldehyde in borate buffer is better. Some algae, especially unarmored forms, are considerably altered by fixation. The reference laboratory should be consulted for proper sample submission.

Treatment

In marine net-pens, reducing feeding or other activities that may bring fish to the surface during blooms may reduce mortalities (Kent, 1992). Algae have also been successfully avoided by pumping water from lower depths, enclosing the pens with a tarpaulin, or culturing fish in pens deep enough to avoid blooms. When feasible, pens can be moved to *clean* sites. The rapid development of many blooms necessitates constant vigilance and rapid response.

Algicides can inhibit many noxious algae in ponds, but care must be taken to avoid oxygen depletion (see *PROBLEM 1*). Bloom recurrence is also a possibility. Relatively small volumes of water, such as for tank culture, can be disinfected and detoxified, using ozonation and activated carbon filtration before adding it to the tank (K. Steidinger, Personal Communication).

PROBLEM 86
Environmental Shock/Delayed Mortality Syndrome (DMS)

Prevalence Index
WF - 2, WM - 2, CF - 2, CM - 2

Method of Diagnosis
Rule-out of other problems combined with the following:
1. Measurement of water quality under old and new conditions
2. History

History
Acute mortality or disease outbreak after large (50% or greater) water change; acute mortality or disease outbreak after transferring fish to a new culture system

Physical Examination
Acute stress response

Treatment
1. Prophylactic antibiotics to reduce opportunistic infections
2. More frequent and smaller water changes in culture systems
3. Reduce stress during transport or other manipulations

COMMENTS
Causes of Environmental Shock
Rapid changes in culture conditions can be dangerous to fish, even if these changes are within the normal physiological range for that species. Thus, if fish are moved to a new aquarium where the pH, hardness, or temperature is quite different from their previous environment, it can cause severe stress. Stress is also imposed by the manipulations involved in the transfer, such as netting the fish; confining them in a transport container; transporting them, with consequent build-up of toxins (e.g., ammonia, CO_2) and changes in pH and temperature; and then exposure to a novel environment.

Pathogenesis
Fish may adversely respond to such stress in several ways. The most severe reaction is peracute mortality. Some highly stress-prone species may die within minutes to hours of capture. If the fish survive the transport and/or transfer to a new environment, they may become sick within several hours to several days after being placed into the new culture system. For example, striped bass are highly stressed by simply confining them in a net for several minutes, even if water quality is optimal. They often develop fungal infections within 24 hours of this acute stress (Noga et al., 1994). This response is often referred to as delayed mortality syndrome or delayed capture mortality syndrome. DMS is associated with opportunistic infections, such as water molds (see *PROBLEM 33*), many bacteria, or ectoparasitic protozoa, which take advantage of the stressed host.

While infections that are caused by delayed mortality syndrome are usually evident within 2 to 5 days of the stressful event, they may not appear until over 1 week later. A critical period of about 2 to 3 weeks after the acute stress is the most likely time that fish will become sick because of DMS; thus, close observation is warranted.

The mechanisms responsible for delayed mortality syndrome are unknown, although some attendant physiological changes resemble the shock response in mammals. Severe exercise can kill fish, but the pathogenesis does not appear similar to capture myopathy of feral mammalian hoofstock. Wild-caught fish are more susceptible to delayed mortality syndrome than captive-bred individuals. This may explain why disease outbreaks are especially common after shipping tropical marine fish. In general, the *hardy* fish species appear to be most resistant to DMS (see Box above), although not entirely immune.

Diagnosis

Diagnosis of DMS is based on the history and clinical signs (i.e., acute mortality with no detectable cause; delayed mortality caused by opportunistic infections). This is obviously a rule-out diagnosis because many other problems have a similar presentation. For example, an acute stress response can occur because of many water quality problems. DMS is differentiated from other water quality problems in that water quality conditions are within the **normal** range for that species. Thus, the stress is caused by an inability to acclimate to conditions within the normal range and is typically potentiated by other stressors (e.g., confinement) (see *ACCLIMATION*, p. 44).

Treatment

If environmental shock is suspected, immediately returning the fish to the previous environmental conditions may be helpful but is usually not feasible. Symptomatic treatment should be used to control morbidity and mortality. Symptomatic treatment

includes using appropriate medications to control opportunistic infections and can also include the use of salt, which acts as an osmoregulatory enhancer, since osmoregulatory dysfunction appears to be a major sequela. Adding calcium also helps (Grizzle et al., 1990).

Prophylaxis

Prevention is especially desirable for DMS becuse of its potentially devastating consequences, as well as lack of specific treatments; this involves the proper handling of fish during manipulations, such as transport. Delayed mortality syndrome is probably one of the major reasons why mortalities are frequently high immediately after shipping fish.

While frequent water changes are useful for maintaining good water quality in aquaria, avoid major changes in environmental conditions. It is usually best to replace 25% or less of the water at any one time to prevent environmental shock, although even larger water changes are tolerated if the fish are acclimated to them.

PROBLEM 87
Traumatic Lesions

Prevalence Index
WF - 1, WM - 1, CF - 2, CM - 2

Method of Diagnosis
Usually rule-out of other problems combined with history and clinical signs

History
One or several (but not all) fish hiding in corners or elsewhere in aquarium; obvious attack of one or more individuals by tankmates; new fish recently introduced into established aquarium; *shy* or *peaceful* fish or smallest fish most affected; normal or more intense coloration in aggressors with faded or otherwise changed color pattern in affected fish; decrease in fish numbers in a rapidly growing population (e.g., fingerlings); large size variation among individuals; fish-eating birds near pond; overcrowding

Physical Examination
Fins ragged or scales missing in submissive individuals; in salmonids, dorsal fin especially damaged or missing, with traumatic wound on dorsum (*soreback*); opportunistic infections; corneal edema or ulceration, especially in large individuals

Treatment
AQUARIUM FISH (AGGRESSION PROBLEMS)
1. Hospitalize attacked individual(s) and treat with antibiotics (topical treatment if small, focal lesion)
2. Remove aggressor(s) from aquarium
3. Change position of rocks and other objects in aquarium

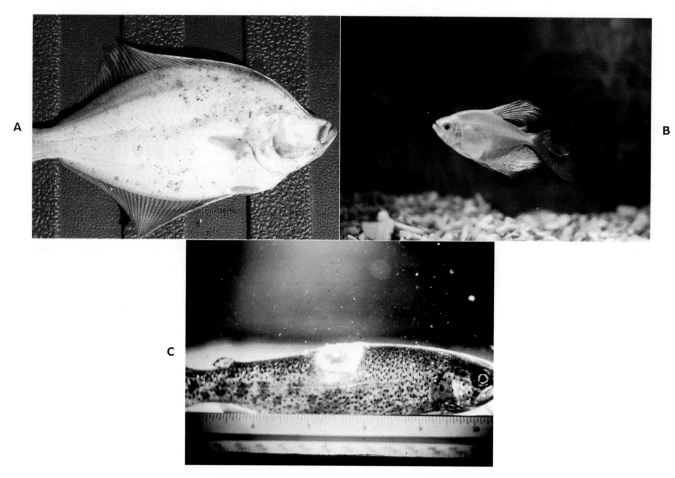

Fig. II-87   **A,** Skin hemorrhage on a flounder after capture by netting (trawling). **B,** Caudal fin damage to a tetra caused by the aggression of tankmates. **C,** Dorsal fin of a rainbow trout that has been completely chewed off by tankmates, leaving an open ulcer (*sore-back*).

[*A* photograph courtesy of H. Moller; *B* photograph courtesy of T. Wenzel; *C* photograph courtesy of C.L. Davis Foundation for Veterinary Pathology.]

4. Reduce (or increase) density
5. Feed lightly, while introducing new fish
6. Place new fish in a clear plastic box for up to several days

OTHER PROBLEMS (DEPENDING UPON ETIOLOGY)
1. Decrease stocking density
2. Increase feeding rate
3. Treat infected wounds if severe
4. Reduce exposure to sunlight
5. Prevent access of fish-eating wildlife

COMMENTS
Causes of Traumatic Lesions
AGGRESSION

Aggression is a common cause of trauma and even mortality in aquarium fish. Some fish, such as large cichlids, are highly prone to be aggressive. Aggression develops out of the instinctual behavior of many fish to form territories. Thus, this is usually not a problem in species that are not territorial (e.g., neon tetras).

However, some species, such as some barbs, tend to nip fins of slower moving species (Fig. II-87, *B*). Aggression-induced lesions can also result from courtship rituals.

Most territorial aquarium species will almost always form dominance hierarchies, unless the fish are crowded to the extent that territories cannot be successfully maintained by any one fish. In the latter case, aggression will not be a problem. However, in most tanks, fish will be in a low enough density to allow dominance hierarchies to form.

Salmonids are territorial and when overcrowded or underfed, will nip fins, especially the dorsal fin. This aggression may result in the entire loss of the fin, with formation of a large open wound on the back (*soreback*) (Fig. II-87, *C*). Channel catfish are relatively nonaggressive, except when sexually mature.

PREDATION
Piscivorous birds, including anhingas, diving ducks, grackles, ospreys, eagles, cormorants, pelicans, herons,

and egrets, can consume extremely large amounts of fish (up to 450 grams [1 pound] of fish per day). Anhingas and cormorants are serious problems in catfish and bait-fish ponds. Herons can also damage fish when attempting to capture them.

Many piscivorous insects will eat fish eggs or larvae. Important predators include the hemipterans (true bugs; e.g., water scorpion [*Ranatra* sp.], water bugs [*Belostoma* spp. and *Lethocerus* spp.], and backswimmer [*Notonecta indica*]), the coleopterans (predaceous diving beetle [*Cybister* sp.]), and the odonates (dragonflies). The true bugs and beetles must breathe air, while the nymph stages of dragonflies have gills. Adult dragonflies feed on larger fish.

Tadpoles are not piscivorous, but rather compete with fish for food. Frogs are highly carnivorous. *Hydra*, a small coelenterate, can kill small fry in aquaria.

CANNIBALISM

Many fish are cannibalistic and will eat their tankmates if given a chance. This can be a serious problem in young, rapidly growing fish (i.e., fry, fingerlings), where there is often a large difference in individual growth rates. The two principal causes of sibling cannibalism are genetic and behavioral (Hecht & Pienaar, 1993). Genetic forms are caused by size variation in a cohort; genotypic differences cause variation in individual growth rates. Behavioral forms are induced by environmental limiting factors. Important food fish aquaculture species displaying cannibalism include walking catfish, snook, barramundi, walleye, striped bass, European sea bass, nebulosus sea trout, chub mackerel, Atlantic cod, European eel, common carp, Northern pike, yellowtail, and dolphin (Hecht & Pienaar, 1993).

CONFINEMENT

Trauma may occur when fish are gathered in a net (Fig. II-87, A) or as a sequela of transport. Close confinement may lead to abrasions from sharp fin spines and puncture wounds. Idiopathic corneal edema, which may lead to ulceration, occurs when some fish are transported (Brandt et al., 1986). Corneal abrasions and ulcerations are common sequelae of trauma, especially in large individuals; this can result not only from fighting, but also from bumping into sharp objects, such as rocks or coral, in an aquarium. Ophthalmic trauma, which can eventually lead to phthisis bulbi, is common in large aquarium fish.

LIGHT

Excessive ultraviolet (UV) radiation causes sunburn in salmonids (Bullock & Roberts, 1979). Common in midsummer in northern latitudes, it is usually seen in small 2- to 3-inch fingerlings that are moved from indoors to outdoors, clear water rearing units. There is low mortality, but there may be high morbidity. Damaging UV radiation can penetrate up to 1 meter in clear water

(Bullock & Roberts, 1979). Excessive light may also cause eye damage (Piper et al., 1982).

Fish exposed rapidly to bright light may be startled. Salmon smolts reared in subdued light may burrow into the base of nets when transferred to net-pens, damaging their heads (e.g., skin loss) (Grant, 1993).

ELECTRICITY

Electrical shock can damage fish from electrofishing (Snyder, 1995) or from electrocution (Langdon, 1988), such as a lightning strike.

Clinical Signs/Diagnosis

Traumatic lesions can grossly mimic lesions with an infectious etiology. The history is extremely important in making a diagnosis of trauma. There should be no pathogens in fresh traumatic lesions, but older lesions are often secondarily infected. Uninfected, traumatic lesions that are caused by aggression often have little hemorrhage (Fig. II-87, B), but there are exceptions. In salmonids, dorsal fin damage caused by aggression (Fig. II-87, C) can appear grossly identical to sunburn lesions.

When cannibalism is occurring, the actual observation of fish feeding on tankmates may be missed. But, cannibalism is strongly suggested by an unexplained decrease in numbers of fish in a healthy population, along with a size variation in the population that is large enough to allow the larger fish to consume the smaller fish. The larger fish often are much larger than the average fish in the population and often will have a full stomach because of constant feeding. Presence of piscivorous birds on or near pond banks and live or dead fish with puncture wounds is strongly suggestive of bird feeding activity.

Treatment

MEDICAL

In aquarium fish, if lesions are small, medical treatment is often unnecessary, so long as the affected fish is isolated and watched closely for secondary wound infections. However, ophthalmic lesions should be treated aggressively to avert blindness. Ophthalmic and other focal lesions can be treated with topical antiseptics or antibiotics (see *PHARMACOPOEIA*). More serious or extensive lesions should be treated with systemic antibiotics. Other medications may also be needed, depending on the type of secondary infections present. In salmonids, infected wounds should be treated for the specific infection.

Environmental

AGGRESSION

In freshwater aquarium fish, aggression can be reduced by choosing compatible tankmates (*community-tank* fish), stocking fish of about the same size (so that one large fish does not bully the others), keeping at least five individuals of one species (so that aggression is not directed against only one submissive individual), and providing adequate hiding places (e.g., rocks, flower pots) for submissive individuals. Also, it may help to feed lightly when introducing a new fish and to place the new fish in a clear plastic box for up to several days, which may accustom the tankmates to the new fish's presence.

The great majority of marine aquarium fish are territorial and thus considerable care should be taken in choosing compatible tankmates. According to Bower (1983), "a (marine) aquarium should contain only one individual of a particular species, of a particular body shape and of a particular color or pattern of colors," to reduce recognition, and thus attack, of tankmates. Aggression in salmonids is remedied by reducing stocking density and/or by increasing feeding rate.

CANNIBALISM

Cannibalism can be reduced by providing more frequent feedings to growing fish, so that individual growth rates are more uniform. Frequent grading should also be done to remove large individuals from the population. Reducing density may also reduce cannibalism.

PREDATION

Covering culture systems with bird netting or other physical barriers (available from aquaculture supply companies) will eliminate bird problems but is often economically unfeasible. Perimeter fencing around ponds can provide protection from wading birds, such as herons. Scare tactics (e.g., dummies, devices that produce loud noises; available from aquaculture supply companies) often work for a while, but then the birds become acclimated. Scare tactics cannot be legally used against threatened or endangered species (e.g., bald eagle). Most piscivorous birds are migratory species, and in the United States and elsewhere are protected by law from being killed. However, farmers in the United States can obtain a depredation permit from the U.S. Fish and Wildlife Service, which allows a limited number of defined species to be killed. This is done to reinforce the effectiveness of the scare tactic that is used as the primary deterrent to bird feeding. Once the permit is issued, the U.S.D.A. Office of Animal Damage Control provides assistance with the control effort. Avault (1995), Stickley (1990), and Littauer (1990) provide more details on controlling birds.

Predaceous insects can be controlled by (Avault, 1995):

1. Reducing aquatic weeds, which provide a breeding habitat
2. Filling ponds with water just before stocking fish larvae to prevent a buildup of predaceous insects
3. Filling ponds at times of the year when insects are less common
4. Stocking larger individuals into ponds, since larger fish are less likely to be eaten

5. Treating ponds with 0.25 ppm methyl parathion several days before adding fish.
6. Treating the pond surface with oil to prevent the insects from breathing. Spray along the pond edge when there is just enough breeze to carry the oil slick across the pond. Since some air-breathing insects can remain under water for over 1 hour, several applications may be needed. Diesel fuel has been most commonly used. However, recent data suggest that other, less toxic oils are at least as effective against backswimmer. Linseed oil, unrefined cottonseed oil, or cod liver oil were all effective when applied at 2.2 gallons per surface acre (21 liters per surface hectare) (Anonymous, 1993). Avault (1995) provides more details on controlling insects. Some tadpoles can be killed with formalin (Helms, 1967). Some gouramies will eat hydra.

MISCELLANEOUS TRAUMATIC LESIONS

Fish with sunburn lesions usually respond quickly to shading. To avoid iatrogenic trauma, routine procedures (e.g., grading, weighing, vaccination) should be done at one time, so that fish can be handled as few times as possible.

DENSITY INDEX

Density is important because, even at densities that are considered adequate in terms of oxygen consumption, fish can get sick (Piper et al., 1982). For example, rainbow trout should be kept at densities measured in pounds/ft³ that are no greater than one-half their length in inches (e.g., 2-inch fish should not be kept at a density > 1 pound/ft³); 4-inch fish should be kept at a density of no more than 2 pounds/ft³, etc.). Thus, a density index can be calculated. This assumes that the density index stays constant as the fish increase in length, but larger fish often tolerate higher densities relative to their length; however, this is still a good rule of thumb. Note that maximum optimal density varies with fish species and culture environment.

PROBLEM 88
Genetic Anomalies

Prevalence Index
WF - 2, WM - 4, CF - 3, CM - 3
Method of Diagnosis
History and clinical signs
History
Excessive inbreeding
Physical Examination
Skeletal abnormalities; cataracts; poor growth; other anomalies may be present
Treatment
Introduce better genetic stock into the population

A 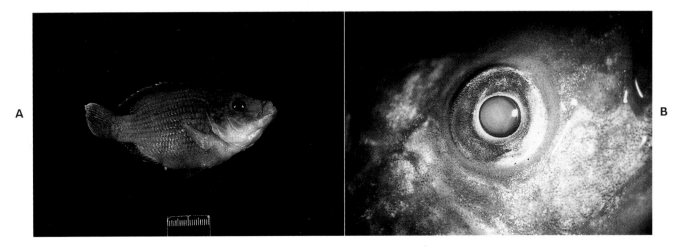 B

Fig. II-88   **A,** Stumpbody in tilapia, an inherited malformation (Tave et al., 1982). Compare with fish having a normal conformation (see Fig. II-53, *B*). **B,** Inherited cataract in Mozambique tilapia.

(*A* photograph by J. Stevens and E. Noga; *B* photograph by D. Wolf and E. Noga.)

COMMENTS
Epidemiology/Clinical Signs
Genetic anomalies are most common in captive bred fish, where such defects can escape natural selection. Twins, cross-bites, pugheads, stumpbody (Fig. II-88, *A*), spinal curvature (see Fig. II-79, *B*), double fins, and opercular deformities are some of the most common anomalies. Ophthalmic defects may also occur (Noga et al., 1981) (Fig. II-88, *B*). Malformations are most likely to appear in young fish and may lead to early death. A certain number of malformations will occur in even normal broods, but the incidence of malformed individuals should be low (often less than 1%). Some anomalies are desirable, such as longer fins or albinism. These traits are often selected for in aquarium fish.

Diagnosis
There are many possible causes for developmental anomalies, and determining a genetic link is often accomplished by ruling out other possible causes: improve the husbandry conditions that may be predisposing to these problems; pay special attention to proper types and amounts of feed (see *PROBLEM 79*), proper density, adequate biological filtration and oxygenation, and frequent water changes. Exposure to teratogenic chemicals, such as malachite green and organophosphates, should also be ruled out.

Treatment
Stocks carrying deleterious genes should be replaced or out-bred to dilute the undesirable gene. See Tave (1993) for details on selecting for or eliminating certain genetic traits.

CHAPTER 20

Problems 89 through 92

Rule-out diagnoses: *Presumptive* diagnosis is based on the absence of other etiologies combined with a diagnostically appropriate history, clinical signs, and/or pathology. *Definitive* diagnosis is not possible since the etiology is unknown (idiopathic)

89. Freshwater hole-in-the-head syndrome
90. Marine hole-in-the-head syndrome
91. Pancreas disease
92. Miscellaneous important idiopathic diseases

PROBLEM 89
Freshwater Hole-in-the-Head Syndrome (Freshwater Head and Lateral Line Erosion, FHLLE)

Prevalence Index
WF - 2
Method of Diagnosis
History and clinical signs
History/Physical Examination
Various numbers of pin-head size to larger depressions, especially near the lateral line of head or flanks; cachexia
Treatment
1. Improve environment and nutrition
2. Appropriate antibiotic

COMMENTS
Epidemiology/Pathogenesis
This important, chronic, idiopathic syndrome primarily affects discus, oscars, and other large South American cichlids (e.g., jurupari). It presents as mild to severe areas of pitting and depigmentation on the skin. Lesions are most prevalent near the lateral line of the head. Lesioned fish can behave normally for quite some time, but eventually become anorexic and lethargic.

Almost all descriptive accounts of this syndrome are based on the popular aquarium literature, and there are no published scientific reports. One hypothesis is that a *Hexamita*-like flagellate, which is present as a latent intestinal infection, spreads by both extension and hematogenously to the gall bladder, peritoneal cavity,

spleen, kidney, and associated vasculature. In later stages, the classical hole-in-the-head lesions appear, first as pinpoint lesions (Fig. II-89, *A*) that may discharge small, white "threads" of material containing the parasites. The lesions then expand and often coalesce, producing large crateriform lesions (Fig. II-89, *B*) that may become secondarily infected with bacteria or fungi. The ultimate cause of death may be secondary microbial infections.

While *Hexamita*-like flagellates are a problem in aquarium fish (see *PROBLEM 69*) and can infect many tissues, their relationship to FHLLE is open to question. Some claim that FHLLE may be caused by a mineral imbalance that results in skeletal damage leading to the pitting lesions. They further speculate that heavy concentrations of flagellates in the intestine can cause maladsorption, leading to the mineral imbalance (Untergasser, 1991).

Clinical impressions indicate that some type of stress, such as overcrowding, poor water quality, or poor nutrition, may predispose fish to FHLLE. Since larger, older, fish are mainly afflicted, FHLLE may be a sequela of decreasing immunocompetence in aging individuals. The common presence of HLLE-type lesions in unrelated fish species (see *PROBLEM 90*) suggests that this may be a nonspecific response to stress.
Diagnosis
Diagnosis of FHLLE is based on the observance of typical, pitting (often symmetrical) lesions associated with the lateral line or flanks (Fig. II-89, *A* and *B*). It is advisable to culture the lesions for bacteria, since some fish respond at least partially to antibiotic therapy (E.J. Noga, Unpublished Data).
Treatment
Most published treatments have focused on controlling *Hexamita*, although there is no proof that this agent is even present in most lesions (Ferguson, 1988; E.J. Noga, Unpublished Data). The environment should always be improved, especially by reducing overcrowding, performing frequent water changes, and providing a varied and balanced diet. Some claim that providing a calcium/phosphorus/vitamin D supplement to the diet can cure fish (Untergasser, 1991).

244

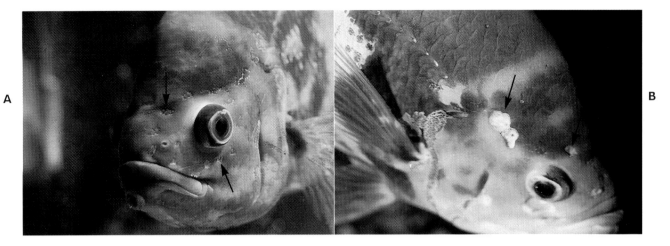

Fig. II-89 A, Oscar with early stage of hole-in-the-head disease (*arrows*). **B,** Oscar with more advanced stage of hole-in-the-head disease (*arrows*).

(*A* and *B* photographs courtesy of T. Wenzel.)

PROBLEM 90
Marine Hole-in-the-Head Syndrome (Marine Head and Lateral Line Erosion, MHLLE)

Prevalence Index
WM - 1
Method of Diagnosis
History and clinical signs
History
Varies with primary cause, but often chronic, low mortalities; various-sized, shallow to deep skin lesions
Physical Examination
Various-sized erosions or ulcerations on the body, often associated with the lateral line canal
Treatment
Improve environment and nutrition

COMMENTS
Epidemiology/Pathogenesis
Marine hole-in-the-head syndrome is probably the most common chronic disease that affects marine aquarium fish, especially tangs (Acanthuridae) and angelfish (Pomacanthidae).

Lesions usually begin on the head as shallow, pinpoint foci that expand in size, depth, and surface area (Fig. II-90, *A*). Advanced lesions may be deep. Lesions often extend to the flanks (Fig. II-90, *B*) and are typically associated with the lateral line. Fish may feed and behave normally, even while they are severely affected. Proposed explanations for the disease include inadequate nutrition, especially ascorbate deficiency (Blasiola, 1989) and toxins released by certain activated carbons (Frakes, 1988). A reovirus has been isolated from one case (Varner & Lewis, 1991) but has not been proven to be the cause. Other cases have been associ-

ated with acid-fast bacterial infection (E. Noga, Unpublished Data), suggesting that this *disease* may actually be a common clinical sign of chronic stress in reef fish.

Interestingly, grossly similar lesions (termed *lateral line necrosis*) have been seen in both feral and cultured Atlantic cod, a cold water species (Fig. II-90, *C*) (Moller & Anders, 1986). Nerve fibers running from the destroyed lateral line to the brain were inflamed, and their medullary ganglia were degenerated (Naeve, 1968).

Diagnosis
Diagnosis of MHLLE is simply based on the observance of typical, pitting (often symmetrical) lesions associated with the lateral line or flanks (Fig. II-90, *A* and *B*). It may be advisable to culture advanced lesions for bacteria.

Treatment
Treatment of MHLLE is purely empirical and relies on elimination of possible initiating causes. This should include a thorough examination for nutritional and environmental stress. Changing the brand of activated carbon used in filters may help (T. Frakes, Personal Communication). Stray voltage is also suspected to be a cause of MHLLE (Johnson, 1993); it may also cause other neurological signs, including disorientation; it is corrected by determining if *stray* voltage is present (i.e., an electrical device is not properly grounded) and eliminating the cause. Instead of trying to find the stray current, a grounding device to correct the problem can be installed (e.g., Solution Ground™, Sandpoint). If such manipulations are unsuccessful, a primary infectious cause should be suspected. Fish can recover from MHLLE but often have permanent scarring (Hemdal, 1989) (Fig. II-90, *C*).

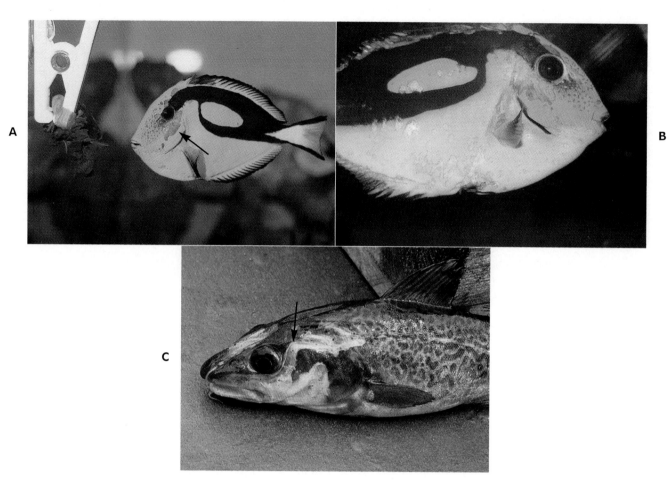

Fig. II-90 **A,** Powder blue tang with mild to moderate MHLLE (*arrow*). **B,** Powder blue tang with severe MHLLE affecting entire body. **C,** Atlantic cod with MHLLE (*arrow*).

(*A* and *B* photographs courtesy of S. Johnson; *C* photograph courtesy of H. Moller.)

PROBLEM 91
Pancreas Disease

Prevalence Index
CM - 3
Method of Diagnosis
1. Rule-out of other problems
2. Histopathology of diagnostic lesions
History/Physical Examination
Anorexia; emaciation; hemorrhages near pancreatic tissue
Treatment
None

COMMENTS
Epidemiology
Pancreas disease is a severe, usually chronic problem that affects sea-cultured salmonids in Europe and the northeast Pacific coast (United States, Canada). Fish usually develop the disease 6 to 12 weeks after transfer to seawater, but outbreaks have occurred after 2 years in seawater. There may be 100% morbidity. While most fish usually recover, they may be "poor doers" and susceptible to other diseases.

Pancreas disease is suspected to be an infectious disease, based on transmission studies (McVicar, 1990), although histopathology lesions are suggestive of a vitamin E-selenium deficiency (Ferguson et al., 1986). However, it is unclear whether the latter may be a secondary effect of the anorexia.

Clinical Signs/Pathogenesis
GROSS LESIONS
Fish are depressed, anorexic, and emaciated. Internally, there are hemorrhages in the pancreas and in pancreatic fat between the pyloric ceca. In some cases, there may be tissue atrophy between the pyloric ceca.

HISTOPATHOLOGY
Active lesions exhibit acute, diffuse necrosis of pancreatic acinar tissue, with inflammation and fibrosis. There may also be necrosis of cardiac myocytes. Recovering fish may have foci of regenerating acinar tissue among the fibrotic lesions.

Diagnosis
Diagnosis is based on the absence of any identifiable etiological agent combined with the characteristic histopathological lesions.

Table II-92 Miscellaneous, important idiopathic diseases of fish.

Disease	Hosts	Geographic range	Morbidity/ mortality	Diagnostic features	References
Infectious salmonid anemia	Salmonids	Norway	Chronic	See *PROBLEM 43*	
Winter kill	Channel catfish; hybrid striped bass	USA	Chronic	See *PROBLEM 33*	
Ulcerative dermal necrosis	Atlantic salmon; brown trout	Great Britain; Ireland; France; Sweden; Portugal	Acute/ subacute/ chronic	Shallow grey area that progresses to deep ulcer; progressive focal pemphigoid to bullous lesions; often secondary bacterial, fungal pathogens; virus-like particles in some lesions	Lounatmaa & Janatuinen, 1978 Roberts, 1989c
Pacific cod ulcerative epidermal hyperplasia	Pacific cod	Bering Sea	Chronic	1 to 50 mm ulcers of raised, circular, ring-shaped lesions; hypertrophied epithelial cells; herpesvirus-associated	McArn et al., 1978 McCain et al., 1979
Atlantic cod ulcus syndrome	Atlantic cod	Baltic Sea	Subacute/ chronic	2 mm papules producing 2 to 18 cm skin ulcers, leading to depigmentation and scarring; iridovirus-associated; peak prevalence in fall; pollution-associated	Larsen & Jensen, 1982
Epizootic ulcerative syndrome (EUS)				See *PROBLEM 34*	
Ambicoloration	Turbot; halibut; other flatfishes	Europe; USA	None	Various-sized areas of skin depigmentation (Fig. II-92, *B*): possibly nutrition-related (e.g., vitamin A); appearance reduces value	Moller & Anders, 1986 Kanazawa, 1993
Gill necrosis	Common carp; eel; trout	Europe; Soviet Union	Acute to chronic	Associated with high unionized ammonia Acute: neurological signs Chronic: gill edema, progressing to epithelial necrosis and hyperplasia; branchitis; iridovirus isolated but unlikely cause; often secondary invaders; diagnosed by measuring blood ammonia and ruling out other causes of gill damage	Kovacs-Gayer, 1984
Red fillet syndrome	Channel catfish	USA	Acute	Punctate to ecchymotic to diffuse pink or red foci in muscle; associated with acute, sublethal hypoxia, such as that caused by environmental hypoxia (*PROBLEM 1*) or PGD (*PROBLEM 59*); appearance causes rejection by processors	Johnson, 1993
Systemic granuloma/ visceral granuloma/ Malawi bloat	Salmonids; gilthead seabream; African rift lake cichlids	USA; Israel; Canada	Chronic	Multiple granulomas in viscera, often surrounding calcium deposits; may be associated with mineral deposition in kidney in salmonids (nephrocalcinosis, see *PROBLEM 80*); cases in gilthead sea bream associated with hypertyrosinemia; nutrition appears to influence disease, but precise cause is unknown; some cases in cichlids associated with protozoan infections (see *PROBLEM 71*) (Fig. II-92, *A*)	Paperna, 1981 Landolt, 1975 Noga, 1986a
Net-pen liver disease (NLD)	Atlantic salmon	Washington, USA; British Columbia, Canada	Chronic	Affects fish in first year at sea, usually summer; mortality to 90%; liver small, friable, yellow; megalocytosis (diagnostic) and other hepatic lesions suggests hepatotoxin as a cause (algal toxin from resident natural foods?)	Kent, 1990

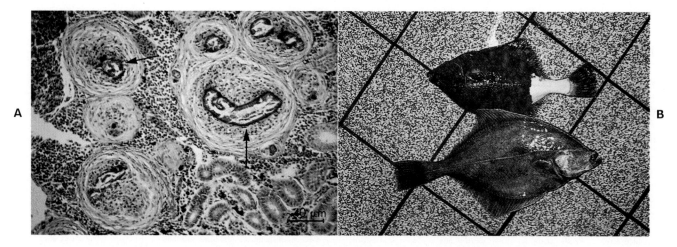

Fig. II-92 A, Visceral granuloma lesion in a salmonid. Note calcification and necrosis (*arrows*) in the center of the granuloma. Von Kossa. **B,** Ambicoloration in a flounder.

(*A* photograph courtesy of C.L. Davis Foundation for Veterinary Pathology; *B* photograph courtesy of H. Moller.)

Treatment

No treatment is available. Reducing stress during the acute phase can lessen mortalities. Feeding fish smaller pellets may reduce the anorexia and overall mortality (Kent, 1992).

PROBLEM 92
Miscellaneous Important Idiopathic Diseases

Prevalence Index
See specific disease
Method of Diagnosis
Rule-out of other problems
History/Physical Examination
See specific disease
Treatment
See specific disease

COMMENTS
See Table II-92

CHAPTER **21**

Problem 93

Egg diseases
93. Egg diseases

PROBLEM 93
Prevalence Index
See specific disease
Method of Diagnosis
See specific disease
History/Physical Examination
See specific disease
Treatment
See specific disease

COMMENTS
See Table II-93

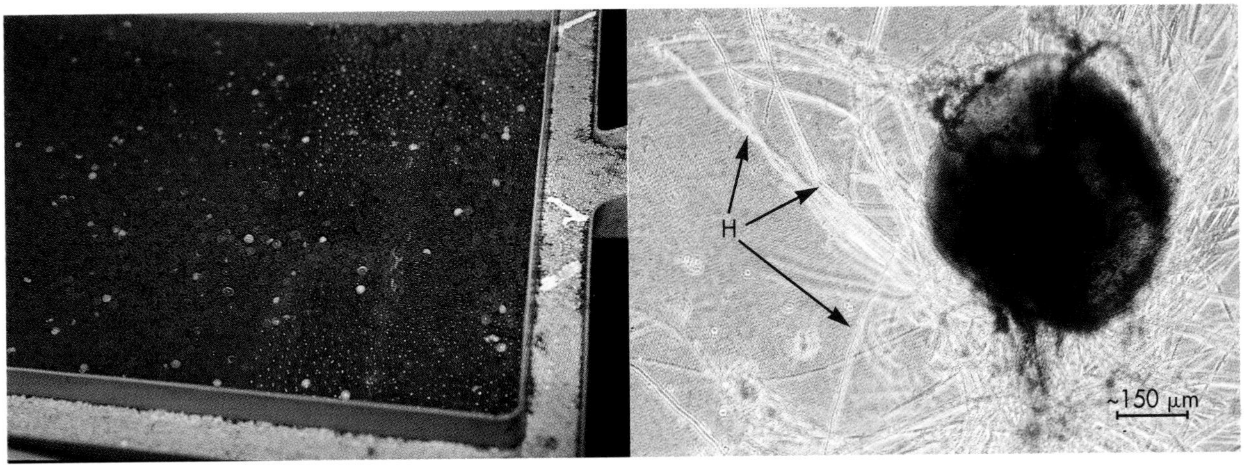

Fig. II-93 **A,** Rainbow trout eggs in an incubator tray. Viable eggs are brown; dead eggs are white because of precipitation of egg protein. **B,** A dead, water mold–infected egg of a Madagascar rainbow fish. Many hyphae (*H*) grow in and through the egg.

Table II-93 Diseases commmonly affecting eggs.

Disease or condition	Host range	Diagnostic clinical signs	Prophylaxis/treatment	References
Gelatinous egg mass	Cyprinids; ictalurids; other species	Eggs stick together; increased secondary bacterial or fungal infection	Treat with sodium sulfite (PHARMACOPOEIA) or other appropriate drug (see Table III-3)	
Dead eggs (bacterial infection, fungal infection, infertile egg)	All fish	Entire egg(s) opaque (Fig. II-93, A and B)	Address pertinent problem	
Polypodium hydriforme infection	Sturgeons; paddlefish	Coelenterate parasite in eggs	None	Raikova, 1994
Icthyoodinium chabellardi infection	Atlantic herring	Dinoflagellate parasite in eggs	None	Noga & Levy (in press)
Soft egg disease	Salmonids	Eggs become soft and flaccid during incubation because perforations in shell allow loss of fluid; may be caused by bacterial or amoebic infestation	Antiseptic treatment may help; maintain good hygiene in hatchery	Warren, 1981
Blue sac disease	Salmonids; other species	Yolk sac swollen and discolored	Reduce/prevent high ammonia or pH change	
Coagulated yolk disease	Salmonids; other species	White foci in the yolk sac	Probably water quality problem	
Smothering	Salmonids; many other species	Eggs covered with debris	Excess turbidity	See PROBLEM 85
Physical shock	Salmonids; probably other species	Movement of eggs between just after fertilization to eyed stage	Avoid moving eggs during this time	Post et al., 1974
Light	Salmonids; probably other species	Too bright, direct sunlight; exposure to short wavelength (blue white) emissions from artificial lighting	Minimize exposure	Leitritz, 1976
Temperature shock	Salmonids; probably other species	Mortality	When acclimating shipped eggs, don't increase temperature >5° C/minute	
Constricted yolk disease	Salmonids	Yolk sac becomes constricted, almost splitting in two	Idiopathic	
Gas bubble disease	Salmonids; many other species	Gas emboli in egg	Prevent gas supersaturation	See PROBLEM 10
Premature hatch	Salmonids; probably other species	Medication of eggs just before hatching	Do not medicate eggs at least 24 hours before hatching (at least 3 days for salmonids)	Post, 1987

PART III

METHODS FOR TREATING FISH DISEASES

CHAPTER **22**

General Concepts In Therapy

When and How to Treat

The isolation or identification of a certain pathogen does not always warrant treatment. The practitioner should assess all relevant variables, including pathogens involved, possible treatment sequelae, mortality rate, dollar value of the population, cost of the treatment, and legal considerations. For example, water-borne antiparasite treatments are often contraindicated if primary viral or bacterial infections are in progress. Caution is also recommended if ponds are treated during hot, summer weather when phytoplankton blooms are dense, since chemical treatment could precipitate a severe oxygen depletion (Allison, 1962).

Cost of treatment versus cost of continued losses is an important consideration for commercial fish producers. If ten 1-kilogram fish are dying daily and if the fish are worth $2.00 per kilogram, a $1200 treatment of potassium permanganate may not be warranted, especially if nonmedical treatments can be used (e.g., reduce stress). In contrast, the owner of a recreational pond or an individual pet fish owner may be willing to spend several hundred dollars to save just a few fish because the animals' importance transcends their commercial value.

Treatment Options in Various Aquaculture Systems

Another important factor influencing treatment is the type of culture system (Table III-1). Culture systems may be classified according to the degree of control that the culturist can exert on the environmental conditions prevailing in the system. The four major types of culture systems follow: aquaria, ponds, cages, and flow-through systems.

Aquaria are the most highly controllable culture systems, since they typically have supplementary methods for maintaining temperature, biological filtration, and oxygen. They are also most amenable to various water-borne treatments because of the relatively small water volume in the system and thus the ease of manipulability.

Ponds, which are more influenced by natural factors such as light, temperature, and rainfall and thus natural

biological cycles (e.g., algal growth, nitrification), are less controllable by the culturist. Also, interventional strategies are more limited compared with aquaria.

Cages or net-pens are even more susceptible to the vagaries of natural environmental changes. Water-borne treatments in such systems are limited. Thus, fish that need to be treated in such systems must usually be either removed from the cage or net-pen and treated in a closed system (e.g., bath treatment), or medications must be delivered orally; this is required because drugs added to water quickly diffuse away and do not maintain therapeutic concentrations and may cause serious damage to other forms of aquatic life.

Raceways and other flow-through systems are the least manipulable systems by virtue of the constant and rapid water turnover. Flow-through systems are even more limited than cages in the ability to use water-borne treatments; similar adverse environmental consequences can follow such treatments.

Treatment of Marine Versus Freshwater Fish

Treatment modalities for marine fish are similar to those for freshwater fish. Important differences in treating marine fish primarily relate to use of water-borne medications (Noga, 1992). The chemistry of saltwater influences the toxicity of many substances. The first important factor to consider is whether the agent is effective in saltwater. Some antibiotics, notably the tetracyclines, and chelate divalent cations (calcium and magnesium) are present in high concentrations in seawater; this can reduce their uptake into the fish, especially if given as a water-borne treatment. The activity of many other therapeutants, such as copper and organophosphates, is affected by seawater. While many of these therapeutants can be used in seawater, the dosage is usually higher than that used in freshwater.

Second, many medications for marine fish are toxic to invertebrates, so their use in aquarium *reef systems* must be avoided. This is especially true for copper, formalin, and organophosphates. Antibiotics, even when they are not directly toxic to invertebrates, may still be harmful. Anemones, corals, and some other invertebrates have

Table III-I   Some characteristics of the major types of fish culture systems.

	Aquaria	Ponds	Cages/net-pens	Raceways and other flow-through systems
Water turnover*	None	None to low	Moderate to high	High
Ability to manipulate environment	Considerable	Some	Little	Virtually none
Water-borne treatments available	Many	Some	Few	Few

*Defined as the amount of water exchange that normally occurs over time (not including water changes intentionally made by the culturist during therapy).

symbiotic bacteria and algae that are required for their survival. If these microorganisms are susceptible to an antibiotic, it could indirectly kill the invertebrate host. For these reasons, it is best to avoid exposure of invertebrates to any fish medications.

Third, drug metabolism (pharmacokinetics) varies tremendously, depending on whether a fish is in saltwater or freshwater. In freshwater, teleost fish are hypertonic relative to their environment and regulate osmotic balance by actively taking up ions, especially via the gills. They also drink almost no water and reabsorb as many ions as possible in the kidney, producing a dilute urine. In full strength seawater, fish face the opposite problem, a hypertonic environment (10 to 14 ppt salinity is close to isosmotic for most species). Thus, fish in full-strength seawater drink large amounts to regain lost water and excrete the excess ions via the gills and kidney (Prosser, 1973b).

Whereas similar types of pathogens affect freshwater and marine fish, relatively few pathogens are transmissible from freshwater to marine fish, or vice versa (i.e., most pathogens affect either marine or freshwater fish, but not both). This is the rationale for why many freshwater pathogens can be treated with salt and many marine pathogens can be treated with freshwater.

Fish Pharmacology

Proper use of therapeutants for fish diseases depends not only on a thorough knowledge of the disease under consideration, but also on the properties of the pharmacological agent used, the species under treatment, and the environmental conditions.

Uptake of Drugs in Relation to Route of Exposure

In contrast to the more traditional routes of administration of therapeutic agents used in treating terrestrial animals, aquatic species are most often treated by adding drugs directly to the water. This mode of therapy is used not only for external problems, such as ectoparasites, but for systemic diseases as well. This method of administration adds another complex variable to the factors that must be considered when attempting to establish the proper therapeutic dose for treating fish under particular circumstances. The following several factors must be considered when treating fish via water-borne administration:

1. The epidermis of fish is not keratinized. Living, dividing cells extend throughout the entire epidermis. This lack of keratinization may increase the ability of drugs to penetrate the epidermis. Conversely, when fish are removed from a therapeutic bath to untreated water, systemic concentrations may decay rapidly because of rapid movement down a concentration gradient.

2. The gill, a highly vascularized organ with a vast blood supply near the epithelial surface, may also be important in drug uptake and excretion.

3. The relative importance of uptake across the gastrointestinal tract in water-borne administration will be influenced by the physiological state and environmental conditions. For example, fish in seawater drink significant amounts of water and may absorb significant amounts of drug via the gastrointestinal tract. Freshwater fish drink little water; thus this route may not be as important in this environment. For example, water-borne uptake of sulfas by rainbow trout in seawater is much greater than uptake in freshwater, probably because of differences in drinking rates (Bergjso & Bergjso, 1978). Conversely, oxytetracycline is less well absorbed in seawater because it chelates divalent cations; the charged complex is not available for uptake across cell membranes. Uptake for many other drugs is less efficient in seawater than in freshwater (Lundestad, 1992).

4. The relative importance of drug uptake across the gastrointestinal versus respiratory versus epidermal epithelium in fish is unknown. Indeed, for many drugs, the relationship between concentration in the water and systemic levels has not been determined and dosage levels are based on empirical data.

5. When drugs are added to the water, their half-life within the fish must be considered, as well as their half-life within the environment. The chemical activity and rate of uptake may be influenced by pH, temperature, light, water hardness, and many other factors (Lundestad, 1992).

6. The water is the life support system of aquatic species and adding any substance to it must be done with full consideration made to the potential consequences of that chemical on environmental quality. For example, formalin, commonly used as a parasiticide, is a strong reducing agent and will rapidly reduce oxygen levels if adequate aeration is not provided. Other drugs, such as methylene blue and certain antibiotics, inhibit the abil-

ity of nitrifying bacteria to detoxify nitrogenous wastes, resulting in the accumulation of these toxic metabolites.

Drug Metabolism in Fish

As in mammals the liver is the primary organ for detoxification of drugs in fish. Available evidence indicates that many qualitative similarities exist in the metabolism of drugs by fish and mammals (James, 1986; Franklin et al., 1980). Fish can carry out many, and possibly all, of the Phase I (oxidation, reduction, and hydrolysis) reactions utilized by mammals to detoxify or activate drugs. Although qualitative differences exist among various fish species, oxidation reactions have been demonstrated in representatives of the most primitive to the most advanced fish groups. These reactions are carried out in the microsomal fraction of liver and require reduced nicotinamide adenine dinucleotide phosphate (NADPH) and oxygen, making them similar to the enzymatic reactions performed by the mammalian mixed function oxidase (MFO) system. Some of the oxidative enzyme systems of fish are inducible by substances, such as DDT,

that are known to induce mammalian enzyme systems. Procarcinogens, such as aflatoxin, can be activated by fish to their active carcinogenic form, producing tumors such as hepatomas in the case of aflatoxin. Some fish can also perform azo- and nitro-reductions, or hydrolyze compounds, such as succinylcholine and organophosphates.

Phase II reactions involve conjugate formation and subsequent excretion via urinary and biliary routes. Fish can conjugate drugs with a number of compounds, including glucuronic acid, glycine, glutathione, acetate, taurine, and sulfate. Excretion appears to be mainly via the urine and bile, but some conjugates are also excreted across the gills.

Fish appear to metabolize drugs at about one tenth the rate in mammals. Also, the temperature optimum for many of these reactions is lower than that of mammals, usually approximating the temperature of the fish's natural environment (see *DEGREE DAYS*, p. 259).

Legal Use of Therapeutants

Policies regarding the enforcement of regulations on the use of therapeutants have changed significantly over the

Table III-2 Drugs that are approved for treating food fish in the United States and their approved uses.*

Drug	Approved labels	FDA(US)-approved use	Tolerance	Comments
Formalin	Formalin-F (Natchez Animal Supply Company, Natchez, Miss.); Paracide-F (Argent Chemical Laboratories, Redmond, Wash.); Parasite-S (Western Chemical, Ferndale, Wash.)	Parasiticide for salmonids, channel catfish, largemouth bass, and bluegill: Tanks and raceways: > 50° F: up to 170 ppm for up to 1 hour < 50° F: up to 250 ppm for up to 1 hour Earthen ponds: 15 to 25 ppm Control water molds on eggs of salmonids and esocids: 1000 to 2000 ppm for 15 minutes in egg treatment tanks	None required	Ponds may be retreated in 5 to 10 days if needed
Sulfadimethoxine/ ormetoprim	Romet-30 and Romet B (Hoffman-LaRoche, Nutley, N.J.)	Antibacterial against *Aeromonas salmonicida* of salmonids and *Edwardsiella ictaluri* of channel catfish; feed 50 mg/kg of fish per day for 5 days	0.1 ppm in salmonids and catfish	Salmonids: 42-day withdrawal time; channel catfish: 3-day withdrawal time
Sulfamerazine	Sulfamerazine in Fish Grade (American Cyanamid, Princeton, N.J.)	Antibacterial against *Aeromonas salmonicida* of rainbow, brook, and brown trout; feed 10 g/100 lb of fish per day for 14 days	Zero tolerance in uncooked, edible tissues of trout	21-day withdrawal time; not currently available
Oxytetracycline hydrochloride	Terramycin for fish (Pfizer, New York, N.Y.)	Antibacterial against *Aeromonas salmonicida*, motile aeromonads, and *Pseudomonas* in salmonids; motile aeromonads and *Pseudomonas* in channel catfish; feed 2.5-3.75 g/100 lb per day for 10 days	0.1 ppm in salmonids and catfish	Water temperature must be > 48.2° F when treating salmonids; water temperature must be > 62° F when treating channel catfish; 21-day withdrawal time
Tricaine methanesulfonate	Finquel (Argent Chemical Laboratories, Redmond, Wash.)	Anesthetic: 15 to 66 ppm for 6 to 48 hours for sedation 50 to 330 ppm for 1 to 40 minutes for anesthesia	None required	21-day withdrawal time

Modified from Schnick et al., 1989, with data supplied by RK Ringer.
*These drugs are approved for use only with the specific commercial formulation listed. Bulk drugs from a chemical company or similar unapproved labels are illegal. Approval is given only for the indications (disease) and methods of administration given.

past several years; the use of therapeutants in fish is receiving increased regulatory scrutiny in the United States and elsewhere (Anonymous, 1992). As is true for other animals, the legal use of drugs in fish is regulated in the United States by the Food and Drug Administration (FDA). This includes all fish, not just those intended for human consumption. All drugs, including animal drugs, must be approved by the FDA (note that pesticides must be registered by the United States Environmental Protection Agency [EPA], and animal biologics/vaccines must be licensed by the United States Department of Agriculture [USDA]). Specific drugs (e.g., formalin, oxytetracycline) are approved for use in specific fish (e.g., channel catfish) and for treating a specific pathogen (e.g., motile aeromonad infection). The precise duration and method of dosing (e.g., in water, in feed) is also indicated. Any other use of an approved drug is considered an extralabel use (see below). The use of drugs in fish is coming under increasing scrutiny, so the practitioner should determine the current status of a drug before recommending its use. Any therapies must also comply with federal or state regulations that govern the discharge of chemically treated effluent into waters (Meyer, 1989).

Tables III-2, III-3, III-4, and III-5 give the current legal status in the United States of many therapeutants

that have been commonly used to treat fish diseases. Note that drugs that are considered "not low regulatory priority" (Table III-4A) or "high regulatory priority" (Table III-4B) should **never** be used in the United States without an INAD exemption (see p. 258). "High regulatory priority" drugs are agents that pose the greatest public health concern and ones in which the FDA is most likely to take regulatory action. Be aware that status of all drugs is in a constant state of flux. Regulations also vary significantly among nations (Michel & Alderman, 1992; Alderman & Michel, 1992).

The Use and Abuse of Drugs in Aquaculture

In the United States, FDA regulates the use of drugs in all fish, regardless of whether they are raised for human consumption (e.g., trout, salmon, catfish) or for other purposes (e.g., as pets).

In those instances where a drug has been approved, legal restrictions on its use are often much narrower than the use to which it has been applied by aquaculturists.

A great many agents have been used to treat diseases in food fish. Few of these drugs are legally approved for use in food fish; to be licensed for use in fish produced for human consumption, a drug must pass rigorous testing

Table III-3   Uses of drugs that are unapproved for treating food fish in the United States but are of low regulatory priority.*

Drug	Use
Hydrogen peroxide	Treating water molds on all species and life stages of fish, including eggs: 250 to 500 mg/l
Acetic acid	Treating ectoparasitic protozoa: 1000 to 2000 ppm for 1 to 2 minutes
Calcium oxide (unslaked lime)	Treating ectoparasitic protozoa of fingerling to adult fish: 2000 mg/l for 5 seconds
Onion (whole form)	Treating crustacean infestations and deterring sea lice from infesting marine fish of all life stages
Garlic (whole form)	Treating helminth and sea lice infestations on marine fish of all life stages
Magnesium sulfate + sodium chloride	Treating monogenean and crustacean infestations on fish of all life stages: 30,000 mg MgSO$_4$ + 7000 mg NaCl/l for 5 to 10 minutes
Sodium chloride	1. Osmoregulatory enhancer to relieve stress and prevent shock: 5000 to 10,000 mg/l for an indefinite period
	2. Treating ectoparasitic protozoa: 30,000 mg/l for 10 to 30 minutes
Potassium chloride	Osmoregulatory enhancer to relieve stress and prevent shock: 10 to 2000 mg/l for an indefinite period
Calcium chloride	Osmoregulatory enhancer to relieve stress and prevent osmotic shock: raise hardness to 150 mg/l as CaCO$_3$
Calcium chloride	Increase calcium to ensure proper egg hardening; raise hardness level by 10 to 20 mg/l as CaCO$_3$
Sodium sulfite	Treating eggs to improve their hatchability: 15% solution for 5 to 8 minutes
Papain	Removing gelatinous matrix of fish egg masses to improve hatchability and reduce disease incidence: 0.2% solution
Fuller's earth	Reducing adhesiveness of eggs and improving hatchability
Urea + tannic acid	Denaturing the adhesive component of fish eggs: add about 400,000 eggs to 5 liters of water with 15 g urea+ 20 g NaCl and incubate for 6 minutes, then transfer eggs to 0.75 g tannic acid in 5 liters of water for another 6 minutes
Ice	Reduce metabolic rate of fish during transport
Carbon dioxide	Anesthetic: 200 to 400 ppm for 4 minutes
Sodium bicarbonate	Anesthetic: 142 to 642 ppm for 5 minutes
Povidone-iodine	Egg disinfectant: 100 mg/l for 10 minutes after water hardening of eggs; 50 mg/l for 30 minutes during water hardening

From MacMillan, 1993.

*Low regulatory priority: Not officially approved by the FDA (US) for the use given, but the FDA (US) is "unlikely to object" to use of these compounds if they are used under the conditions specified. This enforcement position is considered neither approval nor affirmation of the product's safety or efficacy (*Water Farming Journal*, March, 1992, p. 4). These drugs are considered low regulatory priority only if used under the exact condition specified.

Table III-4, A Uses of drugs that are unapproved for treating food fish in the United States and are **not** of low regulatory priority.*

Drug	Use
Benzalkonium chloride; benzethonium chloride (quaternary ammonium compounds)	To treat external bacterial infections (bacterial gill disease)
Copper sulfate	To treat external protozoan, bacterial, or fungal infestations or infections
Sodium chlorite	To treat ectoparasitic protozoa
Potassium permanganate	To treat ectoparasitic protozoa*

From MacMillan, 1993.
*Not low regulatory priority: The FDA (US) has serious concerns about the uses of these compounds when used as described above because of a lack of data about efficacy and/or environmental/human safety.
†FDA (US) is "currently deferring regulatory action against the use of potassium permanganate in food fish."

Table III-4, B Uses of drugs that are unapproved for treating food fish in the United States and are considered high regulatory priority by FDA (US).*

Drug	Use
Chloramphenicol	Antibiotic
Nitrofurazone	Antibiotic
Furazolidone	Antibiotic
Nifurpirinol	Antibiotic
Quinolones	Antibiotic
Fluoroquinolones	Antibiotic
Malachite green	Parasiticide, fungicide
Methylene blue	Fungicide
Acriflavine	Parasiticide
Central nervous system stimulants and depressants (benzocaine, quinaldine sulfate, 2-phenoxyethenol)	Anesthetic; sedative
Hormones and steroids (e.g., human chorionic gonadotropin, pituitary extracts, 17 alpha-methyltestosterone)	Induce reproduction; change sex; induce sterility

*Note that some of these drugs may be used in the United States under an approved INAD.

Table III-5 Chemicals that are not considered to be drugs by the FDA (US) for the uses given.*

Drug	Use
Calcium hydroxide (slaked lime)	To raise pH of water or pond bottom to 10
Calcium carbonate	To alter pH and/or total alkalinity of water
Sodium hydroxide	To raise the pH of water
Tris buffer	To buffer pH changes in freshwater or saltwater
Oxygen	To maintain saturated dissolved oxygen levels in water to ensure fish survival

From MacMillan, 1993.
*Not considered a drug use: compounds that are not regulated by the FDA (US) when used as specified above.

for efficacy in treating a specific disease in a specific species at a specific dosage and route of administration. Extensive data must also be obtained on residue dynamics.

The requirement of current regulations for such rigorous testing for each particular application of a drug has discouraged the pursuit of new drug approvals by pharmaceutical companies, because the relatively small aquaculture market often would not allow them to recoup their expenses. The problem of a lack of legal therapeutants is compounded by the resistance of many of the common pathogens to the presently licensed drugs because of injudicious use of those drugs, especially the antimicrobial agents. However, it is often impossible to avoid repeated use of an antimicrobial agent because of the small number of legally approved antibiotics available.

In the United States the Fish and Wildlife Service has gathered much data necessary for the registration of several drugs considered essential to aquaculture, which has reduced the regulatory burden placed on the developing aquaculture industry in the United States. The FDA has also been asked to consider classifying eggs, fry, small fingerlings, and broodfish as nonfood fish for registration purposes, which, if approved, would allow use of a broader range of compounds on these life stages. At present, however, a food fish in the United States is defined as **any** individual that is used for human consumption at some time in its life. The treatment of nonfood fish, including pet fish, is under much less regulatory scrutiny, but increasing regulatory oversight is also anticipated in this sector.

Many pet fish remedies are still sold as over-the-counter preparations, including numerous antibiotics. Often these preparations have been found to be ineffective at the recommended dosages (Trust, 1972). Also, prolonged exposure to suboptimal concentrations of antibiotics have caused increased incidence of resistant strains of fish-pathogenic bacteria (Dixon et al., 1990). It is the ethical duty of the clinician to use any drug judiciously and to avoid unauthorized use if at all possible.

Legal Use of Unapproved Drugs

INAD Exemptions

Certain unapproved drugs may be used in aquaculture in the United States under certain circumstances by obtaining an investigational new animal drug (INAD) exemption from FDA. An INAD gives the sponsor (i.e., drug user) the authority to buy the unapproved drug and use it for clinical investigation. It also authorizes the slaughter of treated fish for human consumption and assigns an investigational withdrawal period. FDA grants INAD exemptions for the investigational use of drugs. While FDA's purpose in granting an INAD is to generate research data to support eventual FDA approval of the drug, an INAD exemption may also allow, in certain limited situations, legal treatment of fish with an unap-

proved drug. It is important to note that INADs are granted by the FDA's Center for Veterinary Medicine (CVM) with the expectation that data to support an approval of the drug will be generated and submitted to CVM. This data is ultimately intended to generate a New Animal Drug Application (NADA), which FDA will then consider for possible approval of the drug.

Use of EPA-Registered Pesticides

Regarding the use of EPA-registered pesticides for drug purposes (e.g., diquat to treat bacterial gill disease [BGD]), the FDA's position is that the agency will not object to the use of a registered pesticide when used in accordance with the EPA-registered labeling, if the pesticide has a secondary therapeutic benefit, provided that the conditions for which the pesticide is registered actually exist in the treatment situation. An example would be the use of an EPA-registered algicide in a situation where an algae problem actually exists and where the chemical happens to have a secondary therapeutic benefit to the fish (e.g., controls a parasite infestation).

Extra-label Use of Drugs

Drugs approved by the FDA for use in other animals or humans may be used in aquatic species when certain criteria are met. These criteria constitute the FDA's extra-label drug use policy. Note that **only** drugs that are approved by the FDA for some other species can be used in an extra-label manner.

FDA generally allows veterinarians to prescribe any approved drug in an extra-label fashion for nonfood animals (e.g., pet fish). However, in species produced for human consumption, there is much more oversight. For example, several drugs can **never** be used in an extra-label fashion in food-producing animals. They include chloramphenicol, clenbuterol, diethylstilbesterol, all nitroimidazoles (including dimetridazole, metronidazole, and ipronidazole), furazolidone (except for approved topical use, there is no extra-label application for aquatic species), nitrofurazone (except for approved topical use, there is no extra-label application for aquatic species), and all other nitrofurans. Also, use of any drugs that are approved for use in humans is strongly discouraged. Extra-label use does **not** allow the use of an unapproved drug in the feed. Only other routes (e.g., via injection or via water-borne methods) are allowed.

To be used in an extra-label fashion, use of a drug must meet the criteria of the FDA Center for Veterinary Medicine's extra-label use policy, including the following:

1. A careful medical diagnosis is made by an attending veterinarian, within the context of a valid veterinarian client-patient relationship.

2. A determination is made that there is no marketed drug specifically labeled to treat the condition diagnosed or that drug therapy at the dosage recommended by the labeling has been found to be clinically ineffective by the veterinarian in the animals to be treated.

3. Procedures are instituted to ensure that identity of the treated animals is carefully maintained.
4. A significantly extended time period is assigned for drug withdrawal before marketing for human consumption; steps are taken to ensure that the assigned time frames are met and that no illegal residues occur.
5. The prescribed or dispensed extra-label drug (prescription legend or over-the-counter) bears labeling information that is adequate to ensure the safe and proper use of the product.

Examples of drugs listed in the *PHARMACOPOEIA* that could be used in an extra-label manner include fenbendazole (Panacur), levamisole (Levasol), mebendazole (Telmin), monensin (Rumensin), piperazine, praziquantel (Droncit), and some antibiotics.

Legal Withdrawal Times

When food fish are harvested for human consumption, it is the legal responsibility of the person prescribing the treatment (in most countries, the veterinary clinician) to ensure that illegal residues are not present in edible flesh. Withdrawal times are recommended and in many countries legally enforced for some drugs, especially antibiotics. However, these withdrawal times are based on studies mainly performed on fish held in temperate freshwater. The excretion of a drug by a fish can vary greatly with environmental conditions, especially temperature. For example, oxytetracycline persistence in tissues of rainbow trout increases 10% for every 1° C decrease in temperature (Salte & Liestol, 1983). This is intuitively logical, since many metabolic processes in poikilothermic animals generally decrease twofold for every 10° C decrease in temperature (Q_{10} effect; Prosser, 1973a). In practical terms, this led Salte and Liestol (1983) to recommend that for rainbow trout, there should be a 60-day withdrawal time for oxytetracycline-medicated fish kept at over 10° C compared with a 100-day withdrawal time for fish kept at less than 10° C. The excretion rate at less than 10° C for potentiated sulfonamides was so slow that they suggested that this antibiotic not be used when temperatures are this low.

Estimating Withdrawal Time

Because of the variability in drug excretion, especially with temperature, a rule of thumb called *degree days* has been advocated for estimating the required withdrawal time (Debuf, 1991). Degree days are calculated by adding the mean daily water temperatures (measured in degrees Centigrade) for the total number of days measured. Thus, if the mean temperature was 11° C for the 50 days immediately after stopping drug treatment, the degree days would be 550. If the withdrawal time for the

drug used was 500 degree days, the fish would probably be safe to slaughter. Note that there is only limited scientific data on temperature's effect on excretion of most drugs and other factors that affect excretion rate. When they are available, suggested withdrawal times based on degree days are provided in the *PHARMACOPOEIA*. Also provided are legally mandated withdrawal times for drugs used in the United States. The largest problems currently faced with estimating withdrawal times is with antibiotic treatments (see *ANTIBIOTICS*, p. 272).

Legally approved brands of drugs should always be used for therapy (e.g., Table III-2). Stocks purchased from chemical supply firms or from other nonethical sources, including aquarium stores, are not regulated for quality as well as pharmaceutical brands. Also, use of an unapproved drug undermines the market for the approved drug, which discourages the manufacturer from renewing the drug's license and thus jeopardizes the future legal use of the drug.

ROUTES OF DRUG ADMINISTRATION

The three major routes by which fish may be treated are water-borne, oral, and injection. It is often best to withhold food for 24 hours before treatment. Items needed for treatment are simple (Box III-1).

Water-borne

The water-borne route is the most common method of administering treatments to fish and has distinct advantages, such as being relatively nonstressful and easy to administer. However, there are disadvantages. Dosing is often imprecise (too little or too much). Most drugs added to water are unstable and quickly degrade; this method may require repetitive dosing and removal of inactive (and possibly toxic) by-products of the drug with water changes.

Water-borne treatments are mainly used for surface-dwelling (skin and gill) pathogens, including parasites, bacteria, and fungi. Except for **antibiotics** and a few

---

❧ BOX III-1 ❧

EQUIPMENT NEEDED FOR TREATING FISH

Balance
Various-sized beakers (100 to 2000 ml)
Graduated cylinders (50, 250, 1000 ml)
Weighing papers
Spatulas
1, 3, 5, 10, 20 cc syringes
21, 22, 23, 25 GA needles

anthelmintics, virtually all agents act as antiseptics (see *ANTISEPTICS*) and nonspecifically kill pathogens. Thus, they often have a low therapeutic index and must be closely monitored for ichthyotoxicity during treatment. Certain species, such as scaleless fish (e.g., catfish, loaches), are often sensitive to water-borne treatments.

Agents that are intended to treat systemic diseases must reach therapeutic levels in target tissues. **Few drugs administered in water can do so**. Finally, medications can strongly inhibit nitrifying bacteria in aquaria, killing fish with ammonia or nitrite poisoning. Bath treatments are most toxic to biological filters, but some medications (e.g., erythromycin, neomycin, or methylene blue) are toxic even when used as prolonged immersions.

The methods used for water-borne treatment range from high drug concentration–short exposure time (bath) to low drug concentration–long exposure time (prolonged immersion).

If both short- and long-term exposures are probably equally feasible and effective, it is preferable to use a short-duration drug exposure for the following reasons:

1. It is often less expensive because a smaller amount of drug is needed.
2. Drugs do not have to be added to the system that holds the fish; thus, there is less of a problem with side effects, including toxicity to the biological filter, build-up of drug residues or metabolites in the environment (sediment, etc.), and/or development of resistant pathogens. Adequate plans for detoxification/removal/disposal of used therapeutants must be in place before treatment is begun.

It is always advisable to perform a bioassay of a small number of individuals before treating any fish species without a known history of response to the treatment. Most water-borne doses are based on studies of well-established food fish species (e.g., salmonids). When treating other species, idiosyncratic or hypersensitivity reactions can occur. Obviously, bioassay is not feasible before treating an individual pet fish.

Used drugs must be disposed of responsibly. Disposal procedures depend on the type of drug and local government regulations. Proper disposal is especially important for flush and continuous flow treatments (see ACTIVATED CARBONS in *PHARMACOPOEIA*). Know the environmental regulations before using any treatment, especially if effluent may enter public waters.

Methods

Bath

Fish are exposed to a concentrated drug solution for a short time. One to many fish can be treated simultaneously. The concentration required for effective bath treatment is often toxic to nitrifying bacteria; so, when treating fish that are housed in aquaria or other systems that have biological filters, either treatment should be done in a separate container or plans should be made to immediately reseed the treated system with nitrifying bacteria (see *NITRIFYING BACTERIA*) when treatment is finished. All drugs should be completely dissolved and mixed in the treatment water before adding fish, unless this is not possible. In weak individuals or sensitive species, it is best to give multiple treatments of the lower recommended dose rather than a single higher dose.

1. Add water to a clean container (Fig. III-1). Add a maximum of about 5 to 10 g of fish/l of water used for treatment (this will vary with species). Use lower density if a long-term bath (several hours) is anticipated. The amount of water added should be carefully measured, so that an exact drug concentration can be calculated (see step 6). It is desirable to place an airstone in the container and is essential if the fish will be crowded or treated for a long period.
2. Use a syringe or other volumetric container, and add exactly the amount of drug needed for treatment. *Mix well* by swirling. See Boxes III-2, III-3, and III-4 for calculating the amount of drug to add.
3. Net out the fish to be treated, and place them in the treatment solution for several seconds to several hours. The *PHARMACOPOEIA* gives exact times needed for specific drugs. For any treatments over 1 minute, vigorous aeration of the water is mandatory to maintain adequate oxygen levels. Fish should be monitored constantly. If fish become distressed (excitable, attempt to jump out of the water, depressed, lose equilibrium, and/or begin to list to one side), immediately place them in untreated water, even if the full time course of treatment is not complete. Toxicity with bath treatments is most common when antiseptics are used.
4. After exposure to the bath, immediately net out the fish and return them to unmedicated, aerated water. Observe closely over the next several days to see if a second treatment is needed.
5. This procedure can be used to treat large numbers of fish by simply increasing the volume of water used for the bath accordingly.
6. When fish are treated in flow-through systems, the water flow is stopped and the drug is immediately added to the water that holds the fish. If possible, lower the water level before treatment to decrease the amount of drug needed and to allow quicker dilution if toxicity occurs during treatment. Do not add concentrated drug directly onto the fish. If there is a risk of environmental hypoxia during treatment and supplemental aeration is not available, flush or constant-flow treatment may be required instead.

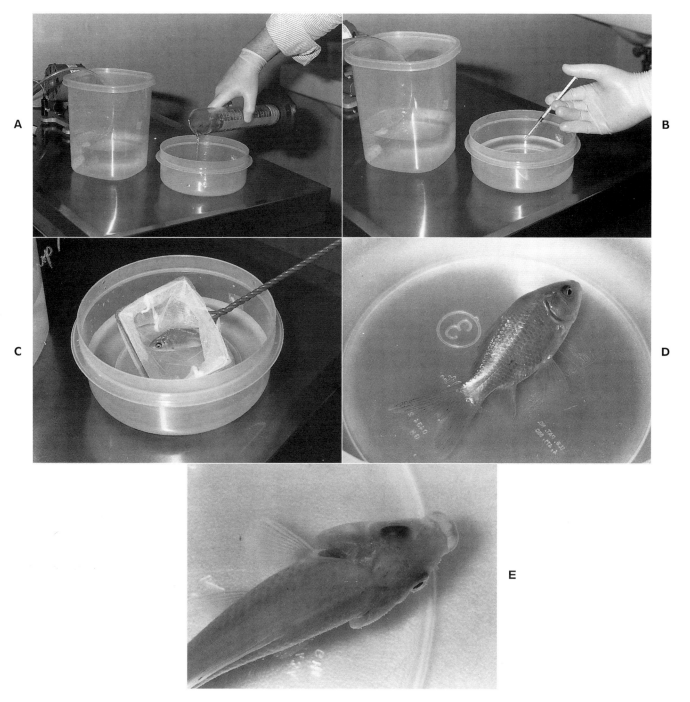

Fig. III-I   Bath method of water-borne treatment. **A,** Adding a known volume of water to a small container, using a graduated cylinder. Note the container with untreated, aerated water nearby. **B,** Adding a known volume of drug to the treatment container, using a syringe. The drug should then be mixed into the water. **C,** Adding the fish to be treated to the treatment container. **D,** Overdose, as indicated by listing of the fish to one side. Fish should be removed immediately if this occurs. **E** Overdose, as indicated by dyspnea (mouth and opercula open wider than normal).

❧ BOX III-2 ❧

SAMPLE CALCULATION NO. 1: PROLONGED IMMERSION TREATMENT WITH A DRY MEDICATION

A fish pond is to be treated with potassium permanganate prolonged immersion. After the permanganate demand of the pond water is determined, the farmer needs to give a dose of 2 mg/l. The pond volume is 3 acre-feet. How many grams of potassium permanganate are needed for treatment?

1. Using Table III-6, convert the concentration of drug to be used to the volumetric units of the culture system to be treated. Since the pond volume was measured in acre-feet, the following is the correct formula to use:

> No. mg/l × 1230 = No. grams/acre-foot
> 2 mg/l × 1230 = No. grams/acre-foot
> = 2460 grams potassium
> permanganate/acre-foot

2. Determine the number of grams of drug needed to treat the pond by using the following formula:

Amount
Drug = volume water × concentration of therapy
(g) × 100/% AI*
= 3 acre-feet × 2460 grams/acre-foot × 100/100
= 7380 grams = 7.38 kg potassium permanganate

3. If the chemical is to be weighed out in pounds, it can be converted to English units by using the conversion chart in Table III-7.

> # kg × 2.2 = # pounds
> 7.38 × 2.2 = 16.2 pounds potassium
> permanganate

---

*% AI = percent active ingredient. Potassium permanganate is considered 100% active.

❧ BOX III-3 ❧

SAMPLE CALCULATION NO. 2: PROLONGED IMMERSION TREATMENT WITH A LIQUID MEDICATION

An aquarium is to be treated with formalin prolonged immersion. The desired dose is 25 ppm. The volume of water in the aquarium is 185 gallons. How much formalin is needed for treatment?

1. Using Table III-6, convert the concentration of drug to be used to the volumetric units of the culture system to be treated. Since the aquarium's volume was measured in gallons, the following is the correct formula to use:

> No. ppm × 0.0038 = No. ml/gallon
> 25 ppm × 0.0038 = No. ml/gallon
> = 0.095 ml formalin/gallon

2. Determine the number of ml of chemical needed to treat the aquarium by using the following formula:

Amount
Drug = volume of water × concentration of drug
(ml) × 100 % AI*
= 185 gallons × 0.095 ml/gallon × 100/100
= 17.6 ml formalin

---

*% AI = percent active ingredient. Formalin is considered 100% active.

❧ BOX III-4 ❧

SAMPLE CALCULATION NO. 3: PROLONGED IMMERSION TREATMENT WITH A COMMERCIAL DRUG SOLUTION

A tank of freshwater pet fish are to be treated with 50 mg/l kanamycin sulfate prolonged immersion. The commercial preparation of kanamycin sulfate contains 250 mg kanamycin sulfate/ml of fluid. The tank has 5 gallons of water. How much of the kanamycin sulfate commercial preparation must be added to the tank?

1. Using Table III-6, convert the concentration of active ingredient to be used to the volumetric units of the culture system to be treated. Since the aquarium's volume is measured in gallons, the following is the correct formula to use:

No. mg/l × 3.785 = No. mg/gallon
50 mg/l × 3.785 = No. mg/gallon
= 189 mg kanamycin sulfate/gallon

2. Determine the mg of active ingredient (AI) needed by using the following formula:

Amount
of AI = volume water × concentration of drug
(mg)   × 100/% AI
= 5 gallons × 189 mg/gallon × 100/100
= 945 mg

3. Determine the amount of commercial preparation needed to treat the tank.

$$\frac{\text{No. mg needed for treatment}}{\text{No. mg/volume of commercial preparation}} = \frac{\text{volume of commercial}}{\text{preparation needed}}$$

$$\frac{945 \text{ mg}}{250 \text{ mg/l}} = \frac{3.8 \text{ ml of commercial}}{\text{preparation needed}}$$

Table III-6   Conversion factors for calculating treatments.

CONVERSION FACTORS FOR DRY MEDICATIONS

No. mg/l	×	3.785	= No. mg/gallon
No. mg/l	×	0.001	= No. grams/liter
No. mg/l	×	0.0038	= No. grams/gallon
No. mg/l	×	1	= No. grams/m³
No. mg/l	×	0.0283	= No. grams/ft³
No. mg/l	×	100,000	= No. grams/hectare-meter
No. mg/l	×	1230	= No. grams/acre-foot

CONVERSION FACTORS FOR LIQUID MEDICATIONS

No. ppm	×	0.001	= No. ml/liter
No. ppm	×	0.0038	= No. ml/gallon
No. ppm	×	1	= No. ml/m³
No. ppm	×	2.83	= No. ml/ft³
No. ppm	×	100,000	= No. ml/hectare-meter
No. ppm	×	1230	= No. ml/acre-feet

Table III-7   Conversion factors from English to metric units.

No. pounds	×	0.454 = No. kilograms
No. kilograms	×	2.20 = No. pounds
No. gallons	×	3.785 = No. liters
No. liters	×	0.264 = No. gallons
No. U.S. fluid ounces	×	0.0296 = No. liters
No. liters	×	33.8 = No. U.S. fluid ounces
No. dry ounces	×	0.0284 = No. kilograms
No. kilograms	×	35.3 = No. dry ounces

Degrees Centigrade = 5/9 (degrees F − 32)
Degrees Fahrenheit = 9/5 (degrees C) + 32

Flush

Flush is a modification of the bath treatment for flow-through systems. Water flow is not stopped, but a high concentration of chemical is added at the inlet and passed through the system as a pulse. The entire dose should be added in 1 to 2 minutes. A measured amount of drug is added to the system upstream and allowed to flush through. Flush has been most widely used in salmonid hatcheries. Flush treatment is only feasible for systems that have enough flow to completely flush out the drug within a predetermined time. Highly toxic treatments should not be applied as flush treatments, since a uniform drug distribution within the system cannot be ensured (Piper et al., 1982). Fish will usually retreat from the drug and then rapidly rush through it, reducing the effective exposure. This can be ameliorated by crowding the fish downstream, where mixing of the

drug will be most thorough and where the fish cannot escape. It is best to use a reduced flow for flush treatment, so the flow can be increased quickly if needed (adverse side effect, hypoxia). The suggested doses may need to be optimized for different systems.

Constant Flow

Constant flow treatments have also been used in flow-through systems when it is not possible to shut off the water long enough to use a bath treatment (i.e., even a temporary halt in water supply might cause fish mortality because of oxygen depletion or waste accumulation). Drugs used in constant flow treatments include **formalin, malachite green, quaternary ammonium compounds**, and **potassium permanganate**. Constant flow treatment is especially good for fungal control on eggs and for treating fish in raceways and small earthen ponds, especially where inflow water turnover rates are less than 1 water change per hour. Treatments are only performed for 1 hour, and "dead spots" must be treated by hand to ensure even chemical concentration (Warren, 1981).

The volume of water flowing into the unit must be accurately determined. A stock solution of the drug treatment is precisely metered into the water to obtain the desired therapeutic concentration. Chemical dosimeters are available for metering but are expensive. Commercial poultry waterers (Agri-Pro Enterprises; Ziggity Systems, Inc.), large carboys with spigots, or intravenous drip bags are inexpensive alternatives (Piper et al., 1982). However, flow rate will change with head pressure in gravity-fed devices, so they need constant monitoring.

Before the metering device is started, enough drug should be added to the water that contains the fish to produce the desired final concentration; this reduces the total amount of drug needed for treatment, by eliminating the time needed to reach therapeutic concentrations. When the treatment period is completed, the inflow of drug is stopped and the unit is flushed with untreated water. Partial draining of the system will help to speed elimination of the drug. See Piper et al. (1982) for more details concerning constant flow treatments.

The amount of drug needed for constant-flow treatments is computed the same as for prolonged immersion treatments, except that the flow rate of the water and treatment time must also be taken into consideration.

Constant-flow treatment is less desirable than bath or prolonged immersion, because of the greater expense and problems with release of toxic chemicals into the environment.

Prolonged Immersion

Fish are left in a low concentration of drug for at least 24 hours. The drug dissipates in the water by natural decay. One advantage to this treatment is that water changes after treatment are usually not mandatory (although still desirable) and many prolonged immersion treatments do not severely impair biological filtration, allowing their use in the system used to maintain the fish.

1. **Aquaria:** Add the drug to either the display tank or a hospitalization tank having biological filtration. **Activated carbon filtration must be stopped during treatment.** Some advocate turning off all filtration during treatment. Reducing filtration rate may be useful, but completely shutting off the filter may kill the nitrifying bacteria after several days.

   During treatment, ammonia, nitrite, and pH should be monitored at least every few days, if possible. The volume of water to be treated is usually fairly easily estimated if the tank size is known. However, a decremental adjustment should be made for objects in the tank that displace water (e.g., gravel, rocks, and coral).

An example is shown in Box III-3. Add a filter that has activated carbon at the end of the treatment to remove residual drug.

2. **Ponds:** Add the drug either at the pond bank or by boat. The proper application of chemicals to fish ponds requires correct calculation of the amount of chemical to be applied. One must always know the exact volume of water to be treated.

Calculation of Pond Treatments

Fertilizers and liming materials are usually applied to ponds on an areal basis (e.g., 2000 kg of agricultural lime/hectare). All other agents must be applied more accurately and are thus calculated on a weight per volume (w/v) basis (e.g., mg/l of copper sulfate) or volume per volume (v/v = ppm). It is satisfactory to estimate the amount needed to treat by +/- 10%, but an overestimate of 10% is wasteful and can be expensive when large ponds are treated (Boyd, 1990).

It is easiest to calculate pond volume in units of *acre-feet* (1 acre-foot of water is equal to 1 surface acre, 1 foot deep) or *hectare-meters* (1 hectare-meter of water is equal to 1 surface hectare, 1 meter deep). If a pond's volume is not known, its dimensions should be measured and its volume calculated. Measure the length and width of the pond at the water line and convert the area to surface acres or surface hectares. One surface acre equals 43,560 ft^2. One surface hectare equals 10,000 m^2. Volume is equal to the product of surface area (acres or hectares) and average depth (feet or meters). Average depth can be calculated by making multiple depth measurements and calculating an average. If maximum depth is known, average depth can usually be estimated to be 40% of the maximum depth (Tucker, 1984); however, this is less accurate than taking multiple depth readings and may be inaccurate in ponds that have highly uneven bottoms. More accurate methods of determining pond volume (e.g., surveying) are available (Boyd, 1990) but are not needed for successfully applying pond treatment, although more accurate estimations may be economically justified for treating large ponds.

Once the volume of water to be treated is known, the amount of drug to apply is calculated as shown in Box III-2. Jensen and Durborow (1984), Piper et al. (1982), and Wellborn (1978) provide more details on calculating treatments.

Application of Drugs to Ponds

Once the exact amount of drug to apply is known, an application method is selected. Application must be uniform to avoid forming "hot spots" of excess drug, which can overdose the fish (Boyd, 1990). Supplemental aeration should be readily available (Noga & Francis-Floyd, 1991).

Large farms can afford specialized chemical applicators. Boat-mounted tanks can be used to spray dissolved drug over the pond. Liquids can also be dispensed through a pipe having small-diameter holes in its underside (Burkhalter et al., Undated). The pipe is hung over the edge of the boat. Solution flow can be regulated either by using a valve on a gravity-fed device or by using a water pump if more uniform release is desired. Drug can be released under the water surface by attaching small vertical tubes of the desired length to the holes in the pipe. Crystals and granules can be spread by using dispensers similar to fertilizer distributors. These dispensers are usually hoppers with adjustable dispensing holes in the bottom. An auger is used to prevent clogging of the holes with coarse particles (Schoenecker & Rhodes, 1965). A simple modification of this device was designed by Boyd (1990). An outboard motor propeller mixes the drug with the water as it is released from the siphon. This type of dispenser is available commercially.

Owners with a single pond usually cannot justify purchasing application equipment. In such cases the drug can be dissolved in a large container of water and applied to the pond surface using a garden sprayer. Otherwise, it can be dispensed with a bucket from a boat. Caution owners about the toxicity of the drug to be handled. It may not be advisable to have owners use this technique for highly toxic drugs (e.g., formalin). Granules can be broadcast by hand or with a small "cyclone" seeder. Crystals can be placed in a burlap bag and towed behind a boat until they have completely dissolved (Boyd, 1990). More details on drug applications are provided by Boyd (1990).

Prolonged Immersion Bioassay

It is especially advisable to perform a bioassay before using some prolonged immersion treatments because prolonged immersion cannot easily be stopped if toxicity develops during treatment. While the safe therapeutic range has been established for most drugs used for commonly cultured food fish (e.g., salmonids, channel catfish), caution is advised when using any drug on a fish species for which no data is available on that species' susceptibility to the drug. Bioassays are also advisable if a particular farm has not previously used copper, since copper's toxicity is often unpredictable.

A bioassay can be performed by placing five or six fish in an aquarium that has treated pond water. Aerate the water to prevent hypoxia. When holding tanks or aquaria are not available, fish can be placed in large polyethylene bags that are filled with pond water and anchored to the pond (Burress, 1975). Fish are seined from the pond and placed in the bags at a density of not more than 1 g/l. The fish should be observed for 1 to 2 days before treatment to be sure that none have died from stress of collection. Fish should not be fed while in the bags. The test drug is added to the bags (it is best to test 3 doses within the desired range), and mortality is compared with fish held in bags without the drug. Fish should be held in the bags for at least 96 hours, unless the drug is known to degrade more quickly.

These procedures can also be used to determine when it is safe to stock fish in a treated pond, such as after liming to disinfect (Boyd, 1990). In the latter case, control fish should be placed in bags that have water from a known nontoxic pond for comparison.

Swab

The swab is not commonly used because few skin diseases are localized enough to allow this to be effective; it is probably most useful in treating local traumatic wounds that are secondarily infected by bacteria or fungi. Dip a cotton swab in a drug solution and gently touch the swab to the lesion, allowing the solution to soak the lesion via capillary action.

Oral Medications

Oral medications are one of the best ways to administer drugs to fish because they are the least stressful yet if consumed in the proper amounts and absorbed by the gastrointestinal tract, they can be very effective. However, they can also be cumbersome if a commercially prepared oral medication is not available. Also, sick fish will often not eat, rendering this therapy useless. Force-feeding can be an option but is not often used (see below). Withholding food for 12 to 24 hours may increase the acceptance of a medicated feed. If fish still refuse the medicated feed after a 24-hour fast, they can be fasted longer if their health status allows this. The dosage can vary within limits, depending on the feeding rate. For example, in the United States oxytetracycline (OTC) can be incorporated into the feed at 2.75 to 3.5 g/100 pounds of feed. At the lower concentration, fish will get 52 mg OTC/kg if eating 1% of their body weight per day. If the fish are eating 3% of their body weight per day, the lower dose can be used. It is usually best to use a feed that has enough medication so that feeding at a rate of 1% of body weight per day will give the needed dosage. This helps to ensure that the fish consume enough medication. The remainder of the daily ration can then be given as a nonmedicated feed.

Methods

1. **Commercially medicated feeds:** Antibiotic-medicated feeds are available for food fish. These feeds can also be fed to aquarium fish directly or can be incorporated into gelatin. A small, crumble-type feed is small enough to be eaten by most aquarium fish. Pellets can also be crushed into smaller pieces for smaller fish by using a mortar and pestle. Medicated feeds for food fish are usually sold only in large quantities (e.g., minimum of 50 pounds for many feeds) but are much less expensive than aquarium medications and, if frozen, will last for well over 1 year in storage. Some commercial aquarium feeds are also medicated with antibiotics, but there is no published data on their efficacy.

❧ BOX III-5 ❧

SAMPLE CALCULATION NO. 4: ORAL MEDICATION

A group of trout are to be fed a medicated diet that contains Tribrissen® (40% active sulfadiazine-trimethoprim). The dose to be used is 50 mg sulfadiazine-trimethoprim/kg of body weight. If the fish are to be fed the medicated diet at a rate of 1% of body weight (BW) of fish/day, how much sulfadiazine-trimethoprim must be added to 100 pounds of feed to provide the correct dosage?

1. Fish are to be fed 50 mg sulfadiazine-trimethoprim/kg BW

   Feeding rate = 1% of BW/day
   = 10 g feed/kg BW/day

   Fish are to be fed 50 mg sulfadiazine-trimethoprim/10 g feed

   = 5000 mg sulfadiazine-trimethoprim/kg feed
   = 5 g sulfadiazine-trimethoprim/kg feed

2. Tribrissen® is 40% sulfadiazine-trimethoprim
   Fish must be fed: 5 g/0.4 = 12.5 g Tribrissen/kg feed

3. If the commercial preparation is to be added to pounds of feed, it can be converted to English units by using the conversion factor in Table III-7:

$$\frac{No.\ g}{No.\ kg} \times \frac{1}{2.2} = \frac{No.\ g}{No.\ lb}$$

   No. g/kg × 0.454 = No. g/lb
   12.5 g Tribrissen/kg feed × 0.454 = No. g Tribrissen/lb feed
   = 5.7 g Tribrissen/lb feed
   = 570 g Tribrissen/100 lb

4. To add to feed, mix with 0.5 kg of soybean oil/25 kg of feed:
   = 0.02 kg of soybean oil/kg of feed
   = 20 g of soybean oil/kg of feed
   = 12.5 g Tribrissen/20 g soybean oil/kg of feed

---

2. **Injection of individual food items:** Injection is a relatively easy way to give oral medications to small numbers of fish. The required dosage is injected into a small fish, which is then fed to the sick fish. This method has limited usefulness, since not all sick fish will accept such preparations, only large fish can be treated, and there is risk of introducing other diseases with the medicated fish.

3. **Loading food with a medication:** Small food items (e.g., brine shrimp) can be "loaded" with therapeutic levels of drug by soaking in a drug solution (For examples, see *SULFADIMETHOXINE-ORMETOPRIM* and *METRONIDAZOLE*).

4. **Preparation of a medicated artificial diet:** The key to making a successful, medicated artificial diet is to prepare one that will be readily eaten by the sick fish; this can often be difficult, since even healthy fish often initially refuse any change in their normal diet. The most common way to prepare a medicated diet for pet fish is to mix food with gelatin and then add the proper dose of medicine just before hardening the gelatin by refrigeration. A key factor in success is palatability. Gelatin is high in calcium and thus may bind some antibiotics, such as tetracyclines and quinolones. However, this has never been reported to be a problem in diet preparations. Three suggested formulae follow:

Gelatin diet for aquarium fish:

1. Dissolve 30 grams of unflavored gelatin in 500 ml of boiling water (= 30 g in 17 United States fluid ounces).
2. Thoroughly suspend about 300 grams of commercial fish feed (Purina Trout Chow® or equivalent) in about 150 ml of water. The feed should be in as fine a suspension as possible.
3. Pour the gelatin solution into the wet food mixture.
4. Mix well, and add more fish feed; try to get as much feed added to the liquid suspension as possible. When the suspension has cooled to room temperature, dissolve the appropriate amount of drug (Boxes III-5 and III-6) in the water, and mix the solution into the food/gelatin mixture.
5. Line a large plastic dish pan with aluminum foil, and pour the food/gelatin mixture into the pan, spreading it evenly over the entire pan to a thickness of about ½ inch (~1 cm).
6. Place the pan in the refrigerator for 2 to 4 hours until it has gelled; then cut it into blocks, place it in an airtight bag, and freeze.
7. Remove bags as needed, cut into appropriately sized square blocks, and feed to fish.
8. Food fish feeds will often taint aquarium water a yellowish-brown. Substituting an aquarium-type pelleted feed or a flake food for the food fish ration will avoid this problem. More complex gel diet formulae are available (Bower, 1983; Spotte, 1992) but are not needed if the above diet is eaten.

Gelatin coating of pellets for large fish (Piper et al., 1982) (Treats 100 pounds of pellets):

1. Slowly dissolve 125 g of gelatin in 3 quarts of boiling water (= 25 g/2.8 liters).
2. Allow the gelatin to cool to room temperature, and then stir the appropriate amount of drug (Table III-5) into the gelatin until there are no lumps.

❧ BOX III-6 ❧

SAMPLE CALCULATION NO. 5: ORAL MEDICATION

The amount of drug that must be added to a feed can be easily calculated by using the dosage (D) of drug to be administered orally and the medication rate (R% of body weight [BW])/day:

D mg/kg BW fed at R% of BW/day requires the addition of the following:

$$\frac{(0.01)(D)}{R} \% \text{ of drug in the feed}$$

or

D mg/lb BW fed at R% of BW/day requires the addition of the following:

$$\frac{(0.022)(D)}{R} \% \text{ of drug in the feed}$$

Example No. 1: If fenbendazole is to be fed at a rate of 25 mg fenbendazole/kg BW/day and the food will be fed at a rate of 1% of body weight/day, the following must be added:

$$\frac{(0.01)(D)}{R} \% = \frac{(0.01)(25)}{1} \%$$

= 0.25% fenbendazole in the diet, or 0.25 g fenbendazole added to every 100 g of feed.

Example No. 2: If the same dosage of fenbendazole is fed as mg/lb (i.e., at a rate of 11 mg fenbendazole/lb BW/day), and the food will be fed at a rate of 1% of body weight/day, the following must be added:

$$\frac{(0.022)(D)}{R} \% = \frac{(0.022)(11)}{1} \%$$

= 0.24% fenbendazole in the diet, or 0.24 g fenbendazole added to every 100 g of feed (the value is slightly different than the result in example No. 1, since the 25 mg/kg dose is slightly greater than 11 mg/lb).

---

3. **Slowly** add the drug-gelatin mixture to the pellets (stir by hand, or use a cement mixer). Stir only long enough to mix (don't break the pellets).

Oil coating of pellets for large fish. Use a wt:wt ratio of 2 to 3 parts oil:100 parts feed (Piper et al., 1982):

1. Heat 2 to 3 pounds (or 2 to 3 kg) of soybean oil to 100° to 120° F (~40° C).
2. **Quickly** mix the drug evenly into the warm oil.
3. **Quickly** pour or spray the drug-oil mixture over 100 pounds (or 100 kg) of pellets (keep exposure of antibiotics to high temperature as short as possible).

Note that lipid carriers may prevent oral uptake of some antibiotics in salmonids, especially macrolides (Austin, 1985). This phenomenon has not been examined in other species.

The amount of drug needed to be placed in a diet is given in the *PHARMACOPOEIA*. Note that normal feeding rates decrease with lower temperature. The method for formulating a medicated feed is shown in Box III-6.

5. **Force-feeding:** Oral medications can be given via stomach tube (Andrews & Riley, 1982).

1. Attach a stomach tube made from a dog catheter (3 mm outer diameter) to a 5 cc syringe, using cyanoacrylate glue (Super Glue®, Loctite). Fill the tube and the syringe with liquid medication. For fish that are larger than 40 to 50 cm long, a larger diameter tube is usually needed (a horse catheter, with 6 mm outer diameter tubing, attached to a 20 cc syringe has been used). Any tube used should have a smooth anterior end to avoid damage to the gastrointestinal mucosa.
2. Anesthetize fish, and place fish in a lateral recumbency on a smooth, nontraumatic surface.
3. Insert the tube into the stomach (or the anterior intestine of cyprinids, since they do not have a stomach).
4. Administer at a rate of about 1.0 to 1.25 ml/kg body weight. Both solutions and suspensions can be administered.
5. Observe closely after recovery for possible regurgitation.

Injection

Injection of drugs has the advantage of delivering a precise dosage. Disadvantages include the stress imposed by capturing the fish and, for aquarium fish, the need to bring the fish to the clinic for every injection, since the owner is usually unable to perform the treatment. The weight of the fish must be closely estimated; this is best done by using a scale and weighing by displacement. A container with aquarium water is placed on a scale. The fish is then added, and the change in weight is determined; however, this is only feasible for small fish, unless a large scale is available. Large fish (> ~200 g) are more easily weighed by placing them directly on the scale. Fish should be sedated during weighing, unless they are weak and it does not appear that they may tolerate sedation. Most veterinary preparations must be diluted considerably in sterile diluent (saline or water) to administer the proper dosage to aquarium fish.

Methods

1. **IP (Intraperitoneal):** Fish should be fasted for 24 hours before injection. Failure to do so runs the risk of causing peritonitis caused by puncture of the stomach or bowel.

   The landmarks for an IP injection are the pelvic fins and the anus. In the more primitive teleosts (e.g., salmonids, goldfish, catfish) the pelvic fins are located in the posterior portion of the body. In the advanced teleosts (i.e., the great majority of fish species), the pelvic fins have evolutionarily migrated anteriorly and the pectoral fins have migrated dorsally. An IP injection can usually be given anywhere from midway between the pectoral and pelvic fins to just anterior to the anus (Akhlaghi et al., 1993) (Fig. III-2, *A*). However, it is best to avoid the area around the pectoral or pelvic girdles.

   The injection should be made near the ventral midline. Fish should be held in dorsal recumbency. A proportionately small-gauge needle (25 GA or less) is recommended for fish ~3 inches to 4 inches (8 to 10 cm), and the needle should not be inserted too far past the body wall to avoid entering the gastrointestinal tract. Presence in the peritoneal cavity is indicated by a lack of resistance to injection and free movement of the end of the needle.

2. **IM (Intramuscular):** This type of injection is best used only on fish greater than 5 inches (13 cm) long. The best site is the dorsal musculature just lateral to the dorsal fin (Fig. III-2, *B*). Only relatively small amounts can be injected (~0.05 ml/50 g of fish). Fish that are not sedated will have tense muscles and thus are more difficult to inject. Injections should be done slowly to allow maximal deposition of material. This route has the disadvantage of causing damage to carcass quality and the potential of forming sterile abscesses. However, it produces a much more reproducible uptake of some drugs and maintains drug levels for a longer time (e.g., see oxytetracycline and flumequine antibiotics) (Nouws et al., 1992).

3. **Dorsal sinus:** This type of injection is mostly used when treating salmonids for bacterial kidney disease (see *PROBLEM 52*). The dorsal sinus runs near the dorsal fin (Fig. III-2, *C*). Because it can be difficult to inject, drugs intended to enter the dorsal sinus

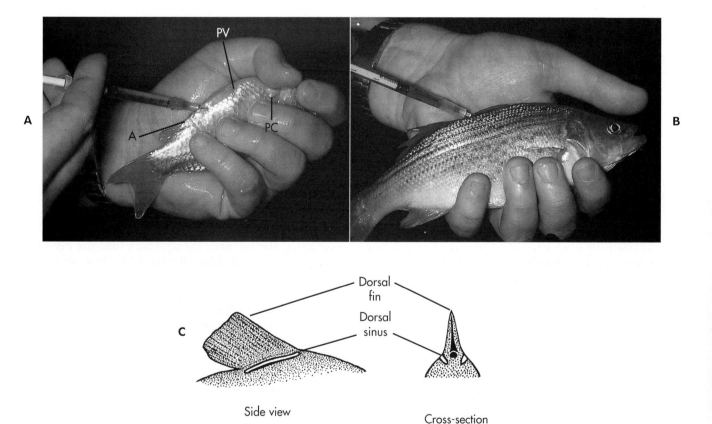

Fig. III-2 Injection of fish. **A,** Site for IP injection. *PC* = pectoral fin; *PV* = pelvic fins; *A* = anus. **B,** Intramuscular injection of fish. The injection should be made lateral to the base of the dorsal fin. **C,** Site for injection into the dorsal sinus.

are often inadvertently deposited subcutaneously (C. Moffitt, Personal Communication).

RECOMMENDED TREATMENTS IN VARIOUS CULTURE SYSTEMS
Aquaria

Treatment in the Display Tank Versus a Hospitalization Tank
Whether to treat in the display tank is of greatest concern when water-borne medications are given, but it is also of concern with oral and injectable preparations. In theory, it is always best to treat a sick fish in a hospitalization tank because (1) it removes contagion from susceptible tankmates; (2) it is easier to deliver medications to the sick individual (e.g., easier to capture the fish if repeated baths or injections are to be given); and (3) it avoids exposing both the (presumptively) healthy fish and the other organisms in the display tank to unnecessary and potentially toxic medications. A smaller amount of drug can often be used because of the relatively small size of the hospitalization tank.

However, in practice, there are several limitations to treatment in a hospitalization tank. Capturing the fish and placing it in a foreign environment can stress the fish (Schreck 1981; Elsaesser & Clem, 1986). It may also be nearly impossible to capture a fish in a large aquarium with many rocks or plantings. Adequate biological filtration must also be provided, so that the fish does not die from ammonia poisoning. Most aquarists do not maintain hospitalization or quarantine tanks that can be used to treat sick fish. If such a tank is to be set up the day that treatment begins, it must be seeded with commercially available **nitrifying bacteria** or gravel or other filter material from a tank that has an established biological filter (see *PROBLEM 4*). There must be an active, functioning biological filter (e.g., in a box, undergravel or other filter; nitrifying bacteria cannot simply be dropped into a bare tank). Note that nitrifiers from freshwater cannot be used to condition marine aquaria (Bower & Turner, 1981); probably because the bacteria are shocked by the rapid salinity change. The converse is also true. Ammonia and nitrite levels must be monitored closely during therapy.

Clinic Hospitalization
If many clients are seen, it may become advisable to set up hospitalization systems. Inpatients can be routinely housed if one has the ability to rapidly set up aquaria that are conditioned with the bacteria needed to detoxify ammonia and nitrite.

To have this ability, conditioned aquaria should be set up. There should be two freshwater and two marine 2½ gallon (10 liter) aquaria (total of four tanks). Each aquarium should have an undergravel filter covered with 3 inches (8 cm) of gravel. One teaspoon of ammonium chloride and 2 teaspoons of sodium bicarbonate should be added to one freshwater and one marine aquarium weekly (to stimulate ammonia oxidizing bacteria); the other two aquaria should receive 1 teaspoon of sodium nitrite weekly (to stimulate nitrite oxidizing bacteria). Ninety percent of the water in each tank should be changed every month.

When a freshwater fish is to be kept for observation and/or treatment, a new aquarium is filled with water, preferably from the tank that held the sick fish. A handful of gravel from both the freshwater ammonia– and freshwater nitrite–conditioned tanks is added to a box filter, which is then added to the tank. The same procedure is followed when a marine fish is to be hospitalized, using instead the gravel from the marine ammonia– and marine nitrite–conditioned tanks to set up a new tank.

These newly set-up tanks will thus have a high concentration of the bacteria needed to detoxify ammonia and nitrite; the sick fish can then be added. Ammonia, nitrite, pH, and temperature should be monitored regularly, until the fish is released.

It is also possible to use commercially available **nitrifying bacteria** (Aquacenter, Argent) to seed new aquaria. However, commercial nitrifier preparations are usually not as active initially as are the bacteria from a well-conditioned aquarium. Thus a slight increase is often seen in ammonia and nitrite when commercial nitrifiers are used. This may stress the treated fish.

While the above methods are effective, they are cumbersome or impractical unless many inpatients are seen. Alternatively, two display aquaria can be maintained, one with healthy freshwater fish and the other with healthy marine fish. The presence of the fish will maintain an active biological filter that can then be used to seed a hospitalization aquarium when needed. Note, however, that there is some risk of exposing treated fish to pathogens carried by subclinically affected fish in the display aquaria.

Ponds

Fish in ponds are best treated using oral medications. However, there are no legally approved oral medications in the United States for treating ectoparasites or fungal infections on fish. Thus, most skin and gill pathogens are controlled by adding drug to the water containing the fish. Since it is impractical to gather up pond fish for bath treatment, prolonged immersion is the method of choice.

Cages

Fish in cages are best treated by using oral medications or bath treatments. Fish in large net-pens often cannot be easily removed and are thus treated with water-borne medication in the pen (e.g., sea lice). In the latter case, the entire pen is enclosed in a tarpaulin, or *skirts* are placed around only the sides of the pen.

Flow-Through Systems

Fish in raceways or other flow-through systems are best treated by using a bath or oral medication. Flush and continuous-flow treatments have also been used in salmonid hatcheries because of the typically high stocking densities and subsequent problems caused by stopping water flow for a particular time period (Piper et al., 1982).

WHICH DOSAGE TO USE

For many drugs in the PHARMACOPOEIA, a range of doses is given. For water-borne treatments, water quality can greatly affect efficacy and ichthyotoxicity. Related pathogens can also vary in susceptibility. If you are unsure about the dose to use, it is usually best to start with the lower recommended dose. If the disease does not respond adequately, repeat the treatment with a higher dose.

For oral medications, dosage varies with feed intake. Fish eating less need a higher percentage of drug in the diet, but there are limits on the legally allowable amount and practical considerations, since some drugs are unpalatable at high doses (e.g., many antibiotics).

CHAPTER 23

PHARMACOPOEIA

The following drug formulations are a compendium of what I consider the most useful agents presently available for treating the major diseases that affect fish. This list is not exhaustive and is not intended to be. Many other recommended treatments are not included either because I believe that a listed treatment is equal if not superior for a given malady or because I believe that the omitted treatment has not yet proven effective. This does not mean that all treatments not included are ineffective; many are useful (see Herwig, 1979; Hoffman & Meyer, 1974; Alderman, 1988 for lists of other treatments); however, I believe that the core list provided will be adequate for tackling the great majority of problems encountered. Indeed, the most important cause of drug **failure** in treating fish is a lack of proper diagnosis, which, when you use this information, you will hopefully remedy. Note that formulations may not be available indefinitely and are dependent on consumer demand, legal/regulatory constraints, and thus manufacturers' continued production.

There is a large body of anecdotal information that purports the efficacy of many drug formulations for treating fish diseases, especially for aquarium fish. Unfortunately, there is an equally great lack of reliable scientific data supporting the use of many remedies. I have avoided recommending the use of such treatments whenever possible. Most scientifically proven treatments are based on work with food fish (e.g., trout). While some treatments require formulating the drug, I have included reliable commercial sources when those are available. Many medications are available over-the-counter in aquarium stores and aquaculture supply firms, including many antibiotics that are usually only available by prescription for ethical veterinary use. The availability of these products varies from country to country. No product should be prescribed without a proper diagnosis.

Regarding over-the-counter aquarium remedies, while many are useful, others are ineffective, and some are even toxic (Trust, 1972). Some remedies are concoctions that contain five or more separate drugs that claim to cure everything from skin flukes to mycobacteriosis.

Some formulations also combine antibiotics (sometimes a bacteriostatic with a bactericidal agent). Obviously, the practitioner should advise the client to avoid such complex mixtures. Also, the lack of demonstrated quality control for many of these over-the-counter aquarium products abrogates recommending their use in many cases.

Not all listed pharmaceutical brands are legally approved for use in fish, and even brands developed for aquaculture are licensed only in certain countries. All treatments can be used for both marine and freshwater fish, unless noted otherwise.

Acetic Acid

Use: Treatment of ectoparasites in freshwater fish
  Smaller fish are more sensitive (Lewbart, 1991)
Water-borne formulations:
  1. Bath
    a. Add 1 to 2 ml of glacial acetic acid/l (= 1000 to 2000 ppm of acetic acid = 3.8 to 7.6 ml/gallon) and treat for 45 seconds to 10 minutes (Schnick et al., 1989; G. Lewbart, Personal Communication). The longer time period may be toxic. Glacial acetic acid is 96% (Japan) to > 99% (United States) acetic acid.

Activated Carbon

Use No. 1: Removal of medications and other organics from water (Dawson et al., 1976); may not remove heavy metals or nitrogenous toxins from the water, unless they are present in an organic form (e.g., chelated copper, chloramine) (Turner & Bower, 1983); note also that some organics are not easily removed (see **COPPER**).

While mainly used in small, closed systems, activated carbon can also be used to remove chemicals or drugs from water in flow-through systems before effluent release into a watershed (Howe et al., 1990; Marking et al., 1990).

Water-borne formulations:
1. Prolonged immersion
   a. Use ~75 g (~250 ml dry volume) of activated carbon (Professional Grade Activated Carbon [Aquarium Pharmaceuticals, Inc.] or equivalent) for every 10 gallons (or every 40 liters) of water for 2 weeks. Carbon may be placed into the filter presently in the tank or added to a separate box filter. Discard the carbon used to remove medication after 2 weeks.

Use No. 2: Removal of colored and other foreign substances from water, keeping aquarium water clear, odor-free, and low in organics
Water-borne formulations:
1. Prolonged immersion
   a. Use ~75 g (~250 ml dry volume) of activated carbon (Professional Grade Activated Carbon [Aquarium Pharmaceuticals, Inc.] or equivalent) for every 10 gallons (or every 40 liters) of water. Replace carbon about monthly.

Acriflavin

Use: Treatment of bacterial, fungal, or parasitic infections/infestations of aquarium fish

This agent has been used frequently in the aquarium trade, but there is a considerable resistance by common fish bacterial pathogens, and there are other, more effective agents for treating fungi and ectoparasites.

Agricultural Lime; See *BUFFERS–PONDS; CALCIUM*

Alum (Aluminum Sulfate, $Al_2[SO_4]_3 \cdot 14H_2O$)

Alum must be mixed into the water to be treated as rapidly and evenly as possible. It is best to dispense it as a solution over the pond. It is dangerous to use in ponds that have low alkalinity, where it can cause a considerable decrease in pH. This pH drop can be counteracted by adding **slaked lime** at the same time. See Boyd (1990) for more details on the use of alum.
Use No. 1: Decreasing turbidity in ponds
Water-borne formulations:
1. Prolonged immersion
   a. Add ~15 to 25 mg alum/l. Alum is more effective and cheaper than **agricultural gypsum** (see *CALCIUM*) but is less safe to use in low-alkalinity waters and has a shorter effective life; however, it is cheaper (Wu & Boyd, 1990).

Use No. 2: Decreasing excessively high pH in ponds
Water-borne formulations:
1. Prolonged immersion
   a. Add 1 mg alum/l for every 1 mg/l of phenolphthalein alkalinity to be removed.

Anesthetics

See *BENZOCAINE, CARBON DIOXIDE, 2-PHENOXYETHANOL, QUINALDINE SULFATE, SODIUM BICARBONATE,* and *TRICAINE* for use of specific agents. See p. 17 for general guidelines for using sedatives/anesthetics.

Antibiotics

Use: Treatment of bacterial infections

Most agents listed are effective against gram-negative bacteria, which are responsible for most fish bacterial diseases. Only a limited number of antibiotics are approved for use in food fish in any single country.

It is best to administer antibiotics orally or by injection. The next best alternative is a bath for antibiotics that are well absorbed via the water. Prolonged immersion treatments are least desirable and are economically unfeasible except in small volumes of water (i.e., aquaria). Most antibiotics used for fish diseases are weakly acidic or weakly basic; thus, pH has an important influence on uptake via water (Endo, 1992).

The elimination rate of antibiotics from fish tissues varies greatly with temperature. Specific withdrawal times that are approved for selected oral antibiotic treatments in the United States are mentioned with specific antibiotics. When specific withdrawal times are not given, a good rule of thumb is 500 degree days. Thus, if the mean daily water temperature after treatment was 10° C, the withdrawal period should be at least 50 days (10 × 50 = 500), while at 25° C, the withdrawal period would be 20 days. This obviously can only be a rough estimate of elimination rate, because temperatures fluctuate diurnally and day-to-day and other factors besides temperature affect elimination rates.

The pharmacokinetics of antibiotics vary tremendously among fish species; thus, doses given are only intended as general guidelines **unless** the formula has been shown to be effective for that particular species (e.g., FDA-approved). Whenever antibiotics are used, it is imperative that the treatment be given for exactly the time period specified. Treating for longer or shorter than recommended leads to treatment failure and/or development of antibiotic-resistant bacterial strains (Aoki, 1992; Lewin, 1992).

Intensive, repeated, use of a single antibiotic unequivocally promotes the development of resistant bacteria (Lewin, 1992; Tsoumas et al., 1989). For example, there is a high prevalence of multiple antibiotic-resistant bacteria in aquarium fish imported to the United States from the Far East, where there is heavy use of prophylactic antibiotics (Dixon et al., 1990). Prophylactic use of antibiotics is highly discouraged. Most bacterial resistance is plasmid mediated, meaning that resistance can be transferred both horizontally and vertically; plasmids typically carry resistance to multiple antibiotics (Lewin, 1992).

Unfortunately, fish diseases often present as rapidly fulminating epidemics, and because of logistical and technological problems and/or lack of knowledge by the owner, it is often not possible to determine the probable efficacy of a treatment before an agent is used. Even knowing the causative agent (e.g., a specific bacterium) may not preclude having to change drug therapy once lab results are received. Once an outbreak becomes established, typically there is significantly higher mortality in a population, even if the antibiotic rapidly reaches therapeutic levels in tissues (Egidius & Andersen, 1979; Pearse et al., 1974). This emphasizes the need for prompt therapy. If the proper therapy is given, fish often respond to treatment (e.g., improve appetite) within 24 hours and should respond within 3 to 5 days.

The pharmacokinetics of most orally administered antibiotic treatments that are listed are fairly well defined. However, most doses given for water-borne and injection routes are empirical, with not much clinical research to optimize or substantiate the dosage. While there is strong evidence that a single treatment with some antibiotics can cure fish of some bacterial infections (Egidius & Andersen, 1979; Pearse et al., 1974; E. Noga, Unpublished Data), fish should be monitored closely to ensure that the treatment is effective. For example, treatment may need to be extended if response is not complete, even though this is not advisable in most cases. However, there is little latitude for legally modifying antibiotic therapy for food fish.

Some antibiotics persist for long periods, especially at low temperature, in the dark, and/or in mud (Jacobsen & Berglind, 1988). These conditions are often found under cages used to culture marine salmonids or in ponds.

The risks to persons handling antibiotics or medicated feeds appear to be low and uncommon, primarily restricted to hypersensitivy reaction to a specific antibiotic (Giroud, 1992).

When antibiotics are used in an extra-label application, it is best to use preparations that do not have carriers, since these may be toxic to fish.

Amoxicillin trihydrate (Vetremox® [Vetrepharm], Aquacil® [PH Pharmaceuticals], or equivalent)
This is a beta-lactam antibiotic.

Oral formulations:
Feed 40 to 80 mg of amoxicillin trihydrate/kg (= 18 to 36 mg/pound) of body weight/day for 10 days
Withdrawal time: 500 degree days (Debuf, 1991)
Ampicillin sodium (Amp-Equine [Smith-Kline], Omnipen [Wyeth-Ayerst], or equivalent)
This is a beta-lactam antibiotic.
Oral formulations:
Feed 50 to 80 mg of ampicillin/kg (= 23 to 36 mg/pound) of body weight/day for 10 days.
Chloramphenicol (Chloromycetin sodium succinate [Parke-Davis], or equivalent)
This antibiotic is poorly absorbed when it is administered through the water (Nusbaum & Shotts, 1981; Gilmartin et al., 1976). This may be because it is unstable in water (Nusbaum & Shotts, 1981), although others have reported it to be water stable (Gilmartin et al., 1976). Chloramphenicol is effective when injected. Chloramphenicol is hazardous to a small percentage of humans, causing an idiosyncratic, aplastic anemia, which is usually fatal. Gloves should be worn during use to avoid contact. Chloramphenicol is highly illegal to use on food animals in some countries, including the United States.
Injectable formulations:
Inject 20 to 50 mg chloramphenicol/kg (= 9 to 23 mg/pound) of body weight IP once weekly for 2 weeks to treat goldfish ulcer disease caused by *Aeromonas salmonicida*.
Enrofloxacin (Baytril® [Miles])
Enrofloxacin is a fluorinated quinolone that is active against *Aeromonas salmonicida* (Bowser et al., 1990) and is also useful for treating aquarium fish (G. Lewbart, Personal Communication). See the general discussion of quinolones under oxolinic acid.
Water-borne formulations:
1. Bath
   a. Add 2 mg of enrofloxacin/l (= 7.6 mg/gallon) and treat for 5 days (G. Lewbart, Personal Communication).
Oral formulations:
1. Feed 10 mg of enrofloxacin/kg (= 4.5 mg/pound) of body weight/day for 10 days. This dose has been experimentally effective against vibriosis in rainbow trout (Dalsgaard & Bjeregaard, 1991).
Injectable formulations:
1. Inject 10 mg of enrofloxacin/kg (= 4.5 mg/pound) of body weight IM or IP every 3 days (G. Lewbart, Personal Communication).
Erythromycin (Erythromycin base [Aurum], Erythro®-200 [Abbott], Erythromycin thiocyanate, or equivalent)
Erythromycin is a macrolide antibiotic that is primarily used for controlling bacterial kidney disease in

salmonids. It is used at several stages in the life cycle, including preventing prespawning adult mortality, decreasing infection in eggs, and treating young fish with clinical disease (Armstrong et al., 1989). It has also been used to treat streptococcosis (Kitao et al. 1987). Prolonged treatment with erythromycin can seriously impair kidney function in salmonids (Hicks & Geraci, 1984). Note that erythromycin is commonly sold as an antibacterial agent for aquarium fish but is *not* recommended as prolonged immersion because of its toxicity to biological filtration.

Use No. 1: Prevention and/or treatment of bacterial kidney disease in salmonids

Oral formulations:

1. Erythromycin is used to prevent and treat clinical BKD (Austin, 1985). Palatability problems have occurred with this treatment.
    a. Feed 100 mg erythromycin thiocyanate/kg (= 45 mg/pound) of body weight/day for 21 days. While Austin (1985) found nearly as good a response after feeding for only 10 days, others have not (C. Moffitt, Personal Communication). Erythromycin thiocyanate is available as a premix (Gallamycin 50P, 11%). The University of Idaho also has an INAD exemption for its use (C. Moffitt, Personal Communication).

Injectable formulations:

1. For treating infected, mature salmonids to prevent mortality, while holding them before spawning, and to reduce infection incidence in eggs
    a. Inject 10 to 20 mg of erythromycin base (Erythro® 100 or 200)/kg (= 9 mg/pound) of body weight via the dorsal sinus or IP 9 to 56 days before spawning. Armstrong et al. (1989) found that the highest drug levels in eggs are achieved by administering the drug 12 to 20 days before spawning, although this difference is not large. Moffitt (1992) found that the best time for injection was 15 to 40 days before spawning.

Use No. 2: Treatment of streptococcosis

Oral formulations:

1. Feed 25 to 50 mg erythromycin/kg (= 11 to 23 mg/pound) of body weight/day for 4 to 7 days (Kitao et al., 1987).

Flumequine

See the general discussion under oxolinic acid. Intramuscular injection produces high antibiotic levels for a reasonably long time (probably several days for most fish) (Nouws et al., 1992). The susceptibility of aquarium fish pathogens to quinolones (Goven et al., 1990) makes this an attractive candidate for treating individual pet fish.

Water-borne formulations:

1. Bath
    a. Add 50 to 100 mg of flumequine/l (= 190 to 380 mg/gallon) of freshwater that has a pH of 6.8 to 7.2 and treat for 3 hours. This has been experimentally effective in treating *Aeromonas salmonicida* (O'Grady et al., 1988). Uptake via bath is less in hard water (O'Grady et al., 1988) and high pH (7-fold less uptake in pH 8.0 water compared to pH 7.0 water). It is probably best to increase the dosage when treating marine fish (Endo, 1992).

Oral formulations:

1. Feed 10 mg of flumequine/kg (= 4.5 mg/pound) of body weight/day for 10 days.

Injectable formulations:

1. Inject 30 mg of flumequine/kg (= 14 mg/pound) of body weight IP. This dose has produced effective serum levels in presmolt Atlantic salmon (held in freshwater) for over 10 days (Scallan & Smith, 1985). IM injection is probably also effective (Nouws et al., 1992).

Furaltadone

See the general discussion under nifurpirinol.

Water-borne formulations:

1. Prolonged immersion
    a. Add 20 to 50 mg of furaltadone/l (= 76 to 190 mg/gallon), and treat fish for 24 hours (Debuf, 1991).

Furazolidone (NF-180, Furox-50, Furazolidone [Aurum], or equivalent)

See the general discussion under nifurpirinol. Furazolidone decays quickly in wet diets (e.g., whole fish, moist salmonid diets).

Water-borne formulations:

1. Prolonged immersion
    a. Add 1 to 10 mg of furazolidone/l (= 3.8 to 38 mg/gallon), and treat fish for at least 24 hours.

Oral formulations:

1. Feed 50 to 100 mg of furazolidone/kg (= 23 to 45 mg/pound) of body weight/day for 10 to 15 days. Palatability problems have occurred at higher oral doses.

Kanamycin sulfate ([Fort Dodge] injectable, [Aurum], or equivalent)

This aminoglycoside antibiotic is relatively stable in water and fairly well-absorbed (Gilmartin et al., 1976) but may not be safe to use for some species.

Water-borne formulations:

1. Prolonged immersion
    a. Add 50 to 100 mg kanamycin sulfate/l (= 190 to 380 mg/gallon) every 3 days for 3 treatments, changing 50% of the water after every treatment.

Oral formulations:
1. Feed 50 mg of kanamycin sulfate/kg (= 23 mg/pound) of body weight/day

Injectable formulations:
1. Inject 20 mg kanamycin sulfate/kg (= 9 mg/pound) of body weight IP every 3 days for 14 days. This dose is toxic to some species. Administering only 10 mg/kg once weekly caused nephrotoxicity (acute tubular necrosis) and liver damage in steelhead trout (McBride et al., 1975).

Nalidixic acid (NegGram® [Upjohn] oral or tablets)

This quinolone inhibits many aquarium fish pathogens (Goven et al., 1990). It may be toxic to some species. See general disussion under oxolinic acid.

Water-borne formulations:
1. Bath
   a. Add 13 mg of nalidixic acid/l of water (= 50 mg of nalidixic acid/gallon), and treat for 1 to 4 hours. Repeat if needed (Lewbart, 1991).

Neomycin sulfate (Neomycin sulfate [Aurum], Biosol® [Upjohn])

This aminoglycoside is commonly sold as an antibacterial for aquarium fish but is difficult to use in prolonged immersions because of its toxicity to biological filtration. Since biological filtration must be removed during treatment to prevent killing the nitrifiers, fish densities must be low enough so that ammonia will not reach toxic levels in the system during treatment.

Water-borne formulations:
1. Prolonged immersion
   a. Add 66 mg of neomycin sulfate/l (= 250 mg/gallon). Repeat every 3 days for up to a total of 3 times.

Nifurpirinol (Furanace, P-7138, Auranace [Aurum], or equivalent)

Nifurpirinol is a nitrofuran. Nitrofurans are an effective group of synthetic antimicrobials. Some are stable in both freshwater and saltwater and are rapidly absorbed by fish (Anonymous, Undated; Nusbaum & Shotts, 1981; Pearse et al., 1974). They are also effective against many of the common pathogens that affect fish (Anonymous, Undated). A single bath treatment is often effective against susceptible organisms (Anonymous, Undated). There have been some palatability problems with oral nitrofurans (Amend, 1972). Unfortunately, nitrofurans are carcinogenic, genotoxic, and mutagenic (Yndestad, 1992) and are strictly illegal for use on fish in some countries, including the United States.

Catfish, loaches, and other scaleless fish are considered sensitive to water-borne nitrofurans, but this varies with species (Anonymous, Undated). Nitrofurans are photosensitive and may be inactivated in bright light. By preventing exposure to light, the half-life is greatly increased.

Water-borne formulations:
1. Bath
   a. Add 1 to 2 mg nifurpirinol/l (= 3.8 to 7.2 mg/gallon), and treat for 5 minutes to 6 hours (Anonymous, Undated; Piper et al., 1982). A wide range of doses have been used. As little as 5 minutes' exposure to a 2 mg/l solution has treated marine fish at 10° C (50 ° F) (Pearse et al., 1974). A 6.5-hour bath is effective against some, but not all channel catfish pathogens (Mitchell & Plumb, 1980). The 96-hour water-borne LC_{50} for nifurpirinol ranges from 0.30 to 2.0 mg/l (Anonymous, Undated).
2. Prolonged immersion
   a. Add 0.10 mg nifurpirinol/l (= 0.40 mg/gallon) and treat for 3 to 5 days (Piper et al., 1982). Prolonged immersion of channel catfish at 0.50 mg/l causes skin damage (Mitchell & Plumb, 1980).

Oral formulations:
Palatability problems have occurred with oral nifurpirinol (Amend, 1972).
1. Feed 4 to 10 mg of nifurpirinol/kg (= 1.8 to 4.5 mg/pound) of body weight twice daily for 5 days (Anonymous, Undated).
2. Feed 0.45 to 0.90 mg of nifurpirinol/kg (= 1 to 2 mg/pound) of body weight/day for 5 days (Piper et al., 1982).

Nitrofurazone (Furacyn® = 9.3% nitrofurazone [Aurum])

See the general discussion under nifurpirinol.

Water-borne formulations:
1. Bath
   a. Add 100 mg nitrofurazone/l (= 380 mg/gallon), and treat for 30 minutes (Anonymous, Undated).
   b. Add 10 mg nitrofurazone/l (= 38 mg/gallon), and treat for 6 to 12 hours. Repeat as needed (Lewbart, 1991).
2. Prolonged immersion
   a. Add at least 2 mg nitrofurazone/l (= 7.6 mg/gallon) and treat for 5 to 10 days. Nitrofurazone is toxic to sac-fry and swim-up fry of channel catfish at 15 mg/l (Piper et al., 1982). Do not use > 5 mg/l for this species (best not to use).

Oxolinic acid (Aqualinic™ [Vetrepharm] or Aquinox™ [Vetrepharm], oxolinic acid [Aurum], or equivalent)

Oxolinic acid is a quinolone, a class of synthetic antimicrobials that are highly effective against many gram-negative bacterial pathogens of fish. Quinolones inhibit bacterial DNA gyrase, thus inhibiting negative supercoiling of the bacterial chromosome. They can be bacteriostatic or bactericidal. They are well absorbed orally (Alderman, 1988).

The widespread use of oxolinic acid has led to the development of a significant amount of chromosomal resistance in organisms from medicated populations (Tsoumas et al., 1989), with cross-resistance against other quinolones. Plasmid-mediated resistance has not yet been reported for any quinolone. A second generation of quinolones, the fluoroquinolones (sarafloxacin, enrofloxacin, flumequine) appear to have additional modes of antibacterial action (Bowser & Babish, 1991).

All quinolones, especially the fluoroquinolones, chelate divalent cations and are thus are inhibited by high hardness and possibly divalent cations in the diet. Water-borne formulations:

There may be less uptake in hard water. There is better uptake at pH < 6.9 (Endo & Onozawa, 1987).

1. Bath
   a. Add 25 mg oxolinic acid/l (= 95 mg/gallon) and treat for 15 minutes. Repeat twice daily for 3 days. This regimen has successfully treated vibriosis in juvenile turbot (Austin et al., 1982).
2. Prolonged immersion
   a. Add 1 mg oxolinic acid/l (= 3.8 mg/gallon), and treat for 24 hours.

Oral formulations:

1. Feed 10 mg of oxolinic acid/kg (= 4.5 mg/pound) of body weight/day for 10 days in freshwater. Up to 30 mg/kg may be needed in seawater. Withdrawal time is 500 degree days (Debuf, 1991).

Oxytetracycline hydrochloride (Terramycin for Fish® [Pfizer], Liquamycin-100® [Pfizer] injectable, Tetraplex® [PH Pharmaceuticals], Microtet® [Microbiologicals])

Tetracyclines are mostly static inhibitors of bacterial protein synthesis that bind to the 30S ribosome. Oxytetracycline is effective against several important fish pathogens. It is probably most useful for treating columnaris disease (see *PROBLEM 37*). Resistance by aeromonads, vibrios, and other bacteria is common. All tetracyclines share virtually identical spectra of antibacterial activity; thus, cross-resistance and susceptibility of bacteria are nearly complete. Transmissible plasmid-mediated bacterial resistance is well documented (Michel & Alderman, 1992).

Oxytetracycline is light-sensitive and will turn dark brown when decomposing. When used as a prolonged immersion, half of the water should be changed immediately if this happens. Degraded tetracyclines are nephrotoxic to humans (Fanconi syndrome). Avoid contact with the degraded drug (wear gloves). A pure preparation of oxytetracycline should be used for prolonged immersion. Do **not** use products that have small amounts of active drug (e.g., products having only 5%

oxytetracycline), since the large amounts of sugar in the these preparations cause a massive bacterial bloom.

Oxytetracycline is fairly stable in water (Nusbaum & Shotts, 1981; Nouws et al., 1992), making it suitable for prolonged immersion. All tetracyclines chelate divalent cations (Ca, Mg), causing their inactivation (Lunestad & Goksoyr, 1990); thus, higher doses should be used in hard water. Magnesium has a higher avidity for oxytetracycline than does calcium. Complexation is probably also responsible for oxytetracycline being less absorbed when it is given as medicated diet to fish in seawater (Lunestad, 1992).

Oxytetracycline is not clinically toxic to lake trout at even 5 times the therapeutic concentration (Marking et al., 1988), but it causes depression of many immune functions at therapeutic doses (Rijkers et al., 1980; van der Heijden et al., 1992). The clinical significance of this immunosuppression is unclear, especially in light of oxytetracycline's long-term success in treating fish pathogens.

Water-borne formulations:

A yellow-brown foam may develop in the water during treatment.

1. Bath
   a. Add 10 to 50 mg oxytetracycline HCl/l (= 38 to 190 mg/gallon), and treat for 1 hour for surface bacterial infections (Bullock & Snieszko, 1970; Piper et al., 1982).
2. Prolonged immersion
   a. Add 10 to 100 mg oxytetracycline HCl/l (= 38 to 380 mg/gallon), and treat for 1 to 3 days (Piper et al., 1982). Use higher doses in hard water. If the fish are still sick, retreat on the third day after a 50% water change before treatment. Keep the tank covered during treatment to prevent photoinactivation.

Oral formulations:

1. Oxytetracycline is palatable
   a. Feed 55 to 83 mg oxytetracycline HCl/kg (= 25 to 37 mg/pound) of body weight/day for 10 days. This dose of Terramycin for Fish® (Pfizer) is approved for treating *Aeromonas*, *Pseudomonas*, and "*Haemophilus*" (*Aeromonas salmonicida*) infections in salmonids and channel catfish in the United States. Withdrawal times are 21 days (United States), 300 to 500 degree days (Debuf, 1991).
   b. Feed 100 mg oxytetracycline HCl/kg (= 46 mg/pound) of body weight/day for 21 days to treat bacterial kidney disease (Kent, 1992).

Injectable formulations:

1. Inject 25 to 50 mg oxytetracycline HCl/kg (= 11 to 23 mg/pound) of body weight IM or IP (Piper et al., 1982). Intramuscular injection produces high antibiotic levels for a reasonably long

time (probably several days for most fish) (Nouws et al., 1992).

Sarafloxacin: This is a fluoroquinolone that has broad-spectrum potency against many fish pathogens, including *Aeromonas salmonicida*, *Vibrio anguillarum*, *Yersinia ruckeri*, and *Edwardsiella ictaluri* (Wilson & MacMillan, 1990; Stamm, 1992). It is presently being tested for future commercial release (Stamm, 1992). See the general discussion under oxolinic acid.

Sulfadiazine-Trimethoprim (Co-trimazine: Sulpha-trim® [Hand/PH], Tribrissen™ 40% powder [Coopers Pitman-Moore], or equivalent)

This is a potentiated sulfonamide consisting of 1 part trimethoprim and 5 parts sulfadiazine. Potentiated sulfonamides inhibit the bacterial dihydrofolate reductase enzyme pathway at two points, causing a synergistic inhibition of folate synthesis. Uptake of water-borne sulfas is much greater in seawater than freshwater (Bergsjo & Bergsjo, 1978). Some sulfas are toxic to fish (Kubota et al., 1970); however, reported toxic side effects with potentiated sulfas are uncommon.

Oral formulations:
1. Feed 30 to 50 mg of sulfadiazine-trimethoprim/kg (14 to 23 mg/pound) of body weight/day for 7 to 10 days. Withdrawal time is 500 degree days (Debuf, 1991).

Injectable formulations:
1. Inject 125 mg of sulfadiazine-trimethoprim/kg (= 60 mg/pound) of body weight IP (Debuf, 1991).

Sulfadimethoxine-Ormetoprim (Romet B® [Hoffman-LaRoche], Romet 30® [Hoffman-LaRoche], Primor® [Hoffman-LaRoche] tablets)

This potentiated sulfonamide is commonly used to treat *Aeromonas* and *Edwardsiella* infections in food fish in the United States. It is available as a premix powder (Romet B®) for incorporation into feed, or it is already incorporated into medicated feed (Romet 30®). It is more expensive than oxytetracycline. For channel catfish, antibiotic should be incorporated into feed at a rate of 1.65%. Higher concentrations in feed are poorly consumed because of the poor palatability of ormetoprim. It is best to incorporate at least 16% fish meal in the feed to ensure palatability (Robinson et al., 1990). See general discussion under *sulfadiazine-trimethoprim*.

Oral formulations:
1. Feed 50 mg of sulfadimethoxine-ormetoprim/kg (= 23 mg sulfadimethoxine-ormetoprim/pound) of body weight/day for 5 days. Withdrawal time for salmonids is 42 days (United States); withdrawal time for channel catfish is 3 days (United States).
2. Produce medicated brine shrimp by placing nauplii (larvae) in a 3 mg/l concentration of Romet-B® in seawater for 4 hours. Rinse in seawater,

using a brine shrimp net, and immediately feed it to fish (Mohney et al., 1990). This procedure may also work with adult brine shrimp and other live feeds. This delivery method is not approved for food fish in the United States.

Sulfamerazine (Sulfamerazine in Fish Grade [American Cyanamid Company])

Sulfamerazine is approved in the United States as an antibacterial against furunculosis in salmonids, but it is virtually useless because of widespread resistance. The product has recently been withdrawn by the manufacturer because of lack of sales. Sulfonamides may be toxic when fed at over 220 mg/kg of body weight/day.

Oral formulations:
1. Feed 220 mg of sulfamerazine/kg (= 100 mg/pound) of body weight/day for 14 days. Withdrawal time is 21 days (United States).

Sulfamethoxazole-Trimethoprim (Co-trimoxazole: Septra® IV [Burroughs Wellcome], or equivalent)

See general discussion under *sulfadiazine-trimethoprim*.

Water-borne formulations:
1. Bath
   a. Add 25 mg of sulfamethoxazole-trimethoprim/l (= 95 mg/gallon) and treat for 6 to 12 hours. Treat until clinical signs are gone (Lewbart, 1991).

Oral formulations:
1. Feed 50 mg of sulfamethoxazole-trimethoprim/kg (= 23 mg/pound) of body weight/day for 10 days (Lewbart, 1991).

Injectable formulations:
1. Inject 50 mg of sulfamethoxazole-trimethoprim/kg (= 23 mg/pound) of body weight IP every day for 7 days (Lewbart, 1991).

Many other antibotics are sold over the counter in aquarium stores or by aquaculture supply firms. In the great majority of cases, their efficacy against treating the diseases that they claim to be useful for are uncertain. Considerable caution is warranted before considering using any of these agents.

Antiseptics

See *ACETIC ACID, CHLORAMINE-T, FORMALIN, HYDROGEN PEROXIDE, POTASSIUM PERMANGANATE, POTENTIATED IODINE, QUATERNARY AMMONIUM COMPOUNDS*. Also see *DISINFECTANTS*.

Bayluscide (Bayer 73 [Bayer])

Use No. 1: Adjunct to TFM to kill lampreys in streams; to survey for lampreys in streams

Bayluscide is the ethanolamine salt of niclosamide (Anonymous, 1989). Niclosamide is used as an anthelmintic for cestodes in mammals. Bayluscide can only be applied to streams by certified government officials (Marking, 1992).

Use No. 2: Control of aquatic snails

This use is not presently approved in the United States, except Puerto Rico, but it is pending in other areas of the United States (Schnick, 1992).

Water-borne formulations:
1. Bath/prolonged immersion
   a. Add 1 pound of Bayluscide/surface acre of water. This is approved by the Florida Department of Agriculture for application to commercial tropical aquarium fish ponds (R. Francis-Floyd, Personal Communication).

Benzocaine (Ethyl Aminobenzoate)

Benzocaine and **tricaine** are both derived from benzoic acid. Benzocaine is used in mammals as a local anesthetic. It is sparingly water soluble, and thus it is best to prepare a stock solution in ethanol, and then add this to the water. Like tricaine, benzocaine solutions should be neutralized. There is faster recovery in warm water. Benzocaine may be more toxic than tricaine for some species. It is no safer or more effective than tricaine, but it is less expensive. Note, however, that in the United States, all ethical sources of benzocaine have complex additives (e.g., lotions, cremes), since benzocaine is approved only as a topical anesthetic for mammals. These preparations are not suitable for fish anesthesia.

Benzocaine's activity may vary considerably with water quality, fish species, fish size, and fish density. Given dosages should be used as general guidelines. The clinical response of the fish should also be used to ascertain the proper dosage (see p. 17).

Use No. 1: Sedation for transporting fish

Water-borne formulations:
1. Bath/prolonged immersion
   a. Add ~10 to 40 mg benzocaine/l (~38 to 150 mg/gallon).

Use No. 2: Anesthesia

Water-borne formulations:
1. Bath
   a. Add ~50 to 500 mg benzocaine/l (= ~190 to 1900 mg/gallon). This concentration will usually cause anesthesia within 60 seconds.
   b. For large fish, a 1 g/l solution of benzocaine can be sprayed onto the gills, using an aerosol pump sprayer. This can be reapplied if needed during a procedure.

Use No. 3: Euthanization

Water-borne formulations:
1. Bath
   a. Add to effect. This usually requires a slightly higher dose than for anesthesia. Fish should be kept in this solution for 10 minutes after all breathing stops to ensure that they are dead.

Buffers: Freshwater Aquaria

Use: Adjusting pH to the proper range in freshwater aquaria. Do not adjust pH more than 0.2 to 0.3 units/day, except in an emergency. Each solution should be added dropwise to the aquarium (start by adding a small amount and measure change in pH after thoroughly mixing; add more as needed).

Water-borne formulations:
1. Prolonged immersion
   a. To *lower* pH, add sodium phosphate (Acidifier [Aquatronics] or equivalent).
   b. To *lower* pH, prepare buffer stock solution by adding 1.0 gram of sodium phosphate monobasic (NaH_2PO_4) to 100 ml of water and 1.0 gram of sodium phosphate dibasic (Na_2HPO_4) to 100 ml of water. Add equal numbers of drops/gallon of both solutions to the tank.
   c. To *raise* pH, add sodium bicarbonate (Alkalizer [Aquatronics] or equivalent).
   d. To *maintain* pH at 7.0, add mixed buffer solution (pH Fixit [Aquatronics], or equivalent).
   e. To *maintain* pH, prepare buffer stock solution by adding 1.0 gram of food-grade sodium bicarbonate (Arm & Hammer Baking Soda, or equivalent) and 1.0 gram of sodium phosphate dibasic (Na_2HPO_4) to 100 ml of water.

Buffers: Marine Aquaria

Use: Adjusting pH to the proper range in marine aquaria

Water-borne formulations:
1. Prolonged immersion
   a. Add a salt mixture of carbonates, borates, and trace elements: AquaLab® I Conditioner pH-Guard™ (Mardel Laboratories). Use as directed.
   b. Add salts of carbonates and borates (Sea Buffer [Aquarium Systems], or equivalent). Use as directed.

Buffers: Ponds
LIMESTONE, AGRICULTURAL LIME, CALCITE, DOLOMITE, SLAKED LIME, UNSLAKED LIME

Use: Adjusting pH and/or alkalinity to proper range in ponds

Agricultural lime (limestone) is *calcite* ($CaCO_3$), *dolomite* ($CaMg[CO_3]_2$), or some combination of both. Do **not** confuse agricultural lime with *slaked lime* or *unslaked lime*, which can also be used for buffering ponds; however, these are much more dangerous to use. Agricultural lime is the safest, cheapest, and most effective liming material for ponds (Boyd, 1990).

To determine the amount of buffer required, mud should be collected from several locations in the pond. About 10 representative, equal-volume samples are usually needed for sampling a 1 ha pond; proportionately more samples are needed in larger ponds (Boyd, 1990). Samples can be shipped to a laboratory for determination of lime requirement. A county extension agent can help to find a suitable lab. About 2000 to 4000 kg/ha (1 to 2 tons/ac) of agricultural limestone will usually be needed; one application usually lasts for several years. Limestone can be applied by shoveling it into the pond from a boat or by placing it along the pond bank and allowing it to wash into the pond. In temperate areas, lime after fertilization ends in late fall or early winter. In the subtropics and tropics, lime a few weeks before fertilization begins in spring. See Sills (1974) and Boyd (1990) for more details on liming ponds.

Water-borne formulations:
    1. Prolonged immersion

Add lime at a rate sufficient to raise the alkalinity to the desired level (usually > 20 mg/l total alkalinity). Ponds that require lime usually need at least 2000 kg/hectare (= 1 ton/acre) (Boyd, 1990). Note that liming rate is calculated based on pond surface area and not on water volume.
        a. Add agricultural lime to effect.
        b. Add slaked lime to effect.
        c. Add unslaked lime to effect.

Calcium

Use No. 1: Adjusting hardness and/or calcium to proper range

Liming with calcite usually will not raise the calcium concentration to more than 45 mg/l hardness (Boyd, 1990). This is satisfactory for most fish species. For species that require harder water, gypsum or calcium chloride must be used. Gypsum is less expensive and more readily available than calcium chloride. Every 1.0 mg/l of calcium that is added to water increases the hardness by 2.5 mg/l as $CaCO_3$.

Water-borne formulations:
    1. Prolonged immersion in aquaria
        a. Add Aqua-cichlids (Aquatronics) mineral mix. Use as directed.
    2. Prolonged immersion in ponds
        a. Add lime (see *BUFFERS: PONDS*).
        b. Add agricultural gypsum at a rate of 1.72 mg pure gypsum/l for every 1.00 mg/l of total hardness required. Gypsum is available in two forms (anhydrite and dihydrate). Anhydrite calcium sulfate ($CaSO_4$) is available as a powder or as granules (land plaster). Dihydrate calcium sulfate ($CaSO_4 \cdot 2H_2O$, damp agricultural gypsum, peanut mixer) is used mainly as a calcium supplement for peanuts. Approximately 50% more of damp gypsum is needed to provide the same amount of calcium as in anhydrite calcium sulfate. However, the anhydrite form is much more expensive than damp agricultural gypsum and is usually used only for small ponds. Determine the percentage of calcium and other minerals in the preparation before using it, and use a neutralized product.
    3. Constant flow in raceways/troughs during egg incubation
        a. Add calcium chloride ($CaCl_2 \cdot 2H_2O$) at a rate of 1.45 mg pure $CaCl_2 \cdot 2H_2O$/l for every 1.00 mg/l of total hardness required.

Use No. 2: Reducing excessively high diurnal pH rise in ponds

Water-borne formulations:
    1. Prolonged immersion
        a. Add a concentration of agricultural gypsum equal to twice the difference between total hardness and total alkalinity to roughly equalize hardness (Boyd, 1990).

Use No. 3: Decreasing turbidity in ponds

Divalent cations, such as calcium, neutralize charged, suspended particles (e.g., clays), causing them to aggregate (flocculate) and thus precipitate (Stumm & Morgan, 1970).

Water-borne formulations:
    1. Prolonged immersion in ponds
        a. Add agricultural lime (see *BUFFERS: PONDS*).
        b. Add agricultural gypsum at a rate of 250 to 500 mg/l. Gypsum is more expensive than alum, but it is safer to use and has a longer lasting effect (Wu & Boyd, 1990).

Carbon Dioxide (Carbonic Acid, CO_2)

In mammals, carbon dioxide causes direct depression of the cerebral cortex, subcortical structures, and vital centers. It also causes direct depression of heart muscle. Similar effects presumably occur in fish. Carbon dioxide is a poor anesthetic or sedative (slow-acting, stressful, lethal after repeated exposures) (Marking & Meyer, 1985). Its major advantage is that it leaves no residue, so fish can be slaughtered immediately for human consumption.

It is essential to maintain high DO (> 5 mg/l). Because of variable results and the difficulty in maintaining proper CO_2 concentrations, it should only be used as a last resort (e.g., when no residues are acceptable or no other anesthetics are available). It is best to measure the free CO_2 (see A.P.H.A., 1992). Do not use CO_2 gas in closed areas ($> 10\%$ causes loss of consciousness in humans).

Also see the general discussion under *SODIUM BICARBONATE* for more information on CO_2 anesthesia.

Note that activity may vary considerably with water quality, fish species, fish size, and fish density. Given dosages should be used as general guidelines, with the clinical response of the fish being used to gauge the proper dosage (see p. 17).

Use No. 1: Sedation/anesthesia

Water-borne formulations:
1. Bath
    a. Produce a CO_2 concentration of 200 to 400 mg/l by bubbling carbon dioxide gas through water (Takeda & Itzawa, 1983). Anesthesia usually occurs within 5 minutes.

Use No. 2: Euthanasia

Water-borne formulations:
1. Bath
    a. Bubble carbon dioxide gas through water until death occurs (no breathing for > 10 minutes).

Chloramine Neutralizer

Use: Removal of chloramine from municipal (tap) water supplies. Chloramine neutralizer can also be used to remove chlorine. Note that ammonia is released by the detoxification of chloramine and must also be removed. Use zeolite to remove ammonia.

Water-borne formulations:
1. Prolonged immersion
    a. Use Super Strength 5-in-1 Water Conditioner™ (Aquarium Pharmaceuticals). Use as directed.

    b. Use Saltwater MarPlex™. Use as directed. For removal of chloramine and ammonia from water used for marine aquaria.
    c. Add sodium thiosulfate (see *CHLORINE NEUTRALIZER*).

Chloramine-T (N-Chloro-4-Methylbenzenesulfonamide Sodium Salt [Wisconsin Pharmacal Company])

Use: Treatment of monogeneans and skin/gill bacterial infections

High doses may be toxic to koi. Do not use with formalin or benzalkonium chloride. Avoid contact with metal or human skin/eye contact. Dose depends on water hardness and pH (Table III-8) (Rach et al., 1988; Bullock et al., 1991).

Water-borne formulations:
1. Bath
    a. Add the appropriate dose of chloramine-T to systems with a 4-hour turnover. Treatment can be repeated every 4 hours for a total of 4 times if needed.

Table III-8   Concentration of chloramine-T to use at various pH and hardness levels.

pH	Dose (mg/l)	
	Soft water	Hard water
6.0	2.5	7.0
6.5	5.0	10.0
7.0	10.0	15.0
7.5	18.0	18.0
8.0	20.0	20.0

Modified from Debuf, 1991.

Chloride

Use: Treatment of nitrite toxicity

Add enough chloride to produce at least a 6:1 ratio (w/w) of $Cl:NO_2$ ions.

$$\text{Amount } Cl^- \text{ needed in mg/l} = (6 \times [NO_2^- \text{ in water}] - [Cl^- \text{ in water}])$$

Note that $[NO_2]$ refers to the amount of nitrite, not the amount of nitrite-nitrogen.

$$\text{Sodium chloride needed (lb)} = \frac{\text{Pond volume}}{\text{(acre-feet)}} \times 4.54 \times \frac{\text{(chloride needed}}{\text{in mg/l)}}$$

PROBLEM 6 describes methods for measuring chloride and nitrite concentrations.

Water-borne formulations:
1. Prolonged immersion
   a. Add rock salt (NaCl) to effect (contains ~60% Cl) (see *SALT*).
   b. Add solar salt to effect (contains ~55% Cl) (see *SALT*).
   c. Add artificial seawater (Instant Ocean®, or equivalent) to effect (contains ~55% Cl).
   d. Add CaCl$_2$ to effect (contains ~64% Cl); 1.0 mg CaCl$_2$/l releases 0.64 mg Cl/l.

Chlorine

Use: Disinfection of utensils and aquaria

Chlorination actually involves the formation of several reactive species that have different disinfecting potencies. Free chlorine residual consists of aqueous molecular chlorine (Cl$_2$), hypochlorous acid (HOCl), and hypochlorite ion (OCl$^-$). Chlorine is less active at high pH (more exists as OCl$^-$, which is less active than other forms). At the pH of most water, hypochlorous acid and hypochlorite ion predominate (also see *PROBLEM 82*).

Chlorination is a better overall disinfectant than **quaternary ammonium compounds** or **potentiated iodine** (see *DISINFECTANTS*); however, it will destroy netting. Prolonged contact will also rapidly corrode metal and damage many plastics (see *QUATERNARY AMMONIUM, FORMALIN*). Chlorination releases volatile chlorine gas, which irritates mucous membranes. Solutions should only be used in a well-ventilated area. Large amounts of organic matter necessitate a higher dosage. Alkaline (> 7.0) pH inhibits chlorination (Boyd, 1990). Use extreme caution around areas that hold fish, since chlorine is highly toxic, even in trace amounts. Items must be well rinsed in water before reuse and should be allowed to stand in aerated water for at least 1 day. Chlorine can also be neutralized with sodium thiosulfate (see *CHLORINE NEUTRALIZERS*). See *DISINFECTANTS* for general guidelines on use.
Water-borne formulations:
1. Prolonged immersion
   a. Add calcium hypochlorite (Ca[OCl])$_2$ = high test hypochlorite = HTH [Olin]) to produce 200 mg/l available chlorine for at least 1 hour to disinfect raceways, small aquaria, and utensils. Calcium hypochlorite is a dry powder. It has a longer shelf life than sodium hypochlorite, but it is more expensive. HTH powder may contain either 15%, 50%, or 65% of available chlorine to produce a solution that has 200 mg/l available chlorine (Leitritz & Lewis, 1976).
      i. Add 1.4 g of 15% available chlorine HTH powder/l (= 2 oz/10.5 gallons).

      ii. Add 0.4 g of 50% available chlorine HTH powder/l (= 1 oz/18 gallons).
      iii. Add 0.32 g of 65% available chlorine HTH powder/L (= 1 oz/23 gallons).
   b. Add 10 ml of commercial household bleach (Clorox® or equivalent = 5.25% sodium hypochlorite)/l (= 35 ml/gallon) for at least 1 hour (= 200 mg/l available chlorine).

Chlorine Neutralizer

Use: Neutralization of chlorine in water

Chemical neutralization of chlorine uses sodium thiosulfate. Seven mg of sodium thiosulfate neutralizes 1 mg of chlorine. Obviously, large amounts must be used when neutralizing chlorine levels used for disinfecting utensils, compared with the relatively low amounts needed to remove chlorine from tap water. Note that some commercial dechlorinating products are unreliable (Kuhns & Borgendale, 1980).
Water-borne formulations:
1. Prolonged immersion for municipal (tap) water
   a. Sodium thiosulfate [Super Strength 5-in-1 Water Conditioner™ (Aquarium Pharmaceuticals) or equivalent]. Use as directed.
2. Prolonged immersion for chlorine-disinfected utensils
   a. Prepare a solution that has enough sodium thiosulfate (Argent, or equivalent) to neutralize the free chlorine in the water. One liter of 200 mg/l available chlorine is neutralized by 1.5 g of sodium thiosulfate.

Chloroquine Diphosphate

Use: Treatment of *Amyloodinium ocellatum*

This drug is effective in treating *Amyloodinium* and is relatively nontoxic to fish. It is used to treat malaria in humans.

Experimentally infested clownfish (*Amphiprion ocellaris*) were freed of *A. ocellatum* infestation after a 10-day exposure to a single treatment of 5 to 10 mg/l chloroquine diphosphate. Chloroquine has no effect on tomont division, but it kills dinospores immediately on their excystment. The therapeutic concentration is nontoxic to fish but is highly toxic to micro- and macroalgae and to various invertebrates (C. Bower, Personal Communication). Chloroquine is expensive.
Water-borne formulations:
1. Prolonged immersion
   a. Add 10 mg chloroquine diphosphate/l (= 40 mg chloroquine diphosphate/gallon). Only one treatment is reportedly needed; however,

monitor closely for 21 days, and retreat if necessary. Add activated carbon if no relapse is apparent after 21 days.

Copper

Use No. 1: Treatment of ectoparasitic protozoa and monogeneans

While copper has been claimed to be effective against columnaris, bacterial gill disease, and water mold infections in cold water species, there are much better treatments available for these problems (Piper et al., 1982). Copper has a low therapeutic index, making it easy to overdose the fish. It is toxic to gill tissue (Cardeilac & Whitaker, 1988) and is immunosuppressive (Hetrick et al., 1979). Copper is also algicidal (also see *PROBLEM 83*).

Copper sulfate (Bluestone, copper sulfate pentahydrate, $CuSO_4 \cdot 5H_2O$)

Water-borne formulations:

1. Prolonged immersion in marine aquaria

Prolonged immersion copper is the most common and well-established method for controlling protozoan ectoparasites on marine aquarium fish (Cardeilhac & Whitaker, 1988). While copper can be used to treat ectoparasites of freshwater aquarium fish, this is not advisable because safer remedies are available. Copper is absorbed and/or inactivated in marine aquaria because of the high levels of calcareous materials (e.g., coral or limestone), which react to form insoluble copper carbonate (Keith, 1981). Copper's solubility is also highly dependent on pH, which controls the solubility of tenorite (CuO), the stable, solid phase of copper above pH 7 (Straus & Tucker, 1993). Cupric ion concentrations decrease dramatically with increasing pH (up to 100-fold with every 1 unit increase in pH). Copper is also bound and inactivated by organic matter.

Free copper ion levels *must* be maintained between 0.15 to 0.20 mg/l. A weaker concentration will not kill parasites, while a stronger concentration may kill the fish. Because of the high alkalinity in marine aquaria, large amounts of copper must first be added to an aquarium to reach this dose. The unpredictable nature of this initial dose requires that copper levels be assessed with a commercial kit (e.g., LaMotte Company, Hach Company, Aquarium Systems) and adjusted as needed. Initially, copper levels should be measured and adjusted twice daily. After several days, copper levels will become more stable and daily monitoring is usually satisfactory. Copper is extremely toxic to invertebrates and many algae. Also, the copper that precipitates out of solution may eventually resolubilize under some conditions, such as if the filter stops working for some reason and thus the pH of the water in the filter begins to drop. This may release toxic levels of free copper. Thus, it is best to treat in a separate hospital tank.

a. Prepare a copper stock solution (Bower, 1983) by adding 1 gram of $CuSO_4 \cdot 5H_2O$ to 250 ml of *distilled* water. Mix thoroughly until all of the crystals have dissolved. This stock solution contains 1 mg of copper/ml. Add enough copper to the aquarium to produce a concentration of 0.15 mg/l (= 0.57 mg/gallon):

#liters to treat × 0.15 = #mg copper needed
= #ml stock needed
#gallons to treat × 0.57 = #mg copper needed
= #ml stock needed

For example, if a 40-liter tank is to be treated with copper, one needs 6 mg of copper and thus must add 6 ml of copper stock solution (40 × 0.15 = 6).

Measure copper immediately to confirm that the proper dosage has been added. Use a copper test kit that measures in increments of at least 0.05 mg/l. Add more copper as needed to maintain a concentration of 0.15 to 0.20 mg copper/l. When more copper is needed, add 0.19 ml/gallon (= 0.05 ml/l) of copper stock to increase the copper concentration by 0.05 mg copper/l. Copper can be quickly removed with activated carbon (Keith, 1982).

2. Prolonged immersion in ponds

Copper sulfate is usually the treatment of choice for protozoan ectoparasites of pond-reared fish. Copper sulfate is approved by the EPA (US) for use in fish ponds as an algicide; however, it has not been approved by the FDA (US) as a drug.

Copper sulfate is relatively economical to use in ponds. It is best to use the finest form of copper sulfate available (i.e., *snow*) since larger-grained forms are more difficult to dissolve (R. Francis-Floyd, Personal Communication). The volumes of different forms of copper sulfate vary, which can affect treatment calculations made on a volume basis rather than a weight basis (Jensen & Durborow, 1984). Only pure forms (100% copper sulfate) of unoxidized (bright blue, not green) copper sulfate should be used.

The free copper ion is the active form of copper. The amount of free copper present in water depends on many factors, but especially total alkalinity. Thus, the amount of copper sulfate to add is determined from the total alkalinity of the water (Jensen & Durborow, 1984):

Total Alkalinity (mg/l)	[$CuSO_4 \cdot 5H_2O$] (mg/l)
20 to 49	0.25 to 0.50
50 to 99	0.50 to 0.75
100 to 149	0.75 to 1.00
150 to 200	1.00 to 2.00

While this information provides useful guidelines, it is preferable to calculate a more accurate dosage based on the following formula (Kleinholz, 1990):

$$\text{Amount } CuSO_4 \cdot 5H_2O \text{ to add (mg/l)} = \frac{\text{Total alkalinity of water (mg/l as } CaCO_3)}{100}$$

It is also advisable to perform a bioassay if copper sulfate has not been used previously in a particular body of water. Many clinicians believe that if the total alkalinity is less than 50 mg/l, copper sulfate is unpredictably toxic and thus contraindicated. Copper should never be used if the alkalinity is less than 20 mg/l. In water with high alkalinity (> 250 mg/l), copper sulfate rapidly precipitates as copper carbonate, and thus a single treatment is insufficient to provide a therapeutic concentration (see prolonged immersion in marine aquaria).

Guidelines for copper treatment in ponds have been based mainly on experience with channel catfish. A bioassay is advisable before treating a species with unknown susceptibility to copper.

 a. Add copper sulfate to effect

Chelated copper
Water-borne formulations:
 1. Prolonged immersion in marine aquaria

Chelated copper compounds consist of copper bound to one of several organic complexing agents, such as citrate, EDTA, or ethanolamine. They have the advantage of being more stable in seawater than copper sulfate, and thus normally require fewer additions of drug.

However, their efficacy and safety have not been thoroughly proven. A special test kit is also needed to measure chelated copper concentrations. It is probably safer to use unchelated copper sulfate. Remove chelated copper with activated carbon at the end of the treatment. Note that some brands of chelated copper are difficult to remove with activated carbon (Keith, 1982), so water changes may be needed instead.

 a. Prepare copper-citrate stock solution (Blasiola, 1978) by adding 2.23 g of $CuSO_4 \cdot 5 H_2O$ and 1.5 g of citric acid to 1 liter of distilled water. This stock solution contains 0.56 mg of copper/ml. Add 1 ml of stock solution/ gallon (= 0.26 ml/l) to produce an initial copper concentration of 0.15 mg/l. Immediately test to be sure that copper is at this concentration. If additional copper is needed, adding 0.33 ml/gallon (= 0.087 ml/l) will add 0.05 mg copper/l. Maintain copper levels at 0.15 to 0.20 mg/l for 14 to 21 days.
 b. Sea Cure Copper Treatment (Aquarium Systems) is to be used as directed.
 c. CopperSafe® (Mardel Laboratories) is a proprietary treatment for freshwater and saltwater parasites. Use as directed.

 2. Prolonged immersion in ponds

Chelated copper is infrequently used for treating freshwater pond fish. Its main advantage is its greater stability in high-alkalinity water. Chelated copper compounds are purportedly less toxic to fish than an equal amount of free copper, also making them potentially useful in low-alkalinity waters (Skea & Simonin, 1979; Straus & Tucker, 1993). However, the safety of chelated copper for treating fish under any conditions is not proven. Concentrations as low as 0.21 mg/l are lethal to some fish species, even in fairly high-alkalinity waters (95 mg/l) (Skea & Simonin, 1979). Chelates are also more costly than copper sulfate. Do not treat with more than 0.15 mg/l total copper, unless the fish species is known to be tolerant of a higher dose. Treatments should only be given once.
 a. Add chelated copper (Cutrine®, Applied Biochemist, or equivalent) (Wellborn, 1979).
 b. Mix two parts copper sulfate with one part citric acid (wt/wt), and spray over the pond (Anonymous, 1989).

Use No. 2: Eradication of snails
Water-borne formulations:
 1. Prolonged immersion in ponds
 a. Use unchelated copper sulfate at the same dosage as for ectoparasites (Use No. 1, Part 2). It may be best to treat at night, since many snails are nocturnal and more susceptible to treatment because they are more active (R. Francis-Floyd, Personal Communication).

Deionized Water (Distilled Water)

Use: Decreasing hardness or salinity
Water-borne formulations:
 1. Prolonged immersion for aquaria
 a. Add deionized water in an amount inversely proportional to the salinity or hardness desired. Several brands of home reverse osmosis (R/O) water treatment units (e.g., Sandpoint, Kent Marine, Spectrapure) are available.

Difluorobenzuron (Dimilin® [Union Carbide Company])

Difluorobenzuron inhibits chitin synthesis and is highly effective against *Lernaea* and other crustacean copepods. But, it is toxic to nontarget crustaceans and not licensed for aquaculture use. Over 76% of the dosage persists after 1 week in water; it is not degraded by pond temperatures > 27° C (80° F) (Hoffman, 1985).
Use: Treatment of copepod ectoparasites

Water-borne formulations:
1. Prolonged immersion
   a. Add 0.03 mg of difluorobenzuron/l (= 0.11 mg/gallon).

Diquat ([Ortho])

Use: Treatment of bacterial gill disease

Diquat is registered by the EPA (US) as a herbicide, but it is also effective against BGD. It is especially useful in earthen ponds; however, it is expensive and has decreased effectiveness in muddy or organically polluted waters (Warren, 1981). Avoid use if the treated water may be used to irrigate crops. Use rubber gloves and a respirator to avoid exposure to the chemical.

Water-borne formulations:
1. Bath
   a. Add 2 ppm of active diquat cation/l, and treat for 1 hour. The commercial preparation is 35.3% active ingredient, so 8.4 ppm of the commercial preparation should be used.

Disinfection (Also See *Chlorine, Formalin, Potentiated Iodine, Quaternary Ammonium Compounds, Slaked Lime, Unslaked Lime*)

Disinfection eliminates virtually all recognized pathogenic microorganisms but not necessarily all microbial forms (e.g., bacterial endospores) on inanimate objects. The effectiveness of disinfection is reduced by large numbers of contaminating organisms, organic matter, and materials that have small crevices that inhibit disinfectant penetration. The type and concentration of germicide and the time and temperature of exposure also affect disinfection. Thus, the exposure times given for various disinfectants are for relatively ideal conditions, and less effective results may occur if, for example, nets are heavily contaminated with debris or there are many pathogens coating a relatively inaccessible crevice.

Disinfectant activity can be divided into several levels: high, intermediate, and low (Tables III-9 and III-10). Note that the disinfectants most commonly used in aquaculture provide only intermediate-level disinfection at best. This is not to say that such disinfectants are not highly effective when used properly, but the clinician should be aware of their limitations. Fortunately, it appears that important pathogens affecting fish appear to be eliminated by proper intermediate-level disinfection, with few exceptions (e.g., *Clostridium*). However, some organisms are especially resistant to certain types of disinfectants at levels used routinely in aquaculture (e.g., *Myxobolus cerebralis* is not totally killed by even

Table III-9 Levels of disinfectant action according to type of microorganism.

Disinfectant level	Killing effect[*]					
	Bacteria			Fungi[†]	Viruses	
	Spores	Tubercle bacillus	Vegetative cells		Nonlipid and small	Lipid and medium size
High	+[‡]	+	+	+	+	+
Intermediate	−[§]	+	+	+	±[‖]	+
Low	−	−	+	±	±	+

Modified from Favero & Bond (1991), with permission.
[*] +, Killing effect can be expected; −, little or no killing effect.
[†] Includes asexual spores but not necessarily chlamydospores or sexual spores.
[‡] Only with extended exposure times are high-level disinfectants capable of killing high numbers of bacterial spores in laboratory tests; they are however, capable of sporicidal activity.
[§] Some intermediate-level disinfectants (e.g., chlorine) may exhibit some sporicidal activity, whereas others (e.g., alcohols or phenolic compounds) have no demonstrated sporicidal activity.
[‖] Some intermediate-level disinfectants, although tuberculocidal, may have limited virucidal activity.

1200 mg/l calcium hypochlorite for 16 hours [Hoffman, 1972]). Disinfection is **not** sterilization; thus, it doesn't guarantee the complete elimination of all pathogens.

Disinfection of water to destroy infectious agents before use in culture systems is usually accomplished by using chlorination, ozonation, or ultraviolet irradiation. Equipment is available from several suppliers (e.g., Engineered Products, Aquaculture Supply, Aquanetics Systems, Inc.). See Piper et al. (1982) and Spotte (1992) for details.

Disinfection refers to the elimination of microorganisms from inanimate objects. Germicides that are used on living tissue (e.g., eggs or fish) are **antiseptics.** Many germicides are used for both purposes (Table III-10).

Use No. 1: Eradication of infectious agents from a contaminated environment

Euthanized fish should be disposed of using standard biohazard guidelines for infectious waste (OSHA or equivalent). Aquaria and everything else that has come in contact with contaminated aquarium water (filters, ornaments, tubing, gravel, etc.) are usually disinfected by using chlorination. If there is a large amount of organic matter in the aquarium, this may require more disinfectant than recommended for "clean" aquaria. In ponds or other large culture systems, slaked or hydrated lime is the method of choice for disinfection.

Use No. 2: Killing of infectious agents in a contaminated water supply

Surface water sources are often contaminated with infectious agents that may cause problems in culture.

Table III-10 Methods of sterilization or disinfection; activity levels of selected liquid germicides.

Method	Use concentration of active ingredient	Disinfectant activity
STERILIZATION		
Hydrogen peroxide	6% to 30%	
Formalin	6% to 8%	
DISINFECTION		
Hydrogen peroxide	3% to 6%	High to intermediate
Formalin	1% to 8%	High to intermediate
Chlorine compounds	500 to 5000 mg of free or available chlorine/liter	Intermediate
Alcohols (ethyl, isopropyl)	70%	Intermediate
Iodophor compounds	30 to 50 mg of free iodine/liter 10,000 ppm available iodine	Intermediate to low
Quaternary ammonium compounds	0.1% to 0.2%	Low
ANTISEPSIS		
Alcohols (ethyl, isopropyl)	70%	
Iodophors	1 to 2 mg of free iodine/liter, 1% to 2% available iodine	

Modified from Favero & Bond (1991), with permission.

Treating incoming water can reduce or eliminate these problems, although it is expensive to treat water in this manner. **Ozone, ultraviolet irradiation,** and **chlorination/dechlorination** have been used (see Piper et al., 1982, and Spotte, 1992, for details).

Euthanasia

An accepted method of euthanasia is one that causes death with minimal discomfort to the animal. In some cases, it may not be possible to use accepted methods. The accepted methods for humane euthanasia of fish include anesthetic overdose (tricaine, benzocaine, or sodium pentobarbital), decapitation, or pithing (Anonymous, 1988; Anonymous, 1993). Although not specifically recommended by AVMA (Anonymous, 1993), quinaldine sulfate and 2-phenoxyethanol are probably also satisfactory for euthanization. Carbon dioxide is approved for use in nonaquatic animals but is less desirable than other anesthetics.

Sodium bicarbonate (baking soda, Alka-Seltzer®, or equivalent) is not an accepted method of euthanasia but is readily available in the home and thus can be used by the client to euthanize a pet in a relatively humane fashion.

When fish are examined for disease, mechanical trauma (decapitation, pithing) is often preferred to chemical overdose because ectoparasites may detach because of the chemical treatment. When chemical overdose is used, be sure that the fish is dead by leaving it in the chemical bath for at least 10 minutes after breathing stops.

1. Anesthetic overdose (see benzocaine, carbon dioxide, quinaldine sulfate, 2-phenoxyethanol, sodium bicarbonate, sodium pentobarbital, and tricaine).
2. Decapitation: Decapitation is assumed to cause rapid unconsciousness by stopping the blood supply to the brain. However, the central nervous system of some poikilothermic vertebrates is tolerant of hypoxic and hypotensive conditions (Cooper et al., 1989); thus, decapitation should be followed by pithing.
3. Pithing: Pithing is an effective and inexpensive means of euthanasia but requires dexterity and skill. It acts by causing trauma to nervous tissue. Double pithing (pithing both the brain and the spinal cord) is recommended to ensure immediate death.

The following methods are not approved as humane forms of euthanasia:

Cranial concussion (stunning): Stunning delivers a single, sharp blow to the head with sufficient force to produce immediate depression of the central nervous system. Stunning renders a fish unconscious but is not a method of euthanasia; thus, it must be followed by a method to ensure death. Cranial concussion can cause iatrogenic gill telangiectasis and thymic hemorrhages (Herman & Meade, 1985).

Cooling: Cooling fish to 4° C (refrigerator temperature) decreases metabolism and facilitates handling but probably does not raise the pain threshold. Rapid freezing is also not considered to be humane, unless preceded by anesthetization.

Rotenone, antimycin, bayluscide, and other poisons are commonly used to kill fish in ponds or other small bodies of water (Marking, 1992) but are not approved methods of euthanasia because they cause considerable distress (e.g., rotenone causes asphyxiation).

Fenbendazole (Panacur® [Hoechst])

Use: Treatment of nonencysted nematodes in the gastrointestinal tract

Water-borne formulations:
1. Prolonged immersion
   a. Add 2 mg fenbendazole/l (= 7.6 mg/gallon) once/week for 3 weeks.

Oral formulations:
1. Feed 25 mg fenbendazole/kg (= 11 mg/pound) of body weight/day for 3 days for aquarium fish (Gratzek & Blasiola, 1992). This is equivalent to a feed that has 0.25% fenbendazole and is fed at a rate of 1% of body weight/day.
2. Feed 50 mg fenbendazole/kg (= 23 mg/pound) of body weight once/week for 2 weeks (Langdon, 1992). This is equivalent to a feed that has 0.50% fenbendazole and is fed at a rate of 1% of body weight/day.
3. Intubate 50 mg fenbendazole/kg (= 23 mg/pound) of body weight (Langdon, 1992a).

Formalin (Formalin-F [Natchez], Paracide-F [Argent])

Formalin-F and Paracide-F are formalin labels approved for food fish use in the United States. Formalin is an aqueous solution of 37% to 40% formaldehyde gas (which equals 100% formalin). Formalin is volatile and irritating. It causes cancer in laboratory rodents and can cause contact hypersensitivity and lung damage in humans; solutions should be tightly sealed during storage and not allowed to contact human skin. Formalin should only be used in well-ventilated areas.

Formalin should be stored in the dark and above 4° C (39° F) to inhibit paraformaldehyde formation, a highly ichthyotoxic white precipitate. Formalin should never be used for treating fish if paraformaldehyde is present. Methanol (12% to 15%) is added to formalin to inhibit paraformaldehyde formation. Formalin should not be mixed with potassium permanganate.

Formalin is an effective parasiticide for bath treatment of most ectoparasitic protozoa and monogeneans. It has moderate-to-weak antibacterial activity. It also has moderate-to-strong activity against water molds on eggs but is not antifungal at doses that are nontoxic to fish.

Formalin is not usually recommended for treating commercial fish ponds because each 5 mg/l of formalin added to a pond chemically removes 1 mg/l of dissolved oxygen from the water (Allison, 1962; Schnick et al., 1989). It is also algicidal, which can further reduce oxygen (Schnick, 1973). Finally, it is usually too costly for use in large ponds. Formalin is also toxic to macrophytes (e.g., aquarium plants).

Formalin can be irritating to the gills, and water should be well aerated during treatment. Formalin is more toxic in soft, acid water and at high temperatures. Some fish are sensitive to formalin, so it is best to do a bioassay before using it on an untested fish species. Idiopathic deaths may occur within 1 to 72 hours of treatment (Warren, 1981). Rainbow trout seem especially susceptible. Typically, fish are piping, have excess mucus and pale color, and die with their mouth agape.

Formalin is contraindicated if fish have been recently stressed (e.g., transported, shipped) or if skin ulcers are present. Used formalin solutions should be diluted to at least 25 ppm before discarding.

Use No. 1: Treatment of protozoan and metazoan ectoparasites

Water-borne formulations:
1. Bath
   a. Add 0.125 to 0.250 ml formalin/l (= 125 to 250 ppm = 0.47 to 0.95 ml formalin/gallon), and treat for up to 60 minutes. This can be repeated two to three times once daily if needed. When temperatures are high (> 21° C [= 70° F] for warm water fish or > 10° C [= 50° F] for cold water fish), do not use > 167 ppm (= 0.167 ml/l = 184 mg/l = 0.63 ml/gallon) (Jensen & Durborow, 1984; Warren, 1981). The maximum dose should only be used every 3 days. Up to 167 ppm can be used on concurrent days (Post, 1983). Formalin is usually contraindicated if the temperature is > 27° C (80° F).
2. Prolonged immersion in aquaria
   a. Add 0.015 to 0.025 ml formalin/l (= 15 to 25 ppm = 16.5 to 27.6 mg/l = 0.06 to 0.09 ml/gallon). For *Ichthyophthirius*, use 25 ppm every other day for 3 treatments (Hoffman & Meyer, 1974). Remove all plants before treatment. Change up to 50% of the water on alternate days. Do not use > 10 ppm for striped bass fingerlings (Piper et al., 1982). The treatment schedule must be prolonged at low temperature (see *PROBLEM 19*).
3. Constant flow
   a. Add 0.015 ml formalin/l (= 15 ppm = 16.5 mg/l = 0.06 ml/gallon) as a constant flow for 24 hours. This can successfully treat ich in trout raceways (J. Hinshaw, Personal Communication).

Use No. 2: Treatment of water mold infection on eggs
Do not treat eggs within 24 hours of hatching. Formalin will concentrate in the shell, killing the embryo (Jensen & Durborow, 1984).

Water-borne formulations:
1. Bath
   a. Add 1 to 2 ml formalin/l (= 1000 to 2000 ppm = 1103 to 2206 mg/l = 3.8 to 7.6 ml/

gallon), and treat eggs for up to 15 minutes. This can be repeated as needed.

b. Add 0.23 ml formalin/l (= 227 ppm = 250 mg/l = 0.87 ml/gallon), and treat eggs for up to 60 minutes. This is experimentally effective in treating infections of rainbow trout eggs (Bailey & Jeffrey, 1989).

Use No. 3: Killing of tadpoles in ponds
Water-borne formulations:
Prolonged immersion

a. Add 0.03 ml formalin/l (= 30 ppm = 0.11 ml/gallon). This dose is most effective for small (2.5 to 5.0 cm [1- to 2-inch]) leopard frog tadpoles. Bullfrogs or larger tadpoles need higher doses that are usually ichthyotoxic (Helms, 1967).

Use No. 4: Disinfectant
Water-borne formulations:
Prolonged immersion

a. Add 27 to 220 ml formalin/l (= 102 to 833 ml/gallon = 1% to 8% formaldehyde [Favero & Bond, 1991]). This can be used as an indefinite soak for nets and other utensils. Keep the solution well covered and in a well-ventilated room. Rinse utensils well before using in aquaria.

Formalin/Malachite Green (Leteux-Meyer Mixture)

Use: Treatment of *Ichthyophthirius multifiliis*

This combination is synergistic for ich. See separate precautions under *FORMALIN* and *MALACHITE GREEN*. Slightly higher doses of either drug are ichthyotoxic (Leteux & Meyer, 1972).
Water-borne formulations:
Prolonged immersion

a. Add 25 ppm formalin + 0.10 mg/l malachite green (= 0.09 ml of formalin + 0.1 ml of malachite green stock [3.7 mg/l stock] solution/gallon). Treat every other day for 3 days. Change up to 50% of the water on alternate days. Remove all plants before treatment. The treatment schedule must be prolonged at low temperature (see *PROBLEM 19*).

Freshwater

Use: Treatment for marine ectoparasites

Freshwater can be used for therapy of clinical cases of marine *Trichodina* and other protozoans, Monogenea, and some crustaceans (Langdon, 1992a).

Water-borne formulations:
1. Bath
   a. Bathe marine fish in dechlorinated freshwater for 3 to 15 minutes. Remove immediately if stressed. This can be repeated weekly for an indefinite number of times. For treating *Caligus elongatus* on euryhaline marine fish, keep fish in freshwater for 20 minutes to kill all parasites (Landsberg et al., 1991).
2. Prolonged immersion
   a. Reduce salinity to freshwater. This is effective but can only be used for treating euryhaline fish (see *HYPOSALINITY*).

Hydrogen Peroxide (H$_2$O$_2$)

Commercial grade hydrogen peroxide is available over-the-counter as a 3% solution (= 30 mg H$_2$O$_2$/ml = 30,000 ppm).

Use No. 1: Treatment of acute environmental hypoxia
Water-borne formulations:
1. Prolonged immersion
   a. Add 0.25 ml of 3% H$_2$O$_2$ solution/l of water to be treated (= 1.0 ml/gallon = 7.5 ppm) (Sterba, 1983).
   b. Add 0.10 ml of 3% H$_2$O$_2$ solution/l (= 0.40 ml/gallon = 3 ppm) to yield 1.0 mg oxygen/l (Maranthe et al., 1975).

Use No. 2: Parasiticide for protozoan ectoparasites
Many fish do not tolerate this treatment.
Water-borne formulations
1. Bath
   a. Add 10 ml of 3% H$_2$O$_2$ solution/l (= 38 ml/gallon = 300 ppm), and treat for 10 to 15 minutes (Sterba, 1983).
   b. Add 19 ml of 3% H$_2$O$_2$ solution/l (= 70 ml/gallon = 570 ppm) and treat for 4 minutes. Use only once (Lewbart, 1991).

Use No. 3: Fungicide for water mold infections of eggs
Water-borne formulations:
1. Bath
   a. Add 0.71 to 1.42 ml of 35% hydrogen peroxide/l (= 2.7 to 5.4 ml/gallon = 250 to 500 ppm; 35% hydrogen peroxide = 350,000 ppm H$_2$O$_2$), and treat for 15 minutes (Dawson et al., 1994). This is a promising treatment for fungal infections. Prophylactic treatments of 250 to 500 ppm H$_2$O$_2$ every other day have protected healthy rainbow trout eggs from fungal infections. This treatment regimen also seems to inhibit fungal growth on infected eggs. However, these results are preliminary and a bioassay should be performed before using it on any fish eggs. When using on food fish in the United States, an appropriate grade

for food fish must be used (e.g., 35% hydrogen peroxide, Eka Noble, Inc.). Wear rubber gloves and eye protection when using this. The cost is comparable to formalin.

Hyposalinity

Use No. 1: Treatment of *Cryptocaryon irritans*
Water-borne formulations:

1. Prolonged immersion
   a. Reduce the salinity of the affected tank by ~5 to 10 ppt/day, using fresh dechlorinated water until the salinity is < 16 ppt (Cheung et al., 1979). Remove all invertebrates before beginning the treatment. Return the tank to normal salinity after 3 weeks. Note that not all marine reef fish may tolerate this salinity. Some fish also tend to become hyperactive.
   b. Reduce the salinity as quickly as possible to 25% of the original salinity for 1 to 3 hours. (For example, if salinity is 40 ppt, reduce to 10 ppt.) Repeat every 3 days for a total of four treatments (Colorni, 1985).

Use No. 2: Treatment of marine ectoparasites
Water-borne formulations

1. Prolonged immersion
   a. Reduce the salinity of the affected system by ~5 to 10 ppt/day, using fresh dechlorinated water until it becomes freshwater. This treatment is effective but can only be used on euryhaline species (i.e., can tolerate freshwater).

Levamisole Hydrochloride (Levasol [Pittman-Moore], Tramisol [Over-the-Counter], or Equivalent)

Use: Treatment of *Anguillicola* and other susceptible nonencysted nematodes.
Levamisole is the levo-isomer of DL-tetramisol. Levamisole has a greater safety margin than the racemic mixture.
Water-borne formulations:

1. Prolonged immersion
   a. Add 10 mg levamisole HCl/l (= 38 mg/gallon) (Butcher, 1993).

Oral formulations:
   a. Feed 2.5 to 10 mg levamisole HCl/kg (= 1.1 to 4.5 mg/pound) of body weight/day for 7 days (Post, 1987). This is equivalent to a feed having 0.025% to 0.100% levamisole and fed at a rate of 1% of body weight/day. Feeding 8 mg levamisole HCl/kg (= 3.6 mg/pound) of

body weight is a proven treatment for *Anguillicola* (Blanc et al., 1992).
Injectable formulations:

1. Inject 8 mg levamisole HCl/kg (= 3.6 mg/pound) of body weight intracardiac (Blanc et al., 1992).

Magnesium Sulfate (MgSO$_4$, Epsom Salts)

Use: Treatment of hexamitosis
Oral formulations

1. Feed 3% magnesium sulfate in the feed for 2 to 3 days. This has been used to successfully treat salmonids (Warren, 1981).

Malachite Green (Malachite Green [Argent] [Marine Enterprises], or Equivalent)

Malachite green is a diarylmethane dye that is the most effective agent known for treating water mold infections of fish and eggs. It is also effective against protozoan ectoparasites. Unfortunately, it is also a **respiratory poison, teratogen,** and **suspected carcinogen** (Meyer & Jorgensen, 1983) and should be handled with appropriate caution. It is illegal to use on food fish in the United States, although it is still legal in some countries. Malachite green appears to persist in tissues for long periods, and repeated treatments cause increased accumulation (Alderman, 1988).

The toxicity of malachite green is highly temperature dependent, increasing with higher temperature (Alderman, 1985). It is more toxic at low pH and is also phytotoxic. It is inactivated (oxidized) by light; tank lights should be turned off during treatment.

Malachite green is toxic to young fry and eggs that are near hatching. It should not be used prophylactically but only on eggs that have fungal infection. It is also reported to be toxic to tetras, catfish, and loaches (halving the suggested concentration may be tolerated, but there is little data on individual species responses). It may also be toxic to small marine fish. Centrarchids seem especially sensitive to malachite green. The 96-hour LC$_{50}$ for bluegill is 0.035 mg/l (Bills et al., 1977). It is toxic to largemouth bass eggs and fry and should not be used on this species (Wright, 1976). Toxicity in fish usually presents as respiratory distress, since it is a metabolic respiratory poison. Treated fish may become anorexic (Post, 1987).

Malachite green will stain all objects, especially plastics. Malachite green is manufactured as a zinc-free oxalate salt (green crystals with a metallic sheen) or as a zinc chloride salt (yellow crystals). The latter is toxic and should not be used. Dye lots vary considerably in potency (Alderman, 1985), although this is usually not considered when calculating doses.

When prolonged immersion is used, remove residual drug with activated carbon 2 days after the last treatment. When malachite green is used in flow-through systems (e.g., treating salmonid eggs), release of drug into the environment should be prevented by treating the effluent with **activated carbon** (Marking et al., 1990).

It is usually best to prepare a stock solution (1.4 g malachite green in 380 ml of water = 3.7 mg/ml). This stock solution will last indefinitely.

Use No. 1: Treating water mold infections and protozoan ectoparasites of freshwater fish
Water-borne formulations:
1. Bath
   a. Add 50 to 60 mg malachite green/l (= 50 to 60 ml of malachite green stock solution/gallon = 13 to 16 ml/liter) and treat for 10 to 30 seconds (Debuf, 1991).
   b. Add 1.0 mg malachite green/l (= 1 ml of malachite green stock solution/gallon = 0.26 ml/liter), and treat for 30 to 60 minutes (Warren, 1981; Debuf, 1991). Use 2.0 mg malachite green/l if the pH is high. For salmonids, treatment can be repeated up to 4 times each week if the temperature is < 14° C (58° F) (Warren, 1981).
2. Prolonged immersion
   a. Add 0.10 mg malachite green/l (= 0.10 ml of malachite green stock solution/gallon = 0.026 ml/liter). Treat three times at 3-day intervals. Remove residual chemical after the last treatment with activated carbon.
   b. Add zinc-free 0.75% malachite green (Marine Enterprises). Use as directed.
3. Swab
   a. Swab a 100 mg malachite green/l solution onto skin lesions. The colored areas on the skin help to monitor healing (Warren, 1981).

Use No. 2: Treating water mold infections of freshwater fish eggs
Water-borne formulations:
1. Bath
   a. Add 10 mg malachite green/l (= 10 ml of malachite green stock solution/gallon = 2.6 ml/liter) for 10 to 30 minutes (Hoffman & Meyer, 1973).
   b. Add 0.50 mg malachite green/l (= 0.50 ml of malachite green stock solution/gallon = 0.13 ml/liter) for 1 hour (Debuf, 1991).
2. Flush
   a. Add 42.5 g malachite green to 1 gallon of water (= 11.2 g/liter). Add 88 ml of this stock to the inflow adjusted to a flow rate of 6 gallons/minute (= 23 liters/min). Return the flow to normal after treating for 1 hour (Warren, 1981).
3. Constant flow
   a. Add 2.2 mg malachite green/l, and treat for 1 hour (Warren, 1981).

Use No. 3: Treatment of proliferative kidney disease
Water-borne formulations:
1. Flush
   a. Add 1 mg malachite green/l, and treat for 1 hour. Treat weekly for 3 weeks (Clifton-Hadley & Alderman, 1987; Debuf, 1991).

Mebendazole (Telmin® [Pittman-Moore], or Equivalent)

Use: Treatment of monogeneans
There is considerable species variation in response. For example, *Pseudodactylogyrus* is effectively treated with 1 mg/l prolonged immersion (Szekely & Molnar, 1987), while *Gyrodactylus elegans* is reportedly susceptible to 0.10 mg/l and *Dactylogyrus vastator* is resistant to even 2 mg/l prolonged immersion (Scott, 1993).
Water-borne formulations:
1. Bath
   a. Add 100 mg mebendazole/l (= 380 mg/gallon) and treat for 10 minutes (Szekely & Molnar, 1987).
2. Prolonged immersion
   a. Add 1 mg mebendazole/l (= 3.8 mg/gallon) and treat for 24 hours (Szekely & Molnar, 1987).

Methylene Blue (Methylene Blue [Aurum] or Equivalent)

Some evidence exists that methylene blue reduces incidence of bacterial and water mold infection of the eggs of freshwater aquarium fish (Herwig, 1979). Methylene blue has also been advocated in the aquarium literature for treating ectoparasites and nitrite toxicity by prolonged immersion; however, other chemicals have stronger evidence of efficacy. Prolonged immersion use of this agent is **not** recommended in systems with biological filtration because it is toxic to nitrifying bacteria (Collins et al., 1975). Note that many over-the-counter aquarium pharmaceuticals contain this ingredient. Methylene blue stains many objects, especially plastics. It is also phytotoxic (van Duijn, 1973). It is best to prepare a stock solution by adding 1.4 g to 380 ml water (= 3.7 mg/ml).

Use No. 1: Preventing infections of freshwater fish eggs
Water-borne formulations:
1. Prolonged immersion
   a. Add 2 mg methylene blue/l (= 2 ml of methylene blue stock solution/gallon = 0.53 ml/liter). Repeat on alternate days for up to a total of three times.

Use No. 2: Treating ectoparasites of freshwater fish
Water-borne formulations:
1. Prolonged immersion
   a. Add 1 to 3 mg methylene blue/l (= 1 to 3 ml of methylene blue stock solution/gallon = 0.26 to 0.79 ml/liter) (Allison, 1966).

Metronidazole (Flagyl® IV [Searle], or Equivalent)

Use: Treatment of hexamitosis and spironucleosis

Metronidazole is a prescription drug for treating intestinal flagellate and anaerobe bacterial infections in humans. It is relatively insoluble in water (maximum solubility ~1 g/100 ml). Make sure that it is dissolved before adding to water or mixing in feed.
Water-borne formulations:
1. Bath
   a. Add 5 mg metronidazole/l (= 19 mg/gallon) and treat for 3 hours. Repeat every other day for three treatments (Gratzek, 1988).
2. Prolonged immersion
   a. Add 6.6 mg metronidazole/l (= 25 mg/gallon), and treat once daily for a total of three times (Gratzek & Blasiola, 1992).
   b. Add 25 mg metronidazole/l (= 95 mg/gallon), and treat every other day for 3 days (Langdon, 1992a).
Oral formulations:
There is evidence that a single oral treatment with metronidazole may be as effective as three water-borne treatments (Whaley & Francis-Floyd, 1991).
   a. Feed 25 mg metronidazole/kg (= 11 mg/pound) of body weight/day for 5 to 10 days. Then reassess clinical condition, and retreat if needed (Gratzek & Blasiola, 1992). This is equivalent to a feed that has 0.25% metronidazole and is fed at a rate of 1% of body weight/day.
   b. Feed 100 mg metronidazole/kg (= 45 mg/pound) of body weight for 3 days (Langdon, 1992a). This is equivalent to a feed that has 1% metronidazole and is fed at a rate of 1% of body weight/day.
   c. Soak brine shrimp in a 1% metronidazole solution in a refrigerator for 3 hours. Feed once (Langdon, 1992a).

Monensin Sodium (Coban® 60 [Elanco], Rumensin® 60 [Elanco])

Use: Treatment of coccidiosis
Oral formulations:
1. Feed 100 mg monensin/kg (= 45 mg/pound) of body weight/day. This treatment is experimentally effective against *Calyptospora*.

Nitrifying Bacteria

Use: Seeding of filters to improve or speed up development of microbiological filtration to detoxify ammonia and nitrite

Note that these preparations consist of live bacteria. Products should not have been exposed to extreme temperatures and should be used before the expiration date. Commercial preparations of nitrifying bacteria often fail because they are sold well beyond the expected shelf life. Freeze-dried preparations have never been shown to be effective; nitrifiers do not appear to survive freeze-drying (Bower & Turner, 1981). One of the best methods of seeding an aquarium with viable bacteria is to use filter material from a healthy aquarium with an active biological filter.
Water-borne formulations:
1. Prolonged immersion
   a. Add Fritz-Zyme No. 7 (Aquacenter) to freshwater aquaria as directed.
   b. Add Fritz-Zyme No. 9 (Aquacenter) to marine aquaria as directed.
   c. Add Cycle Bacteriological Biological Filter Supplement and Organic Sludge Remover (Rolf Hagen Corporation) to freshwater or marine aquaria, as directed.
   d. Add filter material (e.g., floss, gravel) from an aquarium with an active biological filter and healthy fish to a filter to be used in the new aquarium.

Organophosphate (Dichlorvos [= DDVP = 2,2, Dichloroethenyl Dimethylphosphate] Trichlorfon [= 2,2, Trichloro-1-Hydroxyethylphosphonate])

Use: Treatment of monogeneans, leeches, and crustacean ectoparasites (copepods, branchiurans, isopods)

Organophosphates (OPs) are effective treatments for many metazoan ectoparasites, although resistance can be a problem (Goven et al., 1980; Roth et al., 1993). There are many types of OPs. Some are legal to use for treating fish in some countries; most are not.

The two most commonly used OPs in aquaculture are **dichlorvos** (O,O-dimethyl 2-2-dichlorovinyl phosphate or DDVP) and **trichlorfon** (dimethyl-2-2-trichloro-1-hydroxyethylphosphonate). The commercial formulation of dichlorvos is Aquagard [Ciba-Geigy], a 50/50 mixture of DDVP and dibutylphthalate (an emulsifying agent). Trichlorfon is available in several formulations, including Neguvon® ([Miles] or [Bayer]), Dipterex® ([Bayer]), Masoten® ([Bayer] or [Miles]), and Dylox® ([Bayer]) (Roth et al., 1993). Note that OP commercial preparations vary in percentage active ingredient (e.g., Neguvon® is an 8% trichlorfon solution, while Masoten® powder is an 80% trichlorfon formulation).

When it is added to water, trichlorfon degrades to the more toxic DDVP. DDVP degrades more slowly to less toxic by-products. These chemical reactions are influenced by several factors: light, high temperature, aeration, and high pH all speed the chemical reactions (Samuelsen, 1987). For example, in salmon-rearing areas, the half-life of DDVP is typically 5 to 8 days in seawater at 5° C (41° F) (Samuelson, 1987). The half-life of trichlorfon may be over 3 weeks in acid water. In contrast, the half-life of trichlorfon in a typical pond in the southern United States in summer, having a pH of 9.0, is less than 1 day. In such ponds, OP's must be applied in early morning to maintain an effective dose for a long enough time.

Aeration should be provided during bath treatments. Gasping and rolling indicate toxicity and asphyxiation. OPs inhibit acetylcholinesterase (AChE). Some inhibition of brain AChE occurs when fish are treated with OPs. This can lead to overdosing if the same fish are treated even weeks apart. This presents a problem with sea lice control, since multiple treatments are often needed to permanently reduce parasite loads. A 75% to 80% inhibition of brain AChE is lethal or near-lethal to fish (Hoy et al., 1992). Trichlorfon is especially toxic to some larval fish (Flores-Nava & Vizcarra-Quiroz, 1988) and potentially toxic to elasmobranchs and characins.

OPs must be handled with care because they can also induce neurotoxic poisoning in humans. Trichlorfon is a possible teratogen. Avoid inhalation or absorption through the skin.

Water-borne formulations:

1. Bath for sea lice

Dichlorvos and trichlorfon are used for treating salmon with *Lepeophtheirus* and *Caligus* before the stage at which serious skin damage is evident. Use of trichlorfon against sea lice is being superseded by DDVP because of trichlorfon's greater instability in water and thus variable degradation to DDVP. Dilute 1:16 before adding to the cage.

Closely monitor for reinfestation. One may need to retreat up to twice more at 2- to 3-week intervals, since only preadults and adults are killed (need to let chalimus larvae mature) (Pike, 1989; Debuf, 1991).

a. Add 15 to 300 mg trichlorfon/l (= 57 to 1140 mg/gallon), and treat for 15 to 60 minutes at 3° to 18° C (37° to 64° F) (Horsberg et al., 1987). Use the higher dose at the lower temperatures.

b. Add 0.5 to 2.0 mg DDVP/l (= 1.9 to 7.6 mg/gallon), and treat for 30 to 60 minutes. Use the higher dose at the lower temperatures in the range of 3° to 17° C (27° to 63° F) (Pike, 1989). Higher doses are needed for skirted cages versus an enclosed cage because there is more rapid diffusion of chemicals outside of the cage. Withdrawal time is up to 500 degree days (Scott, 1993).

2. Bath for marine capsalid monogeneans

a. Add 2 to 5 mg trichlorfon/l (= 7.6 to 19 mg/gallon), and treat for 60 minutes (Langdon, 1992a).

3. Bath for isopods

a. Add 2 mg trichlorfon/l (= 7.6 mg/gallon), and treat for 60 minutes (Langdon, 1992a).

4. Prolonged immersion for ectoparasites on pond or aquarium fish

a. Add 0.25 mg trichlorfon/l (= 0.94 mg/gallon) (= 0.012 ml Neguvon®/gallon) for freshwater aquaria. Use 0.50 mg trichlorfon/l if temperature is over 80° F (27° C) (Piper et al., 1982). Trichlorfon may not be effective above 80° F (Jensen & Durborow, 1984). Use 0.50 to 1.0 mg trichlorfon/l (= 1.9 to 3.8 mg/gallon) for marine fish. For *Dactylogyrus* and other oviparous monogeneans, give two treatments at 3-day intervals. For marine turbellarians, use 1.0 mg/l every other day for three treatments (Blasiola, 1976). For anchor worms, treat every 7 days for 28 days. OP are only effective against *Lernaea* at 50° to 80° F (10° to 27° C) (temperature range that larvae are produced). For other copepods (except sea lice), other monogeneans, *Argulus,* and leeches, one treatment will usually suffice (Jensen & Durborow, 1984). Another OP, Spotton® [Miles] (20% fenthion solution) has been used successfully to treat *Lernaea* in aquarium fish (JB Gratzek, Personal Communication) and may be useful for other parasites. The dosage of active ingredient to use (i.e., mg/l fenthion) is the same as for trichlorfon.

Peat

Use: Softening and acidifying freshwater

Peat is an anaerobic breakdown product of plant material that consists of a complex mixture of organic acids, resins, waxes, plant hormones, salts, and other compounds. Peat reduces water hardness. By releasing organic acids (e.g., tannins, humic acids) it also lowers and stabilizes the pH in the slightly acidic range, making the water more suitable for acidophilic fish. The lower pH is also bacteriostatic and fungistatic. Peat should be crumbly, since strands of peat have considerable undegraded plant remains that prevent good plant growth (Sterba, 1983).

Water-borne formulations:
1. Prolonged immersion
   a. Add well-pulverized peat to the filter to effect.

2-Phenoxyethanol (Phenoxyethanol, Ethylene Glycol Monophenyl Ether)

Use: Anesthesia/euthanization

2-Phenoxyethanol has the advantage of being inexpensive when it is compared with other anesthetics. However, it has disadvantages, including a narrow safety margin, adverse side effects (long induction time; erratic rapid swimming ["motorboating"] with exposure; hyperactivity during recovery). It may cause liver and kidney damage.

Note that activity may vary considerably with water quality, fish species, fish size, and fish density. Given dosages should be used as general guidelines, with the clinical response of the fish being used to gauge the proper dosage (see p. 17).

Water-borne formulations:
Bath for sedation/anesthesia/euthanasia
Add ~0.10 to 0.40 mg phenoxyethanol/L (~0.025 to 0.010 mg/gallon) for a 2- to 4-minute induction of anesthesia. For euthanization; use about the same dosage. Keep fish in anesthetic for at least 10 minutes after breathing stops.

Piperazine Sulfate (Piperazine 17% [Agrilabs], Piperazine 34% [Agrilabs], Pipfuge [Butler], or Equivalent)

Use: Treatment of nonencysted nematodes in the gastrointestinal tract. Piperazine is a phenothiazine anthelmintic.

Oral formulations:
1. Feed 10 mg piperazine sulfate/kg (= 4.5 mg/pound) of body weight/day for 3 days. This is equivalent to a feed that has 0.10% piperazine sulfate fed at a rate of 1% of body weight/day (Post, 1983).

Potassium Permanganate ($KMnO_4$)

Use No. 1: Treatment of ectoparasites and skin/gill bacterial infections in freshwater

Potassium permanganate is presently undergoing reregistration by the EPA (U.S.) for use as an oxidizing agent. It reduces biological oxygen demand by oxidizing organic matter. It has also been advocated to increase dissolved oxygen levels in ponds; however, there is no evidence for it increasing oxygen at permanganate levels that are nontoxic to fish (Tucker & Boyd, 1977). Potassium permanganate is not approved by FDA (U.S.) as a drug but is an effective external parasiticide and bactericide. It has also been used to treat water molds, but this use has not yet been proven.

Potassium permanganate kills skin and gill pathogens via its strong oxidizing properties (Duncan, 1974). Effective treatment requires 2 mg/l of active chemical: the permanganate ion (MnO_4^-) imparts a light pink tinge to the water. Permanganate ion is reduced to manganese dioxide (MnO_2), which is relatively nontoxic and colorless; thus, the water will revert to being colorless or light tan when the permanganate becomes inactive. This can be tested by placing a sample of the water in a clear glass container. The pink permanganate color can also be seen if the pond water is splashed with an oar or plank to make a wave. Since permanganate reacts with organic matter, the amount needed for effective treatment is higher in organically rich ponds (Tucker & Boyd, 1977). If the light pink tinge begins to decay before 8 to 12 hours has elapsed, more potassium permanganate should be added immediately in 2 mg/l increments, until the light pink color is restored (Jensen & Durborow, 1984). Not more than 6 to 8 mg/l **total** potassium permanganate should be added to a pond. Readjustment to the proper permanganate concentration should be done all at one time to avoid overdosing the fish. Levels of potassium permanganate that exceed approximately 2 mg/l of active ingredient are not considered safe for fish (Plumb, 1979).

A more accurate method of determining the treatment dose is to add 0, 1, 2, 3, 4, 6, 8, 10, and 12 mg/l of potassium permanganate to separate containers that have 1 liter of water each (small aquarium bags are useful). The lowest concentration in which the pink hue remains after 15 minutes is considered the endpoint (Boyd, 1979). The endpoint obtained in this test is multiplied by 2.5 to give a reliable treatment rate for bacterial diseases (Tucker, 1989). For example, if the lowest concentration that retains a pink hue after 15 minutes was 2 mg/l, the total amount of potassium permanganate needed for treatment would be 2 × 2.5 = 5.0 mg/l. Chemically calculating the permanganate demand of the water to be treated (Tucker, 1984) is the most accurate measure of the required permanganate dosage.

Potassium permanganate is toxic in water with high pH, since manganese dioxide may precipitate onto the gills. Thus, it should not be used in seawater. Potassium permanganate should not be mixed with formalin.

Although it is less expensive than formalin, potassium permanganate is still costly to use in large ponds or in those with a high organic content. A source of potassium permanganate may be difficult to locate in some areas, but it may be available from water softening companies if not from farm supply sources. It is considered 100% active.

Water-borne formulations:
1. Bath
   a. Add 1000 mg potassium permanganate/l (= 3,800 mg/gallon) and treat for 10 to 40 seconds (Debuf, 1991).
   b. Add 100 mg potassium permanganate/l (= 380 mg/gallon) and treat for 5 to 10 minutes for fish lice (Kabata, 1985).
   c. Add 5 mg potassium permanganate/l (= 19 mg/gallon) and treat for 30 to 60 minutes (Aldridge & Shireman, 1991; Debuf, 1991).
2. Prolonged immersion in ponds
   a. Add enough potassium permanganate to produce a final concentration of 2 mg/l (= 7.6 mg/gallon) of active (unreduced) potassium permanganate.
3. Flush
   a. Add 2 mg potassium permanganate/l (= 7.6 mg/gallon) for treating cold water bacterial gill disease (Schachte, 1983).

Use No. 2: Oxidation/detoxification of hydrogen sulfide
1. Prolonged immersion
   a. Add enough potassium permanganate to produce a final concentration of 2 mg/l (= 7.6 mg/gallon) of active (unreduced) potassium permanganate.

Potentiated Iodine (Iodophore, Wescodyne® [Ciba-Geigy], Betadine®, Aurodyne® [Aurum], Argentyne® [Argent], or Equivalent)

Different iodine formulations vary in concentration, so the amount of drug added is based on the brand that is used. Some potentiated iodine brands are combined with detergents (e.g., Betadine® Scrub); these should not be used.

Use No. 1: Antisepsis ("disinfection") of eggs to kill *Aeromonas salmonicida*, infectious hematopoietic necrosis virus, viral hemorrhagic septicemia virus, and other surface-dwelling pathogens

Potentiated iodine compounds (PIC) can only kill pathogens on the surface of eggs (not inside the egg). **Rinse** treated ova **thoroughly** in clean water. Do not treat within 5 days of hatching, since this may cause premature hatching and increased mortality (Piper et al., 1982). PIC are also toxic to unfertilized ova and newly hatched fish. A final concentration of about 100 ppm active ingredient (iodine) is usually recommended. In poorly buffered water (< 50 mg/l total alkalinity), add 1 g of sodium bicarbonate/liter (= 3.8 g/gallon) to unbuffered PIC solutions, since PIC will lower the pH and kill eggs. A precipitate may form from bicarbonate treatment, but this will not harm the eggs. Fresh PIC is brown-to-amber. When batches of eggs are treated, the solution should be discarded when it fades to yellow (Warren, 1981). PICs are much more effective than acriflavine or merthiolate (Piper et al., 1982).

Water-borne formulation:
1. Bath (all formulations described below are pre-buffered; therefore, bicarbonate addition is not needed).
   a. Add 3 ml of Wescodyne® ([Ciba-Geigy] 1.6% available iodine solution)/l (= 11 ml/gallon), and treat for 10 minutes (Debuf, 1991).
   b. Add 10 ml of Argentyne® (Argent)/l (= 3.8 ml/gallon), and treat for 10 minutes or use as directed.
   c. Add 20 ml of 0.5% Betadine® solution/l (= 2.6 fluid ounces/gallon). Test before using.
   d. Aurudyne® (Aurum) is to be used as directed.

Use No. 2: Antisepsis of wounds
Water-borne formulations:
   a. Swab a Betadine® solution (= 1% potentiated iodine) on wound. Immediately rinse fish in clean water, and then place it in a recovery tank.

Use No. 3: Disinfecting equipment
See Table III-11 for the range of effectiveness.
Water-borne formulations:
1. Bath/spray
   a. Prepare a solution having 10,000 ppm available iodine (= 30 to 50 mg free iodine). Dip or spray equipment, allowing a contact time of at least 10 minutes before rinsing.

Praziquantel (Droncit® Injection [Miles])

Use: Treatment of adult cestodes, monogeneans, and possibly larval digeneans
Water-borne formulations:
1. Bath for adult cestodes
   a. Add 2 mg praziquantel/l (= 7.6 mg/gallon) for 1 to 3 hours (Moser et al., 1986; Hoffman, 1983; Lewbart & Gratzek, 1990;

Gratzek & Blasiola, 1992). This procedure can be repeated after 1 week if needed.

2. Bath for marine monogeneans
   a. Add 20 mg praziquantel/l (= 76 mg/gallon) for 1.5 hours. Juvenile fish and clupeids are sensitive to this dose, but even higher doses have been used for some other fish species (Schmahl & Tarashewski, 1987; Thoney, 1989).
   b. Add 10 mg praziquantel/l (= 38 mg/gallon) for 3 hours. This is better tolerated than 2a by some fish (Thoney & Hargis, 1991).

3. Prolonged immersion in aquaria for monogeneans
   a. Add 2 mg praziquantel/l (= 7.6 mg/gallon).

4. Prolonged immersion in aquaria for digenean metacercaria
   a. Add 2 to 10 mg praziquantel/l (= 7.6 to 38 mg/gallon) for 24 hours (Krum et al., 1992).

Oral formulations:

1. Oral for adult cestodes
   a. Feed 50 mg praziquantel/kg (= 23 mg/pound) of body weight/day. One day's treatment is usually sufficient. This is equivalent to a feed having 0.50% praziquantel fed at a rate of 1% of body weight/day (Langdon, 1992a).
   b. Intubate 50 mg praziquantel/kg (= 23 mg/pound) of body weight once (Langdon, 1992). This dose has eliminated *Bothriocephalus acheilognathi* from grass carp (Scott, 1993).

2. Oral for digenean larvae
   a. Feed 50 mg praziquantel/kg (= 23 mg/pound) of body weight (Langdon, 1992a). This dose reduces the number of *Diplostomum spacaceum* metacercariae in trout and sculpins (Bylund & Sumari, 1981).

Injectable formulations:

1. Injection for reducing encysted digenean metacercaria parasitosis
   a. Inject 25 mg praziquantel/kg (= 12 mg/pound) of body weight IM once (Lorio, 1989).

Quaternary Ammonium Compounds (QAC, Roccal® [Upjohn], Hyamine 1622, Hyamine 3500)

Quaternary ammonium compounds are disinfectants that have also been used as antiseptics to treat skin and gill infections, such as bacterial gill disease. The QACs used to treat fish diseases include benzalkonium chlorides and benzethonium chlorides. QACs are more toxic at high temperature and in soft water. Quaternary ammonium solutions act as surfactants,

removing excess mucus that contains parasites and bacteria. There are several different formulas of QAC, including powders and liquids. Roccal is a 10% solution of alkyl-dimethyl-benzyl-ammonium chlorides. Some batches of Roccal® are toxic to trout. Hyamine 3500®, a mixture of dodecyl and tetradecyl homologues of alkyl-dimethyl-benzyl-ammonium chlorides, and Hyamine 1622® are both less toxic at therapeutic doses.

When the powder is used to prepare a solution, a respirator should be worn or mixing should be done under a fume hood to avoid inhaling the dust. The powder should be added directly to water (adding water to the powder produces a sticky mass) (Warren, 1981).

Use No. 1: Disinfection of nets and other utensils
Water-borne formulations:
1. Prolonged immersion
   a. Add 5 ml of Roccal®/l (= 19 ml/gallon) as a net dip.

Use No. 2: Treatment of external bacterial infections

Salmon and lake trout appear to be sensitive to Hyamine 3500® and are best treated with Hyamine 1622® (Warren, 1981). Different lots of Roccal® vary in efficacy and ichthyotoxicity; thus, a bioassay should be run before a new lot is used (Piper et al., 1982).

QACs are more toxic in soft water (cut the dose in half). QACs have a low therapeutic index, so the lower dose should be used when in doubt. The homing ability of salmonids may be affected, so QACs should not be used on salmonids that are intended for release into the wild (Scott, 1993).

Water-borne formulations:
1. Bath/prolonged immersion
   a. Add one of the following (Scott, 1993):
   10 mg of active QAC/l (= 38 mg/gallon) and treat for 5 to 10 minutes
   5 mg of active QAC/l (= 19 mg/gallon) and treat for 30 minutes
   2 mg of active QAC/l (= 7.6 mg/gallon) and treat for 60 minutes
   1 mg of active QAC/l (= 3.8 mg/gallon) and treat for several hours
   0.1 to 0.5 mg of active QAC/l (= 0.38 to 1.90 mg/gallon) and treat for 24 hours

Place fish in clean, untreated water immediately after treatment. It is usually best to retreat 2 or 3 times.

Quinaldine Sulfate (Quinate)

This agent appears to have a slightly better therapeutic index than **tricaine**, making it safer to use. Fish under quinaldine anesthesia do not usually stop breathing and thus are not as susceptible to asphyxiation. In some fish, toxicity increases with higher temperature, pH, and hardness. Quinaldine is a *suspected carcinogen* and caution should be exercised in its use. Fish retain a strong reflex response even after total loss of equilibrium, which may be annoying during biopsy or surgical procedures. Some fish (e.g., tilapia) need extremely high doses.

Stock solutions are stable but should be stored in a tightly capped, brown bottle. Like tricaine, quinaldine sulfate acidifies the water (Summerfelt & Smith, 1990). The parent compound (quinaldine) is more cumbersome to use, since it must be dissolved in an organic solvent before adding to water.

Note that activity may vary considerably with water quality, fish species, fish size, and fish density. Given dosages should be used as general guidelines, with the clinical response of the fish being used to gauge the proper dosage (see p. 17).

Use No. 1: Sedation
Water-borne formulations:
1. Bath/prolonged immersion
   a. Add ~1 to 50 mg quinaldine sulfate/l (~4 to 200 mg/gallon).

Use No. 2: Anesthesia
Water-borne formulations:
1. Bath
   a. Add ~2.5 to > 100 mg quinaldine sulfate/l (~10 to > 400 mg/gallon). A proper dosage will usually cause anesthesia within 60 seconds.

Use No. 3: Euthanasia
Water-borne formulations:
1. Bath
   a. This is similar to the anesthetic dose. Keep fish in the solution for at least 10 minutes after breathing stops.

Salt

Many forms of salt can be effectively used for treating ectoparasites. Pure sodium chloride is available in coarse (meat-curing salt or rock salt) and fine (table salt) forms. For small volumes of water, table salt can be used. Noniodized table salt should be used for prolonged immersion. For prolonged immersion, it is best to use a balanced salt mixture, since other important minerals (e.g., Ca, Mg) are then added. One of the most reliable sources of balanced salts are the dry, artificial seawaters (e.g., Instant Ocean®) sold in aquarium stores. However, these can be expensive if large volumes of water are to be treated. An alternative balanced salt is dried seawater, or *solar salt*. Solar salt is available from water-softening companies. Avoid solar salt preparations with anticaking agents, such as sodium ferrocyanide (yel-

low prussiate of soda). Exposure of sodium ferrocyanide to sunlight generates hydrogen cyanide and is highly toxic to fish.

Use No. 1: Treatment of *Ichthyophthirius*
Water-borne formulations:
1. Prolonged immersion in aquaria
   a. Add 2 g salt/l (= 2 ppt = 7.6 g/gallon) to the aquarium. Some freshwater fish, such as many catfish, are sensitive to even low concentrations of salt, so this treatment should be used with caution in those species. This salt level may also be toxic to some plants.

Use No. 2: Treatment of freshwater ectoparasites, columnaris, and bacterial gill disease
Water-borne formulations:
1. Bath
   a. Add 10 to 30 g salt/l (= 10 to 30 ppt = 38 to 114 g/gallon), and treat for up to 30 minutes. The higher doses may only be tolerated for a few minutes. Fish may become excitable when they are first exposed to high salt concentrations. If fish are weak or if they are a salt-sensitive species, use the lower dosage and repeat the next day. Small salmonids (< 5 g) should not be exposed to > 10 ppt salt, while salmonids < 100 g should not be exposed to > 20 ppt salt (Scott, 1993).

A salt bath can remove excess mucus and debris associated with ectoparasite infestations, columnaris, and bacterial gill disease, facilitating the effectiveness of other chemicals against these pathogens (Warren, 1981). It is especially useful in salmonids.

Use No. 3: Prophylaxis or treatment of freshwater ectoparasites and water mold infections
Water-borne formulations:
1. Prolonged immersion in aquaria
   a. Add 1 to 5 g salt/l (= 1 to 5 ppt = 3.8 to 19 g/gallon) (Taylor & Bailey, 1979). Some freshwater fish, such as many catfish, are sensitive to even low concentrations of salt, so the lower dosage should be used with these salt-sensitive species. Virtually all tropical freshwater aquarium fish can be maintained indefinitely in 1 ppt seawater (G. Lewbart, Personal Communication).
   b. Add up to 35 ppt salt for euryhaline fish.

Use No. 4: Increase mineral content for rift lake cichlids
Water-borne formulations:
1. Prolonged immersion
   a. Add mineral mix (Aqua-Cichlids [Aquatronics] or equivalent). Use as directed.

Use No. 5: Increase salinity in brackish or marine aquaria

Note that it is best to allow sea salt mixtures to dissolve overnight before adding to the aquarium, since some salts take time to fully dissolve.

Water-borne formulations:
1. Prolonged immersion
   a. Add artificial seawater, and use as directed.

Use No. 6: Prevention of stress-induced mortality in freshwater fish

Water-borne formulations:
1. Prolonged immersion
   a. Add 3 to 5 ppt solar salt or artificial seawater. A mixture of divalent cations plus sodium chloride is superior to sodium chloride alone in reducing stress-induced mortality (Grizzle et al., 1990).

Sedatives

(See *Anesthetics*)

Slaked Lime (Hydrated Lime, Builder's Lime, Calcium Hydroxide, Ca[OH]₂)

Slaked lime is caustic and caution should be used in handling the powder. **Do not** confuse this with **agricultural lime** (see *BUFFERS: PONDS*), which is most often used for adjusting pH. Slaked lime is a strong alkali and can rapidly raise the pH to over 10, killing all the fish, which is why it is mainly used as a disinfectant.

Use No. 1: Disinfecting ponds

Water-borne formulations:
1. Prolonged immersion
   a. Add slaked lime at a rate of 1784 pounds/acre (= 2000 kg/ha = 18 g/ft²). Best results are obtained when lime is disked into the soil of a drained pond. When it is added directly to water, the pH of the water should be allowed to return to < 8.5 before adding fish (usually takes about 14 days).

Use No. 2: Adjusting pH/alkalinity of ponds (see *BUFFERS: PONDS*)

Use No. 3: Adjusting hardness of ponds (see *CALCIUM*)

Use No. 4: Neutralizing free CO_2 in ponds

Add at least 1.7 mg/l of Ca(OH)₂ for every 1.0 mg/l of CO_2 to be removed (Hansell & Boyd, 1980). This dose is about twice the amount that should theoretically be needed for neutralization because slaked lime is poorly soluble in water. This treatment only removes the CO_2 present in the water. The cause of the hypercarbia should also be corrected. Be careful not to rapidly raise pH or cause ammonia poisoning.

Sodium Bicarbonate (Baking Soda, Na₂HCO₃)

Use No. 1: Raising acidic pH to normal range in aquaria (see *BUFFERS: FRESHWATER AQUARIA*)

Use No. 2: Sedation/anesthesia/euthanasia (also see *CARBON DIOXIDE*)

Sodium bicarbonate produces narcosis via the generation of CO_2 from carbonic acid (H_2CO_3). Carbonic acid anesthesia is effective between pH 6.5 to 8.5 (Post, 1979). Carbonic acid anesthesia is best used for light sedation. Do not use at levels that cause loss of reflex activity or opercular movement (Post, 1979). Some believe that carbonic acid anesthesia should only be used as a last resort because it is easy to overdose and produce a lethal hypercarbia. Concentrated (97% to 98%) sulfuric acid is most commonly used in conjunction with sodium bicarbonate to generate carbonic acid. Concentrated sulfuric acid should be handled with extreme caution. A 10% (wt/vol) sodium carbonate solution can be used to quickly reverse the anesthesia if desired.

Note that activity may vary considerably with water quality, fish species, fish size, and fish density. Given dosages should be used as general guidelines, with the clinical response of the fish being used to gauge the proper dosage (see p. 17).

Water-borne formulations:
1. Bath
   a. Mix 6.75% (wt/vol) sodium bicarbonate with 3.95% (wt/vol) concentrated sulfuric acid to obtain the desired CO_2 concentration (Post, 1979). The volume of each solution that is needed can be calculated as follows:

$$\frac{\text{mg/l } H_2CO_3 \text{ concentration} \times \text{Volume of the anesthetic bath in liters}}{50}$$

For example, if one desires to produce a 200 mg/l carbonic acid concentration in a 40 liter aquarium, one would add the following:

$$\frac{200 \times 40}{50} = 160$$

Therefore, 160 ml of both the sodium bicarbonate and the sulfuric acid solutions would need to be added to the water. Note that acid should always be added to water, not vice versa.

   b. Add 142 to 642 mg sodium bicarbonate/l (= 538 to 2430 mg/gallon). Add concentrated sulfuric acid at a wt:wt ratio of 1.7 mg sodium bicarbonate:1.0 mg sulfuric acid. An appropriate dosage should produce anesthesia in about 5 minutes (Schnick et al., 1989).

c. Add 1 tablet of Alka-Seltzer®, Bromo-Seltzer®, or equivalent/20 liters (= 2 tablets/10 gallons). This method should only be used as a last resort for anesthesia, since the dosage is difficult to control.

d. Make a concentrated solution of sodium bicarbonate by adding ~30 g (10 teaspoons or ¼ cup) of sodium bicarbonate/l (= ~120 g or 40 teaspoons or 1 cup/gallon) of water. Mix well, until virtually all of the powder is dissolved. Add the fish to be euthanized. Leave it in the solution for at least 10 minutes after the fish's breathing has stopped.

Sodium Pentobarbital

Barbiturate euthanasia has the advantages of being rapid and less expensive than fish anesthetics; however, fish must be restrained for the injection, which may be difficult. Barbiturate stocks must also be closely monitored and kept in a secure place because they are regulated narcotics. In the United States, barbiturate use requires preregistration with the Drug Enforcement Administration, which usually takes several months.

Use: Euthanization
Injectable formulations:

1. Inject 60 mg sodium pentobarbital/kg (= 27 mg/pound) of body weight intraperitoneally.

Sodium Phosphate

(See *BUFFERS: FRESHWATER AQUARIA*)

Sodium Sulfite (Na₂SO₃ [Argent], or Equivalent)

Use: Treating eggs to improve hatchability; also see Table III-3 for other methods to reduce adhesiveness
Waterborne formulations:

1. Bath
   a. Add 15% sodium sulfite to eggs of channel catfish, largemouth bass, or smallmouth bass for 5 to 8 minutes. Immediately place eggs in clean water after treatment. Sulfites remove oxygen, and thus are toxic with prolonged exposure (A.P.H.A., 1992).

TFM (Lamprecid [H & S Chemical Company])

Use: Eradication of lamprey larvae

TFM is currently registered by the United States Environmental Protection Agency and is legal to use by authorized individuals.

Tricaine (Tricaine Methanesulfonate [Aurum], MS-222, Finquel® [Argent])

Finquel® is the only tricaine label approved for use in food fish in the United States. Some fish need a higher exposure at lower temperatures for the same effect (Schoettger & Julin, 1967), but tricaine is safer to use at low temperatures. A higher dosage is needed in hard water (Schoettger & Julin, 1967). Crowding fish also increases the required dosage, with up to 10 times the dosage needed because of absorption by the fish (Dupree & Huner, 1984). Tricaine has a narrower safety margin than quinaldine sulfate and is more expensive.

In low-alkalinity water (< 50 mg/l as CaCO₃), sodium bicarbonate should be used to buffer the solution. Otherwise, the pH may drop to 5. This has been shown experimentally to cause acidosis in fish (Houston, 1990). A suggested stock solution is 100 mg/ml. Stock solutions should not be buffered because this causes chemical dissociation of the sulfonate group. Sodium bicarbonate should be added to the working solution at a ratio of about 2 parts sodium bicarbonate:1 part tricaine (wt:wt).

Tricaine solutions are unstable in light, changing to yellow or brown. Stock solutions should be replaced monthly or stored frozen.

Note that activity may vary considerably with water quality, fish species, fish size, and fish density. Given dosages should be used as general guidelines, with the clinical response of the fish being used to gauge the proper dosage (see p. 17). Overdosing is indicated by a recovery time greater than 10 minutes. Induction and recovery is faster at higher temperatures. Tricaine is rapidly cleared by fish and usually no residues are detectable after 24 hours (Houston, 1990).

Use No. 1: Sedation for transporting fish
Water-borne formulations:

1. Bath/prolonged immersion
   a. Add ~10 to 40 mg of tricaine/l (~38 to 150 mg/gallon). This concentration will reduce oxygen uptake and metabolic rate without causing severe depression. Crowded fish may require higher doses. In general, do not use > 100 mg/l for salmonids or > 250 mg/l for warm water fish, unless the fish are crowded.

Use No. 2: Anesthesia
Water-borne formulations:

1. Bath
   a. Add ~50 to 250 mg of tricaine/l (= ~190 to 950 mg/gallon). An optimal concentration

will usually cause anesthesia within 60 seconds.

    b. For large fish a 1 g/liter solution of tricaine can be sprayed onto the gills, using an aerosol pump sprayer. This can be reapplied if needed during a procedure.

Use No. 3: Euthanization

Water-borne formulations:

1. Bath

    a. This is similar to the anesthetic dose. Keep fish in the solution for at least 10 minutes after breathing stops to ensure that they are dead.

Unslaked Lime (Quick Lime, Burnt Lime, Calcium Oxide, CaO)

Unslaked lime is caustic and caution should be used in handling the powder. **Do not** confuse this with **agricultural lime** (see *BUFFERS: PONDS*), which is most often used for adjusting pH. Unslaked lime is an alkali and can rapidly raise the pH to over 10, killing all the fish, which is why it is mainly used as a disinfectant.

Use No. 1: Disinfecting ponds

Water-borne formulations:

1. Prolonged immersion for general disinfection

    a. Add unslaked lime at a rate of ~1500 kg/ha (= 1338 pounds/acre = 14 g/ft^2). Best results are obtained when lime is disked into the soil of a drained pond. When it is added directly to water, the pH of the water should be allowed to return to < 8.5 before fish are added (usually takes about 14 days).

2. Prolonged immersion for eradicating *Myxobolus cerebralis* (Hoffman & Hoffman, 1972)

    a. Add 2500 mg unslaked lime/l, and treat for 6 days.

Use No. 2: Adjusting pH/alkalinity of ponds (see *BUFFERS: PONDS*)

Use No. 3: Adjusting hardness of ponds (see *CALCIUM*)

Vaccines (Biomed, Inc.; Vetrepharm, Ltd.; Aqua Health, Ltd.; Apothekernes Laboratorium A.S.; Aquaculture Vaccines, Ltd.; Micrologix International, Ltd.; or Equivalent)

Vaccines are available for treating several important bacterial diseases of fish, including enteric redmouth disease, vibriosis, Hitra disease, and furunculosis. All are killed vaccines (bacterins). Oral, injectable, and bath preparations are available. Bath preparations are most commonly used and usually give good protection. Injectable preparations, although more labor intensive, give superior protection. Oral vaccines are least effective.

Water Change

Use: Diluting of toxins in closed systems

For aquaria, changing about 10% to 25% of the water every month (or 3% to 5% per week) is usually recommended (Axelrod et al., 1980; Moe, 1992a). Systems with high fish densities may require larger changes. If rapid dilution is needed, do 50% or more, but be cautious about environmental shock (see *PROBLEM 87*).

Zeolite (Clinoptilite)

Use: Removal of ammonia from water

Zeolite is an ion-exchange resin that exchanges ammonia for sodium ions. Clinoptilite is a very active form of zeolite (Marking & Bills, 1982). Under optimal conditions (low hardness, neutral pH, freshwater, 20 × 30 mesh particle size), 1.0 g of zeolite can remove 9 mg of ammonia. More realistic removal rates are around 2 mg ammonia/g zeolite in freshwater (1 pound of zeolite in a 100-gallon tank [or approximately 1 kg in 840 liters] will totally remove 3 mg/l of ammonia). Temperature is not important under aquaculture conditions. High hardness reduces removal by about 50% because of the binding of calcium and magnesium to the resin. Large particle sizes are less efficient, while smaller particles are easily clogged.

At 36 ppt salinity, there is a 95% reduction in zeolite's ability to remove ammonia, but it still can remove dyes and organic matter at the same rate. Zeolite is less effective than activated carbon in removing dyes and organics. It is better than low-grade carbon. Zeolite can also reduce ammonia build-up while shipping fish.

When zeolite becomes saturated with ammonia, it can be reused by placing in a strong, alkaline, NaCl solution (~1 lb salt/3 gallons water [= 1 kg/25 liters] at pH 11 to 12) overnight or by treating with a 200 ppt salt solution for 30 minutes. The resin should be rinsed before reuse. Resins have been regenerated up to 500 times. The brine solution can also be reused (Marking & Bills, 1982).

Water-borne formulations:

1. Prolonged immersion to reduce or prevent ammonia toxicity

When fish are at a density of about 20 to 40 g of fish/l, adding about 20 g of clinoptilite/l of water reduces the total ammonia nitrogen that accumulates after 24 hours by about 75% to 85% (Bower & Turner, 1982a).

a. Ammo® Ammonia Remover (Aquarium Pharmaceuticals). Use as directed.
b. Ammonex® (Argent) bags or loose pieces containing clinoptilite. Use as directed.

LITERATURE CITED

Ahne W: Viral infection cycles in pike (*Esox lucius* L.), *J Appl Ichthyol* 1:90-91, 1985.

Ahne W, Jaing Y, Thomsen I: A new virus isolated from cultured grass carp *Ctenopharyngodon idella*, *Dis Aquatic Org* 3: 181-185, 1987.

Ajello L, McGinnis MR, Camper J: An outbreak of phaeohyphomycosis in rainbow trout caused by *Scolecobasidium humicola*, *Mycopathol* 62:15-22, 1977.

Ajmal M, Hobbs BC: Species of *Corynebacterium* and *Pasteurella* isolated from diseased salmon, trout, and rudd, *Nature* 215:142-143, 1967.

Akhlaghi M, Munday BL, Whittington RL: Comparison of the efficacy of two sites of intraperitoneal injection in fish, *Bull Eur Assoc Fish Pathol* 13:176-178, 1993.

Alabaster JS, Lloyd R: *Water quality criteria for freshwater fish,* ed 2, London, 1982, FAO/Butterworths.

Alderman DJ: Fungal diseases of aquatic animals. In Roberts RJ, editor: *Microbial diseases of fish: society for general microbiology,* Special Publication 9, New York, 1982, Academic Press, pp. 189-242.

Alderman DJ: Malachite green: a review, *J Fish Dis* 8:289-298, 1985.

Alderman DJ: Fisheries chemotherapy: a review. In Muir JF, Roberts RJ, editors: *Recent advances in aquaculture,* vol 3, London, 1988, Croom Helm, pp. 1-61.

Alderman DJ, Clifton-Hadley RS: Malachite green therapy of proliferative kidney disease in rainbow trout field trials, *Vet Rec* 122:103-106, 1988.

Alderman DJ, Feist SW: *Exophiala* infection of kidney of rainbow trout recovering from proliferative kidney disease, *Trans Brit Mycol Soc* 84:157-185, 1985.

Alderman DJ, Michel C: Chemotherapy in aquaculture today. In Michel C, Alderman DJ, editors: *Chemotherapy in aquaculture: from theory to reality,* Paris, 1992, Office International des Epizooties, pp. 3-24.

Alderman DJ, Polglase J: A comparative investigation of the effects of fungicides on *Saprolegnia parasitica* and *Aphanomyces astaci, Trans Brit Mycol Soc* 83:313-318. 1984.

Alderman DJ, Polglase JL: Are fungal diseases significant in the marine environment? In Moss ST, editor: *The biology of marine fungi,* Cambridge, New York, 1986, University Press, pp. 189-198.

Aldridge FJ, Shireman JV: Introduction to fish parasites and diseases and their treatment, *Florida Coop Ext Serv Circ 716,* 1991, p. 14.

Alexander JB, Ingram GA : Noncellular nonspecific defence mechanisms of fish, *Ann Rev Fish Dis* 2:249-280, 1992.

Allen KO, Avault JW, Jr: Effects of brackish water on ichthyophthiriasis of channel catfish, *Prog Fish-cult* 32:227-230, 1970.

Allison R: The effects of formalin and other parasiticides upon oxygen concentrations in ponds, *Proc Ann Conf Southeast Assn Game Fish Comm* 16:446-449, 1962.

Allison R: New control methods for *Ichthyophthirius* in ponds, FAO World Symposium on Warmwater Pond Fish Culture, FR: IX/E-9, 1966.

Alvarez-Pellitero MP, Pereira-Bueno JM, Gonzales-Lanza MC: On the presence of *Chloromyxum truttae* Leger, 1906 in *Salmo trutta fario* from Leon (Duero Basin, NW Spain), *Bull Eur Assn Fish Pathol* 2:4-7, 1982.

Amandi A, Hiu SF, Rohovec JS, Fryer JL: Isolation and characterization of *Edwardsiella tarda* from chinook salmon (*Oncorhynchus tsawyscha*), *Appl Environ Micro* 43:1380-1384, 1982.

Amend DF: Control of infectious hematopoietic necrosis virus by elevating water temperature, *J Fish Res Bd Can* 27:265-270, 1970.

Amend DF: *Efficacy, toxicity, and residues of nifurpirinol in salmonids,* United States Department of Internal Bureau of Sport Fish and Wildlife, Technical Paper No. 62, p. 13, 1972.

Amend DF, McDowell T: Current problems in the control of channel catfish virus, *J World Maricult Soc* 14:261-267, 1983.

Amend DF, McDowell T, Hedrick RP: Characteristics of a previously unidentified virus from channel catfish (*Ictalurus puctatus*), *Can J Fish Aquat Sci* 41:807-811, 1984.

Amend DF, Pietsch JP: Virucidal activity of two iodophores to salmonid viruses, *J Fish Res Bd Can* 29:61-65. 1972.

Amend DF, Smith L: Pathophysiology of infectious hematopoietic necrosis virus disease in rainbow trout (*Salmo gairdneri*): early changes in blood and aspects of the immune response after injection of IHN virus, *J Fish Res Bd Can* 31:1371-1378, 1974.

Amend DF, Yasutake WT, Mead RW: A hematopoietic virus disease of rainbow trout and sockeye salmon, *Trans Am Fish Soc* 98:796-804, 1969.

American Public Health Association (APHA), American Water Works Association, Water Environment Federation: *Standard methods for the examination of water and wastewater,* ed 18, Washington, DC, 1992, APHA.

American Public Health Association (APHA), American Water Works Association, Water Pollution Control Federation: *Standard methods for the examination of water and wastewater,* ed 17, Washington, DC, 1989, APHA.

Amos K, editor: Procedures for the detection and identification of certain fish pathogens, ed 3, Bethesda, Md., 1985, American Fisheries Society, 114 pp.

Anaker RL, Ordal EL: Studies on the myxobacterium *Chondrococcus columnaris.* 1. Serological typing, *J Bacteriol* 78:25-32, 1959.

Anders K, Moller H: Spawning papillomatosis of smelt, *Osmerus eperlanus* L., from the Elbe estuary, *J Fish Dis* 8:233-235, 1985.

Anderson DP, Barney PJ: The role of the diagnostic laboratory in fish disease control, *Ann Rev Fish Dis* 1:41-62, 1991.

Anderson JIW, Conroy DA: The significance of disease in preliminary attempts to raise flatfish and salmonids in sea water, *Bull Off Int Epizoot* 69:1129-1137, 1968.

Andrews C, Exell A, Carrington N: *The manual of fish health,* Morris Plains, N.J., 1988, Tetra Press.

Andrews C, Riley A: Anthelminthic treatment of fish via stomach tube, *Fish Manage* 13:83-84, 1982.

Andrews JW, Matsuda Y: The influence of various culture conditions on the oxygen consumption of channel catfish, *Trans Am Fish Soc* 104:322-327, 1975.

Andrews JW, Murai T, Gibbons G: The influence of dissolved oxygen on the growth of channel catfish, *Trans Am Fish Soc* 102:835-838, 1973.

Angulo FJ et al: Caring for pets of immunocompromised persons, *JAVMA* 205:1711-1718, 1994.

Anonymous: FDA gives "low priority" status to salt, four other aquaculture compounds, *Water Farm J,* March, 1992, p. 4.

Anonymous: *Furanace: a new chemotherapeutic agent for fish disease,* Osaka, Japan, Undated, Dainippon Pharmaceutical Company, Ltd., 57 pp.

Anonymous: *Humane killing of animals,* South Mimms, Potters Bar, Herts, England, 1988, Universities Federation for Animal Welfare.

Anonymous: *National workshop on bacterial kidney disease,* Phoenix, Ariz., 1991.

Anonymous: Report of the AVMA panel on euthanasia, *JAVMA* 202:230-249, 1993.

Anonymous: Treatment of columnaris disease. In *For fish farmers,* No. 86-1, Mississippi State University, 1986, Mississippi Cooperative Extension Service, The University, p. 1-2.

Anonymous: *Using copper sulfate to control algae in water supply impoundments,* Champaign, Ill., 1989, Miscellaneous Publication 11, Illinois State Water Survey, p. 11.

Aoki T: Present and future problems concerning the development of resistance in aquaculture. In Michel C, Alderman DJ, editors: *Chemotherapy in aquaculture: from theory to reality,* Paris, 1992, Office International des Epizooties, pp. 254-262.

Aoki T, Sakaguchi T, Kitao T: Multiple drug-resistant plasmids from *Edwardsiella tarda* in eel culture ponds, *Nippon Suisan Gakkaishi* 53:1821-1825, 1987.

Arakawa CK, Fryer JL: Isolation and characterization of a new subspecies of *Mycobacterium chelonei* from salmonid fish, *Helgolander Meersuntersucheungen* 37:329-342, 1984.

Armstrong RD et al: Erythromycin levels within eggs and alevins derived from spawning broodstock chinook salmon (*Oncorhynchus tshawytscha*) injected with the drug, *Dis Aquat Org* 6:33-36, 1989.

Armstrong RD, Ferguson HW: Systemic viral disease of the orange chromide cichlid *Etroplus maculatus*, *Dis Aquat Org* 7:155-157, 1989.

Austin B: Evaluation of antimicrobial compounds for the control of bacterial kidney disease in rainbow trout, *Salmo gairdneri* Richardson, *J Fish Dis* 8:209-220, 1985.

Austin B, Austin DA: *Bacterial fish pathogens: disease in farmed and wild fish*, Chichester, West Sussex, United Kingdom, 1987, Ellis Horwood Limited, 364 pp.

Austin B, Austin DA: *Bacterial fish pathogens*, ed 2, New York, 1993, Ellis Horwood, 384 pp.

Austin B, Bucke D, Feist S, Rayment J: A false positive reaction in the indirect fluorescent antibody test for *Renibacterium salmoninarum* with a coryneform organism, *Bull Eur Assn Fish Pathol* 5:8-9, 1985.

Austin B et al: Recovery of *Janthinobacterium lividum* from diseased rainbow trout, *Oncorhynchus mykiss* (Walbaum), in Northern Ireland and Scotland, *J Fish Dis* 15:357-359, 1992a.

Austin B, Johnson C, Alderman DJ: Evaluation of substituted quinolones for the control of vibriosis in turbot (*Scophthalmus maximus*), *Aquacult* 29:227-239, 1982.

Austin B, Stobie M: Recovery of *Micrococcus luteus* and presumptive *Planococcus* from moribund fish during outbreaks of rainbow trout (*Oncorhynchus mykiss* Walbaum) fry syndrome (RTFS) in England, *J Fish Dis* 15:203-206, 1992a.

Austin B, Stobie M: Recovery of *Serratia plymuthica* and presumptive *Pseudomonas pseudoalkaligenes* from skin lesions in rainbow trout, *Oncorhynchus mykiss* (Walbaum), otherwise infected with enteric redmouth, *J Fish Dis* 15:541-543, 1992b.

Austin B, Stobie M, Robertson PAW: *Citrobacter freundii*: the cause of gastro-enteritis leading to progressive low-level mortalities in farmed rainbow trout *Oncorhynchus mykiss* Walbaum in Scotland, *Bull Eur Assn Fish Pathol* 12:166-167, 1992b.

Avault Jr JW: Insect and bird predators and pests of fish and crustaceans, *Aquaculture Magazine* 21(2):64-70, 1995.

Avtalion RR et al: Influence of environmental temperature on the immune response of fish. In Aber W, Haas R, editors: *Current topics in microbiology and immunology*, Berlin, 1973, Springer-Verlag, pp. 1-35.

Awad MA, Nusbaum KE, Brady YL: Preliminary studies of a newly developed subunit vaccine for channel catfish virus disease, *J Aquat Animal Health* 1:233-237, 1989.

Awakura T: Studies on the microsporidian infection in salmonid fishes, *Sci Rep Hokkaido Fish Hatch* 29:1-96, 1974.

Axelrod HR, Emmens C, Burgess W, Pronek N, Axelrod G: *Exotic tropical fishes*, Neptune, N.J., 1980, T.F.H., 1302 pp.

Bach R, Chen PK, Chapman GB: Changes in the spleen of channel catfish *Ictalurus punctatus* Rafinesque induced by infection with *Aeromonas hydrophila*, *J Fish Dis* 1:205-218, 1978.

Backman S, Ferguson HW, Prescott JF, Wilcock BP: Progressive panophthalmitis in chinook salmon, *Oncorhynchus tshawytscha* (Walbaum): a case report, *J Fish Dis* 13:345-353, 1990.

Bailey TA: Effects of 25 compounds on 4 species of aquatic fungi (Saprolegniales) pathogenic to fish, *Aquacult* 38:97-104, 1984.

Bailey TA, Jeffrey SM: *Evaluation of 215 candidate fungicides for use in fish culture. Investigations in Fish Control*, No. 99, United States Fish Wildlife Service, 1989, p. 9.

Barbaro A, Francescon A: Parassitosi da *Amyloodinium ocellatum* (Dinophyceae) su larve di *Sparus aurata* allevate in un impianto di riproduzione artificiale, *Oebalia* 11:745-752, 1985.

Barica J, Mathias JA: Oxygen depletion and winterkill risk in small prarie lakes under extended ice cover, *J Fish Res Bd Can* 36:980-986, 1979.

Barnes AC, Lewin CS, Aymes SGB, Hastings TS: Susceptibility of Scottish isolates of *Aeromomas salmonicida* to the antibacterial agent amoxycillin, *ICES CM* F:28, 1991.

Bartholomew JL, Rohovec JS, Fryer JL: Development, use, and characterization of monoclonal and polyclonal antibodies against the myxosporean *Ceratomyxa shasta*, *J Protozool* 36:397-401, 1989.

Bassler G: *Uronema marinum* a new and common parasite on tropical saltwater fishes, *Freshwater Mar Aquar* 6:14:78-79, 1983.

Bauer ON, Nikolskaya NP: *Chilodonella cyprini* (Moroff, 1902), biology and epizootological importance, *Isv Vsesoyuz Nauchno-Issled Inst Ozern Rech Rybn Khoz* 119:116-123, 1957 (In Russian).

Bauer ON, Musselius VA, Strelkov YA: *Diseases of pond fishes* (English translation), Jerusalem, 1973, Israel Program for Scientific Translations, 220 pp.

Bauer ON, Musselius VA, Strelkov YA: *Diseases of pond fishes. Legkaya is pishchevaya promyshlenost* (in Russian), ed 2, Moscow, 1981, 319 pp.

Baxa DV, Kawai K, Kusuda R: Experimental infection of *Flexibacter maritimus* in black seabream (*Acanthopagrus schlegeli*) fry, *Fish Pathol* 22:105-109, 1987.

Baxa-Antonio D, Hedrick RP: Carrier state of enteric septicemia of catfish (ESC), *Am Fish Soc Fish Health Sec Newsltr* 20:1-3, 1992.

Baya AM et al: Association of a *Moraxella* sp. and a reo-like virus, with mortalities of striped bass, *Morone saxatilis*. In Perkins F, Cheng TC, Editors: *Pathology in marine science*, New York, 1990b, Academic Press, pp. 91-100.

Baya AM et al: Phenotypic and pathobiological properties of *Corynebacterium aquaticum* isolated from diseased striped bass, *Dis Aquat Org* 14:115-126, 1992a.

Baya AM et al: Association of *Streptococcus* sp. with fish mortalities in Chesapeake Bay and its tributaries, *J Fish Dis* 13:251-253, 1990a.

Baya AM, Lupiani B, Hetrick FM, Toranzo AE: Increasing importance of *Citrobacter freundii* as a fish pathogen, *FHS/AFS Newsltr* 18(4):4, 1991a.

Baya AM et al: Biochemical and serological characterization of *Carnobacterium* spp. isolated from farmed and natural populations of striped bass and catfish, *Appl Environ Microbiol* 57:3114-3120, 1991b.

Baya AM et al: *Serratia marcescens*: a potential pathogen for fish, *J Fish Dis* 15:15-26, 1992b.

Becker CD, Fujihara MP: *The bacterial pathogen Flexibacter columnaris and its epizootiology among Columbia River fish*, Monograph No. 2, 1978, American Fisheries Society, p. 92.

Becker CD: Flagellate parasites of fishes. In Kreier JP, Editor: *Parasitic protozoa*, vol 1, New York, 1977, Academic Press, pp. 357-416.

Bejerano Y, Sarig S, Horne MT, Roberts RJ: Mass mortalities in silver carp *Hypophthalmichthys molitrix* (Valenciennes) associated with bacterial infection following handling, *J Fish Dis* 2:49-56, 1979.

Bengtsson B-E: Vertebral damage in fish induced by pollutants. In Koeman JH, Strik JJTWA, editors: *Sublethal effects of toxic chemicals on aquatic animals*, New York, 1975, Elsevier, pp. 23-30.

Bennett GW: *Management of artificial lakes and ponds*, New York, 1962, Reinhold.

Bergjso T, Bergjso HT: Absorption from water as an alternative method for the administration of sulfonamides to rainbow trout, *Salmo gairdneri*, *Acta Vet Scand* 19:102-109, 1978.

Berry ES, Shea TB, Gabliks J: Two iridovirus isolates from *Carassius auratus* (L.), *J Fish Dis* 6:501-510, 1983.

Billi JL, Wolf K: Quantitative comparison of peritoneal washes and feces for detecting infectious pancreatic necrosis (IPN) virus in carrier brook trout, *J Fish Res Bd Can* 26:1459-1465, 1969.

Bills TD, Marking LL, Chandler JH: *Malachite green: its toxicity to aquatic organisms, persistence, and removal with activated carbon*, United States Fish and Wildlife Service Investigation in Fish Control, No. 75, 1977, p. 6.

Bjordal A: Wrasse as cleaner fish for farmed salmon, *Prog Underwater Sci* 16:17-28, 1991.

Blanc G, Loussouarn S, Pinault L: Biodisponibilite immediate du levamisole chez l'anguille Europeenne (*Anguilla anguilla* L.) hote definitif des nematodes *Anguillicola* Yamaguti, 1974. In Michel C, Alderman DJ, editors: *Chemotherapy in aquaculture: from theory to reality*, (in French), Paris, 1992, Office International des Epizooties, pp. 468-486.

Blasiola GC: Ectoparasitic turbellaria, *Marine Aquarist* 7:53-58, 1976.

Blasiola GC: Coral reef disease, *O. ocellatum. Marine Aquarist* 7: 50-58, 1978.

Blasiola GC: Description, preliminary studies, and probable etiology of head and lateral line erosion (HLLE) of the palette tang, *Paracanthurus hepatus* (Linnaeus, 1758) and other acanthurids, *Bulletin de l'Institut oceanographique, Monaco,* no special 5: 255-263, 1989.

Blasiola GC: Diseases of ornamental marine fishes. In Gratzek JB, Matthews JR editors: *Aquariology: the science of fish health management,* Morris Plains, N.J., 1992, Tetra Press, pp. 275-300.

Blasiola GC, Jr, Turnier JC: Algal infection of the sevengill shark, *Notorynchus maculatus, J Fish Dis* 2:161-163, 1979.

Blazer VS, Ankley GT, Finco-Kent D: Dietary influences on disease resistance factors in channel catfish, *Dev Comp Immunol* 13:43-48, 1989.

Blazer VS, Wolke RE: An *Exophiala*-like fungus as the cause of a systemic mycosis of marine fish, *J Fish Dis* 2:145-152, 1979.

Bloch B, Mellergaard S, Neilsen E: Adenovirus-like particles associated with epithelial hyperplasias in dab, *Limanda limanda* (L.), *J Fish Dis* 9:281-285, 1986.

Bokeny K, Lewbart G, Piner G: *The occurrence of an Ichthyobodo-like organism on captive Atlantic spadefish, Chaetodipterus faber,* Vallejo, Calif., 1994 (abstract), International Association for Aquatic Animals Medicine, 25th Annual Meeting, p. 163.

Bonami JR, Cousserans F, Weppe M, Hill BJ: Mortalities in hatchery-reared sea bass fry associated with a birnavirus, *Bull Eur Assn Fish Pathol* 3:41, 1983.

Bootsma R, Fijan N, Blommaert J: Isolation and preliminary characterization of the causative agent of carp erythrodermatitis, *Vet Archiv* 6:291-302, 1977.

Bower CE: *The basic marine aquarium,* Springfield, Ill., 1983, Charles C Thomas, p. 269.

Bower CE, Bidwell JP: Ionization of ammonia in seawater: effects of temperature, pH, and salinity, *J Fish Res Bd Can* 35:1012-1016, 1978.

Bower CE, Turner DT: Ammonia removal by clinoptilite in the transport of ornamental freshwater fishes, *Prog Fish-cult* 44:19-23, 1982a.

Bower CE, Turner DT: Accelerated nitrification in new seawater culture systems: effectiveness of commercial additives and seed media from established systems, *Aquacult* 24:1-9, 1981.

Bower CE, Turner DT: Effects of seven chemotherapeutic agents on nitrification in closed seawater culture systems, *Aquacult* 29:331-345, 1982b.

Bower CE, Turner DT, Biever RC: A standardized method of propagating the marine fish parasite, *Amyloodinium ocellatum, J Parasitol* 73:85-88, 1987.

Bower CE, Turner DT, Spotte S: pH maintenance in closed seawater culture systems: limitations of calcareous filtrants, *Aquacult* 23:211-217, 1981.

Bowser PR, Babish JG: Clinical pharmacology and efficacy of fluoroquinolones in fish, *Ann Rev Fish Dis* 1:63-66, 1991.

Bowser PR et al: Methemoglobinemia in channel catfish: methods of prevention, *Prog Fish-cult* 45:154-158.

Bowser PR et al: Isolation of channel catfish virus from channel catfish, *Ictalurus punctatus* (Rafinesque) brood stock, *J Fish Dis* 8:557-561, 1985.

Bowser PR, Schachte JH, Jr, Wooster GA, Babish JG: Experimental treatment of *Aeromonas salmonicida* infections with enrofloxacin and oxolinic acid: field trials, *J Aquatic Animal Health* 2:198-203, 1990.

Boyce NP, Clark WC: *Eubothrium salvelini* (Cestoda: Pseudophyllidea) impairs seawater adaptation of migrant sockeye yearlings (*Oncorhynchus nerka*) from Babine Lake, British Columbia, *Can J Fish Aquatic Sci* 40:821-824, 1983.

Boyce NP, Kabata Z, Margolis L: Investigations of the distribution, detection, and biology of *Henneguya salminicola* (Protozoa, Myxozoa), a parasite of the flesh of Pacific salmon, *Can Tech Rep Fish Aquat Sci,* No. 1405, 1985. 54 pp.

Boyd CE: *Water quality in warmwater fish ponds,* Alabama, 1979. Auburn University, 359 pp.

Boyd CE: *Water quality in ponds for aquaculture,* Alabama, 1990, Alabama Agricultural Experiment Station, Auburn University, 482 pp.

Boyd CE, Romaire RP, Johnston E: Predicting early morning dissolved oxygen concentrations in channel catfish ponds, (Trans Am) *Fish Soc* 107:484-492, 1978.

Bradley TM, DJ Medina, PW Chang, J McClain: Epizootic epitheliotropic disease of lake trout (*Salvelinus namaycush*): history and viral etiology, *Dis Aquatic Org* 7:195-201, 1989.

Brady YJ, Vinitnantharat S: Viability of bacterial pathogens in frozen fish, *J Aquatic Animal Health* 2:149-150, 1990.

Brandal PO, Egidus E: Preliminary report on oral treatment against sea lice, *Lepeophtheirus salmonis,* with Neguvon, *Aquacult* 10:177-178, 1977.

Brandal PO, Egidus E: Treatment of salmon lice (*Lepeophtheirus salmonis* Kroyer, 1838) with Neguvon: description of method and equipment, *Aquacult* 18:183-188, 1979.

Brandt TM, Jones RM, Jr, Koke JR: Corneal cloudiness in transported largemouth bass, *Prog Fish-cult* 48:199-201, 1986.

Bristow GA, Berland B: The effect of long-term, low level *Eubothrium* sp. (Cestoda: Pseudophyllidea) infection on growth of farmed salmon (*Salmo salar* L.). *Aquacult* 98:325-330. 1991.

Brooks AS, Bartos JM: Effects of free and combined chlorine and exposure duration on rainbow trout, channel catfish, and emerald shiners, *Trans Am Fish Soc* 113:786-793. 1984.

Brown CL et al: Maternal triiodothyronine injections cause increases in swim bladder inflation and survival rates in larval striped bass, *Morone saxatilis, J Experiment Zool* 248:168-176, 1988.

Brown EE, Gratzek JB: *Fish farming handbook,* Westport, Conn., 1980, AVI, 391 pp.

Brown EE: *World fish farming: cultivation and economics,* Westport, Conn., 1983, AVI.

Brown EM: *On Oodinium ocellatum brown, a parasite dinoflagellate causing epidemic disease in marine fish,* Proceedings of the Zoological Society of London, Part 3: 583-607, 1934.

Brown EM: A new parasitic protozoan, the causal organism of a white spot disease in marine fish *Cryptocaryon irritans* gen. et sp. n, *Agenda Sci Mtgs Zool Soc,* London, No. 11 (year 1950): 1-2, 1951.

Brown TE, Morley AW, Sanderson NT, Tait RD: Report of a large fish kill resulting from natural acid conditions in Australia, *J Fish Biol* 22:335-350, 1983.

Brownell CL: Water quality requirements for first feeding marine fish larvae: I. ammonia, nitrite and nitrate, *J Exp Mar Biol Ecol* 44:269-283, 1981.

Brugerolle G: Ultrastructural study of the flagellate *Protrichomonas legeri* (Lger 1905) parasite of the stomach of boops (*Box boops*), *Protistologica* 16:353-358, 1980.

Bruno D: Histopathology of bacterial kidney disease in laboratory-infected rainbow trout *Salmo gairdneri* Richardson and Atlantic salmon *Salmo salar* L., with reference to naturally infected fish, *J Fish Dis* 9:523-537, 1986.

Bruno DW, Munro ALS: Immunity in Atlantic salmon *Salmo salar* L., fry following vaccination against *Yersinia ruckeri,* and the influence of body weight and infectious pancreatic necrosis virus (IPNV) on the detection of carriers, *Aquacult* 81:205-211, 1989.

Bruno DW, Munro ALS, Needham EA: Gill lesions caused by *Aeromomas salmonicida* in sea-reared Atlantic salmon, *Salmo salar* L, *ICES CM* F:6, 1986.

Bruno W: Observations on a swim bladder fungal infection of farmed Atlantic salmon, *Salmo salar, Bull Eur Assn Fish Pathol* 9:7-8, 1989.

Buchmann K, Mellergaard S, Koie M: *Pseudodactylogyrus* infections in eels: a review, *Dis Aquatic Org* 3:51-57, 1987.

Buchmann K, Szekely CS, Bjerregaard J: Treatment of *Pseudodactylogyrus* infestations of *Anguilla anguilla.* I. Trials with niclosamide, toltrazuril, phenosulfonphthalein, and rafoxanide, *Bull Eur Assn Fish Pathol* 10:14-17, 1990.

Bucke D: Histopathology. In Austin B, Austin DA, editors: *Methods for the microbiological examination of fish and shellfish,* West Sussex, England, 1989, Ellis Horwood, pp. 69-97.

Bulkley RV: A furunculosis epizootic in Clear Lake yellow bass, *Bull Wild Dis Assoc* 3:322-327. 1969.

Bullock GL, HM Stuckey: Studies on vertical transmission of *Aeromonas salmonicida, Prog Fish-cult* 49:302-303, 1987.

Bullis RA, Noga EJ, Levy MG: Immunological relationship of the fish-pathogenic oomycete *Saprolegnia parasitica,* to other Oomycetes and unrelated fungi, *J Aquatic Animal Health* 2:223-227, 1990.

Bullock AM, Roberts RJ: Induction of UDN-like lesions in salmonids by exposure to ultraviolet light in the presence of phytotoxic agents, *J Fish Dis* 2:439-442, 1979.

Bullock G et al: Observations on the occurrence of bacterial gill disease and amoeba gill infestation in rainbow trout cultured in a water recirculation system, *J Aquatic Animal Health* 6:310-317, 1994.

Bullock GL, Cipriano RC, Snieszko SF: *Furunculosis and other diseases caused by Aeromonas salmonicida,* United States Fish and Wildlife Service, Fish Disease Leaflet 66, 1983.

Bullock GL, Herman RL, Waggy C: Hatchery efficacy trials with Chloramine-T for control of bacterial gill disease, *J Aquat Animal Health* 3:48-50, 1991.

Bullock GL, Hsu T, Shotts EB: *Columnaris disease of fishes,* Washington, DC, 1986, FDL # 72, U.S.D.O.I., F.W.S., Division of Fisheries and Wetlands Research, p. 9.

Bullock GL, Snieszko SF: *Fin rot, coldwater disease, and peduncle disease of salmonid fishes,* Kearneysville, W.Va., 1970, United States Department of the Interior, Division of Fishery Research, Fishery Leaflet No. 462.

Bullock GL, Stuckey HM: *Aeromonas salmonicida* detection in asymptomatically infected trout, *Prog Fish-cult* 37:237-239, 1975.

Burke J, Grischkowsky R: An epizootic caused by infectious hematopoetic necrosis virus in an enhanced population of sockeye salmon (*Oncorhyncus nerka* Walbaum) smolts at Hidden Creek, Alaska, *J Fish Dis* 7:421-429, 1984.

Burkhalter AP et al: *Aquatic weed identification and control manual,* Tallahassee, Fla., Undated, Bureau of Aquatic Plant Research and Control. Florida Department of Natural Resources, 100 pp.

Burkholder JM, Noga EJ, Hobbs C, Glasgow H: New *phantom* dinoflagellate is the causative agent of major estuarine fish kills, *Nature* 358:407-410, 1992.

Burreson EM, Frizzell LJ: The seasonal antibody response in juvenile summer flounder (*Paralichthys dentatus*) to the hemoflagellate *Trypanoplasma bullocki, Vet Immunol Immunopathol* 12:395-402, 1986.

Burress RM: *Development and evaluation of on-site toxicity test procedures for fishery investigations,* United States Fish Wildlife Service, Investigations in Fish Control, 8, 1975, 8 pp.

Busch RA, Lingg AJ: Establishment of an asymptomatic carrier state infection of enteric redmouth disease in rainbow trout (*Salmo gairdneri*), *J Fish Res Bd Can* 32:2429-2432, 1975.

Butcher R: The veterinary approach to ornamental fish. In Brown L, editor: *Aquaculture for veterinarians,* New York, 1993, Pergamon Press, pp. 357-378.

Bychowsky BE: *Monogenetic trematodes: their systematics and phylogeny,* Akad. Nauk. USSR, 1957, p. 509 (English translation by A.I.B.S., Washington, DC, Hargis, WJ, Jr., editor, 1961, Virginia Institution of Marine Science Translation Service 1).

Bylund G, Sumari O: Laboratory tests with Droncit against diplostomiasis in rainbow trout, *Salmo gairdneri* Richardson, *J Fish Dis* 4:259-264, 1981.

Cali A, Takvorian PM, Ziskowski JJ, Sawyer TK: Experimental infection of American winter flounder (*Pseudopleuronectes americanus*) with *Glugea stephani* (Microsporida), *J Fish Biol* 28:199-206, 1986.

Callinan RB: Diseases of native Australian fishes. In *Fish diseases,* Sydney, Australia, 1988, Post Graduate Committee in Veterinary Science, University of Sydney, pp. 459-472.

Campbell AC, Buswell JA: An investigation into the bacterial aetiology of black patch necrosis in Dover sole (*Solea solea* L.), *J Fish Dis* 5:495-508, 1982.

Cann DC, Taylor LY: An evaluation of residual contamination by *Clostridium botulinum* in a trout farm following an outbreak of botulism in the fish stock, *J Fish Dis* 7:391-396, 1984.

Canning EU, Lom J: *The microsporidia of vertebrates,* New York, 1986, Academic Press, 289 pp.

Canning EU, Lom J, Nicholas JP: Genus *Glugea* (Theholan, 1891) (Phylum Microspora): redescription of the type species *Glugea anomala* (Monieq, 1887) and recognition of its sporogonic development within sporphorous vesicles (pansporoblastic membranes), *Protistologica* 18:193-210, 1982.

Cannon LRG, Lester RJG: Two turbellarians parasitic in fish, *Dis Aquat Org* 5:15-22, 1988.

Cardeilhac P, Whitaker B: Copper treatments: uses and precautions, *Vet Clin N Am (Sm Animal Prac)* 18:435-448, 1988.

Carmichael JW: Cerebral mycetoma of trout due to *Phialophora*-like fungus, *Sabouraudia* 5:120-123, 1966.

Carmignani GM, Bennett JP: Rapid start-up of a biological filter in a closed aquaculture system, *Aquacult* 11:85-88, 1977.

Chabot JD, Thune RL: Proteases of the *Aeromonas hydrophila* complex, *J Fish Dis* 14:171-184, 1991.

Chang FH, Anderson C, Boustead NC: First record of a *Heterosigma* (Raphidophyceae) bloom with associated mortality of cage-reared salmon in Big Glory Bay, New Zealand, *NZ J of Marine Freshwater Res* 24:461-469, 1990.

Chen C-RL, Chung YY, Kuo G-H: Studies on the pathogenicity of *Flexibacter columnaris*-1: Effect of dissolved oxygen and ammonia on the pathogenicity of *Flexibacter columnaris* to eel (*Anguilla japonica*), *Rprts Fish Dis Res* 4:57-61, 1982, CAPD Fisheries series No. 8 (Taiwan).

Chen JC, Ting YY, Lin H, Lian TC: Heavy metal concentrations in sea water from grass prawn hatcheries and the coast of Taiwan, *J World Maricult Soc* 16:316-332, 1985.

Chen S-C: Study on the pathogenicity of *Nocardia asteroides* to the Formosa snakehead (*Channa maculata* [Lacepede]), *J Fish Dis* 15:47-53, 1992.

Cheung PJ, Nigrelli RF, Ruggieri GD: Coccidian parasite of blackfish, *Tautoga onitis* (L.): life cycle and histopathology, *Am Zool* 19:1979 (abstract).

Cheung PJ, Nigrelli RF, Ruggieri GD: Studies on the morphology of *Uronema marinum* Dujardin (Ciliata: Uronematidae) with a description of the histopathology of the infection in marine fishes, *J Fish Dis* 3:295-303, 1980.

Chinabut S, Limsuwan C: Histopathological changes in some freshwater fishes found during the disease outbreak: 1982-1983, *Fisheries Gaz* 36:281-289, 1983.

Ching HL, Munday DR: Geographic and seasonal distribution of the infectious stage of *Ceratomyxa shasta* Noble 1950, a myxozoan salmonid pathogen in the Fraser River system, *Can J Zool* 62:1075-1080, 1984a.

Ching HL, Munday, DR: Susceptibility of six Fraser River chinook salmon stocks to *Ceratomyxa shasta* and the effects of salinity on ceratomyxosis, *Can J Zool* 62:1081-1083, 1984b.

Chowdhury MBR, Wakabayashi H: Effects of sodium, calcium, and magnesium ions on the survival of *Flexibacter columnaris* in water, *Fish Pathol* 23:231-235, 1988a.

Chowdhury MBR, Wakabayashi H: Effects of sodium, calcium, and magnesium ions on *Flexibacter columnaris* infection in fish, *Fish Pathol* 23:237-241, 1988b.

Christman RF et al: *Identification of mutagenic by-products from aquatic humic chlorination,* University of North Carolina Water Resource Research Institute's Final Report No. 259, 1991.

Clarridge JE, Musher DM, Fanstein V, Wallace RJ: Extraintestinal human infection caused by *Edwardsiella tarda, J Clin Micro* 11:511-514, 1980.

Clem LW et al: Temperature-mediated processes in teleost immunity: differential effects of *in vitro* and *in vivo* temperature on mitogenic responses of channel catfish lymphocytes, *Dev Comp Immunol* 8:313-322, 1984.

Clifton-Hadley RS, Alderman DJ: The efficacy of malachite green upon proliferative kidney disease, *J Fish Dis* 10:101-107, 1987.

Clifton-Hadley R, Richards RH: Method for the rapid diagnosis of proliferative kidney disease in salmonids, *Vet Rec* 112:609, 1983.

Coles BM, Stroud RK, Sheggeby S: Isolation of *Edwardsiella tarda* from three Oregon sea mammals, *J Wildlife Dis* 14:339-341, 1978.

Colesante RT, Engstrom-Heg R, Ehlinger N, Youmans N: Cause and control of muskellunge fry mortality at Chautauqua Hatchery, New York, *Prog Fish-cult* 43:17-20, 1981.

Collins MT, Dawe DC, Gratzek JB: Immune response of channel catfish under different environmental conditions, *J Am Vet Med Assoc* 169:991-994, 1976.

Collins MT, Gratzek JB, Dawe DL, Nemetz TG: Effects of parasiticides on nitrification, *J Fish Res Bd Can* 32:2033-2037, 1975.

Collins MT, Gratzek JB, Dawe DL, Nemetz TG: Effects of antibacterial agents on nitrification in an aquatic recirculating system, *J Fish Res Bd Can* 33:215-218, 1976.

Collins R: Principles of disease diagnosis. In Brown L, editor: *Aquaculture for veterinarians,* Tarrytown, N.Y., Pergamon Press, 1993, pp. 69-90.

Colorni A: Aspects of the biology of *Cryptocaryon irritans,* and hyposalinity as a control measure in cultured gilt-head sea bream *Sparus aurata, Dis Aquat Org* 1:19-22, 1985.

Colorni A: A systemic mycobacteriosis in the European sea bass *Dicentrarchus labrax, Israeli J Aquacult-Bamidgeh* 44:75-81, 1992.

Colorni A, Ankaous M, Diamant A, Knibb W: Detection of mycobacteriosis in fish using the polymerase chain reaction technique, *Bull Eur Assn Fish Pathol* 13:195-198, 1993.

Colorni A, Diamant A: Ultrastructural features of *Cryptocaryon irritans*: a ciliate parasite of marine fish, *Eur J Protist* 29:425-434, 1993.

Colorni A, Paperna I, Gordin H: Bacterial infections in gilt-head sea bream *Sparus aurata* cultured at Elat, *Aquacult* 23:257-267, 1981.

Colt J: *Computations of dissolved gas concentrations in water as functions of temperature, salinity, and pressure,* Special Publication No. 14, 1984, American Fisheries Society, Bethesda, Md.

Colt J: Gas supersaturation: impact on the design and operation of aquatic systems, *Aquacult Eng* 5:49-85, 1986.

Colt J, Armstrong D: *Nitrogen toxicity to fish, crustaceans and molluscs,* Davis, Calif., 1979, Department of Civil Engineering, University of California, Davis, 30 pp.

Colt J, Bouck GR, Fidler L: *Review of current literature and research on gas supersaturation and gas bubble trauma,* Special Publication No. 1, 1986, B.P.A. and Bioengineering Section, American Fisheries Society.

Colwell RR, Grimes DJ: *Vibrio* diseases of marine fish populations, *Helgolander Meeresuntersuchungen* 37:265-287, 1984.

Cone DK, Odense PH: Pathology of five species of *Gyrodactylus* Nordmann, 1832 (Monogenea), *Can J Zool* 62:1084-1088, 1984.

Cone DK, Wiles M: *Ichthyobodo necator* (Henneguy, 1883) from winter flounder *Pseudopleuronectes americanus* (Walbaum), in the northwest Atlantic Ocean, *J Fish Dis* 7:87-89, 1984.

Conroy D, Solarolo EB: Sensitivity of some acid-fast bacteria of piscine origin to certain chemotherapeutic agents, *J Fish Res Bd Can* 22:243-245, 1965.

Conroy DA: Notes on the incidence of piscine tuberculosis in Argentina, *Prog Fish-cult* 26:89-90, 1964.

Conroy DA: Observaciones sobre casos espontaneos de tuberculosis itica, *Microbiologia Espanola* 19:93-113, 1966.

Cooper JE, Ewbank R, Platt C et al: *Euthanasia of amphibians and reptiles,* London, 1989, UFAW/WSPA.

Cope OB: Interactions between pesticides and wildlife, *Ann Rev Entomol* 16:325-364, 1971.

Crawskaw MT, Sweeting RA: *Myxobolus koi* Kudo, 1919: a new record for Britain, *J Fish Dis* 9:465-467, 1986.

Cruz JM et al: An outbreak of *Plesiomonas shigelloides* in farmed rainbow trout, *Salmo gairdneri* Richardson, in Portugal, *Bull Eur Assn Fish Pathol* 6:20-22, 1986.

Csaba G et al: Septicaemia in silver carp (*Hypophthalmichthys molitrix,* Val.) and bighead (*Aristichthys nobilis* Rich.) caused by *Pseudomonas fluorescens.* In Olah J, Molnar K, Jeney S, Mueller F, editors: *Fish, pathogens and environment in European polyculture,* Szarvas, Hungary, 1981, Fisheries Research Institute, pp. 111-123.

Cusack R, Cone DK: A review of parasites as vectors of viral and bacterial diseases of fish, *J Fish Dis* 9:169-171, 1986.

D'Aoust P-Y, Ferguson HW: The pathology of chronic ammonia toxicity in rainbow trout, *Salmo gairdneri* Richardson, *J Fish Dis* 7:199-205, 1984.

Dalsgaard I, Bjerregaard J: Enrofloxacin as an antibiotic in fish, *Acta Veterinaria Scandinavica* 87(suppl):300-302, 1991.

Daly JG, Stevenson RMW: Importance of culturing several organs to detect *Aeromonas salmonicida* in salmonid fish, *Trans Am Fish Soc* 114:909-910, 1985.

Daniels HV, Boyd CE: Acute toxicity of ammonia and nitrite to spotted seatrout, *Prog Fish-cult* 49:260-263, 1987.

Daoust PY, Ferguson HW: Nodular gill disease: a uniqaue form of proliferative gill disease in rainbow trout *Salmo gairdneri* Richardson, *J Fish Dis* 8:511-522, 1985.

Davies PE, White RWG: The toxicology and metabolism of chlorthalonil in fish, 1: lethal levels for *Salmo gairdneri, Galaxias maculatus, G. truttaceus,* and *G. auratus* and the fate of ^{14}C-TCIN in *S. gairdneri, Aquat Toxicol* 7:93-105, 1985.

Davin WT, Jr, Kohler CC, Tindall DR: Ciguatera toxins adversely affect piscivorous fishes, *Trans Am Fish Soc* 117:374-384, 1988.

Davis HS: A new bacterial disease of freshwater fishes, *Bull US Bur Fish 1921-22* 38:261-280, 1922.

Dawson VK, Marking LL, Bills TD: Removal of toxic chemicals from water with activated carbon, *Trans Amer Fish Soc* 105:119-123, 1976.

Dawson VK, Schnick RA, Rach JJ, Schreier TM: La Crosse Center discovers fungicide for immediate use, *Am Fish Soc Newsltr* 22(1):9, 1994 (Fish Health Section).

Daye PG, Garside ET: Histopathologic changes in surficial tissues of brook trout (*Salvelinus fontinalis*) Mitchill exposed to acute and chronic levels of pH, *Can J Zool* 54:2,140-142;155, 1976.

de Kinkelin P, Hedrick RP: International veterinary guidelines for the transport of live fish or fish eggs, *Ann Rev Fish Dis* 1:27-40, 1991.

de Mateo MM et al: Monoclonal antibody and lectin probes recognize developmental and sporogonic stages of PKX, the causative agent of proliferative kidney disease in European and North American salmonid fish, *Dis Aquat Org* 15:23-29, 1993.

Debuf Y, editor: *The veterinary formulary,* London, 1991, Pharmaceutical Press.

Diamant A: Ultrastructure and pathogenesis of *Ichthyobodo* sp. from wild common dab *Limanda limanda* L., in the North Sea, *J Fish Dis* 10:241-247, 1987.

Diamant A: Morphology and ultrastructure of *Cryptobia eilatica* n. sp (Bodonidae: Kinetoplastida), an ectoparasite from the gills of marine fish, *J Protozool* 37:482-489, 1990.

Diamant A, Issar G, Colorni A, Paperna I: A pathogenic *Cryptocaryon*-like ciliate from the Mediterranean Sea, *Bull Eur Assoc Fish Pathol* 11:122-124, 1991.

Diamant A, McVicar AH: Distribution of X-cell disease in common dab, *Limanda limanda* L., in the North Sea, and untrastructural observations of previously undescribed developmental stages, *J Fish Dis* 12:25-37, 1989.

Dickerson HW, Evans DL, Gratzek JG: Production and preliminary characterization of murine monoclonal antibodies to *Ichthyophthirius multifiliis,* a protozoan parasite of fish, *Am J Vet Res* 47:2400-2404, 1986.

Diggles BK, Roubal FR, Lester RJG: The influence of formalin, benzocaine, and hyposalinity on the fecundity and viability of *Polylabroides multispinosus* (Monogenea; Microcotylidae) parasitic on the gills of *Acanthopagrus australis* (Pisces: Sparidae), *Internat J Parasit* 23:877-884, 1993.

Dixon BA, Yamashita J, Evelyn F: Antibiotic resistance of *Aeromonas* spp. isolated from tropical fish imported from Singapore, *J Aquat Animal Health* 2:295-297, 1990.

Dogel VA, Bykhovski BE: Parasites of fish of the Caspian Sea (Trudy po kompletnon izuchenii Kasp. morya), *Izdat Akad Nauk SSSR* (in Russian), p. 149, 1939, Moskva.

Dorson M, de Kinkelin P, Torchy C, Monge D: Sensibilite du brochet (*Esox lucius*) a differents virus de salmonides (NPI, SHV, NHI) et au rhabdovirus de la perche, *Bull Fr Peche Piscis* 307:91-101, 1987.

Doty MS, Slater DW: A new species of *Heterosporium* pathogenic on young chinook salmon, *Am Midl Nat* 36:663-665, 1946.

Duncan TO: *A review of literature on the use of potassium permanganate (KMnO₄) in fisheries,* 1974, United States Fish and Wildlife Service Report, FWS-LR-74-14, p. 61.

Dupree HK, Huner JV: Transportation of live fish. In Dupree HK, Huner JV, editors: *Third report to the fish farmers,* Washington DC, 1984, United States Fish and Wildlife Service, pp. 165-176.

Durborow RM, Crosby D: Monitoring winter kill conditions can cut losses, *Catfish J* 3:9, 1988.

Dykova I, Lom J: Histopathological changes due to infections with *Cryptobia iubilans* Nohynkova, 1984, in two cichlid fishes, *Z Angew Ichthyol* 1:34-38, 1979a.

Dykova I, Lom J: Histopathological changes in *Trypanosoma danilewskyi* Laveran and Mesnil, 1904 and *Trypanoplasma borreli* Laveran and Mesnil, 1902 infections of goldfish, *Carassius auratus* (L.), *J Fish Dis* 2:381-390, 1979b.

Dykova I, Lom J: Tissue reactions to microsporidian infections in fish, *J Fish Dis* 3:263-283, 1980.

Dykova I, Lom J: Fish coccidia: critical notes on life cycles, classification and pathogenicity, *J Fish Dis* 4:487-505, 1981.

Dykova I, Lom J: Fish coccidia: an annotated list of described species, *Folia Parasitol (Praha)* 30:193-208, 1983.

Dykstra MJ et al: Ulcerative mycosis: a serious menhaden disease of the southeast coastal fisheries of the United States, *J Fish Dis* 12:125-127, 1989.

Dykstra MJ et al: Characterization of the *Aphanomyces* species involved with ulcerative mycosis (UM) in menhaden, *Mycologia* 78:664-672, 1986.

Eaton WD, Kent ML: A retrovirus in chinook salmon (*Oncorhynchus tshawytscha*) with plasmacytoid leukemia and evidence for the etiology of the disease, *Cancer Res* 52:6496-6500, 1992.

Eaton ED, Wingfield WH, Hedrick RP: Prevalence and experimental transmission of the steelhead herpesvirus in salmonid fishes, *Dis Aquat Org* 7:23-30, 1989.

Economon P: Furunculosis in northern pike, *Trans Am Fish Soc* 89:240-241, 1960.

Edwards CJ: Algal infections of fish tissue: a recent record and review, *J Fish Dis* 1:175-179, 1978.

Egidius E, Andersen K: The use of Furanace against vibriosis in rainbow trout *Salmo gairdneri* Richardson in salt water, *J Fish Dis* 2:79-80, 1979.

Egusa S: *Infectious diseases of fish,* New Delhi, India, 1978 (English translation, 1992), Amerind Publishing, 696 pp.

Egusa S: A microsporidian species from yellowtail juveniles, *Seriola quinqueradiata,* with "Beko" disease, *Fish Pathol* 16:187-192, 1982.

Egusa S: Disease problems in Japanese yellowtail, *Seriola quinqueradiata,* culture, a review, *Rapp (pv) Reun Cons Int Explor Mer* 182:10-18, 1983.

Egusa S: *Myxobolus buri* sp. n. (Myxosporea: Bivalvulida) parasitic in the brain of *Seriola quinqueradiata* Temminch et Schlegel, *Fish Pathol* 19:239-244, 1985.

Eklund MW et al: Botulism in juvenile coho salmon (*Oncorhynchus kisutch*) in the United States, *Aquacult* 27:1-11, 1982.

Elliott D, Pascho R, Bullock G: Developments in the control of bacterial kidney disease of salmonid fishes, *Dis Aquatic Org* 6:201-215, 1989.

Elliott DG, Barila TY: Membrane filtration-fluorescent antibody staining procedure for detecting and quantifying *Renibacterium salmoninarum* in coelomic fluid of chinook salmon (*Oncorhynchus tshawytscha*), *Can J Fish Aquatic Sci* 44:206-210, 1987.

Ellis AE: An appraisal of the extracellular toxins of *Aeromomas salmonicida* ssp. *salmonicida,* *J Fish Dis* 14:265-278, 1991.

Ellis AE, Dear G, Stewart DJ: Histopathology of Sekiten- byo caused by *Pseudomonas anguilliseptica* in the European eel *Anguilla anguilla* in Scotland, *J Fish Dis* 6:77-79, 1983a.

Ellis AE, Roberts RJ, Tytler P: The anatomy and physiology of teleosts. In Roberts RJ, editor: *Fish pathology,* London, 1978, Bailliere-Tindall, pp. 13-54.

Ellis AE, Waddell IF, Minter DW: A systemic fungal disease in Atlantic salmon parr, *Salmo salar* L., caused by a species of *Phialophora,* *J Fish Dis* 6:511-523, 1983b.

El-Matbouli M, Hoffmann RW: Effects of freezing, ageing and passage through the alimentary canal of predatory animals on the viability of *Myxobolus cerebralis* spores, *J Aquatic Animal Health* 3:260-262, 1991.

Elsaesser CF, Clem LW: Haematological and immunological changes in channel catfish stressed by handling and transport, *J Fish Biol* 28:511-521, 1986.

Emerson K, Russo RC, Lund RE, Thurston RV: Aqueous ammonia equilibrium calculations: effect of pH and temperature, *J Fish Res Bd Can* 32:2379-2383, 1975.

Emerson CJ, Payne JF, Bal AK: Evidence for the presence of a viral non-lymphocystis type disease in winter flounder, *Pseudopleuronectes americanus* (Walbaum), from the north-west Atlantic, *J Fish Dis* 8:91-102, 1985.

Emmons CW, Binford CH, Utz JP, Kwon-Chung KJ: *Medical mycology,* ed 3, Philadelphia, 1977, Lea & Febiger.

Endo T: Pharmacokinetics of chemotherapeutants in fish and shellfish. In Michel C, Alderman DJ, editors: *Chemotherapy in aquaculture: from theory to reality,* Paris, 1992, Office International des Epizooties, pp. 404-427.

Endo T, Onozawa M: Effects of bath salinity and number of fish on the uptake of oxolinic acid by ayu, *Nippon Suisan Gakkaishi* 53:1493, 1987.

Esch GW, Hazen TC: Thermal ecology and stress: A case history for red-sore disease in largemouth bass. In Thorpe JH, Gibbons JW, editors: *Energy and environmental stress in aquatic systems,* Conf. 77114, United States Department of Energy Series, National Technical Information Service, Springfield, Va., 1978, pp. 331-363.

Esch GW, Hazen TC: *The ecology of Aeromonas hydrophila in Albemarle Sound, North Carolina,* University of North Carolina Water Resources Research Institute Final Report No. 80-153, 1980.

Esch GW, Hazen TC, Dimmock RV, Jr, Gibbons JW: Thermal effluent and the epizootiology of the ciliate *Epistylis* and the bacterium *Aeromonas* in association with centrarchid fish, *Trans Amer Micro Soc* 95:687-693, 1976.

European Inland Fisheries Advisory Committee (E.I.F.A.C.): Water quality criteria for European freshwater fish: extreme pH values and inland fisheries, *Water Res* 3:593-611, 1969.

Evans DL, Gratzek JB: Immune defense mechanisms in fish to protozoan and helminth infections, *Am Zool* 29:409-418, 1989.

Evans WA, Heckmann RA: The life history of *Sanguinicola klamathensis,* *Life Sci* 13:1285-1291, 1973.

Evelyn T: An improved growth medium for the kidney disease bacterium and some notes on the medium, *Bull Off Int Epizoot* 87:511-513, 1977.

Evelyn T, Ketcheson J, Prosperi-Porta L: Further evidence for the presence of *Renibacterium salmoninarum* in salmonid eggs and for the failure of povidone-iodine to reduce the intraovum infection rate in water-hardened eggs, *J Fish Dis* 7:173-182, 1984.

Evelyn TPT: Bacterial kidney disease-BKD. In Inglis V, Roberts RJ, Bromage NR, editors: *Bacterial diseases of fish,* New York, 1993, Halsted Press, pp. 177-195.

Evelyn TPT, Prosperi-Porta L, Ketcheson JE: Persistence of the kidney disease bacterium *Renibacterium salmoninarum,* in coho salmon, *Oncorhynchus kisutcm* (Walbaum) eggs during water-hardening with povidone-iodine, *J Fish Dis* 9:461-464, 1986.

Ewing MS, Kocan KM: *Ichthyophithirius multifiliis* (Ciliophora) development in gill epithelium, *J Protozool* 33:369-374, 1986.

Favero MS, Bond WW: Sterilization, disinfection and antisepsis in the hospital. In Balows A, editor: *Manual of clinical microbiology,* ed 5, Washington, DC, 1991, American Society for Microbiology, pp. 183-200.

Ferguson H: Water quality diseases. In *Fish diseases,* Sydney, Australia, 1988, Proceedings 106, The Post-Graduate Committee in Veterinary Science, University of Sydney, pp. 49-54.

Ferguson HW: *Systemic pathology of fish,* Ames, Iowa, 1989, Iowa State University Press, p. 263.

Ferguson HW, McCarthy DH: Histopathology of furunculosis in brown trout *Salmo trutta* L, *J Fish Dis* 1:165-174, 1978.

Ferguson HW, Moccia RD: Disseminated hexamitiasis in Siamese fighting fish, *J Am Vet Med Assn* 177:854-857, 1980.

Ferguson HW, Needham EA: Proliferative kidney disease in rainbow trout *Salmo gairdneri* Richardson, *J Fish Dis* 1:91-108, 1978.

Ferguson HW, Ostland VE, Byrne P, Lumsden JS: Experimental production of bacterial gill disease in trout by horizontal transmission and by bath challenge, *J Aquatic Animal Health* 3:118-123, 1991.

Ferguson HW, Roberts RJ: Myeloid leucosis associated with sporozoan infection in cultured turbot (*Scophthalmus maximus* L.), *J Comp Pathol* 85:317-326, 1975.

Ferguson HW, Rosendal S, Groom S: Gastritis in Lake Tanganyica cichlids, *Vet Record* 116:687-689, 1985.

Ferguson HW et al: Severe degenerative cardiomyopathy associated with pancreas disease in Atlantic salmon, *Salmo salar* L, *J Fish Dis* 20:95-98, 1986.

Ferguson HW et al: Cranial ulceration in Atlantic salmon *Salmo salar* associated with *Tetrahymena* sp, *Dis Aquat Org* 2:191-195, 1987.

Fickeisen DH, Schneider MH, Montgomery JC: A comparative evaluation of the Weiss saturometer, *Trans Am Fish Soc* 104:816-820, 1975.

Fijan N: The survival of *Chondrococcus columnaris* in waters of different quality, *Bull de l'Office Inter des Epizooties* 69:1159-1166, 1968.

Fijan N: Systemic mycosis in channel catfish, *Bull Wildlife Dis Assn* 5:109-110, 1969.

Fijan N: Infectious dropsy in carp: a disease complex, *Symp Zool Soc Lond* 30:39-51, 1972.

Finn JP, Nielson NO: The effect of temperature variation on the immune response of rainbow trout, *J Comp Pathol* 105:257-268, 1971.

Fletcher GL, Hoyle RJ, Horne DA: Yellow phosphorus pollution: Its toxicity to seawater-maintained brook trout (*Salvelinus fontinalis*) and smelt (*Osmerus mordax*), *J Fish Res Bd Can* 27:1379-1384, 1970.

Flores-Nava A, Vizcarra-Quiroz JJ: Acute toxicity of trichlorphon/(Dipterex) to fry of *Cichlasoma urophthalmus* Gunther, *Aquacult Fish Mgmt* 19:341-345, 1988.

Foissner W, Hoffmann GL, Mitchell AJ: *Heteropolaria colisarum* (Foissner & Schubert, 1977) (Protozoa: Epistylidae) of North American freshwater fishes, *J Fish Dis* 8:145-160, 1985.

Foott JS, Hedrick RP: Seasonal occurrence of the infectious stage of proliferative kidney disease (PKD) and resistance of rainbow trout *Salmo gairdneri* Richardson, to reinfection, *J Fish Biol* 30:477-483, 1987.

Forsythe JW, Hanlon RT, Bullis RA, Noga EJ: *Octopus bimaculoides*: a marine invertebrate host for ectoparasitic protozoans, *J Fish Dis* 14:431-442, 1991.

Fournie JW, Overstreet RM: True intermediate hosts for *Eimeria funduli* (Apicomplexa) from estuarine fishes, *J Protozool* 30:672-675, 1983.

Fouz BI et al: Characterization of *Vibrio damsela* strains isolated from turbot, *Scophthalmus maximus* in Spain, *Dis Aquat Org* 12:155-166, 1992.

Fouz B et al: *Vibrio damsela* strain virulence for fish and mammals, *Am Fish Soc Newsltr (Fish Health Section)* 20, No. 1:3, 1992.

Frakes T: Report on head and lateral line erosion, *SeaScope (Aquarium systems, Mentor, Oh.)* 5:1,3, 1988.

Frakes T, Hoff FH, Jr: Effect of high nitrate-N on the growth and survival of juvenile and larval anemonefish, *Amphiprion ocellaris,* *Aquacult* 29:155-158, 1982.

Francis-Floyd R: Behavioral diagnosis, *Vet Clin N Am, Sm Animal Prac 16,* pp. 303-314, 1988.

Francis-Floyd R: The veterinary approach to game fish. In Brown L, editor: *Aquaculture for veterinarians,* New York, 1993, Pergamon Press, pp. 395-408.

Francis-Floyd R, Beleau MH, Waterstrat PR, Bowser PR: Effect of water temperature on the clinical outcome of infection with *Edwardsiella ictaluri* in channel catfish, *JAVMA* 191:1413-1416, 1987.

Franklin RB, Elcombe CR, Vodicnik MJ, Lech JJ: Comparative aspects of the disposition and metabolism of xenobiotics in fish and mammals, *Fed Proc* 39:3144-3149, 1980.

Frantsi C, Savan M: Infectious pancreatic necrosis virus: temperature and age factors in mortality, *J Wildlife Dis* 7:249-255, 1971.

Fraser GC, RB Callinan, MC Calder: *Aphanomyces* species associated with red spot disease, an ulcerative disease of estuarine fish from eastern Australia, *J Fish Dis* 15:173-181, 1992.

Freeman RS: Ontogeny of cestodes and its bearing on their phylogeny and systematics, *Adv Parasit* 11:481-557, 1973.

Frerichs GN: Mycobacteriosis: nocardiosis. In Inglis V, Roberts RJ, Bromage NR, editors: *Bacterial diseases of fish,* New York, 1993, Halsted Press, pp. 219-234.

Frerichs GN, Millar SD, Roberts RJ: Ulcerative rhabdovirus in fish in southeast Asia, *Nature* 322:216, 1986.

Frerichs GN, Stewart JA, Collins RO: Atypical infection of rainbow trout *Salmo gairdneri* Richardson, with *Yersinia ruckeri,* *J Fish Dis* 8:383-387, 1985.

Fromm PO: A review of some physiological responses of freshwater fish to acid stress, *Environ Biol Fish* 5:79-93, 1980.

Fryer J, Sanders J: Bacterial kidney disease of salmonid fish, *Ann Rev Microbiol* 35:273-298, 1981.

Fryer JL et al: Vaccination for control of infectious diseases in Pacific salmon, *Fish Pathol* 10:155-164, 1976.

Fujihara Y, Kano T, Fukui H: Sulfisozole/trimethoprim as a chemotherapeutic agent for bacterial infections in yellowtail and eel, *Fish Pathol* 19:35-44, 1984.

Fujita S, Yoda M, Ugajin I: Control of an ectoparasitic copepod, *Caligus spinosus* Yamaguti, on the cultured adult yellowtail, *Fish Pathol* 2:122-127, 1968.

Fukuda Y, Kusuda R: Efficacy of vaccination for pseudotuberculosis in cultured yellowtail by various routes of administration, *Bull Japan Soc Sci Fish* 47:147-150, 1981.

Fuller MS, Jaworski A: *Zoosporic fungi in teaching and research,* Athens, Ga., 1987, Southeastern Publishing, 303 pp.

Gaines JL, Jr, Rogers WA: Fish mortalities associated with *Goezia* sp. (Nematoda: Ascaroides) in central Florida, *Proc Ann Conf SE Assoc Game Fish Comm* 25:496-497, 1971.

Galla JF, Hartmann JX: Extension of the host range of channel catfish virus to the walking catfish (*Clarias batrachus* L.), *Fla Sci* 37(suppl 1):1974.

Gaskins JE, Cheung PJ: *Exophiala pisciphila*: a study of its development, *Mycopathologica* 93:173-184, 1986.

Gelev I et al: Identification of the bacterium associated with haemorrhagic septicemia in rainbow trout as *Hafnia alvei,* *Res Microbiol (Institut Pasteur)* 141:573-576, 1990.

Geus A: Nachtragliche Bemerkungen 24r Biologie des Fischpathogenen Dinoflagellater *Oodinium pillularis* Schaperclaus, *Aquarien Terrarien Zoologica* 13:305-306, 1960.

Ghittino P: Nutrition and fish disease. In Halver JE, editor: *Fish nutrition,* ed 2, New York, 1989, Academic Press, pp. 681-713.

Ghittino P, Smith FG, Glenn JS: A case report of Myxosporidia (*Myxidium giardi*) in the dermis of an American eel, *Riv It Piscic Ittiopath* 9:13-17, 1974.

Gilbert JP, Gratzek JB, Brown J: An *in vitro* method for testing the synergistic action of parasiticides using malachite green and formalin as a model system, *J Fish Dis* 2:191-196, 1979.

Gilbertson M: The Niagara labyrinth: the human ecology of producing organochlorine chemicals, *Can J Fish Aquatic Sci* 42:1681-1692, 1985.

Gillespie RB, Baumann PC: Effects of high tissue concentrations of selenium on reproduction by bluegills, *Trans Am Fish Soc* 115:208-213, 1986.

Gilmartin WG, Camp BJ, Lewis DH: Bath treatment of channel catfish with three broad-spectrum antibiotics, *J Wildlife Dis* 12:555-559, 1976.

Giroud JP: Incidents et accidents des antibiotiques. In Michel C, Alderman DJ, editors: *Chemotherapy in aquaculture: from theory to reality,* Paris, 1992, Office International des Epizooties, pp. 141-151.

Glazebrook JS, Heasmann MP, de Beer SM: *Picorna*-like viral particles associated with mass mortalities in larval barramundi, *Lates calcarifer* Bloch, *J Fish Dis* 12:245-249, 1990.

Glaser CA, Angulo FJ, Rooney JA: Animal associated opportunistic infections among persons infected with the human immunodeficiency virus, *Clin Infect Dis* 18:14-24, 1994.

Goede RW, Barton BA: Organismic indices and an autopsy-based assessment as indicators of health and condition of fish, *Am Fish Soc Sym* 8:93-108, 1990.

Goven BA, Gilbert JP, Gratzek JB: Apparent drug resistance to the organophosphate dimethyl (2,2,2-trichloro-1-hydroxyethyl) phosphonate by monogenetic trematodes, *J Wildlife Dis* 16:343-346, 1980.

Grant A: Basic husbandry on fish farms. In Brown L, editor: *Aquaculture for veterinarians,* New York, 1993, Pergamon Press, pp. 31-42.

Gratzek JB: Parasites associated with ornamental fish, *Vet Clin North Am (Small Animal Practice)* 18:375-399, 1988.

Gratzek JB, Blasiola G: Checklists, quarantine procedures, and calculations of particular use in fish health management. In Gratzek JB, Matthews JR, editors: *Aquariology: the science of fish health management,* Morris Plains, N.J., 1992, Tetra Press, pp. 301-315.

Gratzek JB, Shotts EB, Jr, Dawe DL: Infectious diseases and parasites of freshwater ornamental fish. In Gratzek JB, Matthews JR, editors: *Aquariology: the science of fish health management,* Morris Plains, N.J., 1992, Tetra Press, pp. 227-274.

Grier H, Quintero I: *A microscopic study of ulcerated fish in Florida,* Florida Bureau of Marine Research Report WM-164, 1987.

Grimes DJ, Gruber SH, May EB: Experimental infection of lemon sharks, *Negaprion brevirostris* (Poey), with *Vibrio* species, *J Fish Dis* 8:173-180, 1985.

Grischkowsky R, Amend DF: Infectious hematopoietic necrosis virus: prevalence in certain Alaskan sockeye salmon, *Oncorhynchus nerka, J Fish Res Bd Can* 33:186-188, 1976.

Grizzle JM: Effects of hypolimnetic discharge on fish health below a reservoir, *Trans Am Fish Soc* 110:29-43, 1981.

Grizzle JM, Maudlin AC, II, Young D, Henderson E: Survival of juvenile striped bass (*Morone saxatilis*) and Morone hybrid bass (*Morone chrysops* x *Morone saxatilis*) increased by addition of calcium to soft water, *Aquacult* 46:167-171, 1985.

Grizzle JM, Mauldin AC, II, Young D, Henderson E: Effects of environmental calcium on postharvest survival of juvenile striped bass, *J Aquatic Animal Health* 2:104-108, 1990.

Grizzle JM, Schwedler TE, Scott AL: Papillomas of black bullheads, *Ictaluras melas* (Rafinesque), living in a chlorinated sewage pond, *J Fish Dis* 4:345-351, 1981.

Groff JM, McDowell T, Hedrick RP: Sphaerospores observed in the kidney of channel catfish (*Ictalurus punctatus*), *Fish Health Sect Am Fish Soc Newsltr* 17(1):5, 1989.

Gutierrez M, Crespo JP, Arias A: Particulas virus-like en un tumor en boca de dorado *Sparus aurata* L. (virus-like particles in a mouth tumor of gilthead sea bream, *Sparus aurata* L.), *Invest Pesq* 41:331-336, 1977.

Hacking MA, Budd J: *Vibrio* infection in tropical fish in a freshwater aquarium, *J Wildlife Dis* 7:273-280, 1971.

Haines TA: Acid precipitation and its consequences for aquatic ecosystems: a review, *Trans Am Fish Soc* 110:669-707, 1981.

Hall JD: *An ecological study of the chestnut lamprey, Ichthyomyzon castaneus Girard, in the Manistee River, Michigan* (Ph.D. diss., University of Michigan, Ann Arbor, 1963), 106 pp.

Halliday MM: Studies of *Myxosoma cerebralis:* a parasite of salmonids. II. The development and pathology of *Myxosoma cerebralis* in experimentally infected rainbow trout (*Salmo gairdneri*) fry reared at different water temperatures, *Nord Veterinaermed* 25:349-358, 1973.

Hansell DA, Boyd CE: Uses of hydrated lime in fish ponds, *Proc Ann Conf SE Assn Fish Wildlife Agen* 34:49-58, 1980.

Hansen GH, Raa JK, Olafsen JA: Isolation of *Enterobacter agglomerans* from dolphin fish, *Coryphaena hippurus* L, *J Fish Dis* 13:93-96, 1990.

Hanson LA, Grizzle JM: Nitrite-induced predisposition of channel catfish to bacterial diseases, *Prog Fish-cult* 47:98-101, 1985.

Hargis WJ, Thoney DA: *Bibliography of the Monogenea,* Gloucester Point, Va., 1983, Virginia Institute of Marine Sciences.

Harrell LW, Elston RA, Scott TM, Wilkinson MT: A significant new systemic disease of net-pen reared chinook salmon *Oncorhynchus tshawytscha* brood stock, *Aquacult* 55:249-262, 1986.

Harshbarger JC: Pseudoneoplasms in ectothermic animals. In Hoover KL, editor: *Use of small fish in carcinogenicity testing, National Cancer Institute Monograph* 65: 251-273, 1984.

Harshbarger JC, Clark JB: Epizootiology of neoplasms in bony fish from North America, *Sci Total Environ* 94:1-32, 1990.

Harshbarger JC, Spero PM, Wolcott NM: Neoplasms in wild fish from the marine ecosystem emphasizing environmental interactions. In Couch J, Fournie J, editors: *Pathobiology of marine and estuarine organisms,* Boca Raton, Fla., 1993, CRC Press, pp. 157-176,

Hart JS: The circulation and respiratory tolerance of some Florida freshwater fishes, *Proc Fla Acad Sci* 7:221-246, 1944.

Hastein T, Bergsjo T: The salmon lice *Lepeophtheirus salmonis* as the cause of disease in farmed salmonids, *Rivista Italiana Pisciolura e Ittiopatalogia* 11:3-5, 1976.

Hastein T, Bullock GL: An acute septicaemic disease of brown trout (*Salmo trutta*) and Atlantic salmon (*Salmo salar*) caused by a *Pasteurella*-like organism, *J Fish Biol* 8:23-26, 1976.

Hatai K: Fungal pathogens/parasites of aquatic animals. In Austin B, Austin DA, editors: *Methods for the microbiological examination of fish and shellfish,* New York, 1989, John Wiley & Sons, pp. 240-272.

Hatai K, Egusa S: *Candida sake* from the gastro-tympanites of amago, *Oncorhynchus rhodurus, Bull Japanese Soc Sci Fish* 41:993, 1975.

Hatai K, Fujimaki Y, Egusa S, Jo Y: A visceral mycosis in ayu fry, *Plecoglossus altivelis* Temminck & Schlegel, caused by a new species of *Phoma, J Fish Dis* 9:111-116, 1986a.

Hatai K, Kubota SS: A visceral mycosis in cultured masou salmon (*Oncorhynchus masou*) caused by a species of *Ochroconis, J Wildlife Dis* 25:83-88, 1989.

Hatai K, Kubota SS, Kida N, Udagawa S-I: *Fusarium oxysporum* in Red Sea bream *Pagrus* sp, *J Wildlife Dis* 22:570-571, 1986b.

Hatai K, Takahashi S, Egusa S: Studies on the pathogenic fungus of mycotic granulomatosis-IV: Changes of blood constituents in both ayu, *Plecoglossus altivelis* experimentally inoculated and naturally infected with *Aphanomyces piscicida,* *Fish Pathol* 19:17-23, 1984.

Hauck AK: Gas bubble disease due to helicopter transport of young pink salmon, *Trans Am Fish Soc* 115:630-635, 1986.

Hawke JP, Plakas SM, Minton RV, McPherson RM, Snider TG, Guarino AM: Fish pasteurellosis of cultured striped bass (*Morone saxatilis*) in coastal Alabama, *Aquacult* 65:193-204, 1987.

Hawke JP, Thune RL: Systemic isolation and antimicrobial susceptibility of *Cytophaga columnaris* from commercially reared channel catfish, *J Aquatic Animal Health* 4:109-113, 1992.

Hayes MA, Ferguson HW: Neoplasia in teleosts. In HW Ferguson, editor: *Systemic pathology of fish: a text and atlas of comparative tissue responses in diseases of teleosts*, Ames, Iowa, 1989, Iowa State University, pp. 230-247, 1989.

Hazen TC, Fliermans RP, Hirsch RP, Esch GW: Prevalence and distribution of *Aeromonas hydrophila* in the United States, *Appl Envir Micro* 36:731-738, 1978.

Hecht T, Pienaar AG: A review of cannibalism and its implications in fish larviculture, *J World Maricult Soc* 24:246-261, 1993.

Heckmann R: Ivermectin efficacy trials for nematodes parasitic to fish, *Am Fish Soc Fish Health Sec Newsltr* 13(1):6, 1985.

Hedrick RP, Yun S, Wingfield WH: A small RNA virus isolated from salmonid fishes in California, *Can J Fish Aquatic Sci* 48:99-104, 1991.

Hedrick RP et al: Oral administration of Fumagilin DCH protects chinook salmon *Oncorhynchus tschawytscha* from experimentally induced proliferative kidney disease, *Dis Aquatic Org* 4:165-168, 1988.

Hedrick RP, Groff JM, McDowell TS: Hematopoietic intranuclear microspordian infections with features of leukemia in chinook salmon (*Oncorhynchus tschawytscha*), *Dis Aquatic Org* 8:189-197, 1990a.

Hedrick RP et al: Proliferative kidney disease (PKD) among salmonid fish in California USA: a second look, *Bull Eur Assn Fish Pathol* 5:36-38, 1985a.

Hedrick RP, Kent ML. Smith CE: *Proliferative kidney disease in salmonid fishes*, Washington, DC, 1986, U.S.F.W.S. Fish disease Leaflet 74.

Hedrick RP, MacConnell E, DeKinkelin P: Proliferative kidney disease of salmonid fish, *Ann Rev Fish Dis* 3:277-290, 1993.

Hedrick RP, McDowell T, Groff J: Mycobacteriosis from cultured striped bass from California, *J Wildlife Dis* 23:391-395, 1987a.

Hedrick RP, McDowell T, Groff JM, Kent ML: Another erythrocytic virus from salmonid fish? *Am Fish Soc Fish Health Sec Newsltr* 15(2):2, 1987b.

Hedrick RP, McDowell T, Groff JM: *Sphaerospora ictaluri* n. sp. (Myxodsporea: Sphaerosporidae) observed in the kidney of channel catfish, *Ictalurus punctatus* Rafinesque, *J Protozool* 37:107-112, 1990b.

Hedrick RP, Speas J, Kent ML, McDowell T: Adenovirus-like particles associated with a disease of cultured white sturgeon *Acipenser transmontanus*, *Can J Fish Aquatic Sci* 42:1321-1325, 1985b.

Heggberget TG: Effect of supersaturated water on fish in the River Nidelva, southern Norway, *J Fish Biol* 24:65-74, 1984.

Hellawell JM: *Biological indicators of freshwater pollution and environmental management*, New York, 1986, Elsevier.

Helms D: Use of formalin for selective control of tadpoles in the presence of fishes, *Prog Fish-cult* 29:43-47, 1967.

Hemdal J: Marine angelfish: color and style, *Aquar Fish Mag* 8:15-20, 1989.

Henley MW, Lewis DH: Anerobic bacteria associated with mortality in grey mullet (*Mugil cephalus*) and red fish (*Sciaenops ocellata*) along the Texas Gulf Coast, *J Wildlife Dis* 12:448-453, 1976.

Heo GJ, Kasai K, Wakabayashi H: Occurrence of *Flavobacterium branchophila* associated with bacterial gill disease at a trout hatchery, *Fish Pathol* 25:21-7, 1990.

Hepher B: *Nutrition of pond fishes*, New York, 1988, Cambridge University Press, p. 388.

Herman RL: Fish furunculosis 1952 to 1966, *Trans Am Fish Soc* 97:221-230, 1968.

Herman RL, Bullock GL: Pathology caused by *Edwardsiella tarda* in striped bass, *Trans Am Fish Soc* 115:232-235, 1986.

Herman RL, Meade JW: Gill lamellar dilatations (telangiectasis) related to sampling techniques, *Trans Am Fish Soc* 114:911-913, 1985.

Herman RL, Wolf K: *Epitheliocystis infection of fishes*, Washington, DC, 1987, Fish Disease Leaflet #75, United States Department of Interior Fish and Wildlife Service, Division of Fisheries and Wetlands Research, 4 pp.

Herwig N: *Handbook of drugs and chemicals used in the treatment of fish diseases*, Springfield, Ill., 1979, CC Thomas, 272 pp.

Hetrick FM, Knittel MD. Fryer JL: Increased susceptibility of rainbow trout to infectious hematopoietic necrosis virus after exposure to copper, *Appl Environ Microbiol* 37:198-201, 1979.

Hicks BD, Geraci JR: A histological assessment of damage in rainbow trout, *Salmo gairdneri* Richardson, fed rations containing erythromycin, *J Fish Dis* 7:457-465, 1984.

Hill DM: Fish kill investigation procedures. In Nielsen LA, Johnson DL, editors: *Fisheries techniques*, Bethesda, Md., 1983, American Fisheries Society, pp. 261-274.

Hilton LR, Wilson JL: Terramycin-resistant *Edwardsiella tarda* isolated from an epizootic among channel catfish, *Prog Fish-cult* 42:159, 1980.

Hine M: Fish mortalities: cause and effect. In Tierney LD, Akroyd JM, Kilner AR, editors: *Investigating fish kills,* ed 2, Wellington, New Zealand, 1982, Fisheries Management Division, New Zealand Ministry of Agriculture and Fisheries,

Hine PM: *Eimeria anguillae* Leger and Hollande, 1922 parasitic in New Zealand eels, *NZ J Mar Freshwater Res* 9:239-243, 1975.

Hirose H, Sekino T, Egusa S: Note on the egg deposition, larval migration and intermediate hosts of the nematode *Anguillicola crassa* parasitic in the swim bladder of eels, *Fish Pathol* 11:27-31, 1976.

Hiu SF et al: *Lactobacillus piscicola*, a new species from salmonid fish, *Int J Sys Bacteriol* 34:393-400, 1984.

Hjeltnes B, Roberts RJ: Vibriosis. In Inglis V, Roberts RJ, Bromage NR, editors: *Bacterial diseases of fish*, New York, 1993, Halsted Press, pp. 109-121.

Hodson PV, Blunt BR, Whittle DM: Monitoring lead exposure in fish. In Cairns VW, Hodson PV, Nriagu JO, editors: *Contaminant effects on fisheries*, New York, 1984, John Wiley, pp. 87-98.

Hoffman GL: *Parasites of North American freshwater fishes*, Berkeley, 1967, University of California Press.

Hoffman GL: *Annual report, Eastern Fish Disease Laboratory*, Washington, DC, 1972, FR, Bureau of Sport Fish and Wildlife, United States Department of the Interior, 20 pp.

Hoffman GL: Disinfection of contaminated water by ultraviolet irradiation, with emphasis on whirling disease (*Myxosoma cerebralis*) and its effect on fish, *Trans Am Fish Soc* 103:541-550, 1974.

Hoffman GL: *Whirling disease of trout*, Washington, DC, 1976, United States Fish and Wildlife Service, Fish disease leaflet No. 47.

Hoffman GL: Ciliates of freshwater fishes. In Kreier JP, editor: *Parasitic protozoa*, vol 2, New York, 1978, Academic Press, pp. 583-632,

Hoffman GL: Asian tapeworm, *Bothriocephalus acheilognathi*, Yamaguti 1934, in North America, *Fisch und Umvelt* 8:69-75, 1980.

Hoffman GL: Two fish pathogens, *Parvicapsula* sp. and *Mitraspora cyprini* (Myxosporea) new to North America. In Olah J, Molnar K, Jeney Z, editors: *Fish pathogens and environment in European polyculture*, Szarvas, Hungary, 1981, Proceedings International Seminar, Fisheries Research Institution, pp. 184-197.

Hoffman GL: Asian tapeworm *Bothriocephalus acheilognathi*, prevention and control, Stuttgart, Arkansas, 1983, United States Fish and Wildlife Service Leaflet.

Hoffman GL: Anchor parasite (*Lernaea cyprinacea*) control (Fish Health Section), *Am Fish Soc Newsltr* 13(4):4, 1985.

Hoffman GL, Dunbar CE, Brandford A: *Whirling disease of trouts caused by Myxosoma cerebralis in the United States, 1962*, United States Department of Interior Fish and Wildlife Service Special Science Report No. 427.

Hoffman GL, Dunbar CE, Wolf K, Zwillenberg LO: Epitheliocystis, new infectious disease of bluegill (*Lepomis macrochirus*), *Antonie van Leeuwenhoek J Microbiol Serol* 35:146-156, 1969.

Hoffman GL et al: A disease of freshwater fishes caused by *Tetrahymena corlissi* Thompson, 1955, and a key for identification of holtrich ciliates of freshwater fishes, *J Parasitol* 61:217-233, 1975.

Hoffman GL, Hoffman GL Jr: Studies on the control of whirling disease (*Myxosoma cerebralis*). I. The effect of chemicals on spores in vitro, and of calcium oxide as a disinfectant in simulated ponds, *J Wildlife Dis* 8:49-53, 1972.

Hoffman GL, Meyer FP: *Parasites of freshwater fishes,* Neptune City, N.J., 1974, TFH Publications, 224 pp.

Hoffmann GL, Prescott GW, Thompson CB: *Chlorella* parasitic in bluegills, *Prog Fish-cult* 27:175, 1965.

Hoffman GL, Putz RE: Host susceptibility and the effect of aging, freezing, heat, and chemicals on the spores of *Myxosoma cerebralis,* *Prog Fish-cult* 31:35-37, 1969.

Hoffmaster JL et al: Geographic distribution of the myxosporean parasite *Ceratomyxa shasta* Noble 1950, in the Columbia River Basin, *J Fish Dis* 11:97-100, 1985.

Hogans WE, Trudeau DJ: *Caligus elongatus* (Copepoda: Caligoida) from Atlantic salmon (*Salmo salar*) cultured in marine waters of the Lower Bay of Fundy, *Can J Zool* 67:1080-1082, 1989a.

Hogans WE, Trudeau DJ: *Preliminary studies on the biology of sea-lice: Caligus elongatus and Lepeophtheirus salmonis (Copepoda: Caligoida) parasitic on cage-cultured salmonids in the Lower Bay of Fundy,* 1989b, Canadian Technical Report of Fisheries and Aquatic Sciences, No. 1715.

Hojgaard M: Experiences made in Danmarks Akvarium concerning the treatment of *Oodinium ocellatum, Bull l'Institut Oceanographique (Monaco) Numero Spec* 1A:77-79, 1962.

Hollerman WD, Boyd CE: Nightly aeration to increase production of channel catfish, *Trans Am Fish Soc* 109:446-452, 1980.

Holt RA, Piacentini S: *Erythrocytic inclusion body syndrome: (summary report prepared for the Pacific Northwest Fish Health Protection committee),* Corvallis, Ore., 1989, Oregon Deptartment of Fish and Wildlife, Oregon State University.

Holt RA, Rohovec, Fryer JL: Bacterial cold-water disease. In Inglis V, Roberts RJ, Bromage NR, editors: *Bacterial diseases of fish,* New York, 1993, Halsted Press, pp. 3-22.

Hoover DM et al: Enteric cryptosporidiosis in a naso tang, *Naso lituratus* Bloch and Schneider, *J Fish Dis* 4:425-428, 1981.

Hoover KL: Hyperplastic thyroid lesions in fish, *Nat Cancer Inst Monogr* 65:275-289, 1984.

Horlyck JV, Jensen NJ: Electro-induced scoliosis or fracture of the vertebral column in rainbow trout, *Salmo gairdneri* Richardson, 1836, *Bull Eur Assn Fish Pathol* 5:1-2, 1985.

Horsberg TE et al: Diklorvos som avlusningmiddel for fisk. Klinsk utproovning og toksisitetstesting. (Dichlorvos as a fish delousing agent. Clinical trials and toxicity testing), *Norsk Veterinaertidsskrift* 99:611-615, 1987 (In Norwegian).

Horter R: *Fusarium* als Erreger einer Hautmykose bei Karpfen, *Zentralblatt fur Parasitenkunde* 20:355-358, 1960.

Hoshina T: Notes on some myxosporidian parasites on fishes of Japan, *J Tokyo Univ Fish* 39:69-89, 1952.

Houston AH: Blood and circulation. In Schreck CB, Moyle PB, editors: *Methods in fish biology,* Bethesda, Md., 1990, American Fisheries Society, pp. 273-334.

Howe GE, Bills TD, Marking LL: Removal of benzocaine from waters by filtration with activated carbon, *Prog Fish-cult* 52:32-35, 1990.

Hoy T, Horsberg TE: *Chemotherapy of sea lice infestations in salmonids: pharmacological, toxicologic and therapeutic properties of established and potential agents* (Ph.D. diss., Norwegian College of Veterinary Medicine, Oslo, 1991).

Hoy T, Horsberg TE, Wichstroem R: Inhibition of acetylcholinesterase in rainbow trout following dichlorvos treatment at different dissolved oxygen levels. In Michel C, Alderman DJ, editors: *Chemotherapy in aquaculture: from theory to reality,* Paris, 1992, Office International des Epizooties, pp. 206-218.

Hsu Y-L, Chen B-s, Wu J-L: Characteristics of a new reo-like virus isolated from landlocked salmon (*Oncorhynchus masou* Brevoort), *Fish Pathol* 24:37-45, 1989.

Huff JA, Burns CD: Hypersaline and chemical control of *Cryptocaryon irritans* irritans in red snapper, *Lutjanus campechanus,* monoculture, *Aquacult* 222:181-184, 1981.

Hughes GC: Seasonal periodicity of the Saprolegniaceae in the Southeastern United States, *Trans Brit Mycol Soc* 45:519-531, 1962.

Huizinga HW, Esch GW. Hazen TC: Histopathology of red-sore disease (*Aeromonas hydrophila*) in naturally and experimentally infected largemouth bass *Micropterus salmoides* (Lacepede), *J Fish Dis* 2:263-277, 1979.

Hunn J, Godbout R, Arnold CR: Effects of temperature and salinity on egg hatching and larval survival of red drum, *Scienops ocellata,* *NOAA Fish Bull* 79:569-573, 1981.

Hunter VA, Knittel MD, Fryer JL: Stress-induced transmission of *Yersinia ruckeri* infection from carriers to recipient steelhead trout, *Salmo gairdneri* Richardson, *J Fish Dis* 3:467-472, 1980.

Iida Y, Masumura K, Nakai T, Sorimachi M, Matsuda H: A viral disease in larvae and juveniles of the Japanese flounder *Paralichthys olivaceus, J Aquatic Animal Health* 1:7-12, 1989.

Isom BG: Outbreaks of columnaris in Center Hill and Old Hickory Reservoirs, Tennessee, *Prog Fish-cult* 22:43-45, 1960.

Iwata K: Fungal toxins as a parasitic factor responsible for the establishment of fungal infections, *Mycopathol* 65:141-154, 1978.

Izawa K: *Life history of Caligus spinosus Yamaguti, 1939, obtained from cultured yellowtail. Seriola quinqeradiata T. & S (Crustacea: Caligoida),* Reports of the Faculty of Fisheries Prefectural University Mie Tsu 6:127-157, 1969.

Jacobs DL: A new parasitic dinoflagellate from freshwater fish, *Trans Am Microscop Soc* 65:1-17, 1946.

Jacobsen F, Berglind L: Persistence of tetracycline in sediments from fish farms, *Aquacult* 70:375-380, 1988.

Jacobsen MD: Withdrawal times of freshwater rainbow trout, *Salmo gairdneri,* Richardson, after treatment with oxolinic acid, oxytetracycline and trimethoprim, *J Fish Dis* 12:29-36, 1989.

James MO: Overview of in vitro metabolism of drugs by aquatic species, *Vet Human Toxicol* 28(suppl 1):2-8, 1986.

Jeffree RA, Williams NJ: Biological indications of pollution of the Finniss River syatem, especially fish diversity and abundance. In Davie DR, editor: *Rum jungle environmental studies,* Chapter 7, Australian Atomic Energy Commission, Report No. E365, 1975.

Jensen J, Durborow R: *Tables for applying common fish pond chemicals,* Circular ANR-414, Alabama Cooperation Extension Service, Auburn University, Ala., 1984, p. 11.

Jensen NJ, Bloch B: Adenovirus-like particles associated with epidermal hyperplasia in cod (*Gadus morhua*), *Nord Veterinaermed* 32:173-175, 1980.

Johannessen A. 1974. Oppdrett av laksefisk i Norske kystfarvann. Lakselus. Fisken og havet, Ser. B 2: 21-31.

Johnsen BO, Jensen AJ: Infestations of Atlantic salmon, *Salmo salar* by *Gyrodactylus salaris* in Norwegian rivers, *J Fish Biol* 29:233-241, 1986.

Johnson EL: The insidious threat of stray voltage, *Trop Fish Hobbyist* 6:96, 98, 1993.

Johnson KA, Sanders JE, Fryer JL: *Ceratomyxa shasta in salmonids,* Fish Disease Leaflet 58, Washington, DC, 1979, U.S. Dept. of Interior, Fish and Wildlife Service, 11 pp.

Johnson M: The veterinary approach to channel catfish. In L Brown, editor: *Aquaculture for veterinarians,* New York, 1993, Pergamon Press, pp. 249-270.

Johnson SC, Albright LC: Development, growth, and survival of *Lepeophtheirus salmonis* (Copepoda: Caligidae) under laboratory conditions, *J Marine Biol Assoc UK* 71:245-246, 1991a.

Johnson SC, Albright LC: *Lepeophtheirus cuneifer* Kabata: 1974 (Copepoda: Caligidae) from seawater-reared rainbow trout, *Oncorhynchus mykiss* and Atlantic salmon, *Salmo salar*, in the Strait of Georgia, British Columbia, Canada, *Can J Zool* 69:1414-1416, 1991b.

Johnson SK: *Tet disease of tropical fishes and an evaluation of correction techniques*, College Station, 1978, Texas A & M University, Fish Disease Diagnosis Laboratory F12, 7 pp.

Johnson WW, Finley MT: *Handbook of acute toxicity of chemicals to fish and aquatic invertebrates*, Resource Publication, US Department of Interior Fish and Wildlife Service, 137:1-98, 1980.

Johnston TH, Bancroft MJ: The freshwater fish epidemics in Queensland rivers, *Proc Royal Soc Qld* 33:174-210, 1921.

Johnstone AK: *Pathogenesis and life cycle of the myxozoan Parvicapsula sp. infecting marine cultured coho salmon* (Ph.D. diss., University of Washington, 1985), 70 pp.

Jones JB: A redescription of *Caligus patulus* Wilson, 1937 (Copepoda: Caligidae) from a fish farm in the Philippines, *Systematic Parasitol* 2:103-106, 1980.

Jones JB: New Zealand parasitic copepoda; genus *Caligus Muller*, 1985 (Siphonostomatoida: Caligidae), *NZ J Zool* 15:397-413, 1988.

Jones KA, Brown SB, Hara TJ: Behavioral and biochemical studies of onset and recovery from acid stress in arctic char (*Salvelinus alpinus*), *Can J Fish Aquatic Sci* 44:373-381, 1987.

Jorgensen T et al: *Vibrio salmonicida*, a pathogen in salmonids, also causes mortality in net-pen captured cod (*Gadus morhua*), *Bull Eur Assoc Fish Pathol* 9:42-44, 1989.

Joyon L, Lom J: Etude cytologique, systematique et pathologique d'*Ichthyobodo necator* (Henneguy, 1883) Pinto, 1928 (Zooflagelle), *J Protozool* 16:703-719, 1969.

Kabasawa H, Yamada M: The effects of copper sulfate ($CuSO_4$·$5H_2O$) and neguvon on the function of filtering bacteria in a closed circulating seawater system, *Reports Keikyu Aburatsubo Mar, Park Aquarium* 1972:18-22 (In Japanese).

Kabata Z: Incidence of coccidioses in Scottish herring (*Clupea harengus* L.), *J Cons Int Explor Mer* 28:201-210, 1963.

Kabata Z: Parasitic Copepoda of the British fishes, *Ray Soc (London)* 152:1-468, 1979.

Kabata Z: Copepoda (Crustacea) parasitic on fishes: problems and perspectives, *Adv Parasitol* 19:1-71, 1981.

Kabata Z: Diseases caused by metazoans: crustaceans. In *Diseases of marine animals*, vol 4. Part 1. Introduction, Kinne O, editor: Hamburg, FRG, 1984, Biologische Anstalt Helgoland, pp. 321-399.

Kabata Z: *Parasites and diseases of cultured fish in the tropics*, London, 1985, Taylor & Francis.

Kabata Z: Copepoda and Branchiura. In Margolis L, Kabata Z, editors: *Guide to the parasites of fishes of Canada*. Part II. *Crustacea*, Canadian Special Publication, Fisheries Aquatic Science, No.101, 1988, pp 3-27.

Kaige N, Miyazaki T: A histopathological study of white spot disease in Japanese flounder, *Fish Pathol* 20:61-64, 1985.

Kanazawa A: Nutruitional mechanisms involved in the occurrence of abnormal pigmentation in hatchery-reared flatfish, *J World Maricul Soc* 24:162-166, 1993.

Kaper JB, Lockman H, Colwell RR: *Aeromonas hydrophila*: ecology and toxigenicity of isolates from an estuary, *J Appl Bact* 50:359-377, 1981.

Kawakami K, Kusuda R: Efficacy of rifampicin, streptomycin and erythromycin against experimental *Mycobacterium* infection in cultured yellowtail, *Nippon suisan Gakkaishi* 56:51-53, 1990.

Kearn GC: The eggs of monogeneans, *Adv Parasitol* 25:175-273, 1986.

Keith RE: Loss of therapeutic copper in closed marine systems, *Aquacult* 24:355-362, 1981.

Keith RE: Post-therapy removal of copper medications from seawater systems by chemical filtrants, *J Aquariculture Aquatic Sci* 3(1):1-5, 1982.

Kent ML: The life cycle and treatment of a turbellarian disease of marine fish, *Freshwater Mar Aquar Mag* 4:11-13, 1981.

Kent ML: Net-pen liver disease (NLD) of salmonid fishes reared in seawater: species susceptibility, recovery, and probable cause, *Dis Aquatic Org* 8:21-28, 1990.

Kent ML: *Diseases of seawater netpen-reared salmonid fishes in the Pacific Northwest*, Canadian Special Publication Fisheries Aquatic Science, 1992, pp. 76, 116.

Kent ML, Dungan CF, Elston RA, Holt RA: *Cytophaga* sp. (Cytophagales) infection in seawater pen-reared Atlantic salmon *Salmo salar*, *Dis Aquatic Org* 4:173-179, 1988a.

Kent ML et al: Spiral swimming behavior due to cranial and vertebral lesions associated with *Cytophaga psychrophila* infections in salmonid fishes, *Dis Aquatic Org* 6:11-16, 1989.

Kent ML, Hedrick RP: PKX, the causative agent of proliferative kidney disease (PKD) in Pacific salmonid fishes and its affinities with Myxozoa, *J Protozool* 32:254-260, 1985.

Kent ML, Hedrick RP: Development of the PKX myxosporean in rainbow trout *Salmo gairdneri*, *Dis Aquatic Org* 1:169-182, 1986.

Kent ML, Lyons JM: *Edwardsiella ictaluri* in the green knife fish, *Eigenmania virescens*, *Fish Health News* (U.S. Fish and Wildlife Service) 11(1-2):ii, 1982.

Kent ML, Margolis L, Fournie JW: A new eye disease in pen-reared chinook caused by metacestodes of *Gilquinia squali* (Trypanorhyncha), *J Aquatic Animal Health* 3:134-140, 1991.

Kent ML, Olson AC, Jr: Interrelationships of a parasitic turbellarian (*Paravortex* sp.)(Graffillidae, Rhabdocoela) and its marine fish hosts, *Fish Pathol* 21:65-72, 1986.

Kent ML, Sawyer TK, Hedrick RP: *Paramoeba pemaquidensis* (Sarcomastigophora: Paramoebidae) infestation of the gills of coho salmon *Oncorhynchus mykiss* reared in seawater, *Dis Aquatic Org* 5:163-169, 1988b.

Khan RA: Pathogenesis of *Trypanoplasma murmanensis* in marine fish of the northwesterrn Atlantic following experimental transmission, *Can J Zool* 63:2141-2164, 1985.

Khan RA: Developmental stages of *Haemogregarina delagei* Laveran and Mesnil in an elasmobranch, *Raja radiata* Donovan, *Can J Zool* 50:906-907, 1972.

Khan RA, Nag K: Estimation of hemosiderosis in seabirds and fish exposed to petroleum, *Bull Environ Contam Toxicol* 50:125-131, 1993.

Kimura T, Yoshimizu M, Tanaka M: Studies on a new virus (OMV) from *Oncorhynchus masou*. Part I. Characteristics and pathogenicity, *Fish Pathol* 15:143-147, 1981.

Kimura T, Yoshimizu M: Viral diseases of fish in Japan, *Ann Rev Fish Dis* 1:67-82, 1991.

King CH, Shotts EB: Enhancement of *Edwardsiella tarda* and *Aeromonas salmonicida* through ingestion by the ciliated protozoan *Tetrahymena pyriformis*, *FEMS Microbiol Ltrs* 51:85-89, 1988.

Kingsford E: *Treatment of exotic marine fish diseases*, St. Petersburg, Fla., 1975, Palmetto Publishing, 90 pp.

Kinne O, editor: *Diseases of marine animals*, vol IV, Part 1 (Diseases of Pisces), Hamburg, Germany, 1984, Biologische Anstalt Helgoland. 541 pp.

Kitao T: Pasteurellosis. In Inglis V, Roberts RJ, Bromage NR, editors: *Bacterial diseases of fish*, New York, 1993a, Halsted Press, pp. 159-166.

Kitao T: Streptococcal infections. In Inglis V, Roberts RJ, Bromage NR, editors: *Bacterial diseases of fish*, New York, 1993b, Halsted Press, pp. 196-210.

Kitao T et al: Serotyping of *Vibrio anguillarum* isolated from diseased freshwater fish in Japan, *J Fish Dis* 6:175-181, 1983.

Kitao T, Iwata K, Ohta H: Therapeutic attempt to control streptococciosis in cultured rainbow trout, *Salmo gairdneri* using erythromycin, *Fish Pathol* 22:25-28, 1987.

Kleinholz C: *Water quality management for fish farmers,* Langston, Okla., 1990, Extension Facts, Langston University, p. 8.

Knittel MD: Susceptibility of steelhead trout *Salmo gairdneri* Richardson to redmouth infection *Yersinia ruckeri* following exposure to copper, *J Fish Dis* 4:33-40, 1981.

Kodama H et al:*Salmonella arizonae* isolated from a pirarucu, *Arapaima gigas* Cuvier, with septicemia, *J Fish Dis* 10:509-512, 1987.

Kohlmeyer J, Kohlmeyer E: *Marine mycology: the higher fungi,* New York, 1979, Academic Press.

Kovacs-Gayer E: Histopathological differential diagnosis of gill changes with special regard to gill necrosis. In Olah J, Molnar K, Jeney Z, editors: *Fish pathogens and environment in European polyculture,* Szarva, Hungary 1984, Proc International Seminar, Fisheries Research Institute, pp. 219-229.

Kowalski D: Chloramine and wet pets don't mix, *Pets Supplies Mar* 6:46, 48, 1984.

Kraxberger-Beatty T, McGarey DJ, Grier HJ, Lim DV: *Vibrio harveyi* an opportunistic pathogen of common snook, *Centropomus unidecimalis* (Block), held in captivity, *J Fish Dis* 13:557-560, 1990.

Krum H, Gillette D, Lewbart GA: Pathology and treatment of encysted digenean metacercaria in the catfish, *Corydoras schwartzii,* Hong Kong, 1992. Proceedings of the 23rd Annual International Association for Aquatic Animal Medicine Conference, p. 118 (abstract).

Kruse P, Steinhagen D, Korting W, Friedhof KT: Morphometrics and redescription of *Trypanoplasma borreli* Laveran and Mesnil, 1901 (Mastigophora, Kinetoplastida) from experimentally infected common carp (*Cyprinus carpio* L.), *J Protozool* 36:408-412, 1989.

Kubota S, Kojima S, Ishida A: A side-effect of sulfonamides in fish, *Fish Pathol* 4:98-102, 1970.

Kubota SS, Kaige N, Miyazaki T, Miyashita T: Histopathological studies on edwardsiellosis of Tilapia. Part 1. Natural infection, *Bull Fac Fish, Mie Univ* 9:155-165, 1981.

Kudo T, Hatai K, Seino A: *Nocardia seriolae* sp. nov. causing nocardiosis of cultured fish, *Int J System Bacteriol* 38:173-178, 1988.

Kuhns JF, Borgendale K: Studies of the relative dechlorinating abilities of aquarium water conditioners, *J Aquariculture* 1(1):29-34, 1980.

Kuroda N, Hatai K, Kubota SS, Isoda M: A histopathological study of *Ochroconis* infection in yamame salmon: Comparison of fish experimentally injected and those naturally infected with *Ochroconis* sp. (in Japanese), *Bull Nippon Vet Zootech Coll* 35:151-157, 1986.

Kusuda R, Inoue K: Studies on the application of ampicillin for pseudotuberculosis in cultured yellowtails. Part 3. Therapeutic effect of ampicillin on yellowtails artificially infected with *Pasteurella piscicida, Fish Pathol* 12:7-10, 1977.

Kusuda R et al: *Enterococcus seriolicida* sp. nov., a fish pathogen, *Int J Syst Bacteriol* 41:406-409, 1991.

Kusuda R, Ninomiya M, Hamaguchi M, Muraoka A: The efficacy of ribosomal vaccine prepared from *Pasteurella piscicida* against pseudotuberculosis in cultured yellowtail, *Fish Pathol* 23:191-196, 1988.

Kusuda R, Sugiyama A: Studies on the characters of *Staphylococcus epidermidis* isolated from diseased fishes. Part 1. On the morphological, biological and biochemical properties, *Fish Pathol* 16:15-24, 1981.

Kusuda R, Taki H, Takeuchi T: Research into *Nocardia* disease in cultivated yellowtail. Part 2. Properties of *Nocardia kampachi* isolated from yellowtail with branchial node disease, *Bull Jap Soc Sci Fish* 40:369-373, 1974.

Kusuda R, Yokoyama J, Masui T: Bacteriological study on cause of mass mortalities in cultured black sea bream fry, *Bull Japan Soc Sci Fish* 52:1745-1751, 1986.

Lallier R, Boulanger Y, Olivier G: Difference in virulence of *Aeromonas hydrophila* and *Aeromonas sobria* in rainbow trout, *Prog Fish-cult* 42:199-200, 1980.

Lamas J, Anadon R, Devesa S. Toranzo AE: Visceral neoplasia and epidermal papillomas in cultured turbot *Scophthalmus maximus, Dis Aquatic Organ* 8:179-187, 1990.

Landolt ML: Visceral granuloma and nephrocalcinosis of trout. In Ribelin WE, Migaki G, editors: *Pathology of fishes,* Madison, Wisconsin, 1975, University of Wisconsin Press, pp. 793-805.

Landolt ML: The relationship between diet and the immune response of fish, *Aquacult* 79:193-206, 1989.

Landsberg JH, Paperna I: Ultrastructural study of the coccidian *Cryptosporidium* sp. from stomachs of juvenile cichlid fish, *Dis Aquatic Org* 2:13-20, 1986.

Landsberg JH, Paperna I: Intestinal infection by *Eimeria* (s.l.) *vanasi* n. sp. (Eimeridae, Apicomplex, Protozoa) in cichlid fish, *Ann Parasitol Hum Comp* 62:283-293, 1987.

Landsberg JH, Vermeer GK, Richards SA, Perry N: Control of the parasitic copepod *Caligus elongatus* on pond-reared red drum, *J Aquatic Animal Health* 3:206-209, 1991.

Langdon JS: Intestinal infection with a unicellular green alga in the golden perch, *Macquaria ambigua* (Richardson), *J Fish Dis* 9:1259-162, 1986.

Langdon JS: Iron deposition in the gills of fish and crayfish, *Austasia Aquacult* 1:7, 1987a.

Langdon JS: Spinal curvatures and encephalotropic myxosporean *Triangula percae* sp. nov. (Myxozoa: Ortholineidae), enzootic in redfin perch, *Perca fluviatilis* L., in Australia, *J Fish Dis* 10:425-434, 1987b.

Langdon JS: Investigation of fish kills. In *Fish diseases.* Proceedings 106, Post Graduate Committee in Veterinary Science, University of Sydney, Sydney, Australia, 1988, pp. 167-223.

Langdon JS: *Major protozoan and metazoan parasitic diseases of Australian fin fish.* Refresher Course for Veterinarians Procceedings 128, Post Graduate Committee in Veterinary Science, University of Sydney, Australia, 1990, pp. 233-255.

Langdon JS: Major protozoan and metazoan parasitic diseases of Australian finfish. In *Fin fish workshop.* Proceedings 182, Post Graduate Committee in Veterinary Science, University of Sydney, Sydney, Australia, 1992a, pp. 1-26.

Langdon JS: Aust-Asian viral diseases. In *Fin fish workshop.* Proceedings 182, Post Graduate Committee in Veterinary Science, University of Sydney, Sydney, Australia, 1992b. pp. 31-43.

Langdon JS, Gudkovs N, Humphrey JD. Saxon EC: Death in Australian freshwater fishes associated with *Chilodonella hexasticha* infection, *Aust Vet J* 62:409-413, 1985.

Langdon JS, Humphrey JD, Williams LM: Outbreaks of an EHNV-like iridovirus in cultured rainbow trout, *Salmo gairdneri* Richardson, in Australia, *J Fish Dis* 11:93-96, 1988.

Langdon JS, Nowak BS: *Pollutants and biotoxins in fish and consumers.* In Fin Fish Workshop, Proceedings 182, Post Graduate Committee in Veterinary Science, University of Sydney, pp. 165-189.

Langvad F, Pedersen O, Engjom K: A fungal disease caused by *Exophiala* sp. nov. in farmed Atlantic salmon in western Norway. In Ellis AE, editor: *Fish and shellfish pathology,* London, 1985, Academic Press, pp. 323-328.

Larsen JL, Jensen NJ: The ulcus-syndrome in cod (*Gadus morhua*) V. Prevalence in selected Danish marine recipients and a control site in the period 1976-1979, *Nord Veterinaermed* 34:303-312, 1982.

Lawler AR: Dinoflagellate (*Amyloodinium*) infestation of pompano. In Sindermann CJ, editor: *Disease diagnosis and control in North American marine aquaculture,* Amsterdam, 1977a, Elsevier, pp. 257-264.

Lawler AR: Monogenetic trematodes of pompano. In Sindermann CJ, editor: *Disease diagnosis and control in North American marine aquaculture,* Amsterdam, 1977b, Elsevier, pp. 265-267.

Lawler AR: Studies on *Amyloodinium ocellatum* (Dinoflagellata) in Mississippi Sound: natural and experimental hosts, *Gulf Res Rprt* 6:403-413, 1980,

Lawler AR, Ogle JT, Donnes C: *Dascyllus* spp.: new hosts for lymphocystis and a list of recent hosts, *J Wildlife Dis* 13:307-312, 1977.

Lee E G-H, Evelyn TPT: Broodstock erythromycin injection prevents *Renibacterium* vertical transmission, *Am Fish Soc Fish Health Sec Newsltr* 19:1, 1991.

Lee JJ, Hutner SH, Bovee EC: *An illustrated guide to the protozoa*, Lawrence, Kan., 1985, Society of Protozoologists.

Leibovitz L, Riis RC: A viral disease of aquarium fish, *JAVMA* 177:414-416, 1980.

Leitritz C: Trout and salmon culture, *Calif Fish Game Bull* 164, 1976.

Leitritz E, Lewis RC: Trout and salmon and culture (hatchery methods), *Fish Bull*, California Department of Fish and Game, 164, 1976.

Leivestad H: Physiological effects of acid stress on fish. In Johnson RE, editor: *Acid rain/fisheries: proceedings of the international symposium on acidic rain and fishery impacts on Northeast/North America*, Bethesda, Md. 1982, Northeast Division, American Fisheries Society, pp. 157-164.

Leon KA, Bonney WA: Atlantic salmon embryos and fry: effects of various incubation and rearing methods on hatchery survival and growth, *Prog Fish-cult* 41:20-25, 1979.

Leong JC et al: *Biotechnologic advances in fish disease research: short communications of the 1991 International Marine Biotechnology Conference*, vol 2, Dubuque, Iowa, 1993,WC Brown, pp. 573-586.

Leong TS, Wong SY: A comparative study of the parasite fauna of wild and cultured grouper (*Epinephelus malabaricus* Block et Schneider) in Malaysia, *Aquacult* 68:203-207, 1988.

Lester RJG: Metazoan diseases of fish. In *Fish diseases: proceedings 106*, Sydney, Australia, 1988, Post Graduate Committee in Veterinary Science, University of Sydney, pp. 115-124.

Letch CA: Host restriction, morphology and izoenzymes among trypanosomes of some British fishes, *Parasitol* 79:107-117, 1979.

Letch CA: The life cycle of *Trypanosoma cobitis* Mitrophanow, 1883, *Parastiol* 80:163-169, 1980.

LeTendre GC, Schneider CP, Ehlinger NF: Net damage and subsequent mortality from furunculosis in smallmouth bass, *NY Fish Game J* 19:73-82, 1972.

Leteux F, Meyer FP: Mixtures of malachite green and formalin for controlling *Ichthyophthirius* and other protozoan parasites of fish, *Prog Fish-cult* 34:21-26, 1972.

Lewbart GA, Gratzek JB: *The use of praziquantel in the elimination of intestinal cestodes from the red snakehead*, Vancouver, B.C., 1990, 21st Annual Meeting International Association of Aquatic Animal Medicine, pp. 11-13.

Lewbart GL: Medical management of disorders of freshwater tropical fish, *Compend Contin Ed Prac Vet* 13:109-116, 1991.

Lewin CS: Mechanisms of resistance development in aquatic microorganisms. In Michel C, Alderman DJ, editors: *Chemotherapy in aquaculture: from theory to reality*, Paris, 1992, Office International des Epizooties, pp. 288-301.

Lewis DH, Grumbles LC, McConnell S, Flowers AI: *Pasteurella*-like bacteria from an epizootic in menhaden and mullet in Galveston Bay, *J Wildlife Dis* 6:160-162, 1970.

Lewis DH, Udey LR: *Meningitis in fish caused by an asporogenous anaerobic bacterium*, Fish Disease Leaflet No. 56, United States Fish and Wildlife Service, 1978, 5 pp.

Lewis WM, Morrios DP: Toxicity of nitrite to fish: a review, *Trans Am Fish Soc* 115:183-195, 1986.

Lewis WM, Summerfelt RC: A myxosporidian, *Myxobolus notemigoni* sp. n., parasite of the golden shiner, *J Parasitol* 50:386-389, 1964.

Lightner D et al: A renal mycosis of an adult hybrid red tilapia *Oreochromis mossambique* X *O. honorum*, caused by the imperfect fungus, *Paecilomyces marquandii*, *J Fish Dis* 11:437-444, 1988.

Lio-Po G, Sanvictores E: Studies on the causative organism of *Oreochromis niloticus* (Linnaeus) fry mortalities. Part I. Primary isolation and pathogenicity experiments, *J Aquatic Trop* 2:25-30, 1987.

Littauer GA: *Control of bird predation at aquaculture facilities: strategies and cost estimates*, Southern Regional Aquaculture Center Publication No. 402, US Department of Agriculture, 1990.

Liu CI, Tsai SS: *Edwardsiellosis in pond-cultured eel in Taiwan*, CAPD Fisheries Series No. 3, Reports on Fish Disease Research 3:109-115, 1980.

Lom J: The adhesive disc of *Trichodinella epizootica*: Ultrastructure and injury to the host tissue, *Folia Parasitol (Praha)* 20:193-202, 1973a.

Lom J: The mode of attachment and relations to the host in *Apiosoma piscicola* Blanchard and *Epistylis lwoffi* Faure-Fremiet, ectocommensals of freshwater fishes, *Folia Parasitol (Praha)* 20:105-112, 1973b.

Lom J: Diseases caused by Protista. In Kinne O, editor: *Diseases of marine animals*, vol 4, Hamburg, FRG, 1984, Pisces, Biological Anstalt Helgoland, pp. 114-168.

Lom J, Corliss JO: Observations on the fine structure of two species of the peritrich ciliate genus Scyphidia and on their mode of attachment to their host, *Trans Am Microsc Soc* 87:493-509, 1968.

Lom J, Dykova I: Pathogenicity of some protozoan parasites of cyprinid fishes, *Symp Biol Hung* 23:99-118, 1984.

Lom J, Dykova I, Kirting W, Klinger H: *Heterosporis schuberti* n. sp., a new microsporidian parasite of aquarium fish, *Eur J Protistol* 25:129-135, 1989.

Lom J, Dykova I: *Protozoan parasites of fishes: development in aquaculture and fisheries science*, vol 26, New York, 1992, Elsevier, 315 pp.

Lom J, Lawler AR: An ultrastructural study on the mode of attachment in dinoflagellates invading the gills of Cyprinodontidae, *Protistologica* 9:293-309, 1973.

Lom J, Nigrelli RF: *Brooklynella hostilis*, n.g., n.sp., a pathogenic cyrtophorine ciliate in marine fishes, *J Protozool* 17:224-232, 1970.

Lom J, Pike AW, Feist SW: Myxosporean stages in rete mirabile in the eye of *Gasterosteus aculeatus* infected with *Myxobilatus gasterostei* and *Sphaerospora elegans*, *Dis Aquatic Org* 11:67-72, 1991b.

Lom J, Schubert G: Ultrastructural study of *Piscinoodinium pillulare* (Schaperclaus, 1954) Lom, 1981 with special emphasis on its attachment to the fish host, *J Fish Dis* 6:411-428, 1983.

Lorio WJ: Experimental control of the metacercariae of the yellow grub *Clinostomum marginatum* in channel catfish, *J Aquatic Animal Health* 1:269-271, 1989.

Lounatmaa K, Janatuinen J: Electron microscopy of an ulcerative dermal necrosis (UDN)-like salmon disease in Finland, *J Fish Dis* 1:369-375, 1978.

Love M et al: *Vibrio damsela*, a marine bacterium, causes skin ulcers on the damselfish *Chromis punctipinnis*, *Science* 214:1139-1140, 1981.

Lovell RT: Fish culture in the United States, *Science* 206:1368-1372, 1979.

Lovell RT: Nutrition and feeding. In Brown EE, Gratzek JB, editors: *Fish farming handbook*, Westport, Conn., 1980, AVI Publishing, pp. 207-236.

Lovell RT: *Nutrition and feeding of fish*, New York, 1989, AVI Van Nostrand Reinholt, 260 pp.

Lundbjorg LE, Ljungberg O: Attack of *Caligus* sp. in salmon and rainbow trout in brackish water floating cage management, *J Nordisk Veterinaer Medicin* 29:20-21, 1977.

Lunestad BT: Fate and effects of antibacterial agents in aquatic environments. In Michel C, Alderman DJ, editors: *Chemotherapy in aquaculture: from theory to reality*, Paris, 1992, Office International des Epizooties, pp. 152-161.

Lunestad BT, Goksoyr J: Reduction in the antibacterial effect of oxytetracycline in seawater by complex formation with magnesium and calcium, *Dis Aquatic Org* 9:67-72, 1990.

Lupiani B et al: New syndrome of mixed bacterial and viral etiology in cultured turbot *Scophthalmus maximus*, *J Aquatic Animal Health* 1:197-204, 1989.

MacDonnell MT, Colwell RR: Phylogeny of the Vibrionaceae and recommendations for two new genera, *Listonella* and *Shewanella*, *Sys Appl Microbiol* 6:171-182, 1985.

MacFarlane RD, Bullock GL, McLaughlin JJA: Effects of five metals on susceptibility of striped bass to *Flexibacter columnaris*, *Trans Am Fish Soc* 115:227-231, 1986.

MacKenzie K, Liversidge JM: Some aspects of the biology of the cercaria and metacercaria of *Stephanostomum baccatum* (Nicoll, 1907) Manter, 1934 (Digenea: Acanthocolpidae), *J Fish Biol* 7:247-256, 1975.

MacMillan JR: Infectious diseases. In Tucker CS, editor: *Channel catfish culture*, Elsevier, Amsterdam, 1985, pp. 405-496.

MacMillan JR: Biological factors impinging upon control of external protozoan fish parasites, *Ann Rev Fish Dis* 1:119-131, 1991.

MacMillan JR, Jr: President's message, *Fish Health Sec Am Fish Soc Newsltr* 21(1):15-19, 1993.

MacMillan JR, Mulcahy D, Landolt M: Viral erythrocytic necrosis: some physiological consequences of infection in chum salmon (*Oncorhynchus keta*), *J Fish Res Bd Can* 37:799-804, 1980a.

MacMillan JR, Mulcahy D, Landolt ML: Cytopathology and coagulopathy associated with viral erythrocytic necrosis in chum salmon, *J Aquatic Animal Health* 1:255-262, 1989b.

MacMillan JR, Wilson C, Thiyagarajah A: Experimental induction of proliferative gill disease in specific-pathogen-free channel catfish, *J Aquatic Animal Health* 1:245-254, 1989.

Macri B, Panebiaco A, Costa AL. Midili S: Patologia da lieviti in pesci maini. Part II. Studi sull'agent eziologico, sugli aspetti anatomoistopatologici e su alcune considerazioni di ordini sonitario ed ispettivo, *Summa* 1:89-94, 1984.

Magarinoz B et al: Phenotypic, antigenic, and molecular characterization of *Pasteurella piscicida* strains isolated from fish, *Appl Environ Microbiol* 58:3316-3322, 1992.

Maisse G, Dorson M, Torchy C: Ultraviolet inactivation of two pathogenic salmonid viruses (IPN virus and VHS virus), *Bull F. Piscicult* 278:34-40, 1980.

Major RD, McCraren JP, Smith CE: Histopathological changes in channel catfish (*Ictalurus punctatus*) experimentally and naturally infected with channel catfish virus disease, *J Fish Res Bd Can* 32:563-567, 1975.

Malins DC et al: Chemical pollutants in sediments and diseases of bottom-dwelling fish in Puget Sound, Washington, *Environ Sci Technol* 18:705-713, 1984.

Mallatt J: Fish gill structural changes induced by toxicants and other irritants: a statistical review, *Can J Fish Aquatic Sci* 42:630-648, 1985.

Malsberger RG, Lautenslager G: Fish viruses: rhabdovirus isolated from a species of the family Cichlidae, *Fish Health News* 9:i-ii, 1980.

Maranthe VB, Huilgol NV, Patil SG: Hydrogen peroxide as a source of oxygen supply in the transport of fish fry, *Prog Fish-cult* 37:117, 1975.

Marincek M: Development d'*Eimeria subepithelialis* (Sporozoa, Coccidia) parasite de la carpe, *Acta Protozool* 12:195-215, 1973.

Marking LL: *Gas supersaturation in fisheries: causes, concerns and cures*, Washington, DC, 1987, Fish Wildlife Leaflet No. 9, United States Fish and Wildlife Service, p. 10.

Marking LL: Evaluation of toxicants for the control of carp and other nuisance fishes, *Fisheries* 17:6-12, 1992.

Marking LL, Bills TD: Factors affecting the efficiency of clinoptilite for removing ammonia from water, *Prog Fish-cult* 44:187-189, 1982.

Marking LL, Howe GE, Crowther JR: Toxicity of erythromycin, oxytetracycline and tetracycline administered to lake trout in water baths, by injection, or by feeding, *Prog Fish-cult* 30:197-201, 1988.

Marking LL, Leith D, Davis J: Development of a carbon filter system for removing malachite green from hatchery effluents, *Prog Fish-cult* 52:92-99, 1990.

Marking LL, Meyer FP: Are better anesthetics needed in fisheries? *Fisheries* 10:2-5, 1985.

Markiw ME, Wolf KE: *Myxosoma cerebralis*: trypsinization of plankton centrifuge harvests increases optical clarity and spore concentration, *Can J Fish Aquatic Sci* 37:2225-2227, 1980.

Markiw ME, Wolf K: *Myxosoma cerebralis* (Myxozoa: Myxosporea) etiologic agent of salmonid whirling disease requires tubificid worm (Annelida:Oligochaeta) in its life cycle, *J Protozool* 30:561-564, 1983.

Martinez-Murcia AJ, Esteve C, Garay E, Collins MD: *Aeromonas allosaccharophila* sp. nov., a new mesophilic member of the genus *Aeromonas*, *FEMS Microbiol Letrs* 91:199-206, 1992.

Matthews RA, Matthews BF: Cell and tissue reaction of turbot *Scophthalmus maximus* (L.) to *Tetramicra brevifilum* gen. n., sp.n. (Microspora), *J Fish Dis* 3:495-515, 1980.

Mawdesley-Thomas LE: Neoplasia in fish. In Ribelin WE, Migaki G, editors: *The pathology of fishes*, Madison, 1975, University of Wisconsin Press, pp. 805-870.

Mawdesley-Thomas LE: Some tumors of fish. In Mawdesley-Thomas LE, editor: *Diseases of fish*, London, 1972, Symposium of the Zoological Society of London, 30:191-284.

Mayer KS, Mayer FL: Waster transformer oil and PCBersity toxicity to rainbow trout, *Trans Am Fish Soc* 114:869-886, 1985.

McAllister PE, Herman RL: Epizootic mortality in hatchery-reared lake trout *Salvelinus namaycush*, caused by a putative virus possibly of the herpesvirus group, *Dis Aquatic Org* 6:113-119, 1989.

McAllister KW, McAllister PE: Transmission of infectious pancreatic necrosis virus from carrier striped bass to brook trout, *Dis Aquatic Org* 4:101-104, 1988.

McAllister PE, Owens WJ. Ruppenthal TM: Detection of infectious pancreatic necrosis virus in pelleted cell and particulate components from ovarian fluids of brook trout *Salvelinus fontinalis*, *Dis Aquatic Org* 2:235-237, 1987.

McArn GE, McCain B, Wellings SR: Skin lesions and associated virus in Pacific cod (*Gadus macrocephalus*) in the Bering Sea, *Fed Proc* 37:937, 1978.

McBride J, Strasdine G, Fagerlund UHM: Acute toxicity of kanamycin to steelhead trout (*Salmo gairdneri*), *J Fish Res Bd Can* 32:554-558, 1975.

McCain BB, Gronlund WD, Myers MS, Wellings SR: Tumours and microbial diseases of marine fishes in Alaskan waters, *J Fish Dis* 2:111-130, 1979.

McCarthy DH: *A study of the taxonomic status of some bacteria currently assigned to the genus Aeromonas*. Ph.D. Thesis, 1978, Council of National Academic Awards, United Kingdom.

McCarthy DH, Roberts RJ: Furunculosis in fish—the present state of our knowledge. In Droop MR, Jannasch HW, editors: *Advances in aquatic microbiology*, New York, Academic Press, 1980, pp. 293-341.

McCraren JP, Landolt ML, Hoffman GL, Meyer FP: Variation in response of channel catfish to *Henneguya* sp. infections (Protozoa:Myxosporidea), *J Wildlife Dis* 11:2-7, 1975.

McDowell T, Hedrick RP, Kent ML, Elston RA: Isolation of a new virus from Atlantic salmon (*Salmo salar*), *Am Fish Soc Fish Health Sec Newsltr* 17(2):7, 1989.

McFadden TW: Furunculosis in nonsalmonids, *J Fish Res Bd Can* 27:2365-2370, 1970.

McGlamery MH, Jr, Gratzek JB: Stunting syndrome associated with young channel catfish that survived exposure to channel catfish virus, *Prog Fish-cult* 36:38-41, 1974.

McIntosh D, Austin B: Recovery of an extremely proteolytic form of *Serratia liquefaciens* as a pathogen of Atlantic salmon, *Salmo salar*, in Scotland, *J Fish Dis* 13:765-772, 1990.

McKee JE, Wolf HW, editors: *Water quality criteria*, ed 2, Sacramento, Calif., 1963, State of California, State Water Quality Control Board, Publication No. 3-A, p. 548.

McKenzie RA, Hall WTK: Dermal ulceration of mullet (*Mugil cephalus*), *Australian Vet J* 52:230-231, 1972.

McKnight IJ, Roberts RJ: The pathology of infectious pancreatic necrosis. 1. The sequential histopathology of the naturally occurring condition, *Br Vet J* 132:76-86, 1976.

McVicar AH: *Ichthyophonus* infections of fish. In Roberts RJ, editor: *Microbial diseases of fish*, London, 1982, Society for General Microbiology, Special Publication No. 9, Academic Press, pp. 243-269.

McVicar AH: Infection as a primary cause of pancreas disease in farmed Atlantic salmon, *Bull Eur Assn Fish Pathol* 10:84-87, 1990.

Meade JW: Allowable ammonia for fish culture, *Prog Fish-cult* 47:135-145, 1985.

Melhorn H, Schmahl G, Haberkorn A: Toltrazuril effective against a broad spectrum of protozoan parasites, *Parasitol Res* 75:64-66, 1988.

Mellergard S, Bloch B: Herpesvirus-like particles in angelfish, *Pterophyllum altum, Dis Aquatic Org* 5:151-155, 1988.

Meyer FP: Parasites of freshwater fishes. Part 2. *Protozoa 3, Ichthyophthirius multifiliis.* Washington, DC, 1974, Fish Disease Leaflet No. 2, United States Department of the Interior, U.S.F.W.S.

Meyer FP: Incidence of disease in warmwater fish farms in the south-central United States, *Marine Fish Rev* 40:38-41, 1978.

Meyer FP: Solutions to the shortage of approved fish therapeutants, *J Aquatic Animal Health* 1:78-80, 1989.

Meyer FP, Bullock GL: *Edwardsiella tarda,* a new pathogen of channel catfish (*Ictalurus punctatus*), *Appl Microbiol* 25:151-156, 1973.

Meyer FP, Collar JD: Description and treatment of *Pseudomonas* infection white catfish, *Appl Microbiol* 12:201-203, 1964.

Meyer FP, Jorgensen TA: Teratological and other effects of malachite green on the development of rainbow trout and rabbits, *Trans Am Fish Soc* 112:818-824, 1983.

Meyer FP, Robinson JA: Branchiomycosis: a new fungal disease of North American fishes, *Prog Fish-cult* 35:74-77, 1973.

Meyers SP, Baslow MH, Bein SJ, Marks CE: Studies on *Flavobacterium piscicida* Bein. Part 1. Growth, toxicity, and ecological considerations, *J Bacteriol* 78:225-230, 1959.

Meyers TR: Serological and histopathological responses of rainbow trout, *Salmo gairdneri* Richardson, to experimental infection with the 13p$_2$ reovirus, *J Fish Dis* 6:277-292, 1983.

Meyers TR, Hendricks JD: A summary of tissue lesions in aquatic animals induced by controlled exposure to environmental contaminants, chemical agents and potential carcinogens, *Mar Fish Rev* 44:1-17, 1982.

Michel C et al: *Heterosporis finki,* a microsporidian parasite of the angel fish *Pterophyllum scalare*: patholgy and ultrastucture, *Dis Aquatic Org* 7:103-109, 1989.

Michel C, Alderman DJ, editors: *Chemotherapy in aquaculture: from theory to reality,* Paris, 1992, Office International des Epizooties, p. 567.

Michel C, Faivre B, Kerouault R: Biochemical identification of *Lactobacillus piscicola* strains from France and Belgium, *Dis Aquatic Org* 2:27-30, 1986.

Miller RW, Chapman WR: *Epistylis* and *Aeromonas hydrophila* infections in fishes from North Carolina reservoirs, *Prog Fish-cult* 38:165-168, 1976.

Minchew CD: Five new species of *Henneguya* (Protozoa: Myxosporidia) from ictalurid fishes, *J Protozool* 24:213-220, 1977.

Mitchell AJ: Parasites and diseases of striped bass. In McCraren JP, editor: *The aquaculture of striped bass: a proceedings,* University of Maryland Sea Grant Publication No. UM-SG-MAP-84-01, pp 177-204, 1984.

Mitchell AJ: Agricultural pesticides in fish production, *Aquacult Mag* 21(2):54-59, 1995.

Mitchell AJ, Plumb JA: Toxicity and efficacy of Furanace on channel catfish, *Ictalurus punctatus* (Rafinesque) infected experimentally with *Aeromonas hydrophila, J Fish Dis* 3:93-99, 1980.

Mitchum DL, Moore TD: Efficacy of Di-N-Butyl tin oxide on an intestinal fluke, *Crepidostomum farionis,* in golden trout, *Prog Fish-cult* 31:143-148, 1966.

Mix MC: *Cancerous diseases in aquatic animals and their association with environmental pollutants: a critical review of the literature,* Corvallis, Ore., 1985, Final Report for the American Petroleum Institute, Oregon State University, 239 pp.

Miyazaki T et al: Histopathology associated with two viral diseases of larval and juvenile fishes: epidermal necrosis of Japanese flounder *Paralichthys olivaceus* and epithelial necrosis of black seabream *Acanthopagrus sclegeli, J Aquatic Animal Health* 1:85-93, 1989.

Miyazaki T, Egusa S: Studies on mycotic granulomatosis in freshwater fishes. Part 1. The goldfish (in Japanese), *Fish Pathol* 7:15-25, 1972.

Miyazaki T, Egusa S: Histopathological studies of edwardsiellosis of the Japanese eel (*Anguilla japonica*). Part 1. Suppurative interstitial nephritis form, *Fish Pathol* 11:33-44, 1976a.

Miyazaki T, Egusa S: Histopathological studies of edwardsiellosis of the Japanese eel (*Anguilla japonica*). Part 1. Suppurative interstitial hepatitis form, *Fish Pathol* 11:67-76, 1976b.

Mo TA, Poppe TT, Iversen L: Systemic hexamitosis in salt-water reared Atlantic salmon, *Bull Eur Assn Fish Pathol* 10:69-70, 1990.

Moccia RD, Leatherland JR, Sonstgard RA: Increasing frequency of thyroid goiters in coho salmon (*Oncorhynchus kisutch*) in the Great Lakes, *Science* 198:425-426, 1977.

Moe, MA, Jr: *The marine aquarium handboook: beginner to breeder,* Plantation, Fla., 1992a, Green Turtle Publications, p. 320.

Moe, MA, Jr: *The marine aquarium reference: systems and invertebrates,* Plantation, Fla., 1992b, Green Turtle Publications, p. 512.

Moffitt CM: Oral and injectable applications of erythromycin in salmonid fish culture, *Vet Human Toxicol* 33(suppl 1):49-53, 1991.

Moffitt CM: Survival of juvenile chinook salmon challenged with *Renibacterium salmoninarum* and administered oral doses of erythromycin thiocyanate for different durations, *J Aquatic Animal Health* 4:119-125, 1992.

Mohney LL, Lightner DV, Williams RR, Bauerlein M: Bioencapsulation of therapeutic quantities of the antibacterial Romet-30 in nauplii of the brine shrimp *Artemia* and the nematode *Panagrellus redivivus, J World Aquatic Soc* 21:186-191, 1990.

Moller H, Anders K: *Diseases and parasites of marine fishes,* Kiel, Germany, 1986, Verlag Moller, p. 365.

Molnar K: Data on the octomitosis (spironucleosis) of cyprinids and aquary fishes, *Acta Vet Acad Sci Hung* 24:99-106, 1974.

Molnar K: *Myxobolus pavloskii* (Akhmerov, 1954) (Myxosporidia) infection in the silver carp and bighead, *Acta Vet Acad Sci Hung* 17:207-216, 1979.

Molnar K: Biology and histopathology of *Thelohanellus nikolskii* Akhmerov, 1955 (Myxosporea, Myxozoa), a protozoan parasite of the common carp (*Cyprinus carpio*), *Z Parasitenkd* 68:269-277, 1982.

Molnar K: Recent achievements in the chemotherapy of myxosporean infections of fish, *Acta Vet Hungarica* 41:51-58, 1993.

Molnar K, Fischer-Scheri T, Baska F, Hoffmann RW: Hoferellosis in goldfish *Carassius auratus* and gibel carp *Carassius auratus gibelio, Dis Aquatic Org* 7:89-95, 1989.

Molnar K, Hanek G: Seven new *Eimeria* spp. (Protozoa, Coccidia) from freshwater fishes of Canada, *J Protozool* 21:489-493, 1974.

Moore AA, Eimers ME, Cardella MA: Attempts to control *Flexibacter columnaris* epizootics in pond-reared channel catfish by vaccination, *J Aquatic Animal Health* 2:109-111, 1990.

Moore AR, Li MF, McMenemy M: Isolation of a picorna-like virus from smelt, *Osmerus mordaxx* (Mitchill), *J Fish Dis* 11:179-184, 1988.

Moravec F: Some remarks on the biology of *Capillaria ptrophylii* Heinze, 1933, *Folia Parasitol* 30:129-130, 1983.

Moravec F, Colnar M, Rehulka J: *Capillostrongyloides ancistri* sp. n. (Nematoda: Capillaridae) a new pathogenic parasite of aquarium fishes, *Folia Parasitol* 34:157-161, 1987.

Morrison C, Hoffman GL, Sprague V: *Glugea pimephales* Fantham, Porter and Richardson, 1941, n. comb. (Microsporidia, Glugeidae) in the fathead minnow, *Pimephales promelas, Can J Zool* 63:380-391, 1985.

Morrison CM, Cone DK: A possible marine form of *Ichthyobodo* sp. on haddock *Melangrammus aeglefinus* (L.) in the northwest Atlantic Ocean, *J Fish Dis* 9:141-142, 1986.

Morrison CM, Cornick JW, Shum G, Zwicker B: Histopathology of atypical *Aeromomas salmonicida* infection in Atlantic cod, *Gadus morhua* L, *J Fish Dis* 7:477-494, 1984.

Morrison CM, Poynton SL: A new species of *Goussia* (Apicomplexa, Coccidia) in the kidney tubules of the cod, *Gadus morhua* L, *J Fish Dis* 12:533-560, 1989.

Moser M, Sakanari J, Heckmann R: The effects of praziquantel on various larval and adult parasites from freshwater and marine snails and fish, *J Parasitol* 72:175-176, 1986.

Mueller KW, Watanabe WO, Head WD: Effect of salinity on hatching in *Neobenedenia melleni*, a monogenean ectoparasite of seawater-cultured tilapia, *J World Maricult Soc* 23:199-204, 1992.

Muhvich AG, Reimschuessel R, Lipsky MM, Bennett RO: *Fusarium solani* isolated from newborn bonnethead sharks *Sphyrna tiburo* (L.), *J Fish Dis* 12:57-62, 1989.

Mulcahy D: Control of mortality caused by infectious hematopoetic necrosis virus. In Leong JC, Barile TY, editors: *Proceedings of a workshop on viral diseases of salmonid fishes in the Columbia River basin, Portland, Ore., October 7, 8, 1982*, pp. 51-71, 1983.

Mulcahy D, Fryer JL: Double infection of rainbow trout fry with IHN and IPN viruses, *Fish Health News* 5:5-6, 1976.

Mulcahy D, Klaybor D, Batts WN: Isolation of infectious hematopoietic necrosis virus from from a leech (*Piscicola salmositica*) and a copepod (*Salmincola* sp.), ectoparasites of sockeye salmon *Oncorhynchus nerka*, *Dis Aquatic Org* 8:29-34, 1990.

Mulcahy D, Pascho RJ: Adsorption to fish sperm of vertically transmitted fish viruses, *Science* 225:333-335, 1984.

Mulcahy D, Pascho R, Jenes CK: Comparison of in vitro growth characteristics of ten isolates of infectious hematopoietic necrosis virus, *J Gen Virol* 65:2199-2207, 1984.

Munday BL: Amoebic gill disease of salmonids. In *Fish diseases,* Sydney, Australia, 1988, Proceedings 106, Post Graduate Committee in Veterinary Science, University of Sydney, pp. 111-112.

Munro ALS, Hastings TS: Furunculosis. In Inglis V, Roberts RJ, Bromage NR, editors: *Bacterial diseases of fish,* New York, 1993, Halsted Press, pp. 122-142.

Muroga K, Nakai T, Sawada T: Studies on red spot disease of cultured eels. Part 4. Physiological characteristics of the causative bacterium *Pseudomonas anguilliseptica*, *Fish Pathol* 12:33-38, 1977.

Muroga K, Takahashi S, Yamanoi H: Non-cholera *Vibrio* isolated from diseased ayu, *Bull Japan Soc Sci Fish* 45:829-834, 1979.

Murray CN, Riley JP: The solubility of gases in distilled water and sea water. Part 2. Oxygen, *Deep-sea Res* 16:311-320, 1969.

Murty AS: *Toxicity of pesticides to fish,* vol 1, Boca Raton, Fla., 1986a, CRC Press.

Murty AS: *Toxicity of pesticides to fish,* vol 2, Boca Raton, Fla., 1986b, CRC Press.

Myers TR et al: Comparison of the enzyme-linked immunosorbent assay (ELISA) and the fluorescent antibody test (FAT) for measuring the prevalences and levels of *Renibacterium salmoninarum* in wild and hatchery stocks of salmonid fishes in Alaska, USA, *Dis Aquatic Org* 16:181-189, 1993.

Naeve H: Die Endigung afferenter Fasern der Seitenliniennerven im Mittelhirn des Dorsches Gadus morhua, *Mar Biol* 1:257-262, 1968.

Nagel ML, Summerfelt RC: Apparent immunity of goldfish to *Pleistophora ovariae, Proc Oklahoma Acad Sci* 57:61-63, 1977.

Nash G, Nash M, Schlotfeld HJ: Systematic amoebiasis in cultured European catfish, *Silurus glanis* L, *J Fish Dis* 11:15-23, 1988.

National Research Council: *Nutrient requirements of warm water fishes and shellfishes,* Washington, DC, 1983, National Academy of Sciences, 102 pp.

National Research Council: *Nutrient requirements of cold water fishes,* Washington, DC, 1981, National Academy of Sciences.

Needham DJ: Practitioner's approach to a fish case. In *Fish diseases: proceedings no.106,* Sydney, Australia, 1988, The Post-Graduate Committee in Veterinary Science, University of Sydney, pp. 419-428.

Neish GA, Hughes GC: *Fungal diseases of fishes,* Neptune, N.J., 1980, TFH Publications.

Nepszy SJ, Budd J, Dechtiar AA: Mortality of young-of-the-year rainbow smelt (*Osmerus mordax*) in Lake Erie associated with occurrence of *Glugea hertwigi, J Wildlife Dis* 14:233-239, 1978.

Nevins MJ, Johnson WW: Acute toxicity of phosphate ester mixtures to invertebrates and fish, *Bull Environ Contam Toxicol* 19:250-256, 1978.

Nie DS, Pan JP: Diseases of grass carp (*Ctenopharyngodon idella* Valenciennes, 1844) in China, a review from 1953 to 1983, *Fish Pathol* 20:323-330, 1985.

Nieto TP et al: Isolation of *Serratia plymuthica* as an opportunistic pathogen in rainbow trout, *Salmo gairdneri* Richardson, *J Fish Dis* 13:175-177, 1990.

Nigrelli RF: The morphology, cytology, and life history of *Oodinium ocellatum* Brown, a dinoflagellate parasitic on marine fishes, *Zoologica* 21:129-164, 1936.

Nigrelli RF: Further studies on the susceptibility and acquired immunity of marine fishes to *Epibdella melleni*, a monogenetic trematode, *Zoologica NY Zool Soc* 22:185-191, 1937.

Nigrelli RF: Mortality statistics for specimens in the New York Aquarium, 1939, *Zool NY* 25:525-552, 1940.

Nigrelli RF: Two diseases of the neon tetra, *Hyphessobrycon innesi, Aquarium J (San Francisco)* 24:203-208, 1953.

Nigrelli RF, Hutner SH: The presence of a myxobacterium, *Chondrococcus columnaris* (Davis) Ordal and Rucker (1944), on *Fundulus heteroclitus* (Linn.), *Zoologica* 30:101-104, 1945.

Nigrelli RF, Ruggieri G: Enzootics in the New York Aquarium caused by *Cryptocaryon irritans* Brown 1951 (= *Ichthyophthirius marinus* Sikama, 1961), a histophagous ciliate in the skin, eyes and gills of marine fishes, *Zool NY* 51:97-107, 1966.

Nigrelli RF, Vogel H: Spontaneous tuberculosis in fishes and other cold-blooded vertebrates with special reference to *Mycobacterium fortuitum* Cruz from fish and human lesions, *Zoologica* 48:131-144, 1963.

Noble GA, Noble ER: *Monocercomonas molae* n. sp., a flagellate from the sunfish *Mola mola, J Protozool* 13:257-259, 1966.

Noga EJ: Diet-associated systemic granulomatous disease in African cichlids, *J Am Vet Med Assn* 189:1145-1147, 1986a.

Noga EJ: The importance of *Lernaea cruciata* (LeSeuer) in the initiation of skin lesions in largemouth bass *Micropterus salmoides* (Lacepede) in the Chowan River, North Carolina, *J Fish Dis* 9:295-302, 1986b.

Noga EJ: Propagation in cell culture of the dinoflagellate *Amyloodinium*, an ectoparasite of marine fishes, *Science* 236:1302-1304, 1987.

Noga EJ: Biopsy and rapid postmortem techniques for diagnosing diseases of fish, *Vet Clin N Am (Sm Animal Prac)* 18:401-426, 1988.

Noga EJ: A synopsis of mycotic diseases of marine fishes and invertebrates. In Perkins FO, Cheng TC, editors: *Pathology in marine science,* New York, 1990, Academic Press, pp. 143-160.

Noga EJ: Important problems in marine aquarium fishes. In Kirk RW, Bonagura JD, editors: *Current veterinary therapy xi: small animal practice,* Philadelphia, Penn., 1992, WB Saunders, pp. 1202-1203.

Noga EJ: Fungal and algal diseases of temeratte freshwater and estuarine fishes. In Stoskopf MK, editor: *Fish medicine,* Philadelphia, 1993a, WB Saunders, pp. 278-283.

Noga EJ: Fungal diseases of marine and estuarine fishes. In Couch JA, Fournie JW, editors: *Pathobiology of marine and estuarine organisms,* Boca Raton, Fla., 1993b, CRC Press, pp. 85-110.

Noga EJ: Water mold infections of freshwater fishes: recent advances, *Ann Rev Fish Dis* 3:291-304, 1993c.

Noga EJ, Berkhoff HA: Pathological and microbiological features of *Aeromonas salmonicida* infection in the American eel (*Anguilla rostrata*), *Fish Path* 25:127-132, 1990.

Noga EJ, Bullis RA, Miller GC: Epidemic oral ulceration in largemouth bass (*Micropterus salmoides*) associated with the leech *Myzobdella lugubris, J Wildlife Dis* 26:132-134, 1990a.

Noga EJ, Dykstra MJ: Oomycete fungi associated with ulcerative mycosis in Atlantic menhaden, *J Fish Dis* 9:47-53, 1986.

Noga EJ et al: Kidney biopsy: a nonlethal method for diagnosing *Yersinia ruckeri* infection (enteric redmouth disease) in rainbow trout (*Salmo gairdneri*), *Am J Vet Res* 49:363-365, 1988b.

Noga EJ et al: *Determining the relationship between water quality and ulcerative mycosis in Atlantic menhaden,* Albemarle-Pamlico Estuarine Study Final Report No. 92-15, 1993a, 42 pp.

Noga EJ et al: A new ichthyotoxic dinoflagellate: cause of acute mortality in aquarium fishes, *Vet Rec* 133:96-97, 1993b.

Noga EJ et al: Novel toxic dinoflagellate causes epidemic disease in estuarine fishes, *Marine Pollut Bull* (in press).

Noga EJ et al: Quantitative comparison of the stress response of striped bass (*Morone saxatilis*) and hybrid bass (*Morone saxatilis* x *Morone chrysops* and *Morone saxatilis* x *Morone americana*), *Am J Vet Res* 55:405-409, 1994.

Noga EJ, Francis-Floyd R: *Medical management of channel catfish: the environment.* Compendium on Continuing Education for the Practicing Veterinarian 13:160-166, 1991.

Noga EJ, Levine JF, Dykstra MJ, Hawkins JH: Pathology of ulcerative mycosis in Atlantic menhaden *Brevoortia tyrannus, Dis Aquatic Org* 4:189-197, 1988a.

Noga EJ, Levy MG: Dinoflagellate parasites of fish. In Woo PTK, editor: *Fish diseases I: protozoan and metazoan infections,* Oxon, England, CAB International (in press).

Noga EJ, Wolf D, Cardeilhac PT: Cataract in cichlid fish, *J Am Vet Med Assn* 179:1181-1182, 1981.

Noga EJ, Wright JF, Pasarell L: Some unusual features of mycobacteriosis in the cichlid fish *Oreochromis mossambicus, J Comp Pathol* 102:336-344, 1990b.

Nouws JFM, Grondel JL, Boon JH, van Ginneken VJTh: Pharmacokinetics of antimicrobials in some fresh water fish species. In Michel C, Alderman DJ, editors: *Chemotherapy in aquaculture: from theory to reality,* Office International des Epizooties, pp. 437-447, 1992.

Nusbaum KE, Shotts EB, Jr: Absorption of selected antimicrobic drugs from water by channel catfish, *Ictalurus punctatus, Can J Fish Aquatic Sci* 38:993-996, 1981.

Oestmann DJ: Environmental and disease problems in ornamental marine aquariums, *Comp Contin Educ Prac Vet* 7:558-664, 1985.

O'Grady P, Moloney M, Smith PR: Bath administration of the quinolone antibiotic flumequine to brown trout *Salmo trutta* and Atlantic salmon *S. salar, Dis Aquatic Org* 4:27-33, 1988.

O'Halloran J, Cornick J, Zwicker B, Griffiths S: Cross-Canada disease report: Atlantic Canada, *Can Vet J* 33:406-407, 1992.

Odense PH, Logan VH: Prevalence and morphology of *Eimeria gadi* (Fiebiger, 1913) in the haddock, *J Protozool* 23:564-571, 1976.

Ogawa K, Andoh H, Yamaguchi M: Some biological aspects of *Paradeontacylix* (Trematoda: Sanguinicolidae) infection in cultured marine fish *Seriola dumerli, Gyobo Kenkyu* 28:177-180, 1993.

Ohtsuka H, Nakai T, Muroga K, Jo Y: Atypical *Aeromonas salmonicida* isolated from diseased eels, *Fish Pathol* 19:101-107, 1984.

Olah L, Farkas: Effect of temperature, pH, antibiotics, formalin, and malachite green on the growth and survival of *Saprolegnia* and *Achlya* parasitic on fish, *Aquacult* 13:273-288, 1978.

Olson DP et al: Strawberry disease in rainbow trout, *Salmo gairdneri* Richardson, *J Fish Dis* 8:103-111, 1985.

Olufemi B: The aspergilli as pathogens of cultured fishes, *Rec Adv Aquaculture* 2:193-218, 1985.

Osadchaya EF: Fish diseases caused by rhabdoviruses in the Ukraine. In *Proceedings of an international seminar on fish, pathogens and environment in European polyculture,* Szarvas, Hungary, 1981, pp. 36-47.

Oseko N, Yoshimizu M, Gorie S, Kimura T: Histopathological study on diseased hirame (Japanese flounder; *Paralichthys olivaceus*) infected with *Rhabdovirus olivaceus* (hirame rhabdovirus; HRV), *Fish Pathol* 23:117-123, 1988.

Ostland VE et al: Case report: Granulomatous peritonitis in fish associated with *Fusarium solani, Vet Rec* 121:595-596, 1987.

Ostland VE et al: Bacterial gill disease of salmonids: relationship between the severity of gill lesions and bacterial recovery, *Dis Aquatic Org* 9:5-14, 1990.

Otis EJ: Lesions of coldwater disease in steelhead trout (*Salmo gairdneri*): the role of *Cytophaga psychrophila* extracellular products. Master's thesis, University of Rhode Island, 1984.

Otte E: Eine mykose bei einem Stachelrochen (*Trigon pastinaceae*), *Wiener Tierarzliche Monaksschrift* 51:171-175, 1964.

Overstreet RM: Coccidiosis of killifishes. In Sindermann CJ, Lightner DV, editors: *Disease diagnosis and control in North American marine aquaculture,* New York, 1988, Elsevier, pp. 373-376.

Pagenkopf GK: Gill surface interaction model for trace-metal toxicity to fishes: role of complexation, pH, and water hardness, *Environ Sci Technol* 17:342-347, 1983.

Palmer R et al: Preliminary trials on the efficacy of ivermectin against parasitic copepods of Atlantic salmon, *Bull Eur Assn Fish Pathol* 7:47-54, 1987.

Panasenko NM, Jukhimenko SS, Kaplanova NF: On the infection rate of Far East salmon of the genus *Oncorhynchus* with the parasitic copepod *Lepeiophtheirus salmonis* in the liman of the Amun, *Parazitologiya* 20: 327-329, 1986.

Paperna I: Parasites and diseases of the grey mullet (Mugilidae) with special reference to the seas of the Near East, *Aquacult* 5:65-80, 1975.

Paperna I: Study of *Caligus minimus* (Otto, 1821) (Caligidae Copepoda) infections of the sea bass, *Dicentrarchus labrax* (L.) in Bardawil lagoon, *Annales de Parasitologie humaine et comparee (Pariah)* 55:686-706, 1980.

Paperna I: Reproduction cycle and tolerance to temperature and salinity of *Amyloodinium ocellatum* (Brown, 1931) (Dinoflagellida), *Annales de Parasitologie Humanine et Comparee* 59:7-30, 1984.

Paperna I: Solving parasite-related problems in cultured marine fish, *Int J Parasitol* 17: 368-376, 1987.

Paperna I: Diseases caused by parasites in the aquaculture of warm water fish, *Ann Rev Fish Dis* 1:155-194, 1991.

Paperna I, Colorni A, Ross B, Colorni B: *Diseases of marine fish cultured in Eilat mariculture project based at the Gulf of Aqaba, Red Sea,* European Mariculture Society Special Publication 6:81-91, 1981.

Paperna I, Diamant A, Overstreet RM: Monogenean infestations and mortality in wild and cultured Red Sea fishes, *Helgolander Meeresunters* 37:445-462, 1984.

Paperna I, Hartley AH, Cross RHM: Ultrastructural studies on the plasmodium of *Myxidium giardi* (Myxosporea) and its attachment to the epithelium of the urinary bladder, *Intl J Parasitol* 17:817-819, 1987.

Paperna I, Landsberg JH, Feinstein N: Ultrastructure of the macrogamont of *Goussia cichlidarum* Landberg and Paperna, 1985, a coccidian parasite in the swimbladder of cichlid fish, *Ann Parasitol Hum Comp* 61:511-520, 1986.

Paperna I, Overstreet R: Parasites and diseases of mullets (Mugilidae) In Oren OH, editor: *Aquaculture of grey mullets,* Cambridge, Mass., 1981, Cambridge University Press, pp. 411-493.

Paperna I, SabnaiI, Zachary A: Ultrastructural studies in piscine epitheliocystis: evidence for a pleomorphic development cycle, *J Fish Dis* 4:459-472, 1981.

Paperna I, Van As JG: The pathology of *Chilodonella hexasticha* (Kiernik) infections in cichlid fishes, *J Fish Biol* 23:441-450, 1983.

Paperna I, Zwerner D: Parasites and diseases of striped bass, *Morone saxatilis* (Walbaum), from the lower Chesapeake Bay, *J Fish Biol* 9:267-287, 1976.

Parker JC: Studies on the natural history of *Ichthyophthirius mulfifiliis* Fouquet 1876, an ectoparasitic ciliate of fish. Master's thesis, Department of Zoology, University of Maryland, 1965, pp. 83.

Pascho RJ, Elliott DG, Mallett RW, Mulcahy D: Comparison of five techniques for the detection of *Renibacterium salmoninarum* in adult sockeye salmon, *Trans Am Fish Soc* 116:882-890, 1987.

Paterson WB, Desser SS: The biology of two *Eimeria* species (Protista: Apicomplexa) in their mutual fish host in Ontario, *Can J Zool* 60:764-775, 1982.

Pauley GB, Nakatani RE: Histopathology of gas-bubble disease in salmon fingerlings, *J Fish Res Board Can* 24:867-870, 1967.

Pazos F, Santos Y, Nunez S, Toranzo AE: Increasing occurrence of *Flexibacter maritimus* in the marine aquaculture of Spain, *Fish Health Sec Am Fish Soc Newsltr* 21(3):1, 1993.

Pearce, M: *Epizootic ulcerative syndrome technical report,* Northern Territory (Australia) Department of Primary Industry and Fisheries Fishery Report No. 22, December, 1987, through September, 1989, p. 82.

Pearse L, Pullin RSV, Conroy DA, McGregor D: Observations on the use of Furanace for the control of *Vibrio* disease in marine flatfish, *Aquacult* 3:295-302, 1974.

Pellerdy L, Molnar K: Known and unknown eimerian parasites of fishes in Hungary, *Folia Parasitol (Prague)* 15:97-105, 1968.

Perkins FO: Phylogenetic considerations of the problematic thraustochytriaceous–labyrinthulid-*Dermocystidium* complex based on observations of fine structure, *Veroff Inst Meeresforsch Bremerh* 5 (suppl):45-63, 1974.

Petrochenko VI, Skrjabin KI, editor: *Acanthocephala of domestic and wild animals,* Washington, DC, 1971, Israel Program for Scientific Translations, Ltd., National Science Foundation.

Petrushevski GK, Shulman SS: The parasitic diseases of fishes in the natural waters of the USSR. In Dogiel VA, Petrushevski GK, Polyanski YI, editors: *Parasitology of fishes,* London, 1961, p. 384 (English translation by Kabata Z, Oliver and Boyd, Edinburgh, 1970).

Pfeil-Putzien C: Experimental transmission of spring viremia of carp through carp lice (*Argulus foliaceus*), *Zentralblatt fur Veterinarmedizin* 258:319-323, 1978 (in German).

Pickering AD, Willoughby LG: Epidermal lesions and fungal infection on the perch, *Perca fluviatilis* L., in Windermere, *J Fish Biol* 11:349-354, 1977.

Pierotti P: Su di particolare episodiodi micosi in *Tinca tinca*, *Atti Soc Ital Sci Vet* 25:361-363, 1971.

Pike AW: Sea lice: Major pathogens of farmed Atlantic salmon, *Parasitol Today* 5:291-297, 1989.

Pillay TVR: *Aquaculture: principles and practices,* Oxford, England, 1993, Fishing News Books.

Piper RG et al: *Fish hatchery management,* Washington, DC, 1982, United States Department of the Interior, Fish and Wildlife Service, p. 517.

Plumb JA: Survival of channel catfish virus in chilled, frozen and decomposing channel catfish, *Prog Fish-cult* 35:170-172, 1973.

Plumb JA, editor: Principal diseases of farm-raised catfish, Southern Cooperative Series No. 225, Auburn University, Alabama, 1979, 92 pp.

Plumb JA: Epizootiology of channel catfish virus disease, *Mar Fish Rev* 40:26-29, 1978.

Plumb JA: Relationship of water quality and infectious diseases in channel catfish, *Symp Biol Hung* 23:189-199, 1984.

Plumb JA: *Edwardsiella* septicemia. In Inglis V, Roberts RJ, Bromage NR, editors: *Bacterial diseases of fish,* New York, 1993, Halsted Press, pp. 60-79.

Plumb JA, Bowser PR, Grizzle JM, Mitchell AJ: Fish viruses: a double-stranded RNA icosahedral virus from a North American cyprinid, *J Fish Res Bd Can* 36:1390-1394, 1979.

Plumb JA, Chappell J: Susceptibility of blue catfish to channel catfish virus, *Proc Ann Conf Southeast Assn Fish Wildlife Ag* 32:680-685, 1978.

Plumb JA et al: *Streptococcus* sp. from marine fishes along the Alabama and northwest Florida coast of the Gulf of Mexico, *Trans Am Fish Soc* 103:358-361, 1974.

Plumb JA, Horowitz SA. Rogers WA: Feed-related anemia in cultured channel catfish (*Ictalurus punctatus*), *Aquacult* 51:175-179, 1986.

Plumb JA, Liu PR, Butterworth CE: Folate-degrading bacteria in channel catfish feeds, *J Appl Aquacult* 1:33-43, 1991.

Plumb JA, Quinlan EE: Survival of *Edwardsiella ictaluri* in pond water and bottom mud, *Prog Fish-cult* 48:212-214, 1986.

Plumb JA, Sanchez DJ: Susceptibility of five species of fish to *Edwardsiella ictaluri*, *J Fish Dis* 6:261-266, 1983.

Plumb JA, Thune RL, Klesius PH: Detection of channel catfish virus in adult fish, *Dev Biol Standard* 49:29-34, 1981.

Poirier A, Baudin-Laurencin F, Bodennec G, Quentel C: Intoxication experimentale de la truite arc-en-ciel, *Salmo gairdneri* Richardson, par du gas-oil moteur: modifications haematologiques, histologie, *Aquacult* 55:115-137, 1986.

Polglase JL: Thraustochytrids as potential pathogens of marine animals, *Bull Brit Mycol Soc* 16(suppl 1):5, 1981.

Porter D: Mycoses of marine organisms: an overview of pathogenic fungi. In Moss ST, editor: *The biology of marine fungi*, New York, 1986, Cambridge University Press, pp. 141-153.

Post G, Powers DV, Kloppel TM: Survival of rainbow trout eggs after receiving physical shocks of known magnitude, *Trans Am Fish Soc* 103:711-716, 1974.

Post GW: Carbonic acid anesthesia for aquatic organisms, *Prog Fishcult* 41:142-143, 1979.

Post GW: *Textbook of fish health*, Neptune City, N.J., 1983, TFH Publications, 256 pp.

Post GW: *Textbook of fish health*, ed 2, Neptune City, N.J., 1987, TFH Publications, 288 pp.

Price RL: Incidence of *Pleistophora cepedianae* (Microsporidia) in gizzard shad (*Dorosoma cepedianum*) on Carlyle Lake, Illinois, *J Parasitol* 68:1167-1168, 1982.

Pritchard NH, Malsberger RG: A cytochemical study of lymphocystis tumors in vivo, *J Exp Zool* 169:371-380, 1968.

Probasco D, Noga E, Khoo L: Fibrosarcoma in a goldfish, *J Small Exotic Animal Med* 2:173-175, 1994..

Prosser CL: Temperature. In Prosser CL, editor: *Comparative animal physiology*, vol 1, Philadelphia, 1973a, WB Saunders, pp. 362-428.

Prosser CL: Water, osmotic balance, hormonal regulation. In Prosser CL, editor: *Comparative animal physiology*, vol 1, Philadelphia, 1973b, WB Saunders, pp. 1-78.

Pulsford A, Matthews RA: An ultrastructural study of *Myxobolus exiguus* Thelohan, 1895 (Myxsporea) from grey mullet, *Crenimugil labrosus* (Risso), *J Fish Dis* 5:509-526, 1982.

Putz RE: *Parasites of freshwater fish. II. Protozoa. I. Microsporidea of fish*, Washington, D.C., 1964. Fishery Leaflet No. 571, United States Department of the Interior, pp. 1-4.

Putz RE, Hoffman GL, Dunbar CE: Two new species of *Pleistophora* (Microsporidea) from North American fish with a synopsis of Microsporidea of freshwater and euryhaline fishes, *J Protozool* 12:228-236, 1965.

Pyle SW, Shotts EB: DNA homology studies of selected flexibacteria associated with fish disease, *Can J Fish Aquat Sci* 38:146-151, 1981.

Pyle SW, Shotts EB: A new method of differentiating *Flexibacteria* from cold-water and warmwater fish, *Can J Fish Aquatic Sci* 37: 1040-1042, 1980.

Rach JJ, Bills TB, Marking LL: *Effects of physical and chemical factors on the toxicity of chloramine-T,* United States Fish and Wildlife Service Research Information Bulletin, 1988, pp. 88-69.

Rae GH: On the trail of the sea louse, *Fish Farmer* 2:22-23, 25, 1979.

Raikova EV: Life cycle, cytology, and morphology of *Polypodium hydriforme*, a coelenterate parasite of the eggs of acipenseriform fishes, *J Parasitol* 80:1-22, 1994.

Ransom DP, Lannan CN, Rohovec JS, Fryer JL: Comparison of histopathology caused by *Vibrio anguillarum* and *Vibrio ordalii* and three species of Pacific salmon, *J Fish Dis* 7:107-115, 1984.

Reichenbach HH: Cytophagales. In Stanley JT, Bryant MP, Pfennig N, Holt JG, editors: *Bergey's manual of systematic bacteriology*, vol 3, Baltimore, 1989, Williams & Wilkins, pp. 2015-2050.

Reichenbach-Klinke HH: *Some aspects of mycobacterial infections in fish.* Symposium of the Zoological Society of London No. 30, 1972, pp. 17-24.

Reichenbache-Klinke HH: Uber einige bisher ubekannte Hyphomyceten bei Verscheidenen Suswasser und Meeresfischen, *Mycopath Mycol Appl* 7:333-368, 1956.

Reichenbache-Klinke HH: *Fish pathology,* Neptune City, N.J., 1973, TFH Publications.

Reid W, Anderson D: *Regional fishery management investigations: region 3 stream investigations,* Idaho Department of Fish and Game Report, 1982, pp. 17-26.

Rensel JE: Severe blood hypoxia of Atlantic salmon (*Salmo salar*) exposed to the marine diatom *Chaetoceros concavicornis.* In Smayda T, Shimizu Y, editors: *Toxic phytoplankton blooms in the sea,* New York, 1993, Elsevier, pp. 625-630.

Reyes XP, Bravo SS: Nota sombre una copepodosis en salmones de cultivo, *Investigaciones Marinas Valparaiso* 11:55-57, 1983.

Richard J: *Sea lice in North America: experiences and concerns,* Report to the British Columbia Aquaculture Research and Development Council, 1991.

Richards RH, Buchanan JS: Studies on *Herpesvirus scophthalmi* infection of turbot *Scophthalmus maximus* (L.): histopathological observations, *J Fish Dis* 1:251-258, 1978.

Richards RH, Holliman A, Helagson S: *Exophiala salmonis* infection in Atlantic salmon, *Salmo salar* L, *J Fish Dis* 1:357-368, 1978.

Richards RH, Pickering AD: Changes in serum parameters of *Saprolegnia*-infected brown trout, *Salmo trutta* L, *J Fish Dis* 2:197-206, 1979.

Riggs SR et al: *Heavy metal pollutants in organic-rich muds of the Pamlico River estuarine system: their concentration, distribution, and effects upon benthic environments and water quality.* Final Report to the Albemarle/Pamlico Estuarine Study, Raleigh, N.C., 1989, p. 108.

Rijkers GT, Teunissen AG, Van Oosterom AG, van Muisiwinkel R: The immune system of cyprinid fish: the immunosuppressive effect of the antibiotic oxytetracycline in carp (*Cyprinus carpio*), *Aquacult* 19:177-189, 1980.

Roald SO, Hastein T: Infection with an *Acinetobacter*-like bacterium in Atlantic salmon (*Salmo salar*) broodfish. In Ahne W, editor: *Fish diseases: third COPRAQ session,* Berlin, 1980, Springer-Verlag, pp. 154-156.

Roberts RJ: Pathophysiology and systemic pathology of teleosts. In Roberts RJ, editor: *Fish pathology,* London, 1989a, Bailliere-Tindall, pp. 56-134.

Roberts RJ: Rugged species near the top in farming, *Fish Farm Int* August, 1989b, p. 6.

Roberts RJ: The mycology of teleosts. In *Fish pathology,* ed 2, London, 1989c, Bailliere-Tindall, pp. 320-326.

Roberts RJ: Motile aeromonad septicemia. In Inglis V, Roberts RJ, Bromage NR, editors: *Bacterial diseases of fish,* New York, 1993, Halsted Press, pp. 143-156.

Roberts RJ, Bullock AM: Nutritional pathology. In Halver JE, editor: *Fish nutrition,* ed 2, New York, 1989, Academic Press, pp. 423-473.

Roberts RJ et al: *Field and laboratory investigations into ulcerative fish diseases in the Asia-Pacific region,* FAO, Tech. Rep FAO Proj TCP/RAS/4508, Bangkok, 1986, p. 214.

Roberts RJ, Horne MT: Bacterial meningitis in farmed rainbow trout *Salmo gairdneri* affected with chronic pancreatic necrosis, *J Fish Dis* 1:157-164, 1978.

Roberts RJ, McKnight IJ: The pathology of infectious pancreatic necrosis. II. Stress-mediated recurrence, *Brit Vet J* 132:209-214, 1976.

Roberts RJ, Willoughby LG, Chinabut AS: Mycotic aspects of epizootic ulcerative syndrome (EUS) in Asian fishes, *J Fish Dis* 16:169-183, 1993.

Robinson EH, Brent JR, Crabtree JT, Tucker CS: Improved palatability of channel catfish feeds containing Romet-30^R, *J Aquatic Animal Health* 2:43-48, 1990.

Robohm RA: *Pasteurella piscida.* In Anderson DP, Dorson M, Daborget P, editors: *Antigens of fish pathogens,* Collection Foundation Marcel Merieux, Lyon, 1983, pp. 161-175.

Rogers CJ, Austin B: Oxolinic acid for control of enteric redmouth disease in rainbow trout, 112:83, 1982.

Rogers WA: Protozoan parasites. In Plumb JA, editor: *Principal diseases of farm-raised catfish,* Southern Cooperative Research Series No. 225, Alabama Agricultural Experimental Station, Auburn University, Alabama, 1979, pp. 28-37.

Rohde K: Diseases caused by metazoans: Helminths. In Kinne O, editor: *Diseases of marine animals,* vol 4, Hamburg, Germany, 1984, Pisces, Biological Anstalt Helgoland, pp. 193-320.

Rose AS, Ellis AE, Munro ALS: The infectivity of different routes of exposure and shedding rates of *Aeromonas salmonicida* subsp. *salmonicida* in Atlantic salmon, *Salmo salar* L., held in seawater, *J Fish Dis* 12:573-578, 1989.

Ross AJ, Earp BJ, Wood JW: *Mycobacterial infections in adult salmon and steelhead trout returning to the Columbia River basin and other areas in 1957,* United States Fish and Wildlife Service, Special Scientific Report on Fisheries 332, 1959, p. 34.

Ross AJ, Johnson HE: Studies of transmission of mycobacterial infections in chinook salmon, *Prog Fish-cult* 24:147-149, 1962.

Ross AJ, Yasutake WT, Leek S: *Scolecobasidium humicola,* a fungal pathogen of fish, *J Fish Res Bd Can* 30:994-995, 1975.

Roth M, Richards RH, Sommerville C: Current practices in the chemotherapeutic control of sea lice infections in aquaculture: a review, *J Fish Dis* 16:1-26, 1993.

Ruangpan L, Kabata Z: An invertebrate host for *Caligus* (Copepoda, Caligidae)? *Crustaceana* 47:219-220, 1984.

Rucker RR: A streptomycete pathogenic to fish, *J Bacteriol* 58:659-664, 1949.

Rucker RR: Redmouth disease of rainbow trout (*Salmo gairdneri*), *Bull L'Office Int Epizoot* 65:825-830, 1966.

Russell PH: Lymphocystis in wild plaice *Pleuronectes platessa* (L.) and flounder *Platichthys flesus* (L.) in British coastal waters: a histopathological and serological study, *J Fish Biol* 6:771-778, 1974.

Russo RC: Ammonia, nitrite and nitrate. In Rand GM, Petrocelli SR, editors: *Fundamentals of aquatic toxicology,* Hemisphere, New York, 1985, pp. 455-471.

Rychlinski RA, Deardorff TL: *Spirocamallanus*: a potential fish health problem, *Freshwater Mar Aquar* Feb, pp. 22-23, 1982.

Saeed MO, Alamoudi MM, Al-Harbi A-H: A *Pseudomonas* associated with disease in cultured rabbitfish *Siganus rivulatus* in the Red Sea, *Dis Aquatic Org* 3:177-180, 1987.

Salte R, Liestol K: Drug withdrawal from farmed fish: depletion of oxytetracycline, sulfadiazine, and trimethoprim from muscular tissue of rainbow trout (*Salmo gairdneri*), *Acta Vet Scand* 24:418-430, 1983.

Samuelsen OB: Aeration rate, pH and temperature effects on the degradation of trichlorphon to DDVP and the half-lives of trichlorphon and DDVP in sea water, *Aquacult* 66:373-380, 1987.

Sanders JE, Fryer JL, Leith DA, Moore KD: Control of the infectious protozoan *Ceratomyxa shasta* by treating hatchery water supplies, *Prog Fish-cult* 34:13-17, 1972.

Sano T: Viral diseases of cultured fishes in Japan, *Fish Pathol* 10:221-226, 1976.

Sano T, Fukuda H: Principal microbial diseases of mariculture in Japan, *Aquacult* 67:59-69, 1987.

Sano T, Fukuda N, Okamoto N, Kaneko F: Yamame tumor virus: lethality and oncogenicity, *Bull Japan Soc Sci Fish* 49:1159-1163, 1983.

Sano T, Morita N, Shima N, Akimoto M: A preliminary report on pathogenicity of cyprinid herpesvirus, *Bull Eur Assn Fish Pathol* 10:11-13, 1990.

Sano T, Okamoto N, Nishimura T: A new viral epizootic of *Anguilla japonica* Temminck and Schlegel, *J Fish Dis* 4:127-139, 1981.

Sato N, Yamane N, Kawamura T: Systemic *Citrobacter freundii* infection among sunfish *Mola mola* in Matsushima aquarium, *Bull Japan Soc Sci Fish* 48:1551-1557, 1982.

Scallan A, Smith PR: Control of asymptomatic carriage of *Aeromonas salmonicida* in Atlantic salmon smolts with flumequine. In Ellis AE, editor: *Fish and shellfish pathology,* New York, 1985, Academic Press, pp. 119-127.

Scarano G, Saroglia MG: Recovery of fish from functional and haemolytic anemia after brief exposure to a lethal concentration of nitrite, *Aquacult* 43:421-426, 1984.

Scarano G, Saroglia MG, Gray RH, Tibaldi E: Hematological response of sea bass *Dicentrarchus labrax* to sublethal nitrite exposures, *Trans Am Fish Soc* 113:360-364, 1984.

Schachte JA: Coldwater disease. In Meyer FP, Warren JW, Carey TG, editors: *A guide to integrated fish health management in the Great Lakes basin,* Special Publication No. 83-2, Great Lakes Fishery Commission, Ann Arbor, Mich., 1983, pp. 193-197.

Schaperclaus W: Der Colisa-Parasit, ein neuer Krankheitserreger bei Aquarienfischen, *Die Aquarien- und Terrarienzeitschrift* 4:169-171, 1951.

Schaperclaus W: *Fischkrankheiten (fish diseases),* vol 1, New Delhi, 1991a, Amerind Publishing, p. 594.

Schaperclaus W: *Fischkrankheiten (fish diseases),* vol 2, New Delhi, 1991b, Amerind Publishing, p. 1398.

Schiewe MH, Novotny AJ, Harrell LW: Botulism of salmonids, *Dev Aquacult Fish Sci* 17:336-338, 1988.

Schiewe MH, Trust TJ, Crosa JH: *Vibrio ordalii* sp. nov.: a causative agent of vibriosis in fish, *Current Microbiol* 6:343-348, 1981.

Schmahl G, El Toukhy A, Ghaffar FA: Transmission electron microscopic studies on the effects of toltrazuril on *Glugea anomala,* Moniez, 1887 (Microsporidia) infecting the three-spined stickleback *Gasterosteus aculeatus, Parasitol Res* 76:700-706, 1990.

Schmahl G, Melhorn H, Haberkorn A: Symposium triazinone (toltrazuril) effective against fish-parasitizing Monogenea, *Parasitol Res* 75:67-68, 1988.

Schmahl G, Taraschewski H: Treatment of fish parasites. II. *Parasitol Res* 341-351, 1987.

Schmidt GD: *CRC handbook of tapeworm identification,* Boca Raton, Fla., 1986, CRC Press.

Schneider JA: The killing of Rush Creek, *Water Spectrum* 12:38-43, 1979.

Schnick RA: *Formalin as a therapeutant in fish culture,* United States Fish and Wildlife Service, Report No. FWS-LR-74-15, 1973, p. 131.

Schnick RA: Registration status report for fishery compounds, *Fisheries* 17:12-13, 1992.

Schnick RA, Meyer FP, Gray DL: *A guide to approved chemicals in fish production and fishery resource management,* United States Fish and Wildlife Service, and University of Arkansas Cooperative Extension Service, MP 241-89, Little Rock, 1989.

Schnick RA, Meyer FP, Walsh DF: Status of fishery chemicals in 1985, *Prog Fish-cult* 48:1-17, 1986.

Schoenecker W, Rhodes W: Potassium permanganate dispenser, *Prog Fish-cult* 27:55-56, 1965.

Schoettger RA, Julin AM: *Efficacy of MS-222 on as an anesthetic on four salmonids,* United States Fish and Wildlife Service Investment in Fish Control 13, 1967.

Schreck CB: Stress and compensation in teleostean fishes: response to social and physical factors. In Pickering AD, editor: *Stress and fish,* New York, 1981, Academic Press, pp. 295-322.

Schultz M, May EB, Kraeuter JL, Hetrick FM: Isolation of infectious pancreatic necrosis virus from an epizootic occurring in cultured striped bass, *Morone saxatilis* (Walbaum), *J Fish Dis* 10:29-34, 1984.

Schwedler TE, Tucker CS, Beleau CS, Beleau MH: Non-infectious diseases. In Tucker CS, editor: *Channel catfish culture,* Elsevier, Amsterdam, 1985, pp. 497-541.

Scott AL, Rogers WA: Histological effects of prolonged sublethal hypoxia on channel catfish, *Ictalurus punctatus* (Rafinesque), *J Fish Dis* 3:305-316, 1980.

Scott P: Therapy in aquaculture. In Brown L, editor: *Aquaculture for veterinarians,* New York, 1993, Pergamon Press, pp. 131-152.

Scott WW, O'Bier Jr AH: Aquatic fungi associated with diseased fish and fish eggs, *Prog Fish-cult* 24:3-15, 1962.

Scott WW, Warren CO: Studies of the host range and chemical control of fungi associated with diseased tropical fish, *Va Agricul Exp Sta Blacksburg Tech Bull* 24:171, 1964.

Seymour R, Fuller MS: Collection and isolation of water molds (Saprolegniaceae) from water and soil. In Fuller MS, Jaworski A, editors: *Zoosporic fungi in teaching and research,* Athens, Ga., 1987, Southeastern Publishing, pp. 125-127.

Shah KL, Tyagi BC: An eye disease in silver carp, *Hypophthalmichthys molitrix,* held in tropical ponds, associated with the bacterium *Staphylococcus aureus, Aquaculture* 55:1-4, 1986.

Shaharom-Harrison FM et al: Epizootics of Malaysian cultured freshwater pond fishes by *Piscinoodinium pillulare* (Schaperclaus, 1954) Lom, 1981, *Aquacult* 86:127-138, 1990.

Shields RJ, Goode RP: Host rejection of *Lernaea cyprinacea* L. (Copepoda), *Crustaceana* 35:301-307, 1978.

Shields RJ, Sperber RG: Osmotic relationships of *Lernaea cyprinacea* L, *Crustaceana* 26:157-171, 1974.

Shilo M: The toxic principles of *Prymnesium parvum.* In Carmichael WW, editor: *The water environment: algal toxins and health,* New York, 1981, Plenum Press, pp. 22-47.

Shimura S, Inoue K, Kudo M, Egusa S: Studies on effects of parasitism of *Argulus coregoni* (Crustacea: Branchiura) on furunculosis of *Oncorhynchus masou* (Salmonidae), *Fish Pathol* 18:37-40, 1983.

Shiomitsu K, Kusuda R, Osuga H, Munekiyo M: Studies on chemotherapy of fish disease with erythromycin. II. Its clinical studies against streptococcal infection in cultured yellowtails, *Fish Pathol* 15:17-23, 1980.

Short JW, Thrower FP: Toxicity of tri-N-butyl-tin to chinook salmon, *Oncorhynchus tshawytscha,* adapted to seawater, *Aquacult* 61:193-200, 1987.

Shotts EB, Blazer VS, Waltman WD: Pathogenesis of experimental *Edwardsiella ictaluri* infections in channel catfish (*Ictalurus punctatus*), *Can J Fish Aquatic Sci* 43:36-42, 1986.

Shotts EB, Rimler R: Medium for the isolation of *Aeromonas hydrophila, Appl Micro* 26:550-553, 1973.

Shotts EB, Talkington FD, Elliot DG, McCarthy DH: Aetiology of an ulcerative disease in goldfish, *Carassius auratus* (L.): characterization of the causative agent, *J Fish Dis* 3:181-186, 1980.

Shotts EB, Teska JD: Bacterial pathogens of aquatic vertebrates. In Austin B, Austin DA, editors: *Methods for the microbiological examination of fish and shellfish,* New York, 1989, John Wiley & Sons, pp. 164-186.

Shotts EB, Tsu TC, Waltman WD: Extracellular proteolytic activity of *Aeromonas hydrophila* complex, *Fish Pathol* 20:37-44, 1985.

Shotts EB, Vanderwork VL, Cambell LN: Occurrence of R factors associated with *Aeromonas hydrophila* isolates from aquarium fish and waters, *J Fish Res Bd Can* 33:736-740, 1976.

Shulman SS, Jankovski AV: Phylum Ciliates-Ciliophora Doflein, 1901. In Shulman SS, editor: *Parasitic protozoa,* vol 1. In Bauer ON, editor: *Key to parasites of freshwater fishes of U.S.S.R.,* vol 140 of *Keys to the fauna of the U.S.S.R.,* Nauka, Leningrad, 1984, pp. 252-280 (in Russian).

Sills JB: *A review of the literature on the use of lime (Ca[OH]₂, CaO, CaCO₃) in fisheries,* United States Fish and Wildlife Service, Washington, DC, 1974, p. 30.

Simon RC, Schill WB: Tables of sample size requirements for detection of fish infected by pathogens: three confidence levels for different infection prevalence and various population sizes, *J Fish Dis* 7:515-520, 1984.

Sindermann CJ: *Principal diseases of marine fish and shellfish,* ed 2, vol 1, New York, 1990, Academic Press.

Sitja-Bobadilla A, Alvarez-Pellitero P: *Sphaerospora testicularis* sp. nov. (Myxosporea: Sphaerosporidae) in wild and cultured sea bass, *Dicentrarchus labrax* (L.), from the Spanish Mediterranean area, *J Fish Dis* 13:193-203, 1990.

Skea JC, Simonin HA: Evaluation of Cutrine for use in fish culture, *Prog Fish-cult* 41:171-174, 1979.

Smart GR: Aspects of water quality producing stress in intensive fish culture. In Pickering AD, editor: *Stress and fish,* New York, 1981, Academic Press, pp. 277-293.

Smayda TJ: Novel and nuisance phytoplankton blooms in the sea: evidence for a global epidemic. In Graneli E, Sundstrom B, Edler L, Anderson DM, editors: *Toxic marine phytoplankton,* New York, 1990, Elsevier, pp. 29-40.

Smith AC, Ramos F: Occult haemoglobin in fish skin mucus as an indicator of early stress, *J Fish Biol* 9:537-541, 1976.

Smith JE, editor: *Torrey Canyon pollution and marine life,* Marine Biological Association, Cambridge, UK, 1968, Cambridge University Press.

Smith SA, Noga EJ: General parasitology. In Stoskopf MK: *Fish medicine,* Philadelphia, 1993, WB Saunders, pp. 132-148.

Smith SA, Noga EJ, Bullis RA: *Mortality in Tilapia aurea due to a toxic dinoflagellate bloom,* Proceedings of the Third International Collectors of Pathological Marine Aquaculture, Gloucester Point, Va., 1988, pp. 167-168.

Smith SA, Noga EJ, Levy MG, Gerig TM: Effect of serum from *Oreochromis aureus,* immunized with dinospores of *Amyloodinium ocellatum,* on the motility, infectivity and growth of the parasite in cell culture, *Dis Aquatic Organ* 15:73-80, 1993.

Smith SA, Levy MG, Noga EJ: Detection of anti-*Amyloodinium ocellatum* antibody from cultured hybrid striped bass during an epizootic of amyloodiniosis, *J Aquatic Animal Health* 6:79-81, 1994.

Snieszko SF, Bullock GL, Hollis E, Boone JG: *Pasteurella* species from an epizootic of white perch (*Roccus americanus*) in Chesapeake Bay tidewater areas, *J Bacteriol* 88:1814-1815, 1964.

Snieszko SF: The effects of environmental stress on outbreaks of infectious diseases of fishes, *J Fish Biol* 6:197-208, 1974.

Snyder DE: Impacts of electrofishing on fish, *Fisheries* 20(1):26-27, 1995.

Solangi MA, Overstreet RM: Biology and pathogenesis of the coccidium *Eimeria funduli* infecting killifishes, *J Parasitol* 66:513-526, 1980.

Sommerville C: A comparative study of the tissue response to invasion and encystment by *Stephanochasmus baccatus* (Nicoll, 1907) (Digenea: acanthocolpidae) in four species of flatfish, *J Fish Dis* 4:53-68, 1981.

Sonstegard RA, Sonstegard KS: Herpesvirus-associated epidermal hyperplasia in fish (carp). In de The G, Henle W, Rapp F, editors: *Proceedings of an international symposium on oncogenes and herpesviruses,* International Agency Research Cancer-Science Publications No. 24, 1978, pp. 863-868, 1978.

Sorensen EM: *Metal poisoning in fish,* Boca Raton, Fla., 1991, CRC Press, p. 383.

Sorimachi M: Pathogenicity of ICD virus isolated from Japanese eel, *Bull Nat Res Inst Aquacult* 6:71-75, 1984.

Sorimachi M, Egusa S: A histopathological study of ICDV infection of Japanese eel, *Anguilla japonica, Bull Nat Res Inst Aquacult* 12:87-92, 1987.

Sorimachi M, Hara T: Characteristics and pathogenicity of a virus isolated from yellowtail fingerlings showing ascites, *Fish Pathol* 19:231-238, 1985.

Speare DJ et al: Pathology of bacterial gill disease: ultrastructure of branchial lesions, *J Fish Dis* 14:1-20, 1991.

Spotte S: *Fish and invertebrate culture,* New York, 1979a, John Wiley & Sons, p. 179.

Spotte S: *Seawater aquariums,* New York, 1979b, John Wiley & Sons, p. 413.

Spotte S: *Captive seawater fishes: science and technology,* New York, 1992, John Wiley & Sons, p. 942.

Sprague V, Hussey KL: Observations of *Ichthyosporidium giganteum* (Microspordia) with particular reference to the host-parasite relations during merogony, *J Protozool* 27:169-175, 1980.

Stadtlander C, Kirchoff H: Gill organ culture of rainbow trout, *Salmo gairdneri* Richardson: an experimental model for the study of pathogenicity of *Mycoplasma mobile* 163 K, *J Fish Dis* 12:79-86, 1989.

Stamm J: In vitro activity and resistance development for sarafloxacin (A-56620): an aquaculture antibacterial. In Michel C, Alderman DJ, editors: *Chemotherapy in aquaculture: from theory to reality,* Paris, 1992, Office International des Epizooties, pp. 333-339.

Starliper CE, Shotts Jr EB, Hsu T, Schill WB: Genetic relatedness of some gram-negative yellow pigmented bacteria from fishes and aquatic environments, *Microbios* 56:181-198, 1988.

Steffens W: *Principles of fish nutrition,* Chichester, 1989, Ellis Horwood, p. 384.

Steidinger KA, Baden D: Toxic marine dinoflagellates. In Spector DL, editor: *Dinoflagellates,* New York, 1984, Academic Press, pp. 201-261.

Steinhagen D, Kirting W, van Muiswinkel WB: Morphology and biology of *Goussia carpelli* (Protozoa: Apicomplexa) from the intestine of experimentally infected common carp *Cyprinus carpio, Dis Aquatic Org* 6:93-98, 1989.

Sterba G: *The aquarium encyclopedia.* Poole, Dorset, U.K., 1983, Blandford Books, p. 605 (Translated by Lexicon der Aquaristik Ichthyologie).

Stevenson JP: *Trout farming manual,* ed 2, Oxford, England, 1987, Fishing News Books, 259 pp.

Stevenson R, Flett D, Raymond BT: Enteric redmouth (ERM) and other entobacterial infections of fish. In Inglis V, Roberts RJ, Bromage NR, editors: *Bacterial diseases of fish,* New York, 1993, Halsted Press, pp. 80-106.

Stickley Jr AR: *Avian predators on southern aquaculture,* Southern Regional Aquaculture Center Publication No. 400, US Department of Agriculture, Washington, DC, 1990, US Government Printing Office.

Stirling HP, editor: *Chemical and biological methods of water analysis for aquaculturists,* Stirling, Scotland, 1985, Institute of Aquaculture.

Stoskopf MK: Taking the history, *Vet Clin N Am Small Animal Prac* 16:283-291, 1988.

Straus DL, Tucker CS: Acute toxicity of copper sulfate and chelated copper to channel catfish *Ictalurus punctatus, J World Aquacult Soc* 24:390-395, 1993.

Studnicka M, Siwicki A: The nonspecific immunological response in carp (*Cyprinus carpio* L.) during natural infection with *Eimeria subepithelialis, Mamigdeh Israeli J Aquacult* 42:18-21, 1990.

Stumm W, Morgan JJ: *Aquatic chemistry,* New York, 1970, John Wiley & Sons, p. 583.

Styer EL, Harrison LR, Burtle GJ: Experimental production of proliferative gill disease in channel catfish exposed to a myxozoan-infected oligochaete, *Dero digitata, J Aquatic Animal Health* 3:288-291, 1991.

Sugimoto N, Kashiwaga S, Matsuda T: Pathogenic relation between columnaris disease in cultured eel and the formula feeds, *Bull Japan Soc Sci Fish* 47:716-725, 1981.

Summerfelt RC, Smith LS: Anesthesia, surgery and related techniques. In Schreck CB, Moyle PB, editors: *Methods for fish biology,* Bethesda, Md., American Fisheries Society, 1990, pp. 213-272.

Sundstrom B, Edler L, Granelli E: The global distribution and harmful effects of phytoplankton. In Granelli E, Sundstrom B, Edler L, Anderson DM, editors: *Toxic marine phytoplankton,* New York, 1990, Elsevier, pp. 537-541.

Svendsen YS, Haug T: Effectiveness of formalin, benzocaine and hypo- and hypersaline exposures against adults and eggs of *Entobdella hippoglossi* (Muller), an ectoparasite on Atlantic halibut (*Hippoglossus hippoglossus* L.), laboratory studies, *Aquaculture* 94:279-289, 1991,

Svobodova Z, Groch L: Zaberni onemocneni vyvolane invazi *Sphaerospora molnari, Bul VURH Vodnany* 22:13-17, 1986.

Swingle HS: Relationship of pH of pond waters to their suitability for fish culture, *Proc Pacific Sci Congr* 10:72-75, 1961.

Swingle HS: *Methods of analysis for waters, organic matter and pond bottom soils used in fisheries research,* Auburn, Ala., 1969, Auburn University.

Szekely C, Molnar K: Mebendazole is an efficacious drug against pseudogyrodactyolsis in the European eel (*Anguilla anguilla*), *J Appl Ichthyol* 3:183-186, 1987.

Tacon AGJ: *Nutritional fish pathology,* FAO Fisheries Technical Paper No. 330, Rome, 1992, Food and Agriculture Organization of the United Nations, p. 75.

Takahashi S, Egusa S: Studies on *Glugea* infection of the ayu, *Plecoglossus altivelis.* III. Effect of water temperature on the development of xenoma of *Glugea plecoglossi, Japanese J Fish* 11:195-200, 1977.

Takeda T, Itzawa Y: Examination of possibility of applying anesthesia by carbon dioxide in the transportation of live fish, *Bull Japan Soc Sci Fish* 49:725-732, 1983.

Tave D: *Genetics for fish hatchery managers,* ed 2, New York, 1993, Van Nostrand Reinhold, p. 415.

Tave D, Bartels JE, Smitherman RO: Stumpbody *Sarotherodon aureus* (Steindachner) (=*Tilapia aurea*) and tail-less *S. nilotica* (L.) (=*T. nilotica*): two vertebral anomalies and their effects on body length, *J Fish Dis* 5:487-494, 1982.

Taylor PW, Johnson MR: Antibiotic resistance in *Edwardsiella ictaluri, Am Fish Soc Fish Health Sec Newsltr* 19(2):3-4, 1991.

Taylor SG, Bailey JE: *Saprolegnia:* control of fungus on incubating eggs of pink salmon by treatment with seawater, *Prog Fish-cult* 41:181-183, 1979.

TeStrake D, Lim DV: *Bacterial and fungal studies of ulcerative fish in the St. Johns' River,* Report of Contract WM 138 to Florida Department of Environmental Regulation, 1987.

Thoesen JC, editor: *Suggested procedures for the detection and identification of certain fish and shellfish pathogens,* ed 4, version 1, Bethesda, Md., 1994, Fish Health Section/American Fisheries Society.

Thompson Jr JC: A redescription of *Uronema marinum* and a proposed new family, Uronematidae, *Va J Sci* 15:80-87, 1963.

Thompson Jr CJ, Moewus L: *Miamiensis avidus* n.g., n. sp., a marine facultative parasite in the ciliate order Hymenostomatida, *J Protozool* 11:378-381, 1964.

Thoney DA: The effects of trichlorphon, praziquantel, and copper sulphate on various stages of the monogenean *Benedeniella posterocolpa,* a skin parasite of the cownose ray, *Rhinoptera bonasus, J Fish Dis* 13:385-389, 1990.

Thoney D: The effects of various chemicals on monogeneans parasitizing the skin of elasmobranchs. In *American Association of Zoological Parks and Aquariums Annual Proceedings,* Wheeling, W. Va., 1989, The association, pp. 217-222.

Thoney DA, Hargis Jr WJ: Monogenea (Platyhelminthes) as hazards for fish in confinement, *Ann Rev Fish Dis* 1:133-153, 1991.

Thurston RV, Chakonmakos C, Russo RC: Effect of fluctuating exposures on the acute toxicity of ammonia to rainbow trout (*Salmo gairdneri*) and cutthroat trout (*S. clarki*), *Water Res* 15:911-917, 1981.

Tiffney WN: The host range of *Saprolegnia parasitica, Mycologia* 31:310-321, 1939a.

Tiffney WN: The identification of certain species of the Saprolegniaceae parasitic to fish, *J Elisha Mitch Sci Soc* 55:134-151, 1939b.

Tiner JD: Birefringent spores differentiate *Encephalitozoon* and other Microsporidia from Coccidia, *Vet Path* 25:227-230, 1988.

Todaro F et al: Gas ophthalmus in black sea bream *Spondyliosoma cantharus* caused by *Sarcimomyces crustaceus, Mycopathologia* 81:95-98, 1983.

Tomasso JR: Comparative toxicity of nitrite to freshwater fishes, *Aquatic Tox* 8:129-137, 1986.

Tomasso JR et al: Inhibition of nitrite-induced methemoglobinemia in channel catfish (*Ictalurus punctatus*), *J Fish Res Bd Can* 36:1141-1144, 1980.

Tompkins JA, Tsai C: Survival time and lethal exposure time for the blacknose dace exposed to free chlorine and chloramines, *Trans Am Fish Soc* 105:313-321, 1976.

Tookwinas S: Larviculture of seabass (*Lates calcarifer*) and grouper (*Epinephelus malabaricus*) in Thailand: advances in tropical aquaculture, Tahiti, February 20-March 4, 1989, *AQUACOP IFREMER Actes de Colloque* 9:645-659, 1990.

Toranzo A, Hetrick FM: Comparative stability of two salmonid viruses and poliovirus in fresh, estuarine and marine waters, *J Fish Dis* 5:223-231, 1982.

Toranzo AE, Baya AM, Romalde JL, Hetrick FM: Association of *Aeromonas sobria* with mortalities of adult gizzard shad, *Dorosoma capedianum* LeSueur, *J Fish Dis* 12:439-448, 1989.

Toranzo AE et al: Molecular factors associated with virulence of marine vibrios isolated from striped bass in Chesapeake Bay, *Infect Immun* 39:1220-1227, 1983.

Traxler G, Bell G: Pathogens associated with impounded Pacific herring *Clupea harengus pallasi,* with emphasis on viral erythrocytic necrosis (VEN) and atypical *Aeromonas salmonicida, Dis Aquatic Org* 5:93-100, 1988.

Treasurer J, Cox D: The occurrence of *Aeromonas salmonicida* in wrasse (Labridae) and implications for Atlantic salmon farming, *Bull Eur Assoc Fish Pathol* 11:208-210, 1991.

Tripathi YR: Monogenetic trematodes from fishes of India, *Indian J Helminthol* 9:1-49, 1959.

Trust T: Inadequacy of aquarium antibacterial formulations for the inhibition of potential pathogens of freshwater fish, *J Fish Res Bd Can* 29:1425-1430, 1972.

Tsoumas A, Alderman DJ, Rogers CJ: *Aeromonas salmonicida:* development of resistance to 4-quinolone antimicrobials, *J Fish Dis* 12:492-507, 1989.

T'sui WH, Wang CH: On the *Pleistophora* infection in eel. I. Histopathology, ultrastructure and development of *Pleistophora anguillarum* in eel, *Anguilla japonica, Bull Inst Zool Acad Sin Taiwan* 27:159-166, 1988.

Tucker CS: Potassium permanganate demand of pond waters, *Prog Fish-cult* 46:24-28, 1984.

Tucker CS: Water quality. In Tucker CS, editor: *Channel catfish culture,* Amsterdam, 1985, Elsevier, pp. 135-227.

Tucker CS: *Calcium needs for catfish egg hatching and fry survival,* Mississippi Cooperative Extension Service Reference No. 87-2, 1987, pp. 1-2.

Tucker CS: Method for estimating potassium permanganate disease treatment rates for channel catfish on ponds, *Prog Fish-cult* 51:24-26, 1989.

Tucker CS, Boyd CE: Relationship between potassium permanganate treatment and water quality, *Trans Am Fish Soc* 106:481-488, 1977.

Tucker CS, Floyd RF, Beleau MH: Nitrite-induced anemia in channel catfish, *Ictalurus punctatus* (Rafinesque), *Bull Environ Contam Toxicol* 43:295-301, 1989.

Tucker CS, Francis-Floyd R, Beleau MH: Acute toxicity of saponified castor oil to channel catfish, *Ictalurus punctatus,* under laboratory and field conditions, *Bull Environ Contam Toxicol* 37:297-302, 1986.

Tucker L, Boyd CE, McCoy EW: Effects of feeding rate on water quality, production of channel catfish, and economic returns, *Trans Am Fish Soc* 109:446-452, 1979.

Tully O, Morrissey D: Concentrations of dichlorvos in Beirtreach Bui Bay, Ireland, *Marine Pollut Bull* 20:190-191, 1989.

Tung MC et al: An acute septicemic infection of *Pasteurella* organism in pond-cultured Formosa snakehead (*Channa maculata* Lacepede), *Fish Pathol* 20:143-148, 1985.

Turnbull JF: Bacterial gill disease and fin rot. In Inglis V, Roberts RJ, Bromage NR, editors: *Bacterial diseases of fish,* New York, 1993a, Halsted Press, pp. 40-58.

Turnbull JF: Epitheliocystis and salmonid rickettsial septicemia. In Inglis V, Roberts RJ, Bromage NR, editors: *Bacterial diseases of fish,* New York, 1993b, Halsted Press, pp. 237-254.

Turner DT, Bower CE: Removal of some inorganic and organic substances from freshwater and artificial seawater by two commercial filtrants, *J Aquaricult Aquatic Sci* 3:57-63, 1983.

Udey LR, Young E, Sallman B: Isolation and characterization of an anaerobic bacterium, *Eubacterium tarantellus* sp. nov., associated with striped mullet *Mugil cephalus* mortality in Biscayne Bay, Florida, *J Fish Res Bd Can* 34:402-409, 1977.

US Environmental Protection Agency and Association of Metropolitan Water Agencies: *Disinfection by-products in U.S. drinking water,* vol 1, Report, Pasadena, Calif., 1989, James M. Montgomery Consulting Engineers.

US Environmental Protection Agency: *Water quality standards criteria digest,* Washington, D.C., 1979-1980, US Government Printing Office.

US Environmental Protection Agency: *Water quality criteria, 1972,* (EPA R3.73.003), Washington, DC, 1973, US Government Printing Office.

US Environmental Protection Agency: *Methods for chemical analysis of water and wastes,* Environmental Monitoring and Support Laboratory, Office of Research and Development, EPA-600/4-79, U.S.E.P.A., Cincinnati, Oh., 1979.

US Environmental Protection Agency: *Handbook for sampling, and sample preservation of water and wastewater,* EPA-600/4-82-029, Cincinnati, Oh., 1982, Environmental Monitoring and Support Laboratory.

US Department of Agriculture: *Aquaculture: situation and outlook, publication aqua VII,* Rockville, Md., 1991, Economic Research Service, p. 43.

Untergasser D: *Handbook of fish diseases,* Neptune City, N.J., 1989, Tropical Fish Hobbyist Publications, p. 160.

Untergasser D: *Discus health,* Neptune City, N.J., 1991, Tropical Fish Hobbyist Publications, p. 416.

Urawa S, Kato T: Heavy infestions of *Caligus orientalis* (Copepoda: Caligidae) on caged rainbow trout, *Oncorhynchus mykiss,* in brackish water, *Gyobyo Kenkyu* 26:161-162, 1991.

Urawa S, Kusakari M: The survivability of the ectoparasitic flagellate *Ichthyobodo necator* on chum salmon fry (*Oncorhynchus keta*) in seawater and comparison to *Ichthyobodo* sp. on Japanese flounder (*Paralichthys olivaceus*), *J Parasitol* 76:33-40, 1990.

Vallejo AN, Ellis AE: Ultrastructural study of the response of eosinophil granule cells to *Aeromonas salmonicida* extracellular product and histamine liberations in rainbow trout *Salmo gairdneri* Richardson, *Dev Comp Immunol* 13:133-148, 1989.

Van As JG, Basson L: Host specificty of trichodinid parasites of freshwater fish, *Parasitol Today* 3:88-90, 1987.

van Duijn C: Tuberculosis in fishes, *J Small Animal Prac* 22:391-411, 1981.

van Duijn Jr C: *Diseases of fishes,* ed 3, 1973, Springfield, Ill., Charles C. Thomas.

van der Heijden, van Muiswinkel WB, Grondel JL, Boon JH: Immunomodulating effects of antibiotics. In Michel C, Alderman DJ, editors: *Chemotherapy in aquaculture: from theory to reality,* Paris, 1992, Office International des Epizooties, pp. 219-230.

Varner PW, Lewis DH: Characterization of a virus associated with head and lateral line erosion syndrome in marine angelfish, *J Aquatic Animal Health* 3:198-205, 1991.

Ver LMB, Chiu YN: The effect of paddlewheel aerators on ammonia and carbon dioxide removal in intensive pond culture. In Maclean JL, Dizon LB, Hosillos LV, editors: *The first Asian fisheries forum,* Manila, Philippines, 1986, Asian Fisheries Society, pp. 97-100,

Vestergard-Jorgensen PE: Egtved virus: occurrence of inapparent infections with virulent virus in free-living rainbow trout, *Salmo gairdneri* Richardson, at low temperature, *J Fish Dis* 5:47-55, 1982.

Vestergard-Jorgensen PE: A study of viral disease in Danish rainbow trout, their diagnosis and control, Ph.D. diss., Royal Danish Veterinary and Agricultural University, Copenhagen, 1974.

Vinyard WC: Epizoophytic algae from molluscs, turtles, and fish in Oklahoma, *Proc of Oklahoma Acad Sci* 34:63-65, 1953.

Voelker FA et al: Amebiasis in goldfish, *Vet Pathol* 14:247-255, 1977.

Wada S et al: Histopathological findings of tiger puffer, *Takifugu rubripes,* artificially infected with "Kuchijiro-sho," *Fish Pathol* 21:101-104, 1986.

Wada S et al: Histopathology of *Aphanomyces* infection in dwarf gourami (*Colisa lalia*), *Fish Pathol* 29:229-237. 1994.

Wakabayashi H: Columnaris disease. In Inglis V, Roberts RJ, Bromage NR, editors: *Bacterial diseases of fish,* New York, 1993, Halsted Press, pp. 23-39.

Wakabayashi H, Hikida M, Masumura K: *Flexibacter maritimus* sp. nov., a pathogen of marine fishes, *Int J Sys Bacteriol* 36:396-398, 1986.

Wakabayashi H, Huh GJ, Kimura N: *Flavobacterium branchophila* sp. nov., a causative agent of bacterial gill disease of freshwater fishes, *Int J Sys Bacteriol* 39:213-216, 1989.

Walczak EM, Noga EJ, Hartmann JX: Properties of a vaccine for channel catfish virus disease and a method of administration, *Dev Biol Std* 49:419-429, 1981.

Walters GR, Plumb JA: Environmental stress and bacterial infection in channel catfish, *Ictalurus punctatus* Rafinesque, *J Fish Biol* 17:177-185, 1980.

Waltman WD, Shotts EB Jr: A medium for the isolation and differentiation of *Yersinia ruckeri,* *Can J Fish Aquat Sci* 41:804-806, 1984.

Waltman WD, Shotts EB: Antimicrobial susceptibility of *Edwardsiella ictaluri,* *J Wildlife Dis* 22:173-177, 1986.

Waltman WD, Shotts EB, Hsu TC: Biochemical and enzymatic characterization of *Edwardsiella tarda* from the United States and Taiwan, *Fish Pathol* 21:1-8, 1986.

Warren JW: *Diseases of hatchery fish,* Ft. Snelling, Twin Cities, Minn., 1981, US Fish and Wildlife Service, p. 91.

Waterman B, Dethlefsen V: Histology of pseudobranchial tumors in Atlantic cod (*Gadus morhua*) from the North Sea and the Baltic Sea, *Helgo Wiss Meresunters* 35:231-242, 1982.

Weatherley AH: Effects of superabundant oxygen on thermal tolerance of goldfish, *Biol Bull* 139:229-238, 1970.

Wedemeyer GA, Meyer FP, Smith L: *Diseases of fishes: environmental stress and fish diseases,* Book 5, Neptune City, N.J., 1976, TFH Publications, p. 192.

Wedemeyer GA, Nelson NC, Yasutake WT: Potentials and limits for the use of ozone as a fish disease control agent, *Ozone Sci Eng* 1:295-318, 1979.

Wedemeyer GA, Yasutake WT: Prevention and treatment of nitrite toxicity in juvenile steelhead trout (*Salmo gairdneri*), *J Fish Res Bd Can* 35:822-827, 1978.

Wellborn TL: *Calculation of treatment levels for control of fish diseases and aquatic weeds,* Information Sheet No. 673, Extension Service of Mississippi State University, 1978, p. 2.

Wellborn TL: Control and therapy. In Plumb JA, editor: *Principal diseases of farm raised catfish,* Auburn University, Ala., 1979, Southern Cooperative Series No. 225, pp. 61-85.

Wellborn Jr TL, Morgan R, Guyton GW: *Agriculture chemical toxicity to selected aquatic animals: bluegill, channel catfish, rainbow trout, crawfish, and freshwater shrimp,* Publication No. 1455, Mississippi State, Miss., 1984, Mississippi Cooperative Extension Service, p. 24.

Wellings SR: Neoplasia and primitive vertebrate phylogeny: echinoderms, prevertebrates and fishes, a review, *Nat Cancer Inst Monogr* 31:59-128, 1969.

Wellings SR, McCain BB, Miller BS: Epidermal papillomas in Pleuronectidae of Puget Sound, Washington, *Prog Experimental Tumor Res* 20:155-174, 1976.

Westin DT, Olney CE, Rogers BA: Effects of parenteral and dietary organochlorines on survival and body burdens of striped bass larvae, *Trans Am Fish Soc* 114:125-136, 1985.

Whaley J, Francis-Floyd R: A comparison of metronidazole treatments of hexamitiasis in angelfish, *Proc Int Assn Aquatic Animal Med,* pp. 110-114, 1991.

White AW: Dinoflagellate toxins as probable cause of an Atlantic herring (*Clupea harengus*) kill, and pteropods as an apparent vector, *J Fish Res Bd Can* 34:2421-2424, 1977.

White AW: Paralytic shellfish toxins and finfish. In Ragelis EP, editor: *Seafood toxins,* Washington, DC, 1981, American Chemical Society, pp. 171-180.

Whittington ID: The egg bundles of the monogenean *Diochus remorae* and their attachment to the gills of the remora, *Echeneis naucrates, Int J Parasitol* 20:45-49, 1990.

Wiles M, Cone D, Odense PH: Studies on *Chilodonella cyprini* and *C. hexasticha* (Protozoa: ciliata) by scanning electron microscopy, *Can J Zool* 63:2483-2487, 1985.

Wilkie DW, Gordin H: Outbreak of cryptocaryoniasis in marine aquaria at Scripps Institute of Oceanography, *Calif Fish Game* 55:227-236, 1969.

Wilkinson HW, Thacker LG, Facklam RR: Nonhemolytic Group B streptococci of human, bovine and ichthyic origin, *Infect Immun* 7:496-498, 1973.

Wilson JC, MacMillan JR: Evaluation of two aryl-fluoroquinolones against bacterial pathogens of channel catfish, *J Aquatic Animal Health* 1:222-226, 1990.

Wilson RP, editor: *CRC handbook of nutrient requirements of fish,* Boca Raton, Fla., 1992, CRC Press, p. 248.

Winfree RA: Tropical fish: their production and marketing in the United States, *World Aquacult* 20:24-30, 1989.

Winsor DK, Bloebaum AP, Mathewson JJ: Gram-negative aerobic, enteric pathogens among intestinal microflora of wild turkey vultures (*Cathartes aura*) in west central Texas, *Appl Environ Micro* 42:1123-1124, 1981.

Winton JR: Recent advances in detection and control of infectious hematopoietic necrosis virus in aquaculture, *Ann Rev Fish Dis* 1:83-93, 1991.

Winton JR, Lannan CN, Fryer JL, Kimura T: Isolation of a new reovirus from chum salmon in Japan, *Fish Pathol* 15:155-162, 1981.

Winton JR, Lannan CN, Ransom DP, Fryer JL: Isolation of a new virus from chinook salmon (*Oncorhynchus tshawytscha*) in Oregon, U.S.A., *Fish Pathol* 20:373-380, 1985.

Wise DJ, Tomasso JR, TM Brandt: Ascorbic acid inhibition of of nitrite-induced methemoglobinemia in channel catfish, *Prog Fish-cult* 50:77-80, 1988.

Wise JA, Bowser PR, Boyle JA: Detection of channel catfish virus in asymptomatic adult channel catfish, *Ictalurus punctatus* (Rafinesque), *J Fish Dis* 8:485-493, 1985.

Witschi WA, Ziebel CD: Evaluation of pH shock on hatchery-reared rainbow trout, *Prog Fish-cult* 41:3-5, 1979.

Wolf K, Markiw ME, Hiltunen JK: Salmonid whirling disease: *Tubifex tubifex* (Muller) identified as the essential oligochaete in the protozoan life cycle, *J Fish Dis* 9:83-85, 1986.

Wolf K: *The viruses and viral diseases of fish,* Ithaca, N.Y., 1988, Cornell University Press.

Wolf K, Markiw ME: Biology contravenes taxonomy in the Myxozoa: new discoveries show alternation of invertebrate and vertebrate hosts, *Science* 225:1449-1552, 1984.

Wolf K, Smith CE: *Herpesvirus salmonis:* pathological changes in parenterally infected rainbow trout, *Salmo gairdneri* Richardson fry, *J Fish Dis* 4:445-458, 1981.

Wolke RE: Pathology of bacterial and fungal disease affecting affecting fish. In Ribelin WE, Migaki G, editors: *Fish pathology,* Madison, 1975, University of Wisconsin Press, pp. 33-116.

Wolke RE: Piscine macrophage aggregates: a review, *Ann Rev Fish Dis* 2:91-108, 1992.

Wolke RE, Stroud RK: Piscine mycobacteriosis. In Montali RJ, editor: *Mycobacterial infections of zoo animals,* Washington, DC, 1978, Smithsonian Institute Press, pp. 269-275.

Woo PTK: *Cryptobia* and cryptobiosis in fishes, *Advan Parasitol* 26:199-237, 1987.

Wood CC, Rutherford DT, McKinnell S: Identification of sockeye salmon *Oncorhynchus nerka* stocks in mixed-stock fisheries in British Columbia, Canada, and southeast Alaska, USA, using biological markers, *Can J Fish Aquatic Sci* 46:2108-2120, 1989.

Wood EM, Yasutake WT: Histopathology of fish III: peduncle (*cold water*) disease, *Prog Fish-cult* 18:58-61, 1956.

Wood JW: *Diseases of Pacific salmon: their prevention and treatment,* ed 2, State of Washington Department of Fisheries Hatchery Division, 1974, p. 82.

Wood JW: *Diseases of Pacific salmon,* ed 2, Seattle, Wash., 1976, Washington Department of Fisheries.

Wood JW, Ordal EJ: Tuberculosis in Pacific salmon and steelhead trout, *Fish Commiss Oregon Contrl* 25:1-38, 1958.

Wooster GA, Hsu H-M, Bowser PR: Nonlethal surgical procedures for obtaining tissue samples for fish health inspections, *J Aquatic Animal Health* 5:157-164, 1993.

Wooten R: The parasitology of teleosts. In Roberts RJ, editor: *Fish pathology,* London, 1989, Bailliere-Tindall, pp. 242-288.

Wootten R, Smith JW. Needham EA: *Aspects of the biology of the parasitic copepods Lepeophtheirus salmonis and Caligus elongatus on farmed salmonids, and their treatment.* Proceedings of the Royal Society of Edinburgh 81B:185-197, 1982.

Wright LD: Effect of malachite green and formalin on the survival of largemouth bass eggs and fry, *Prog Fish-cult* 38:155-157, 1976.

Wu R, Boyd CE: Evaluation of calcium sulfate for use in aquaculture ponds, *Prog Fish-cult* 52:26-31, 1990.

Wyatt LE, Nickelson II R, Vanderzant C: *Edwardsiella tarda* in freshwater catfish and their environment, *Appl Environ Micro* 38:710-714, 1979.

Yamaguti S: *Parasitic copepoda and branchiura of fishes,* New York, 1963, Interscience Publishers, p. 1104.

Yamaguti S: *Monogenetic trematodes of Hawaiian fishes,* Honolulu, Hawaii, 1968, University of Hawaii Press.

Yamamoto T, Arakawa CK, Batts WN, Winton JR: Comparison of infectious hematopoietic necrosis virus in natural and experimental infections of spawning salmonids by infectivity and immunochemistry. In Ahne W, Kurstak E, editors: *Viruses of lower vertebrates,* New York, 1989, Springer-Verlag, pp. 411-429.

Yamamoto T, Kelly RK, Nielsen O: Epidermal hyperplasias of northern pike (*Esox lucius*) associated with herpesvirus and C-type particles, *Arch Virol* 79:255-272, 1984.

Yamamoto T, Kelly RK, Nielsen O: Epidermal hyperplasia of walleye, *Stizostedion vitreum vitreum* (Mitchill), associated with retrovirus-like C-type particle: prevalence, histologic and electron microscopic observations, *J Fish Dis* 8:425-436, 1985.

Yanohara Y, Kaegi N: Studies on metacercaria of *Centrocestus forasnus* (Nishigori, 1924). I. Parasitism of metacercariae in gills of young rearing eels, and abnormal deaths of host, *Fish Pathol* 17:237-241, 1983.

Yasutake W: Fish viral diseases: clinical, histopathological, and comparative aspects. In Ribelin WE, Migaki G, editors: *The pathology of fishes,* Madison, 1975, University of Wisconsin Press, pp. 247-269.

Yasutake WT: Histopathology of yearling sockeye salmon (*Oncorhynchus nerka*) infected with infectious hematopoietic necrosis (IHN), *Fish Pathol* 14:59-64, 1978.

Yasutake WT, Rasmussen CJ: Histopathogenesis of experimentally induced viral hemorrhagic septicemia in fingerling rainbow trout (*Salmo gairdneri*), *Bull Off Int Epizoot* 69:977-984, 1968.

Yasutake WT, Wood EM: Some myxosporidia found in Pacific Northwest salmonids, *J Parasitol* 43:633-642, 1957.

Yndestad M: Public health aspects of residues in animal products: fundamental considerations. In Michel C, Alderman DJ, editors: *Chemotherapy in aquaculture: from theory to reality,* Paris, 1992, Office International des Epizooties, pp. 494-510.

Yokoyama H, Ogawa K, Wakabayashi H: Involvement of *Branchiura sowerbyi* (Oligochaeta: Annelida) in the transmission of *Hoferellus-carassii* (Myxosporea: Myxozoa), the causative agent of kidney enlargement disease (KED) of goldfish *Carassius auratus, Gyobo Kenkyu* 28:135-139, 1993.

Yoshikoshi K, Inoue K: Viral nervous necrosis in hatchery-reared larvae and juveniles of Japanese parrotfish, *Oplegnathus fasciatus, J Fish Dis* 13:69-77, 1990.

Yoshimizu M, Sami M, Kimura T: Survivability of infectious pancreatic necrosis virus in fertilized eggs of masu and chum salmon, *J Aquatic Animal Health* 1:13-20, 1989.

Yoshinaga T, Nakazoe J-I: Isolation and in vitro cultivation of an unidentified ciliate causing scuticociliatosis in Japanese flounder (*Paralichthys olivaceus*), *Gyobo Kenkyu* 28:131-134, 1993.

Yu K-Y, MacDonald RD, Moore AR: Replication of infectious pancreatic necrosis virus in trout leucocytes and detection of the carrier state, *J Fish Dis* 5:401-410, 1982.

Yun S, Hedrick RP, Wingfield WH: A picorna-like virus from salmonid fishes in California, *Am Fish Soc Fish Health Sec Newsltr* 17(2):5, 1989.

Fish Disease Diagnosis Form

Date: _____   Case No.: _____

Name: _____

Address:_____ Phone: _____

_____

HISTORY

Freshwater: _____   Marine: _____   System size: _____ gal (l)/ac (ha)

Species affected: _____

Species in system: _____

No. fish in system: _____   No. fish and % affected: _____(%)

Average fish size: _____ in (cm)/oz (g)

Age(s) of affected fish: _____

When morbidity started: _____   When mortality started: _____

When morbidity ended: _____   When mortality ended: _____

How long has system been set up? _____   Temperature: _____

Types of life support present: _____

Any new introductions? Y __   N __   If yes, when and what? _____

_____

Water source: _____   Pipes: metal ___   plastic ___

Water appearance (cloudy, colored?): _____

History of routine maintenance, including water changes and water quality checks:

_____

_____

Behavioral changes? Y __   N __   Describe: _____

Respiratory rates: (normal _____   faster _____   slower _____)

Appearance of fish: _____

Appetite (normal ___   less ___   more ___): _____

Other clinical signs: _____

_____

CLINICAL WORK-UP

Water quality

DO: _____ mg/l   Temp: _____   pH: _____

Ammonia: TAN _____ mg/l   UIA _____ mg/l

Nitrite: _____ mg/l   Salinity: _____ ppt

Chloride: _____ mg/l   Hardness: _____ mg/l

Alkalinity: _____ mg/l   Nitrate: _____ mg/l

Water samples preserved for further analysis: _____

Physical exam

Behavior: _____   Respiration (depth and rate): _____

Skin: _____

Gills: _____

Biopsies and Cultures

Skin Biopsy: _____

Gill Biopsy: _____

Blood smears taken? Y ____ N ____   Results: _____

Bacterial cultures taken? Y ____   N ____

Organs cultured: Kidney _____   Other _____

Results of cultures: _____

Necropsy

Peritoneal cavity/visceral fat: _____

Gonads: _____

Liver/gall bladder: _____

Stomach/intestines: _____

Spleen: _____

Swim bladder: _____

Kidney: _____

Heart: _____

Brain: _____

Other: _____

Tissues preserved for histology or other further analysis: _____

Problems identified   Recommended treatment(s)

1. _____   1. _____

2. _____   2. _____

3. _____   3. _____

Results of treatment: _____

Suppliers

The following includes addresses of companies whose products were mentioned in the text. Note that this is only a partial listing of suppliers. The *Buyer's Guide* issue of *Aquaculture Magazine* (P.O. Box 2329, Asheville, NC 28802) provides a comprehensive listing of aquaculture-related products, including equipment for measuring water quality, and specialized disease diagnostic services.

Abbott Laboratories
Veterinary Division,
P.O. Box 68,
Abbott Park,
North Chicago, IL 60064

Agri Laboratories, Ltd.
6221 North K Highway,
P.O. Box 3101,
St. Joseph, MO 64505

Agri-Pro Enterprises
Box 27,
Iowa Falls, IA 50126

American Cyanamid Company
One Cyanamid Plaza,
Wayne, NJ 07470

Apothekernes Laboratorium A.S.
P.O. Box 158,
Skoyen, 0212,
Oslo, Norway

Applied Biochemists, Inc.
6120 West Douglas Avenue,
Milwaukee, WI 53218

Aqua Health, Ltd.
West Royalty Highway,
Industrial Park,
Charlottetown, Prince Edward Island,
C1E 1BO, Canada

Aquacenter
166 Seven Oaks Road,
Leland, MS 38756

Aquaculture Supply
33418 Old Saint Joe Road,
Dade City, FL 33525

Aquaculture Vaccines, Ltd. (AVL)
24-26 Gold Street,
Saffron Walden,
Essex, CB10 1EJ, United Kingdom

Aquanetics Systems, Inc.
5252 Lovelock Street,
San Diego, CA 92110

Aquarium Pharmaceuticals, Inc.
P.O. Box 218,
Chalfont, PA 18914

Aquarium Systems, Inc.
8141 Tyler Boulevard,
Mentor, OH 44060

Aquatic Ecosystems, Inc.
2056 Apopka Boulevard,
Apopka, FL 32703

Aquatronics
P.O. Box 6028,
Zuma Station,
Malibu, CA 90265

Argent Chemical Laboratories
8702 152nd Avenue N.E.,
Redmond, WA 98052

Aurum Aquaculture Ltd.
P.O. Box 2042,
Bothell, WA 98041

Baxter Diagnostics, Inc.
1430 Waukegan Road,
McGaw Park, IL 60085-6787

Bayer
c/o Sterling Health USA,
90 Park Avenue,
New York, NY 10016

Becton-Dickinson
Cockneysville, MD 21030

Biomed, Inc.
1720-130th Avenue, N.E.,
Bellevue, WA 98005-2203

Burroughs-Wellcome, Ltd.
3030 Cornwallis Road,
Research Triangle Park, NC 27709

The Butler Company
5000 Bradenton Avenue,
Dublin, OH 43017-0753

Carolina Biological Supply Company
2700 York Road,
Burlington, NC 276215-3398

Chemetrics, Inc.
Route 28,
Calverton, VA 22016-0214

Ciba-Geigy Animal Health
P.O. Box 18300,
Greensboro, NC 27419-8300

Cole-Parmer Instrument Company
7425 North Oak Park Avenue,
Niles, IL 60714

Coopers Pittman-Moore
421 East Hawley Street,
Mundelein, IL 60060

Diagxotics
27 Cannon Road,
Wilton, CT 06897

Eka Noble, Inc.
1519 Johnson Ferry Road,
Marietta, GA 30062

Elanco Products Company
Lilly Corporate Center,
Indianapolis, IN 46285

Engineered Products
P.O. Box 30,
Philomath, OR 97370

Fisher Scientific
711 Forbes Avenue
Pittsburg, PA 15219-4785

Fort Dodge Laboratories
800 Fifth Street,
Fort Dodge, IA 50501

Fritz Chemical Company
P.O. Drawer 17040,
Dallas, TX 75217

H & S Chemical Company, Inc.
Cincinnati, OH 45202

Hach Company
P.O. Box 389,
Loveland, CO 80539

Rolf C. Hagen, Inc.
50 Hampden Road,
Mansfield, MA 02048

Hoechst-Roussel
Agri-Vet Company,
Sommerville, NJ 08876

Hoffman-LaRoche
Roche Animal Health and Nutrition, Hoffman-LaRoche, Inc.
340 Kingsland Street,
Nutley, NJ 07110

Kent Marine
1377 Barclay Circle,
Suite K,
Marietta, GA 30060

Kirkegaard and Perry Laboratories, Inc.
2 Cessna Court,
Gaithersburg, MD 20879

LaMotte Company
P.O. Box 329,
Rt. 213 North,
Chestertown, MD 21620

Mardel Laboratories, Inc.
1958 Brandon Court,
Glendale Heights, IL 60139

Marine Enterprises International, Inc.
8800 A Kelso Drive,
Baltimore, MD 21221-3125

Micrologix International, Ltd.
6761 Kirkpatrick Crescent,
Victoria, British Columbia,
V8X 3X1, Canada

Miles, Inc.
Agricultural Division, Animal Health Products,
Box 390,
12707 West 63rd Street,
Shawnee, KS 66201

Nachez Animal Supply Company
201 John R. Junkin Drive,
Nachez, MS 39120

Northwest Distribution Company
8804 220th Street, S.W.,
Edmonds, WA 98026

Olin Corporation
120 Long Ridge Road,
Stamford, CT 06904

Ortho Pharmaceutical Corporation
Raritan, NJ 08869

Parke-Davis
201 Tabor Road,
Morris Plains, NJ 07950

Pfizer, Inc.
Animal Health Division,
235 East 42nd Street,
New York, NY 10017

Pitman-Moore, Inc.
421 East Hawley Street,
Mundelein, IL 60060

Sandpoint Aquarium Products
1365B Interior Street,
Eugene, OR 97402

G.D. Searle & Company
Box 5110,
Chicago, IL 60680-5110

SmithKline Beecham Animal Health
812 Springdale Drive,
Exton, PA 19341

SpectraPure
738 South Perry Lane,
Suite 1,
Tempe, AZ 85281

Tetra Sales USA
3001 Commerce Street,
Blacksburg, VA 24060

The Upjohn Company
Animal Health Division,
7000 Portage Road,
Kalamazoo, MI 49001

Union Carbide Company
Old Ridgebury Road,
Danbury, CT 06817

Vetrepharm Ltd.
Unit 15, Industrial Estate,
Sandleheath, Fordingbridge,
Hants 5PG 1PA Great Britain

Wisconsin Pharmacal Company
P.O. Box 198,
Jackson, WI 53037

Wyeth-Ayerst Laboratories
P.O. Box 8299,
Philadelphia, PA 19101

Yellow Springs Instruments, Inc.
P.O. Box 279,
Yellow Springs, OH 45387

Ziggity Systems, Inc.
P.O. Box 1169,
Middlebury, IN 46540

APPENDIX III

Dangerous Aquatic Animals

The vast majority of fish kept in home aquaria are innocuous. However, the practitioner should be aware of those select species that may be dangerous. The greatest potential for harm is from poisonous species. These include some catfish, such as *Ictalurus* spp., *Plotosus* spp., *Notropus*, and *Heteropneustes* that have poison associated with their sharp dorsal and pectoral spines, or can inflict a locally painful wound. Of more serious concern are the scorpionfish and weaverfish, which can inflict painful wounds that, depending on the species and severity, may require medical attention. The most commonly maintained member of this group are the lionfish (*Pterois* and *Dendrobates* spp.), which have numerous specialized fin spines capable of delivering poison. The most dangerous scorpionfish is the stonefish (*Synganus* sp.), which has a dangerous and rapidly lethal toxin. Fortunately, it is rarely seen in hobbyists' tanks.

Some fish can inflict painful bites if they are not handled carefully, such as the moray eels (Muraenidae). Some freshwater fish can produce a powerful electrical current. The electric catfish can produce a mild jolt, but the electric eel (*Electrophorus electricus*) can produce a powerful surge. Some rays have barbs on their tail fins that can be whipped into an unsuspecting handler.

APPENDIX IV

Scientific Names of Fishes Mentioned in the Text

Common name	Scientific name
Amberjack	*Seriola dumerli*
Anabantids (family)	Anabantidae
Anemonefish, clown	*Amphiprion ocellaris*
Anemonefish, sebae	*Amphiprion sebae*
Anemonefish (family)	Amphiprionidae
Angelfish, deep	*Pterophyllum altum*
Angelfish, French	*Pomacathus paru*
Angelfish, freshwater	*Pterophyllum scalare*
Angelfish, semicirculatus	*Pomacanthus semicirculatus*
Angelfish, marine (family)	Pomacanthidae
Archerfish	*Toxotes jaculator*
Atherinid, boyeri	*Atherina boyeri*
Ayu	*Plecoglossus altivelis*
Barb, lineatus	*Barbus lineatus* (= *Puntius lineatus*)
Barb, rosy	*Barbus conchonius* (= *Puntius conchonius*)
Barb, tiger	*Barbus tetrazona* (= *Capoeta tetrazona*)
Barbel	*Barbus barbus*
Barbs	*Barbodes, Capoeta, Puntius, Barbus*
Barbs (family)	Cyprinidae
Barramundi	*Lates calcarifer*
Bass, Australian sea	see barramundi
Bass, hybrid striped	*Morone saxatilis* × *Morone chrysops*
Bass, largemouth	*Micropterus salmoides*
Bass, Mediterranean sea	*Dicentrarchus labrax*
Bass, percichthyid (family)	Percichthyidae
Bass, smallmouth	*Micropterus dolomieui*
Bass, striped	*Morone saxatilis*
Bass, white	*Morone chrysops*
Bluefish	*Pomatomus saltatrix*
Bluegill	*Lepomis machrochirus*
Bream, white	*Blicca bjoerkna*
Bream, yellowfin	*Acanthopagrus australis*
Bream	*Abramis brama*
Bullhead, black	*Ictalurus melas*
Bullhead, brown	*Ictalurus nebulosus*
Bullhead, yellow	*Ictalurus natalis*
Burbot	*Lota lota*
Butterflyfish, freshwater	*Pantodon buchholzi*
Butterflyfish, marine (family)	Chaetodontidae
Carangids (family)	Carangidae
Carp, bighead	*Hypophthalmichthys molitrix*
Carp, black	*Mylopharyngodon piceus*
Carp, common	*Cyprinus carpio*
Carp, Crucian	*Carassius carassius*
Carp, grass	*Ctenopharyngodon idella*

Common name	Scientific name
Carp, silver	*Hypophthalmichthys nobilis*
Carps (family)	Cyprinidae
Catfish, ancistrid	*Ancistrus* spp.
Catfish, blue	*Ictalurus furcatus*
Catfish, bullhead	See bullhead
Catfish, channel	*Ictalurus punctatus*
Catfish, corydoras	*Corydoras* spp.
Catfish, European	see sheatfish
Catfish, hardhead sea	*Arius felis*
Catfish, pimelodella	*Pimelodella* spp.
Catfish, plecostomus	*Plecostomus* spp.
Catfish, saltwater	*Plotosus anguillaris*
Catfish, walking	*Clarias batrachus*
Catfish, white	*Ictalurus catus*
Catfish, labyrinth (family)	Clariidae
Catfish, suckermouth (family)	Loricaridae
Catfish, bullhead (family)	Ictaluridae
Cavallas (family)	Carangidae
Char, arctic	*Salvelinus alpinus*
Characins (family)	Characidae
Chebachek	*Pseudorasbora parva*
Chub	*Coregonus zenithicus*
Cichlid, chromide	*Etroplus maculatus*
Cichlid, convict	*Cichlasoma nigrofasciatum*
Cichlid, firemouth	*Herichthys meeki* (= *Cichlasoma meeki*)
Cichlid, jewel	*Hemichromis bimaculatus*
Cichlid, Ramirez's dwarf	*Apistogramma ramirezi*
Cichlid, Rio Grande	*Cichlasoma cyanoguttatum*
Cichlid, severum	*Cichlasoma severum*
Cichlid, zilli	*Tilapia zilli*
Cichlids, African Rift Lake	*Cynotilapia, Callochromis, Cyphotilapia, Eretmodus, Haplochromis, Iodotropheus, Julidochromis, Lamprologus, Labeotropheus, Melanochromis, Petrotilapia, Pseudotropheus, Tropheus* spp.
Cichlids	Cichlidae
Cisco	*Coregonus artedii*
Clariids (family)	Walking catfish
Clupeids (family)	Herring, sardines, menhaden
Coalfish	See sablefish
Cod, Atlantic	*Gadus morhua*
Cod, Pacific	*Gadus macrocephalus*
Cods (family)	Gadidae
Crevalle, jack	*Caranx hippos*
Croaker, Atlantic	*Micropogonias undulatus*
Ctenopoma	*Ctenopoma* spp.
Cunner	*Tautoglabrus adspersus*
Cyclopterids (family)	Lumpfish, snailfish
Cyprinids (family)	Carps, barbs
Dab	*Limanda limanda*
Damselfish, bicolor	*Pomacentrus partitus*
Damselfish, blacksmith	*Chromis punctipinnis*
Damselfish, blue	*Chromis* sp.
Damselfish, domino	*Dacyllus tricmaculatus*
Damselfish (family)	Pomacentridae
Danio, devario	*Danio devario*
Danio, zebra	*Brachydanio rerio*
Danios	*Brachydanio* spp., *Danio* spp.
Discus	*Symphysodon discus*

Common name	Scientific name
Dolphin	*Coryphaena hippurus*
Drum, red	*Sciaenops ocellatus*
Drums (family)	Sciaenidae
Eel, American	*Anguilla rostrata*
Eel, European	*Anguilla anguilla*
Eel, Japanese	*Anguilla japonica*
Eel, swamp	*Fluta alba*
Eels, anguillid (family)	Anguillidae
Eels, true (family)	Anguillidae
Flatfishes (order)	Pleuronectiformes
Flounder, Japanese	*Paralichthys olivaceus*
Flounder, southern	*Paralichthys lethostigma*
Flounder, winter	*Pseudopleuronectes americanus*
Flounders, lefteye (family)	Bothidae
Four-eyes	*Anableps anableps*
Fundulids	*Fundulus* spp. killifish
Gasterosteids (family)	Sticklebacks
Gibel	*Carassius auratus gibelio*
Gobies (family)	Gobiidae
Goby, yellowfin	*Acanthogobius flavimanus*
Goldfish	*Carassius auratus auratus*
Gourami, dwarf	*Colisa lalia*
Gourami, three-spot	*Trichogaster trichopterus*
Gouramies (family)	Belontiidae
Gouramies, kissing (family)	Helostomatidae
Grayling	*Thymallus thymallus*
Graylings (family)	Thymallidae
Greenling, spotbelly	*Hexagrammos agrammus*
Grouper, malabaricus	*Epinephelus malabaricus*
Grouper, red	see redspotted grouper
Grouper, redspotted	*Epinephelus akaara*
Groupers (family)	Serranidae
Grunters (family)	Teraponidae
Gudgeon	*Pseudorasbora parva*
Guppy	*Poecilia reticulata*
Haddock	*Melanogrammus aeglefinus*
Halibuts, bastard (family)	Paralichthyidae
Herring, Atlantic	*Clupea harengus harengus*
Herring (family)	Clupeidae
Ictalurids (family)	Bullhead catfish
Ide, golden	*Leuciscus idus*
Jacks (family)	Carangidae
Jacopever	*Sebastes schlegeli*
Jacopever, fox	*Sebastes vulpes*
Jawfish (family)	Opistognathidae
Jurupari	*Geophagus jurupari*
Killifish (family)	Cyprinodontidae
Knifefish, green	*Eigenmannia virescens*
Koi	*Cyprinus carpio*
Lamprey, American sea	*Petromyzon marinus dorsatus*
Lampreys (family)	Petromyzontidae
Loach, clown	*Botia macracanthus*
Loach, kuhlii	*Acanthophthalmus kuhlii*
Loaches (family)	Cobitidae
Lookdown	*Selene vomer*
Mackerel, chub	*Scomber japonicus*
Luderick	*Girella tricuspidata*
Mackerel, jack	*Trachurus japonicus*
Mackerels (family)	Scombridae

Common name	Scientific name
Menhaden, Atlantic	*Brevoortia tyrannus*
Menhaden, gulf	*Brevoortia patronus*
Milkfish	*Chanos chanos*
Minnow, blue	*Fundulus grandis*
Minnow, fathead	*Pimephales promelas*
Mollies (family)	Poeciliidae
Molly, black	*Poecilia sphenops*
Mono	*Monodactylus sebae*
Mosquitofish	*Gambusia affinis*
Mudskipper	*Periophthalmus* sp.
Mullet, grey	*Mugil capito*
Mullet, striped	*Mugil cephalus*
Mullets (family)	Mugilidae
Mummichog	*Fundulus heteroclitus*
Muskellunge	*Esox masquinongy*
Opistognathids (family)	Opistoganthidae
Oscar	*Astronotus ocellatus*
Oval fish	*Navodan modestus*
Paradisefish	*Macropodus opercularis*
Paradisefishes (family)	Belontiidae
Parrotfish, Japanese	*Oplegnathus faciatus*
Parrotfishes (family)	Scaridae
Perch, climbing	*Anabas testudineus*
Perch, Eurasian	*Perca fluviatilis*
Perch, European	*Perca fluviatilis*
Perch, golden	*Macquaria ambigua*
Perch, redfin	*Perca fluviatilis*
Perch, silver	*Bairdiella chrysura*
Perch, white	*Morone americana*
Perch, yellow	*Perca flavescens*
Perches, freshwater (family)	Percidae
Pike, northern	*Esox lucius*
Pike-perch	*Stizostedion lucioperca*
Pikes (family)	Esocidae
Pinfish	*Lagodon rhomboides*
Piranha	*Serrasalmus* spp.
Piranha, spotted	*Serrasalmus rhombeus*
Pirarucu	*Arapaima gigas*
Plaice	*Pleuronectes platessa*
Platyfish	*Xiphophorus maculatus*
Platys (family)	Xiphiidae
Platys	*Xiphophorus* sp.
Pleuronectids (family)	Pleuronectid flatfishes
Poecilids (family)	Poeciliidae
Poecilids (family)	Mollies, platies, swordtails
Pollock	*Pollachirus virens*
Pompano	*Trachinotus carolinus*
Pompano (family)	*Carangidae*
Porgy	*Stenotomus versicolor*
Puffer, tiger	*Tahifugu rubripes*
Pumpkinseed	*Lepomis gibbosus*
Rabbitfish	*Siganus cahaliculatus*
Rabbitfish, rivulatus	*Siganus rivulatus*
Rainbowfish, Australian	*Melanotaenia* spp.
Rainbowfish, Madagascar	*Bedotia geayi*
Rainbowfish (family)	Melanotaenidae
Redfish	See red drum
Roach	*Rutilus rutilus*
Rockfish, black	*Sebastes inermis*

Common name	Scientific name
Rudd	*Scardinius erythrophthalmus*
Sablefish	*Anoplopoma fimbria*
Sailfish	*Istiophorus platypterus*
Salmon, amago	*Oncorhynchus rhodurus*
Salmon, Atlantic	*Salmo salar*
Salmon, chinook	*Oncorhynchus tshawytscha*
Salmon, coho	*Oncorhynchus kisutch*
Salmon, kokanee	*Oncorhynchus nerka*
Salmon, masou	*Oncorhynchus masou*
Salmon, Pacific	*Oncorhynchus gorbuscha, O. keta, O. kisutch, O. nerka,* and *O. tshawytscha*
Salmon, pink	*Oncorhycnchus gorbuscha*
Salmon, silver	See coho salmon
Salmon, sockeye	See kokanee salmon
Salmon, yamame	See masou salmon
Salmonids (family)	Salmon and trouts
Salmonids (family)	Salmonidae
Sardines (family)	Clupeidae
Scat	*Scatophagus* sp.
Sculpin, sunrise	*Pseudoblennius cottoides*
Sea bream, black	*Mylio macrocephalus*
Sea bream, cantharus black	*Spondyliosoma cantharus*
Sea bream, crimson	*Evynnis japonicus*
Sea bream, gilthead	*Sparus aurata*
Sea bream, pagrus	*Pagrus major*
Sea bream, red	*Chrysophrys major*
Sea bream, schlegeli black	*Acanthopagrus schlegeli*
Sea bream, young black	*Acanthopagrus schlegeli*
Seahorse	*Hippocampus hudsonius*
Sea trout	*Cynoscion regalis*
Sea trout, silver	*Cynoscion nothus*
Shad, gizzard	*Dorosoma cepedianum*
Shark, bonnethead	*Sphyrna tiburo*
Shark, brown	See sandbar shark
Shark, lemon	*Negraprion brevirostris*
Shark, sandbar	*Carcharinus plumbeus*
Shark, smooth dogfish	*Mustelus canis*
Shark, spiny dogfish	*Squalus acanthias*
Sharks, dogfish (order)	Squaliformes
Sheatfish	*Siluris glanis*
Shiner, emerald	*Notemigonus atherinoides*
Shiner, golden	*Notemigonus crysoleucas*
Shiners	*Notropis* spp.
Siamese fighting fish	*Betta splendens*
Silver dollar	*Metynnis argenteus*
Silverside	*Menidia* sp.
Silversides (family)	Atherinidae
Smelt, rainbow	*Osmerus mordax*
Smelts	*Osmerus* spp.
Smelts (family)	Osmeridae
Snakehead, Formosa	*Ophicephalus maculatus*
Snakehead, striped	*Ophicephalus striatus*
Snakeheads	*Ophicephalus* spp.
Snapper, gray	*Lutjanus griseus*
Snook	*Centropomus unidecimalis*
Snook, common	See snook
Sole, English	*Parophrys vetulus*
Soles (family)	Soleidae
Spadefish, Atlantic	*Chaetodipterus faber*

Common name	Scientific name
Spot	*Leiostomus xanthurus*
Stickleback, brook	*Culaea inconstans*
Stickleback, ten-spined	*Pungitius pungitius*
Stickleback, three-spined	*Gasterosteus aculeatus*
Sticklebacks (family)	Gasterosteidae
Stingray	*Dasyatis* sp.
Stingrays (family)	Dasyatidae
Sturgeon, baeri	*Acipenser baeri*
Sturgeon, white	*Acipenser transmontanus*
Sucker, white	*Catostomus commersoni*
Suckers (family)	Catostomidae
Sunfish, green	*Lepomis cyanellus*
Sunfish, marine	*Mola mola*
Sunfishes, freshwater (family)	Centrarchidae
Swordtails (family)	Xiphiidae
Tang, naso	*Naso lituratus*
Tang, yellow	*Zebrasoma flavescens*
Tang, powder blue	*Paracanthurus hepatus*
Tangs (family)	Acanthuridae
Tautog	*Tatutoga onitis*
Tench	*Tinca tinca*
Tetra, neon	*Hyphessobrycon innesi*
Tetras (family)	Characidae
Tetras	*Cheirodon, Crenuchus, Hemigrammus, Hyphessobrycon, Megalamphodus, Moenkhausia, Paracheirodon* spp.
Tilapia, blue	*Tilapia aurea*
Tilapia, Nile	*Tilapia nilotica*
Tilapia, nilotica	See Nile tilapia
Tilapias	*Oreochromis* spp., *Tilapia* spp., *Sarotherodon* spp.
Tomcod, Atlantic	*Microgadus tomcod*
Topminnows	*Fundulus* sp., *Cyprinodon* sp.
Triggerfish, vidua	*Melichthys vidua*
Triggerfish, sargassum	*Xanthichthys ringens*
Trout, brook	*Salvelinus fontinalis*
Trout, brown	*Salmo trutta*
Trout, cutthroat	*Oncorhynchus clarki*
Trout, golden	*Oncorhynchus aguabonita*
Trout, Kamloops	*Oncorhynchus mykiss kamloops*
Trout, lake	*Salvelinus namaycush*
Trout, rainbow	*Oncorhynchus mykiss*
Trout, steelhead (marine)	*Oncorhynchus mykiss*
Turbot	*Scophthalmus maximus*
Walleye	*Stizostedion vitreum vitreum*
Weatherfish, oriental	*Misurgunus anguillicaudatus*
Weatherfishes (family)	Cobitidae
Whitefish, muksun	*Coregonus muksun*
Whitefish, peled	*Coregonus peled*
Whitefishes (family)	Coregonidae
Wrasse, C. melops	*Crenilabrus melops*
Wrasse, C. ocellatus	*Crenilabrus ocellatus*
Wrasses (family)	Labridae
Yellowtail	*Seriola quinqueradiata*

Definitions of Terms

Acute Having severe clinical signs or a short course

Agonal Pertaining to the death struggle; occurring at the time of or just before death

Algicidal Lethal to algae

Anorexic/anorexia Lack or loss of appetite for food

Anoxia Total lack of oxygen

Antemortem Before death

Antiseptic A substance that prevents the growth or development of a microorganism on living tissue

Asepsis Freedom from infection; aseptic (adj.)

Autolysis Spontaneous disintegration of cells or tissues by the body's own enzymes, as occurs after death; autolyze (verb)

Bacteremia Bacterial infection of the blood

Bilateral Affecting both sides

Biofiltration Process by which specific bacteria detoxify nitrogenous wastes (ammonia, nitrite) using oxygen; biofilter (noun)

Branchial Pertaining to the gill

Cachexia General ill health and malnutrition

Cathartic An agent that causes evacuation of intestinal contents

Chondrodysplasia The abnormal formation of cartilage

Chronic Persists for a long time

Clinical hypoxia Clinical signs associated with hypoxia, such as labored breathing and piping

Clinical signs Any evidence of disease observed by the clinician (e.g., reddening of the body, abnormal swimming)

Community tank An aquarium that has peaceful, compatible, easily maintained species of fish

Conditioned Refers to an aquaculture system that has a stable and functioning biofilter

Congestion Abnormal accumulation of blood in a body part

Conspecific Individual that is in the same species

Cyst 1: A developmental stage in some protozoan parasites; 2: Any closed epithelium-lined cavity

Dematiaceous A family of imperfect fungi having hyphae and/or conidia that are brownish or black colored

Depression A lowering or decrease in activity; depressed (adj.)

Diagnosis Determination of the nature of a case of a disease; diagnostic (adj.)

Differential diagnosis The determination of which one of several diseases may be producing the clinical signs

Dyspnea Labored or difficult breathing; dyspneic (adj.)

Ecchymosis A hemorrhagic spot, larger than a petechia, in the skin or mucous membrane

-emia An affliction of the blood (e.g., bacteremia is a bacterial infection in the blood)

Epithelium The cellular covering of external and internal body surfaces

Erosion A shallow or superficial loss of epithelium; shallower than an ulcer

Etiology The science that deals with causes of disease; etiologic, etiological (adj.)

Euryhaline Capable of tolerating a wide range of salinity

Eutrophic An ecosystem that has a large input of nutrients

Exophthalmos Abnormal protrusion of the eye; exophthalmic (adj.)

Facultative Not obligatory

Fistula An abnormal passage from an organ to the body surface

Fluctuant Movable and compressible

Focus 1: The chief center of a morbid process; 2: A discrete area having a morbid process; focal (adj.)

Fomite An inanimate object or material on which disease-producing agents may be conveyed

Fontanelle One of the membrane-covered spaces that remain at the junction of the sutures of the incompletely ossified skull in some immature animals

Gangrene Death of tissue; gangrenous (adj.)

Hemorrhage The escape of blood from vessels; bleeding; hemorrhagic (adj.)

History The events preceding and associated with a disease outbreak; also known as subjective data

Holotrichous Cilia distributed evenly over the body; usually refers to protozoa

Hyperemia An excess of blood in a body part

Hyperplasia Abnormal increase in the number of normal cells in normal arrangement in an organ or tissue, which increases the organ's or the tissue's volume

Hypertrophy Enlargement of an organ or its part caused by an increase in the size of its cells

Hyphema Hemorrhage in the anterior chamber of the eye

Hypoxia Deficiency of oxygen, such as reduction of oxygen in tissues below physiologically required levels

-iasis A condition or state; e.g., parasitiasis is the state of being parasitized; also see -osis

Iatrogenic Resulting from the actions of a clinician, usually referring to an adverse effect

Idiopathic Occurring without known cause

In toto Entirely; totally

Infection Invasion and multiplication of organisms in body tissues

Infestation Subsistence on the surface of the skin or gills, without invasion into these tissues

Inflammation A protective tissue response to injury, which serves to destroy, dilute, or wall off both the injurious agent and the injured tissues

Intensive culture system A culture system designed to hold a large amount of fish in a small amount of water; e.g., aquarium, raceway

-itis Inflammation of a tissue or organ (e.g., splenitis is inflammation of the spleen)

Keratinized Formation of a horny, outer layer on the skin, typically found in terrestrial vertebrates (mammals, reptiles)

Latent Dormant or concealed

LC50/LD50 The concentration or dose of a chemical that causes 50% mortality in a specified period of time (e.g., the 96-hour LC50 is the concentration of a chemical that will kill 50% of the individuals after 96 hours' exposure to the chemical)

Lesion Any pathological or traumatic discontinuity of tissue or loss of function of a part

Lethargy Drowsiness or indifference

Macroalgae Macrophytes that are members of the algae

Macronucleus In ciliate protozoa, the larger of two types of nucleus in each cell, which controls nonreproductive functions

Macrophyte A large macroscopically visible aquatic plant (e.g., hydrilla, cryptocorynes, hair algae, and kelp are macrophytes, while dinoflagellates, diatoms, and other microscopic plants are not)

Mesohaline Refers to brackish water between ~5 to 18 ppt salinity

Morbidity 1: The condition of being diseased; 2: The sickness rate; the ratio of sick to well animals in a population

Moribund In a dying state

Mucous membrane The tissue lining various canals and cavities of the body; also see epithelium

Necrosis Death of individual cells or groups of cells, or of localized areas of tissue; necrotic (adj.)

Obligate Characterized by the ability to survive only in a particular environment (e.g., obligate pathogen)

Ocular Pertaining to the eye

Oligohaline Refers to slightly brackish water (between ~0.5 to 5 ppt salinity)

Operculum The bony covering of the gill

Opportunistic Capable of adapting to the tissue or host other than the normal one, or, capable of taking advantage of an immunocompromised host; said of microrganisms and parasites

-osis Disease, morbid state; e.g., parasitosis is being sick from parasite infection or infestation; also see -iasis

Parasitemia Parasite infection of the blood

Paratenic host A host that is not absolutely required for completion of a parasite's life cycle (i.e., is not an obligate host); transport host (syn.)

Parenchyma The essential or functional elements of an organ, as distinguished from its stroma or framework

Paresis Slight or incomplete paralysis

Pathognomonic Specifically distinctive or characteristic of a disease or pathologic condition

Pathology The branch of medicine that studies the changes in body tissues and organs that are caused by disease

Peracute Very acute

Pericardium The sac enclosing the heart

Peritoneum The membrane that lines the wall of the abdominal cavity and covers the viscera

Peritonitis Inflammation of the peritoneum

Petechia A minute red spot caused by escape of a small amount of blood; petechial (adj.)

pH The negative logarithm of the hydrogen ion concentration, expressed on a scale of 0 to 14, values < 7 being increasingly acidic (more hydrogen ion), values > 7 being increasingly basic (less hydrogen ion), and 7 being neutral

Pharmacokinetics The study of quantifying how an administered drug becomes distributed throughout various tissues and excreted from the body

Phytoplankton Microscopic plants found in the water column (e.g., microscopic algae, such as diatoms, dinoflagellates, and green algae)

Piping The act of fish gulping air at the surface of the water

Poikilothermy The state of having a body temperature that varies with the temperature of the environment; poikilothermic (adj.)

Polyhaline Refers to brackish water approaching full strength seawater (~18 to 30 ppt salinity)

Postmortem After death

Prepatent Period before being evident

Primary infection The infectious agent that is responsible for initiating damage to tissue; also see secondary infection

Recrudescence Recurrence of clinical signs after temporary abatement

Secondary infection An infectious agent that invades the tissue after another agent has initially damaged the tissue; also see opportunistic; primary infection

Septicemia Toxin in the blood; often refers to the presence of bacterial toxin

Sequela A morbid condition following or occurring as a consequence of another condition or event

Serosanguineous   Composed of serum and blood

Sessile   Attached

Sexual dimorphism   Characteristics that distinguish male from female

Shimmies   Swimming in one place in a slow, weaving fashion; usually associated with some skin ectoparasite infestation

Stenohaline   Unable to withstand a wide variation in salinity

Systemic   Pertaining to or affecting the body as a whole (e.g., versus only affecting the skin or gills)

Theront   The infective stage of certain parasitic protozoa (e.g., *Ichthyophthirius*)

Tissue   A group or layer of similarly specialized cells that together perform certain specialized functions

Tomont   The dividing stage of certain parasitic protozoa (e.g., *Ichthyophthirius*)

Toxicosis   Any diseased condition caused by poisoning

Trophont   The attached, fish-feeding stage of certain parasitic protozoa (e.g., *Ichthyophthirius, Amyloodinium*)

Trophozoite   General term for the feeding stage of a parasitic protozoan

Ulcer/ulceration   A local defect on the surface of an organ or tissue, usually produced by sloughing of necrotic tissue

Unilateral   Affecting only one side

Vascularized   To be supplied with blood vessels

Vascular plant   The evolutionarily advanced plants that have a specialized conduction system, which includes xylem and phloem; such plants include almost all of the commonly propagated aquarium plants, as well as many aquatic pond weeds (e.g., hydrilla); the other major group of aquatic plants is the algae

Viremia   Virus infection of the blood

Viscera   Plural of viscus

Viscus   Any large interior organ in any of the great body cavities (e.g., pericardial and abdominal cavities of fish), especially those in the abdomen

Zoonosis   A disease of animals that can be transmitted to man; zoonotic (adj.)

Index

Intestine — cont'd
cestode infection in, 170
features of, 39
furunculosis diagnosed with culture of, 145
wet mount of, 38f
Intraerythrocytic viral disease, 138
Investigational new animal drug, 258
Iodine
potentiated, treatment of fish with, 293
requirements of, for fish, 222
Ion exchange filter, toxic metals removed with, 230
IPN; *see* Infectious pancreatic necrosis
Ipronidazole, prevention of use for food fish of, 258
Iron
metal poisoning from, 227
poisoning from, 230
requirements of, for fish, 222
Isopod
families of, 86
infestation by, 86-87
organophosphate for treatment of, 291
Ivermectin, nematodes controlled with, 167

K

Kanamycin
enteric septicemia treated with, 147
mycobacteriosis treated with, 158
treatment of fish with, 274
KED; *see* Kidney enlargement disease
Kidney
bacterial kidney disease and, 155
biopsy of, 28
copper toxicosis and, 227
dorsal approach to, during postmortem, 30-34
features of, 41
furunculosis diagnosed with culture of, 145
necrosis of
bacterial infection as cause of, 139
channel catfish viral disease indicated by, 207
infectious hematopoietic necrosis associated with, 212
viral hemorrhagic septicemia associated with, 214
neoplasms in, 203f
proliferative kidney disease and, 182
swelling of, kidney enlargement disease indicated by, 182
ventral approach to, during postmortem, 34-35
Kidney bloater, 181-182
Kidney disease, antibiotics for, 273-274
Kidney enlargement disease, 181-182
Killifish, description of, 3

Koi
anchor worm infestation in, 83
description of, 3
furunculosis in, 143-146
optimal and tolerable water temperature ranges for, 60t
sleeping sickness in, 135
Krill, fish feed with, 223

L

Lamella, swollen, proliferative gill disease indicated by, 179
Lamprey
American, infestation by, 78
Bayluscide for killing of, 277
furunculosis in, 143-146
infectious pancreatic necrosis in, 210
infestation by, 77-78
sodium sulfite for eradication of, 297
Larvae, diet of, 223
Latex gloves, fish biopsy and, 14
Lead, metal poisoning from, 227
Leech
infestation by, 78
organophosphate for treatment of, 290-291
trypanosomes transmitted by, 134-135
Lepeophtheirus, infestation by, 83
Lernaea, infestation by, 83
Lernaea cyprinacea, infestation by, 83
Lernaeagiraffa, infestation by, 83
Lernaeidae, infestation by, 80
Lernaeopodid parasites, infestation by, 83
Lernaeopodidae, infestation by, 80
Lernanthropidae, infestation by, 80
Lesion
bacteria as cause of, 21
chronic inflammatory, causes of, 22
deep, atypical water mold infection indicated by, 121
eye, disease indicated by, 14
gill
causes of, 131-133
columnaris infection indicated by, 124
water mold as cause of, 119
in liver, gas supersaturation associated with, 77
in muscle, gas supersaturation associated with, 77
necrotic, furunculosis indicated by, 145
skin
causes of, 21-22, 131-133
columnaris infection indicated by, 124
culturing of, during postmortem, 35
red-sore disease and, 141